Ulcerative Colitis: Symptoms, Diagnosis and Treatment

Ulcerative Colitis: Symptoms, Diagnosis and Treatment

Edited by Freya Carter

hayle medical

New York

Hayle Medical,
750 Third Avenue, 9th Floor,
New York, NY 10017, USA

Visit us on the World Wide Web at:
www.haylemedical.com

ISBN: 978-1-63241-912-5

Cataloging-in-Publication Data

Ulcerative colitis : symptoms, diagnosis and treatment / edited by Freya Carter.
p. cm.
Includes bibliographical references and index.
ISBN 978-1-63241-912-5
1. Ulcerative colitis. 2. Symptoms. 3. Ulcerative colitis--Diagnosis.
4. Ulcerative colitis--Treatment. I. Carter, Freya.
RC862.C63 U53 2020
616.344 7--dc23

Table of Contents

Preface

Ulcerative colitis is an inflammatory bowel disorder characterized by inflammation and ulcers of the colon and rectum. Various factors can contribute to the development of this disease, like immune system dysfunction, changes in the gut bacteria, genetics and environmental factors. Diarrhea mixed with blood and mucus, anemia, weight loss, abdominal pain, etc. may be observed. Extra-intestinal symptoms like painful arthritis may also occur. Depending on the extent of the disease, ulcerative colitis may be distal or extensive. A complete blood count, liver function tests, stool culture, endoscopy, sigmoidoscopy, biopsy, etc. aid in determining if a patient has ulcerative colitis. A therapeutic regime is designed such that remission is first induced, by achieving mucosal healing of the colitis and providing relief of symptoms. This is followed by treatment aimed at maintaining remission and preventing complications. The surgical removal of the large intestine is also an effective strategy if medication fails to control extra-intestinal symptoms, or if frank perforation, exsanguinating hemorrhage or carcinoma occur. This book contains some path-breaking studies in the diagnosis and treatment of ulcerative colitis. It outlines the signs and symptoms of ulcerative colitis in detail. A number of latest researches have been included to keep the readers up-to-date with the global concepts in this medical condition.

After months of intensive research and writing, this book is the end result of all who devoted their time and efforts in the initiation and progress of this book. It will surely be a source of reference in enhancing the required knowledge of the new developments in the area. During the course of developing this book, certain measures such as accuracy, authenticity and research focused analytical studies were given preference in order to produce a comprehensive book in the area of study.

This book would not have been possible without the efforts of the authors and the publisher. I extend my sincere thanks to them. Secondly, I express my gratitude to my family and well-wishers. And most importantly, I thank my students for constantly expressing their willingness and curiosity in enhancing their knowledge in the field, which encourages me to take up further research projects for the advancement of the area.

Editor

Preface

1

CCL25/CCR9 Interactions Regulate the Function of iNKT Cells in Oxazolone-Induced Colitis in Mice

Siying Zhu[1,2]⁹, Yuntao Bing[2]⁹, Xiaobing Wang[1,2], Qiao Yu[2], Yipeng Wang[1], Shufang Xu[1,2], Lu Song[1,2], Xintao Wang[1,2], Bing Xia[1,2], Youqing Zhu[1,2]*, Rui Zhou[1,2]*

1 Department of Gastroenterology/Hepatology, Zhongnan Hospital of Wuhan University, Wuhan, Hubei, P. R. China, **2** The Hubei Clinical Center & Key Laboratory of Intestinal & Colorectal Diseases, Wuhan, Hubei, P. R. China

Abstract

Background: Natural killer T (NKT) cells share phenotypic and functional properties with both conventional natural killer cells and T cells. These cells might have an important role in the pathogenesis of ulcerative colitis (UC). The interaction of chemokine ligand 25 (CCL25) with chemokine receptor 9 (CCR9) is involved in gut-specific migration of leukocytes and induces regulatory T cells (Tregs) to migrate to the intestine in chronic ileitis.

Methodology/Findings: In UC patients, NKT receptor CD161, CCL25, and CCR9 expression levels were evaluated by qRT-PCR. A murine model of oxazolone-induced colitis was induced in BALB/c mice. The mRNA levels of NK1.1, CCL25 and CCR9, and pro-inflammatory cytokines in mice were evaluated. The CCR9 expression on Type I or invariant NKT (iNKT) cells, and the iNKT cells chemotaxis are observed according to flow cytometry. NKT receptor CD161, CCL25 and CCR9 expression levels were significantly increased in UC patients. And, the mRNA expression levels of NK1.1, CCL25 and CCR9 were increased in oxazolone-induced colitis in mice. The production of pro-inflammatory cytokines was significantly increased, especially interleukin 4 (IL-4), IL-10 and IL-13. We observed significantly increased CCR9 expression on iNKT cells. Furthermore, we found an increased iNKT population and enhanced chemotaxis during oxazolone-induced colitis.

Conclusions/Significance: Our study suggests that CCL25/CCR9 interactions may promote the induction and function of iNKT cells during oxazolone-induced colitis. These findings may have important implications for UC treatment and suggest a role for CCR9 inhibitors.

Editor: Maria Leite de Moraes, CNRS, France

Funding: This work was supported by National Natural Science Foundation of China (No. 81100266). The funders had no role in study design, data collection and analysis, decision to publish, or preparation of the manuscript.

Competing Interests: The authors have declared that no competing interests exist.

* E-mail: zhourui8310@126.com (RZ); uqing_zhu@sina.com (YZ)

⁹ These authors contributed equally to this work.

Introduction

Ulcerative colitis (UC) and Crohn's disease (CD) are clinical subtypes of inflammatory bowel disease (IBD) and are chronic, relapsing immune-mediated disorders of the gastrointestinal tract with unknown etiology [1]. Nevertheless, UC and CD differ from one another both clinically and pathologically [2]. UC is characterized by a T-helper type 2 (Th2) immune responses with contiguous mucosal inflammation in the rectum and colon that cause epithelial barrier dysfunction and lead to ulceration [3]. There are several murine models of mucosal inflammation that mimic human IBD, including a model of hapten-induced colitis in which oxazolone (4-ethoxymethylene-2-phenyl-2-oxazoline-5-one) is delivered intrarectally to rodents. This model is driven by the production of Th2 cytokines and reproduces many UC features [4,5].

Natural killer T (NKT) cells share phenotypic and functional properties with both conventional natural killer cells and T cells. NKT cells recognize the foreign or microbial lipid antigens presented by the non-classical major histocompatibility complex (MHC) molecule CD1d [6]. There are distinct NKT-cell subsets and other types of T cell that resemble NKT cells. NKT cells include CD1d-dependent NKT cells (type I and II) and CD1d-independent NKT-like cells [7]. CD1d-dependent NKT cells are divided into 2 subsets based on differences in T cell receptor (TCR) characteristics [8]. Type I or invariant NKT (iNKT) cells are composed of an invariant TCR α-chain (Vα14-Jα18 in mice and Vα24-Jα18 in humans) paired with a limited set of TCR β-chain. These cells are present in both human and mouse intestines [9]. iNKT cells recognize the marine sponge-derived glycolipid α-galactosylceramide (α-GalCer) in mureine and humans. However, Type II NKT cells are other populations of CD1d-dependent NKT cells, which respond to lipid antigens are broadly. Type II NKT cells exhibit much more TCR sequence diversity and do not respond to α-GalCer, compared to iNKT cells [6]. The most commonly described subset is the iNKT subset [8]. iNKT cells most likely play an important role in the pathogenesis of UC and asthma [10–12].

Chemokine ligand 25 (CCL25, TECK) is highly expressed by the intestinal epithelium and thymus, and regulates trafficking of gut-specific memory/effector T cells via upregulation of the integrin homing receptor α47 and chemokine receptor 9 (CCR9) [13,14]. CCR9 has been associated with IBD and other inflammatory disorders of the intestine, such as celiac disease and primary sclerosing cholangitis [15–17]. CCX282-B is an orally bioavailable CCR9 antagonist that can delay disease progression in moderate to severe Crohn's Disease patients [18]. However, the role of CCL25/CCR9 interactions in the regulation of NKT cells during colitis has not been studied. In the present study, we evaluated the role of CCL25/CCR9 interactions in the regulation of NKT cells in a model of oxazolone-induced colitis.

Materials and Methods

Ethics Statement

All specimen study was approved by the Medical Ethical Committee of the Zhongnan Hospital of Wuhan University and conducted according to the principles expressed in the Declaration of Helsinki. A written informed consent was obtained from all patients and healthy individuals participating in this study. The individual in this manuscript has given written informed consent (as outlined in PLOS consent form) to publish these case details. All animal procedures were performed in strict accordance with the recommendations in the Guide for the Care and Use of Laboratory Animals of Wuhan University. The protocols were approved by the Committee on the Ethics of Animal Experiments of Wuhan University. All of the surgeries were performed under sodium pentobarbital anesthesia, and all efforts were made to minimize suffering.

Patients and Specimens

For this study, 10 consecutive UC patients (5 men and 5 women, aged 21–79 years) were enrolled from January 2012 to January 2013. The diagnosis of UC was based on clinical, endoscopic, radiological and histological findings according to the Lennard-Jones (1989) criteria [19]. The level of disease activity was assessed according to the Truelove and Witt activity index [20]. A total of 10 age- and sex-matched healthy controls were also enrolled in the study. The controls were healthy volunteers unrelated to the patients. Colonic biopsy specimens were obtained from the UC patients and healthy controls by elective colonoscopy.

Animals

Specific pathogen-free 6- to 8-wk-old BALB/c male mice weighing 20–25 g were purchased from the Experimental Animal Center of Wuhan University. All mice were maintained in plastic cages with free access to pellet food and water. The animals were housed at 21±2°C and kept on a 12-h light/dark cycle. The animals were acclimated to these conditions for at least 5 days before the start of the experiment. Animals were randomly allocated to three groups using a random numbers table. Each group contained 15 animals. Animals were humanely sacrificed if they reached a predetermined experimental end point (i.e., loss of ≥20% body weight and significant deterioration of body conditions).

Induction of Colitis

Oxazolone (4-ethoxymethylene-2-phenyl-2-oxazolin-5-one) was obtained from Sigma-Aldrich (St. Louis, MO, USA). Oxazolone (OXA) colitis was induced as previously described [21]. To pre-sensitize mice, a 2×2 cm field of the abdominal skin was shaved, and 150 μl of a 3% (w/v) solution of OXA in 100% ethanol (ETOH) was applied. Seven days later, 150 μl of 2% OXA in 50% ETOH was administered intrarectally with a polyethylene catheter inserted 3 cm into the colon of the OXA mice. The ETOH mice were treated intrarectally with 150 μl of 50% ETOH alone. The control mice were treated without OXA or ETOH. The mice were autopsied 2 days post-oxazolone treatment and sacrificed by cervical dislocation under anesthesia. All of the surgeries were performed under sodium pentobarbital anesthesia, and efforts were made to minimize suffering.

Evaluations of Colitis Severity

Mice were examined daily for body weight, stool consistency, hematochezia and rectal bleeding to grade the clinical colitis severity. The clinical disease activity index (DAI) was determined based on weight loss, stool consistency, hematochezia and rectal bleeding using standard protocols [22,23], as shown in Table 1. The animal survival rate was monitored during the experiment, and colon length was measured after the autopsy.

Histological Assessment of Colitis

Colons were collected on day 2 post-oxazolone administration and fixed in 10% neutral buffered formalin. After paraffin embedding, 5-μm sections were cut and stained with hematoxylin and eosin. The stained sections were examined for evidence of colitis by a blinded reviewer. The histology damage score was calculated on a 12-point scale: loss of architecture, 0–3; inflammatory infiltrate, 0–3; goblet cell depletion, 0 or 1; ulceration, 0 or 1; edema, 0 or 1; muscle thickening, 0–2; and presence of crypt abscesses, 0 or 1 [24].

Myeloperoxidase (MPO) Assay

MPO activity was assayed according to the MPO assay kit manufacturer's instructions (Jiancheng BioEngineering, Nanjing, China). Briefly, MPO is an enzyme found in granulocytes. We assessed MPO activity using a kinetic assay in which H_2O_2 is degraded by the MPO released from the samples of colon [25]. The change in absorbance at 460 nm was measured with a Life Science UV/Vis Spectrophotometer DU 530 (Beckman Coulter, USA). The data are presented as units per milligram of tissue, where 1 unit is equal to the amount of MPO required to degrade 1 μmol of H_2O_2 per minute at 25°C.

Quantitative Real-time Polymerase Chain Reaction (qRT-PCR)

RNA was extracted from colonic biopsy specimens and colon tissue samples using TRIzol reagent (Invitrogen, USA) according to the manufacturer's protocol. Total RNA quantification was performed with a Nanodrop^{TM} spectrophotometer (Thermo Scientific, USA). cDNA was synthesized using an iScript^{TM} cDNA synthesis kit (Bio-Rad, USA). DNA amplification was performed with an iQ5 quantitative PCR System (Bio-Rad, USA) and SYBR® Green Master Mix (Toyobo, Japan) using 50 ng RNA. CD161, CCL25 and CCR9 mRNAs were quantified from the colonic biopsy specimens of UC patients and healthy controls. β-actin was used to normalize expression. For the colon tissue samples from mice, NK1.1, CCL25 and CCR9 mRNAs were quantified using β-actin mRNA for normalization. The gene-specific primers are listed in Table 2. The cycle threshold (Ct) indicated the fractional cycle number at which the PCR product was first detected above a fixed threshold. The relative mRNA levels were determined using the $2^{-\Delta\Delta CT}$ method.

Table 1. Scoring system for disease activity index (DAI) in the study.

Score	Weight loss (%)	Stool consistency	Hematochezia	Rectal bleeding
0	0	Normal	None	Absent
1	1–10	Loose stool	Hemaoccult positive	Present
2	11–20	Diarrhea	Gross blood	N/A
3	≥20	N/A	N/A	N/A

ELISA Assays

Tumor necrosis factor alpha (TNF-α), interferon gamma (IFN-γ), interleukin 17 (IL-17), IL-14, IL-13 and IL-10 were assayed by antibody sandwich ELISA in colon lysates using a mouse ELISA immunoassay kit (Beijing Dakewe Biotech Co. LTD., China). Total protein was extracted from tissues using a Total Protein Extraction Kit (Beijing Tiangen Biotech Co. LTD., China) in accordance with the manufacturer's protocol.

Isolation of Lamina Propria Lymphocytes (LPLs)

LPL suspensions were obtained as previously described [26]. The colons were flushed and opened longitudinally. To remove intra-epithelial lymphocytes and epithelial cells, intestinal pieces were incubated in HBSS without Ca^{2+}/Mg^{2+} supplemented with 2 mM EDTA, 10 mM HEPES, 5% FCS and 1 mM DTT twice for 15 min at 37°C with shaking at 250 rpm. The intestinal pieces were digested in HBSS with Ca^{2+}/Mg^{2+}, 5% FCS, 1.5 mg/ml Collagenase VIII (Sigma-Aldrich, USA) and 0.1 mg/ml DNase I (Thermo Scientific, USA) for 45 min at 37°C with shaking at 250 rpm. The LPLs were purified using 40% and 80% Percoll gradients (Sigma-Aldrich, USA) by centrifuging at 1,000×g for 20 min at 20°C without brakes. The LPLs were washed and resuspended in fluorescence-activated cell sorting (FACS) buffer or culture medium (RPMI 1640 containing 5% FCS).

Flow Cytometry

All staining procedures were performed in Staining Buffer (eBioscience, USA) at 4°C. Single-, double-, or triple-color flow cytometric analyses were performed on a FACS Calibur (BD Biosciences, USA). The data were analyzed using FlowJo software version 7.6.1 (Treestar, Ashland, OR, USA). The peridinin chlorophyll protein-Cy5.5 (PerCP-Cy5.5)-conjugated anti-TCRβ antibody (eBioscience, USA) and phycoerythin (PE)-conjugated α-GalCer-loaded CD1d tetramer (ProImmune, UK) were used as cell surface markers of iNKT cell subpopulations [12]. Additionally, fluorescein isothiocyanate (FITC)-conjugated anti-CCR9 antibody (eBioscience, USA) was used for surface receptor staining. For each marker, the threshold of positivity was defined beyond the nonspecific binding observed in the presence of a relevant isotype control antibody.

In vitro Chemotaxis Assays

The chemokine-dependent migration of LPLs was measured using an *in vitro* 2-chamber migration assay with Transwell Boyden chambers (BD Biosciences, USA) followed by flow cytometry

Table 2. The gene-specific primer list in the study.

Primer names	Primer sequences (5′-3′)
Human:	
CD161-F	TAATGCCACCTTCCTCTG
CD161-R	GAATAATCCCAGCACAGC
CCL25-F	CCACCACAACACGCAGAC
CCL25-R	GATGGAGCCCAGAAATGAG
CCR9-F	TTCCGCTTATTCCTTGGT
CCR9-R	CTAGGGAGCAGACAGACG
β-actin-F	TCAGCAAGCAGGAGTATG
β-actin-R	GTCAAGAAAGGGTGTAACG
Mice:	
NK1.1-F	TGGATTGCTGTTTCCGTCTG
NK1.1-R	TATTGTCAACCCACCACCTT
CCL25-F	CCAAGGTGCCTTTGAAGACT
CCL25-R	TCCTCCAGCTGGTGGTTACT
CCR9-F	CCAGGAAATCTCTGGTCTGC
CCR9-R	CTGTGGAAGCAGTGGAGTCA
β-actin-F	GCTGTATTCCCCTCCATCGT
β-actin-R	GCCATGTTCAATGGGGTACT

analysis [27]. The chemotaxis assays were performed in pre-warmed migration buffer (RPMI 1640 containing 1% FCS). Primary LPLs were seeded at a density of 1×10^5 per well into the upper chamber. A total of 600 µl of migration buffer alone or supplemented with 500 ng/ml recombinant mouse CCL25 protein (Reprokine Research Immunity, USA) was added to the lower chamber. The chambers of cells were incubated for 6 hours at 37°C in an incubator with 5% CO_2. The cells in the lower chambers were centrifuged, fixed in 500 µl Fixation Buffer (eBioscience, USA) and counted using a FACS Calibur (BD Biosciences, USA). The results were expressed as a chemotactic index (CI), which is the ratio between the number of migrating cells in the sample and in the medium control.

Statistical Analysis

All data are presented as the mean ± SEM or SD. The statistical significance of differences between experimental groups was analyzed using one-way analysis of variance (ANOVA) for overall comparisons or Student's unpaired *t*-test for individual comparisons. Differences with $p<0.05$ were considered significant. The correlations of CD161 or NK1.1 expression with the CCL25 and CCR9 expression levels, and the correlation between CCL25 and CCR9 were tested using Pearson's correlation coefficient. Statistical analysis was conducted using SPSS 17.0 software (SPSS for Windows version 17.0, USA).

Results

Increased Expression of CD161, CCL25 and CCR9 in UC Patients

A recent study demonstrated that NKT cells were originally determined based on their expression of NK-like markers such as CD161 (NK1.1) marker in UC [28]. Compared to the healthy controls, UC patients had mRNA levels of CD161, CCL25 and CCR9 that were significantly increased by 3-fold (0.11±0.04 vs. 0.04±0.02, $p=0.037$), 31-fold (4.05±3.57 vs. 0.13±0.21, $p=0.001$) and 46-fold (10.56±2.87 vs. 0.23±0.32, $p<0.001$), respectively (Figure 1A, B, C). The level of CD161 mRNA expression was significantly positively correlated with the levels of the CCL25 ($r=0.529$, $p=0.008$) and CCR9 ($r=0.900$, $p<0.001$) mRNA expression (Figures 1D and E). As shown in Figure 1F, the level of CCR9 mRNA expression was significantly positively correlated with the levels of CCL25 mRNA expression ($r=0.528$, $p=0.008$) in all of the colonic biopsy specimens tested. These results showed that CD161, CCL25 and CCR9 expression levels were remarkably increased in UC patients and suggest that CCL25/CCR9 interactions have a positive correlation with NKT cells in the pathogenesis of UC.

Oxazolone Induce Acute Forms of UC-like Colitis in BALB/c Mice

To examine the correlation between CCL25/CCR9 interactions and NKT cells, we used oxazolone-induced colitis in mice. Mice treated with oxazolone developed a rapid-onset colitis marked by weight loss and reduced survival rate. Mice were evaluated daily to assess the DAI (Table 1).

The difference in body weight for each mouse was determined daily by comparing the current weight with the weight on day 0. On day 1 and day 2, the body weights of the ETOH mice were significantly decreased by 12% (96.87±1.96 vs. 110.61±4.41%, $p<0.001$) and 21% (91.53±0.90 vs. 115.76±3.77%, $p<0.001$), respectively, compared to the control mice. The OXA mice had lost approximately 8% (89.37±2.46 vs. 96.87±1.96%, $p<0.001$) of their weight by day 1 and 9% (84.64±3.02 vs. 91.53±0.90%, $p<0.001$) on day 2 compared to the ETOH mice (Figure 2A). As shown in Figure 2B, the numbers of dead mice were 0 (0/15), 1 (14/15) and 3 (12/15) for the control mice, ETOH mice and OXA mice, respectively. The stool consistency, hematochezia and rectal bleeding of the mice were monitored beginning on day 0. As shown in Figure 2C, the ETOH mice and OXA mice had significantly elevated clinical scores compared to the control mice. Compared to the ETOH mice, the clinical scores of the OXA mice increased significantly by 1.7-fold (1.70±0.48 vs. 1.00±0.00, $p<0.001$) and 1.6-fold (1.90±0.32 vs. 1.20±0.42, $p<0.001$) on day 1 and day 2, respectively. It is clear that the body weight loss, mortality rates and clinical scores for the OXA mice were more than for the ETOH mice.

The Macroscopic Clinical Signs and MPO Activity during Oxazolone-induced Colitis

The colons of the OXA mice showed histologic features similar to those of human UC, including crypt hyperplasia, crypt loss, cryptitis and neutrophil infiltration and mononuclear cells into the lamina propria. These histologic features were less evident in the ETOH mice (Figure 3A). Consistent with these findings, the histological scores were elevated in the OXA mice compared with the ETOH mice. The data are presented in Figure 3B (OXA, 6.20±1.48 vs. Control, 0.20±0.42, $p<0.001$; OXA, 6.20±1.48 vs. ETOH, 0.80±0.79, $p<0.001$).

The shortening of the colon that occurs due to ulceration and inflammation is an indicator of colitis severity in colitis mice [29]. As shown in Figure 3C, we observed shorter colons in the OXA mice than in the ETOH mice (8.58±1.20 vs. 11.05±0.70 cm, $p<0.001$). However, there was no significant reduction in colon length in the ETOH mice (11.05±0.70 vs. 11.87±0.57 cm, $p=0.067$) compared to the control mice. In the OXA mice, MPO activity was significantly increased by 6-fold (2.27±0.59 vs. 0.40±0.13 U/mg tissue, $p<0.001$) compared with the control mice. Additionally, MPO was significantly increased by 4-fold (2.27±0.59 vs. 0.56±0.20 U/mg tissue, $p<0.001$) in OXA mice compared with the ETOH mice (Figure 3D). These results suggested that the OXA mice had acute UC-like colitis, which was determined based on histological appearance, histological scores, colon length and MPO activity.

Increased Expression Levels of NK1.1, CCL25 and CCR9 are Found in Oxazolone-induced Colitis

A low-level of expression for CCL25 and CCR9 has been detected in the large intestine [30]. To determine whether colitis affects the expression levels of NK1.1, CCL25 and CCR9, we analyzed the mRNA expression levels using qPCR. Compared to the control mice, the expression levels of NK1.1, CCL25 and CCR9 in OXA mice were significantly increased by 3-fold (3.94±0.75 vs. 1.14±0.40, $p<0.001$), 2-fold (1.04±0.45 vs. 0.42±0.16, $p=0.001$) and 5-fold (6.15±2.07 vs. 1.15±0.50, $p<0.001$), respectively. As shown in Figure 4A, B, C, the expression levels of NK1.1, CCL25 and CCR9 were all increased by 2-fold (3.94±0.75 vs. 1.68±0.64, $p<0.001$; 1.04±0.45 vs. 0.45±0.15, $p<0.001$; 6.15±2.07 vs. 2.49±0.73, $p<0.001$) compared to the ETOH mice. However, the expression levels of NK1.1, CCL25 and CCR9 were not increased in the ETOH mice (1.68±0.64 vs. 1.14±0.40, $p>0.05$; 0.45±0.15 vs. 0.42±0.16, $p>0.05$; 2.49±0.73 vs. 1.15±0.50, $p>0.05$) compared to the control mice. As shown in Figures 4D and E, the level of NK1.1 mRNA expression was significantly positively correlated with the levels of the CCL25 ($r=0.677$, $p=0.001$) and CCR9 ($r=0.819$, $p<0.001$) mRNA expression in all of the colonic biopsy specimens tested.

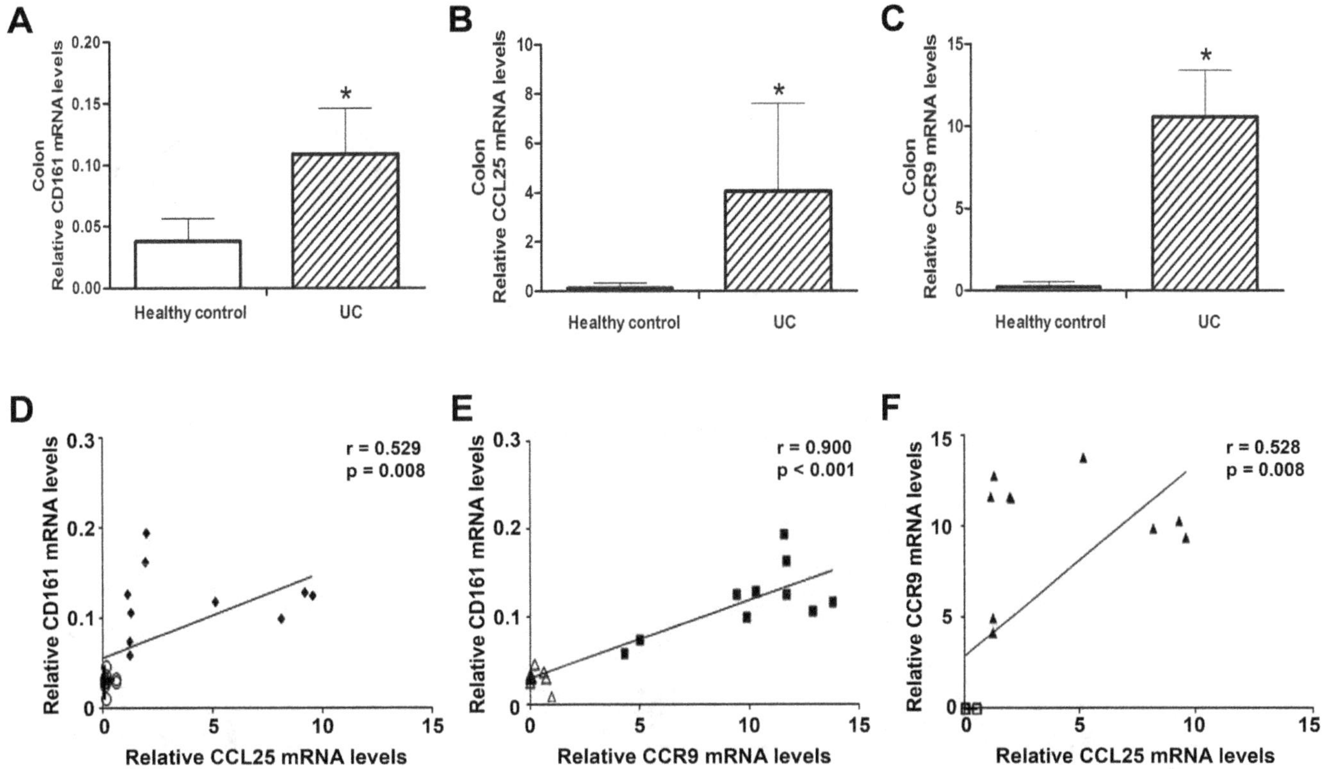

Figure 1. Expression of CD161, CCL25 and CCR9 in UC and healthy controls. The mRNA levels of CD161 (**A**), CCL25 (**B**) and CCR9 (**C**) were significantly increased in the UC patients compared to the healthy controls. n = 10 per group, *$p<0.05$ versus the healthy controls. **D and E.** CD161 mRNA expression was positively correlated with CCL25 mRNA and CCR9 mRNA expression. **F.** The mRNA level of CCR9 had a positive correlation with the mRNA level of CCL25. Each data point represents one colonic biopsy specimen in each panel, and each panel includes data from all colonic biopsy specimens in our experiments. Different symbols are used for UC patients and healthy controls in each panel. Data were analyzed by Pearson's correlation coefficient.

The level of CCR9 mRNA expression was significantly positively correlated with the level of CCL25 mRNA expression ($r = 0.495$, $p = 0.023$) (Figures 4F). These results show that NK1.1, CCL25 and CCR9 expression levels increased in the OXA mice, suggesting that CCL25/CCR9 interactions are correlated with NKT cells during colitis.

Production of Pro-inflammatory Cytokines during Oxazolone-induced Colitis

To assess tissue inflammation, we analyzed the Th1/Th2/Th17 cytokines in intestinal tissue homogenates. As shown in Figure 5, the production of TNF-α, IFN-γ, IL-17, IL-4, IL-10 and IL-13 in OXA mice was significantly increased compared to the control and ETOH mice.

The production of TNF-α in OXA mice was increased by 5-fold (3003.79±732.95 vs. 613.23±133.16 pg/ml, $p<0.001$) and 3-fold

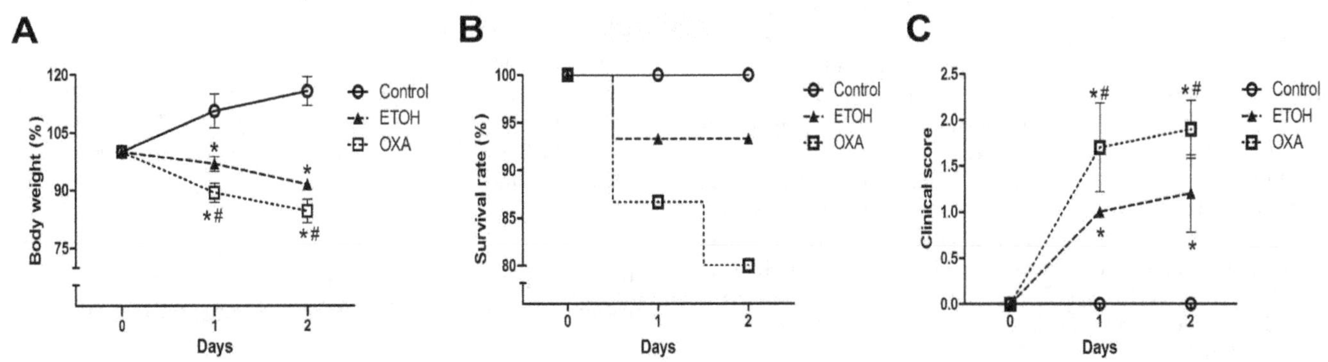

Figure 2. Changes in body weight, survival rate and clinical scores during oxazolone-induced colitis. A. The OXA mice lost the more body weight on day 2 compared to the ETOH mice. **B.** An 80% survival rate was observed in the OXA mice. **C.** The clinical scores of the OXA mice were significantly increased compared to the ETOH mice. n = 15 per group, *$p<0.05$ versus the control mice, and $^{\#}p<0.05$ versus the ETOH mice.

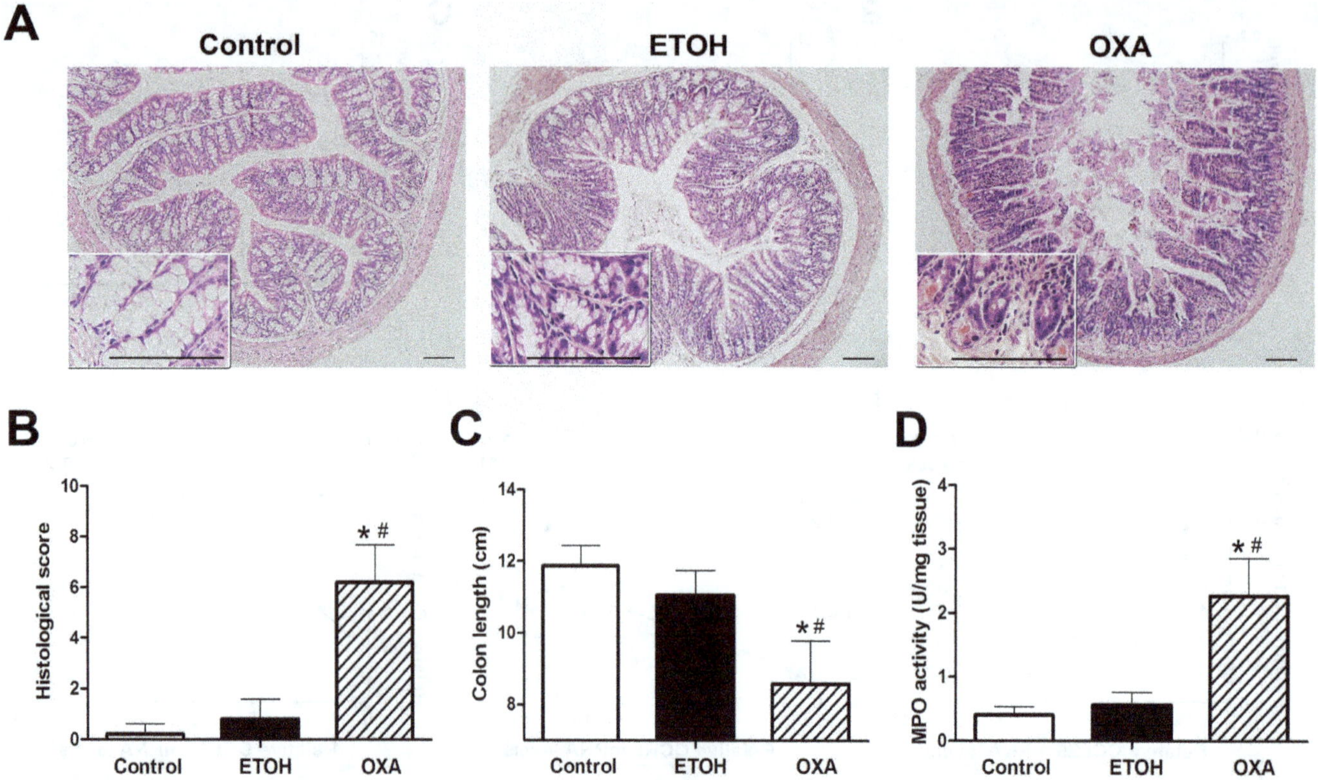

Figure 3. Changes in histological scores, colon length and MPO activity during oxazolone-induced colitis. A. Tissue slices were inspected by a certified pathologist, and the inflammation severity of colonic tissues from surviving mice in each group was scored and documented. Cross-sections represent the transverse colon. Image magnifications are 100-fold and 400-fold. Scale bar, 100 μm. **B.** The histological scores were higher in the OXA mice during colitis. **C.** The colon length of the OXA mice was significantly shorter than the ETOH mice. **D.** The MPO activity was significantly increased in the OXA mice compared to the ETOH mice. n = 10 per group, *$p<0.05$ versus the control mice, and $^{\#}p<0.05$ versus the ETOH mice.

(3003.79±732.95 vs. 1099.23±306.68 pg/ml, $p<0.001$), compared to the control and ETOH mice, respectively (Figure 5A). In the OXA mice, IFN-γ was increased by 6-fold (44637.53±14115.58 vs. 7543.80±1819.68 pg/ml, $p<0.001$) and 4-fold (44637.53±14115.58 vs. 12593.29±2589.37 pg/ml, $p<0.001$), compared to the control and ETOH mice, respectively, (Figure 5B). However, IL-17 was increased by 4-fold (2794.40±945.04 vs. 623.94±185.79 pg/ml, $p<0.001$) and 2-fold (2794.40±945.04 vs. 1209.65±134.73 pg/ml, $p<0.001$), respectively, compared to the control and ETOH mice (Figure 5C). Oxazolone strongly enhanced the production of IL-4, IL-10 and IL-13. The levels of IL-4, IL-10 and IL-13 were all increased by 7-fold (419.78±166.71 vs. 62.12±19.35 pg/ml, $p<0.001$; 5662.00±1544.00 vs. 773.65±179.00 pg/ml, $p<0.001$; 435.97±133.24 vs. 59.76±12.18 pg/ml, $p<0.001$) compared to the control mice, and by 4-fold (419.78±166.71 vs. 114.72±39.20 pg/ml, $p<0.001$; 5662.00±1544.00 vs. 1259.74±400.02 pg/ml, $p<0.001$; 435.97±133.24 vs. 110.72±22.25 pg/ml, $p<0.001$) compared to the ETOH mice (Figure 5D, E, F). These results indicated the levels of IL-4, IL-10 and IL-13 in the OXA mice were remarkably high compared to the ETOH mice, while the levels of TNF-α, IFN-γ and IL-17 changing little.

Highly Increased Frequency of Colonic iNKT Cells and CCR9 Expression during Oxazolone-induced Colitis

We investigated the recruitment of iNKT cells and expression of CCR9 by flow cytometry in LPL populations extracted from the colon of mice in three independent experiments. We observed that iNKT cells (TCRβ$^+$ α-GalCer-loaded CD1d tetramer$^+$ cells) were recruited in the colons of OXA mice (2.41%) and ETOH mice (0.18%) (Figure 6A). As shown in Figure 6A, CCR9 expression by the colon iNKT cells of OXA mice (50.5%) was increased compared to the colon iNKT cells of ETOH mice (26.1%). The percentage of iNKT cells was significantly increased by 8-fold (2.05±0.46 vs. 0.26±0.16%, $p<0.001$) in the OXA mice compared to the ETOH mice (Figure 6B). As shown in Figure 6C, the CCR9 expression levels on iNKT cells were higher in the OXA mice (2-fold, 58.87±14.01 vs. 29.90±5.32%, $p=0.001$) compared to the ETOH mice. Interestingly, CCR9 expression on iNKT cells and the levels of iNKT cells were significantly increased during colitis. These results suggested CCL25/CCR9 interactions might promote the induction of iNKT cells during colitis.

Highly Increased Chemotaxis of Colonic iNKT Cells Towards CCL25 during Oxazolone-induced Colitis

To analyze the functionality of the chemokine receptors expressed by iNKT cells, we performed a chemotaxis assay to determine the ability of iNKT cells to migrate toward CCL25 (500 ng/ml). As shown in Figure 7A, the percentages of iNKT

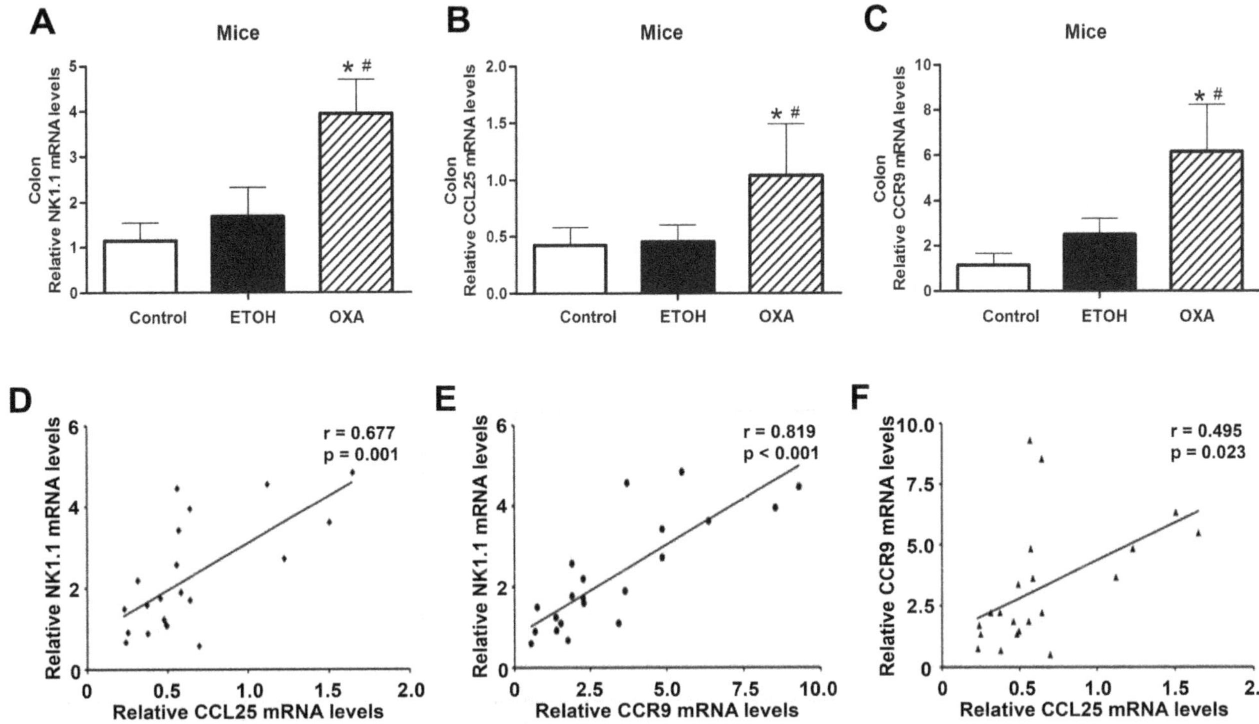

Figure 4. Expression levels of NK1.1, CCL25 and CCR9 during oxazolone-induced colitis. The mRNA levels of NK1.1 (**A**), CCL25 (**B**) and CCR9 (**C**) were significantly increased in the OXA mice compared to the ETOH mice. n = 10 per group, *$p<0.05$ versus the control mice, and #$p<0.05$ versus the ETOH mice. **D and E.** NK1.1 mRNA expression had positive correlations with CCL25 mRNA and CCR9 mRNA expression. **F.** The mRNA expression of CCR9 was significantly positively correlated with CCL25 mRNA expression. Each data point represents one colonic biopsy specimen in each panel, and each panel includes data from all colonic biopsy specimens in our experiments. Data were analyzed by Pearson's correlation coefficient.

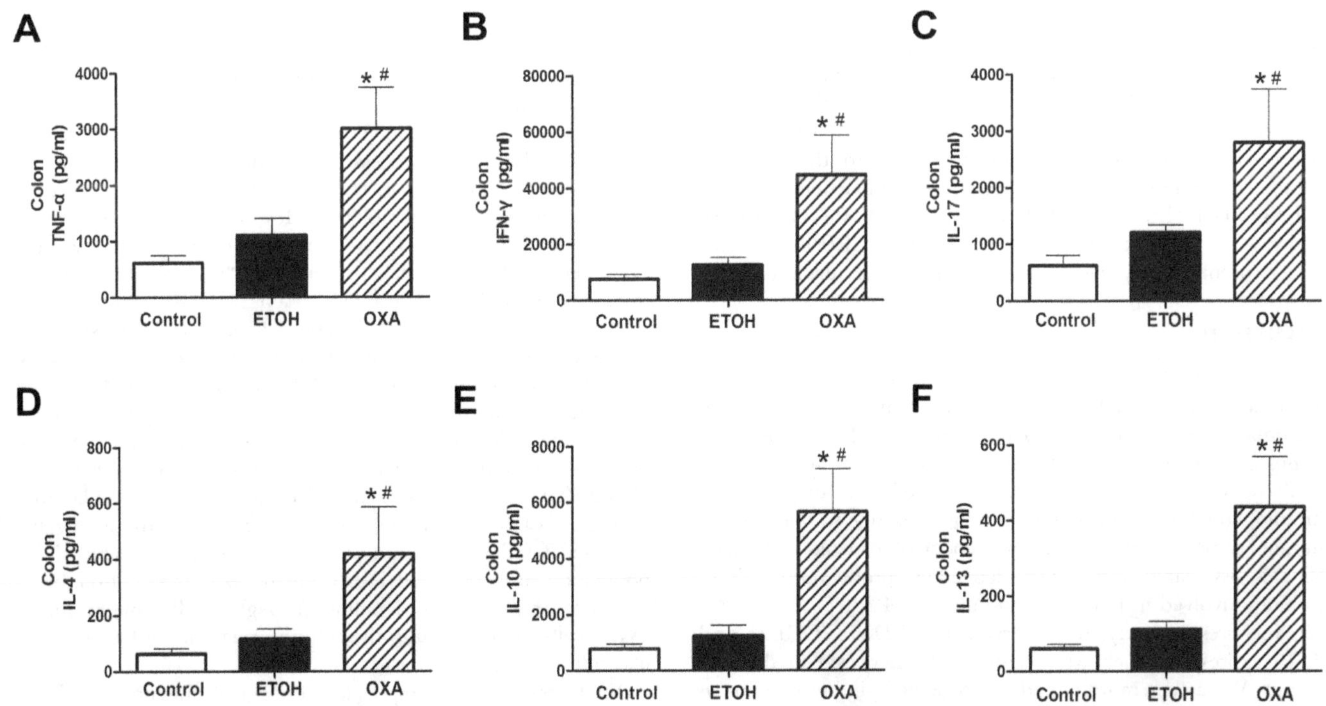

Figure 5. Production of TNF-α, IFN-γ, IL-17, IL-4, IL-10 and IL-13 during oxazolone-induced colitis. The levels of TNF-α (**A**), IFN-γ (**B**), IL-17 (**C**), IL-4 (**D**), IL-10 (**E**) and IL-13 (**F**) were significantly increased in the OXA mice compared to the ETOH mice. n = 10 per group, *$p<0.05$ versus the control mice, and #$p<0.05$ versus the ETOH mice.

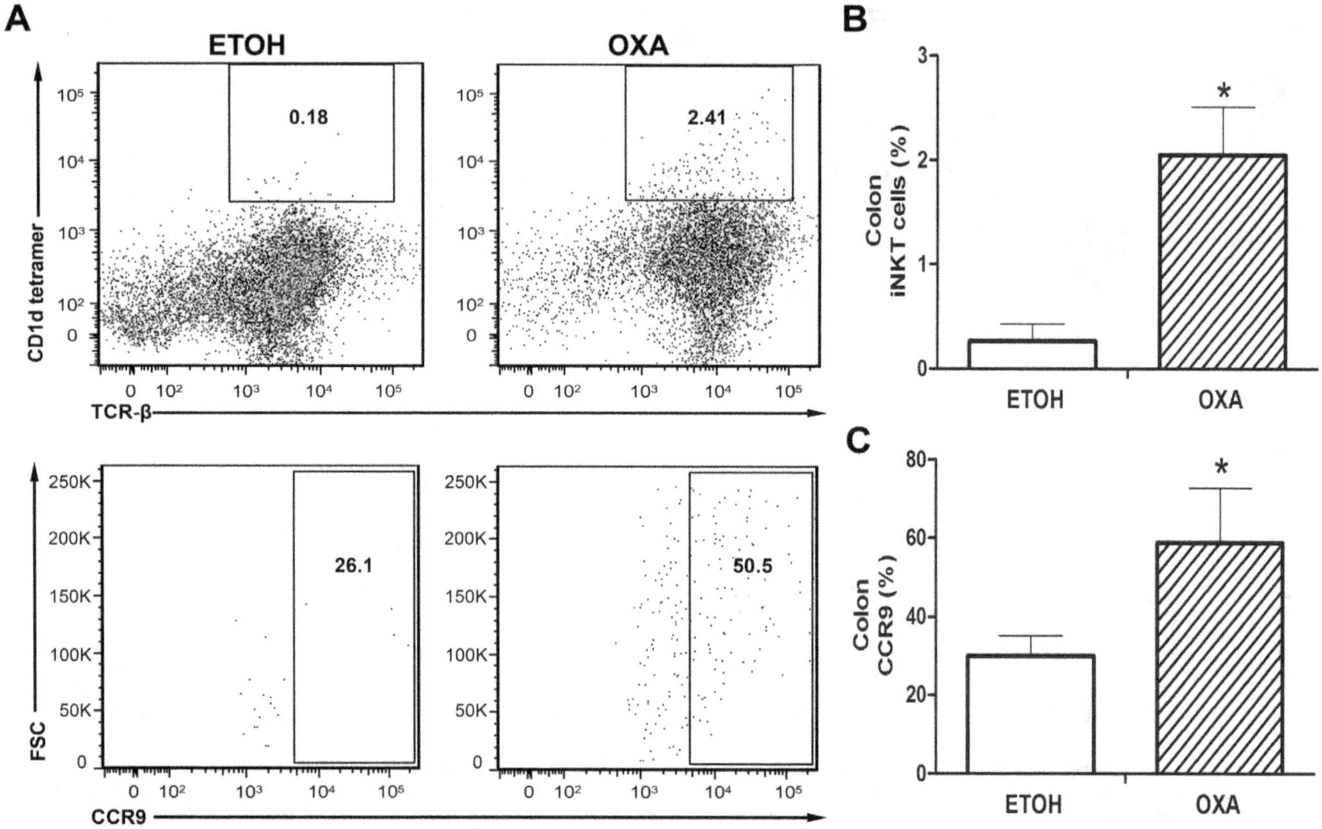

Figure 6. Frequency of colonic iNKT cells and CCR9 expression during oxazolone-induced colitis. The recruitment of iNKT cells and CCR9 expression on iNKT cells in LPL populations extracted from the colon of mice in three independent experiments by flow cytometry. **A.** The frequency of iNKT cells and CCR9 expression on iNKT cells in the OXA mice and ETOH mice. **B.** The percentage of iNKT cells was significantly increased in the OXA mice. **C.** Increased expression of CCR9 on iNKT cells was observed in the OXA mice. n = 3 per group, *$p<0.05$ versus the ETOH mice.

cells specifically migrating to CCL25 were increased in the LPLs from both ETOH and OXA mice. After chemotaxis to CCL25, the percentage of iNKT cells was increased by 4-fold (5.45±0.70 vs. 1.29±0.27%, $p = 0.029$) in the LPLs from OXA mice (Figure 7B). More iNKT cells migrated toward the chamber containing recombinant CCL25 than to the compartment without CCL25 (30.64±1.61 vs. 2.02±0.65, $p<0.001$) in the OXA mice (Figure 7C). These results suggested CCL25/CCR9 interactions might promote iNKT cell migration to the colon during colitis.

Discussion

Although the exact etiology of IBD is unclear, it is know that altered immunological functions can contribute to the mucosal inflammation of the intestinal tract [31]. iNKT cell development is thymus dependent, but iNKT cells are found in the liver, spleen, lymph nodes and intestines [12]. iNKT cells are an important immunoregulatory population of lymphocytes able to polarize the immune response [12]. A murine model of oxazolone-induced colitis is associated with CD1d-dependent production of Th2 cytokines involved in mucosal inflammation [4,32].

In the present study, we observed that CD161, CCL25 and CCR9 expression levels were significantly increased in the UC patients. We used a murine model of oxazolone-induced colitis to investigate the potential regulatory roles of CCL25/CCR9 interactions in NKT cells and the underlying mechanisms involved. We found that the expressions of NK1.1, CCL25 and CCR9 were significantly increased during oxazolone-induced colitis. Importantly, we demonstrated that human UC and UC-like colitis upregulated the expression of NKT, CCL25 and CCR9 in both humans and mice.

Chemokines are small heparin-binding proteins that play roles in multiple biological processes, including leukocyte chemotaxis [33]. Most chemokines can recognize several receptors, and one receptor binds many chemokines. However, the CCR9 receptor only binds CCL25 [34]. The combination of chemokine receptors expressed on the cell surface provides an "address" for leukocyte migration to different sites [35]. CCL25/CCR9 interaction is involved in gut-specific migration of leukocytes, suggesting this chemokine/receptor pair is non-promiscuous [36]. Wermers et al. recently demonstrated that chemokine CCL25 could induce Tregs to migrate to the intestine in chronic ileitis through its receptor CCR9 [37]. Although the induction of regulatory molecules occurs via common pathways, little is known about the roles of CCL25/CCR9 interactions in iNKT trafficking and regulation of immune responses in the colon. We observed significantly increased CCR9 expression on iNKT cells, an increased iNKT population and increased iNKT chemotaxis. It is reasonable to speculate that CCL25 signaling through CCR9 might induce iNKT cells to migrate into the colon during human UC and UC-like colitis.

NKT cells have complicated biological functions and can rapidly produce large amounts of Th1, Th2 and regulatory cytokines [38]. It has been shown that iNKT cells play an important role in the pathogenesis of UC and secrete large amounts of pro-inflammatory cytokines such as IL-4 and IL-13

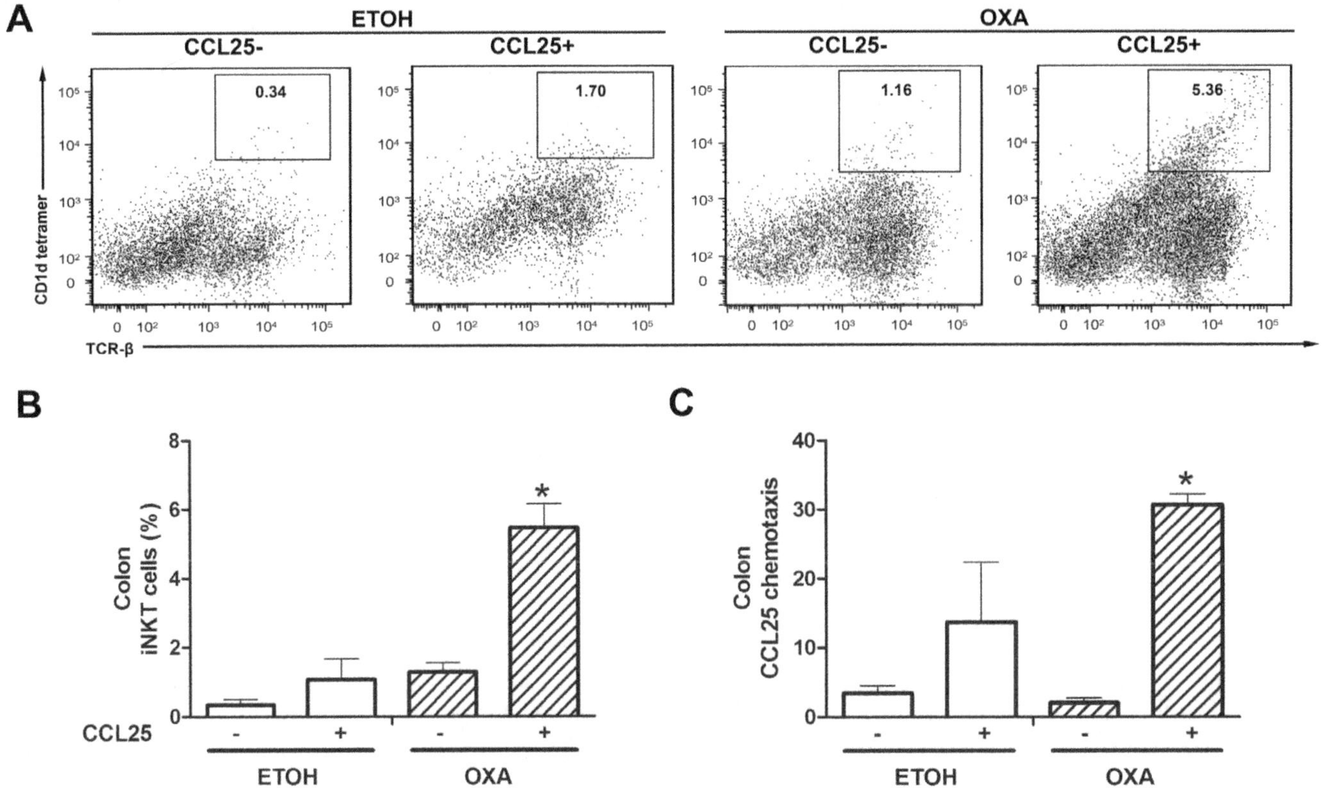

Figure 7. Chemotaxis of colonic iNKT cells towards CCL25 during oxazolone-induced colitis. The chemotaxis of colonic iNKT cells toward CCL25 was evaluated by a chemotaxis assay. **A.** After CCL25 treatment, the percentage of iNKT cells was determined in the LPLs from the OXA and ETOH mice. **B.** After chemotaxis to CCL25, the percentage of iNKT cells was significantly increased in the LPLs from the OXA mice. **C.** Colonic CCL25 chemotaxis was significantly increased in the LPLs from the OXA mice. n = 3 per group, $^{*}p<0.05$ versus the ETOH mice.

upon activation [10,11]. Mouse NKT cells have been recognized as immunosuppressive cells that produce Th2 cytokines or IL-10 [39]. Our interpretation that the results are a consequence of a highly inflammatory response in OXA mice is supported by our data in two ways. First, there was a pronounced accumulation of iNKT cells. Second, there was increased expression of the pro-inflammatory cytokines, especially IL-4, IL-10 and IL-13. The increased expression of these pro-inflammatory cytokines has also been described for human UC [40].

We demonstrated significantly increased CCR9 expression on iNKT cells, an expanded iNKT population and increased chemotaxis of iNKT cells during oxazolone-induced colitis. It is our hypothesis that CCL25/CCR9 interactions promote the induction and function of iNKT cells during oxazolone-induced colitis. However, it is yet to be tested the role of CCL25/CCR9 interactions in iNKT cells migrating into the colon. CCR9- or CCL25-deficient animals or antibody-mediated neutralization of these factors are needed in future studies to definitively define the function and mechanism of CCL25/CCR9 interactions in the regulation of iNKT cells during oxazolone-induced colitis.

In conclusion, this study has shown that CCL25/CCR9 interactions may promote the induction and function of iNKT cells during oxazolone-induced colitis. These findings expand our understanding of the underlying mechanism of CCL25/CCR9 interactions in the regulation of iNKT cells during human UC and UC-like colitis. This study has provided further evidence that CCR9-inhibitors could be a potential therapeutic strategy for patients with UC.

Acknowledgments

We want to thank the members of the Animal Care Committee of Wuhan University for the staff at the animal facility for their helpfulness and good animal care. We thank editors in American Journal Experts for the valuable contribution to edit and revise the manuscript.

Author Contributions

Conceived and designed the experiments: SYZ YTB YQZ RZ. Performed the experiments: SYZ YTB XBW QY YPW. Analyzed the data: SYZ YTB XBW QY. Contributed reagents/materials/analysis tools: SYZ YTB SFX LS XTW. Wrote the paper: SYZ YTB BX YQZ RZ.

References

1. Molodecky NA, Soon IS, Rabi DM, Ghali WA, Ferris M, et al. (2012) Increasing incidence and prevalence of the inflammatory bowel diseases with time, based on systematic review. Gastroenterology 142: 46–54.
2. Fuss IJ, Heller F, Boirivant M, Leon F, Yoshida M, et al. (2004) Nonclassical CD1d-restricted NK T cells that produce IL-13 characterize an atypical Th2 response in ulcerative colitis. J Clin Invest 113: 1490–1497.
3. Galitovskiy V, Qian J, Chernyavsky AI, Marchenko S, Gindi V, et al. (2011) Cytokine-induced alterations of alpha7 nicotinic receptor in colonic CD4 T cells mediate dichotomous response to nicotine in murine models of Th1/Th17- versus Th2-mediated colitis. J Immunol 187: 2677–2687.
4. Heller F, Fuss IJ, Nieuwenhuis EE, Blumberg RS, Strober W. (2002) Oxazolone colitis, a Th2 colitis model resembling ulcerative colitis, is mediated by IL-13-producing NK-T cells. Immunity 17: 629–638.
5. Boirivant M, Fuss IJ, Chu A, Strober W. (1998) Oxazolone colitis: A murine model of T helper cell type 2 colitis treatable with antibodies to interleukin 4. J Exp Med 188: 1929–1939.

6. Liao CM, Zimmer MI, Wang CR. (2013) The functions of type I and type II natural killer T cells in inflammatory bowel diseases. Inflamm Bowel Dis 19: 1330–1338.
7. Godfrey DI, MacDonald HR, Kronenberg M, Smyth MJ, Van Kaer L. (2004) NKT cells : what's in a name ? Nat Rev Immunol 4: 231–237.
8. Juno JA, Keynan Y, Fowke KR. (2012) Invariant NKT cells: regulation and function during viral infection. PLoS Pathog 8: e1002838.
9. Montbarbon M, Pichavant M, Langlois A, Erdual E, Maggiotto F, et al. (2013) Colonic inflammation in mice is improved by cigarette smoke through iNKT cells recruitment. PLoS One 8: e62208.
10. Cohen NR, Garg S, Brenner MB. (2009) Antigen Presentation by CD1 Lipids, T Cells, and NKT Cells in Microbial Immunity. Adv Immunol 102: 1–94.
11. Akbari O, Stock P, Meyer E, Kronenberg M, Sidobre S, et al. (2003) Essential role of NKT cells producing IL-4 and IL-13 in the development of allergen-induced airway hyperreactivity. Nat Med 9: 582–588.
12. Olszak T, An D, Zeissig S, Vera MP, Richter J, et al. (2012) Microbial exposure during early life has persistent effects on natural killer T cell function. Science 336: 489–493.
13. Stenstad H, Ericsson A, Johansson-Lindbom B, Svensson M, Marsal J, et al. (2006) Gut-associated lymphoid tissue-primed $CD4^+$ T cells display CCR9-dependent and -independent homing to the small intestine. Blood 107: 3447–3454.
14. Wurbel MA, Malissen M, Guy-Grand D, Malissen B, Campbell JJ. (2007) Impaired accumulation of antigen-specific CD8 lymphocytes in chemokine CCL25-deficient intestinal epithelium and lamina propria. J Immunol 178: 7598–7606.
15. Papadakis KA, Prehn J, Moreno ST, Cheng L, Kouroumalis EA, et al. (2001) CCR9-positive lymphocytes and thymus-expressed chemokine distinguish small bowel from colonic Crohn's disease. Gastroenterology 121: 246–254.
16. Eksteen B, Gran AJ, Miles A, Curbishley SM, Lalor PF, et al. (2004) Hepatic endothelial CCL25 mediates the recruitment of $CCR9^+$ gut-homing lymphocytes to the liver in primary sclerosing cholangitis. J Exp Med 200: 1511–1517.
17. Olaussen RW, Karlsson MR, Lundin KE, Jahnsen J, Brandtzaeg P, et al. (2007) Reduced chemokine receptor 9 on intraepithelial lymphocytes in celiac disease suggests persistent epithelial activation. Gastroenterology 132: 2371–2382.
18. Walters MJ, Wang Y, Lai N, Baumgart T, Zhao BN, et al. (2010) Characterization of CCX282-B, an orally bioavailable antagonist of the CCR9 chemokine receptor, for treatment of inflammatory bowel disease. J Pharmacol Exp Ther 335: 61–69.
19. Lennard-Jones JE. (1989) Classification of inflammatory bowel disease. Scand J Gastroenterol 170: 2–16.
20. Truelove SC, Witts LJ. (1955) Cortisone in ulcerative colitis; final report on a therapeutic trial. Br Med J 2: 1041–1048.
21. Wirtz S, Neufert C, Weigmann B, Neurath MF. (2007) Chemically induced mouse models of intestinal inflammation. Nat Protoc 2: 541–546.
22. Boirivant M, Strober W, Fuss IJ. (2005) Regulatory cells induced by feeding TNP-haptenated colonic protein cross-protect mice from colitis induced by an unrelated hapten. Inflamm Bowel Dis 11: 48–55.
23. Kihara N, de la Fuente SG, Fujino K, Takahashi T, Pappas TN, et al. (2003) Vanilloid receptor-1 containing primary sensory neurones mediate dextran sulphate sodium induced colitis in rats. Gut 52: 713–719.
24. Hunter MM, Wang A, Hirota CL, McKay DM. (2005) Neutralizing anti-IL-10 antibody blocks the protective effect of tapeworm infection in a murine model of chemically induced colitis. J Immunol 174: 7368–7375.
25. Hunter MM, Wang A, McKay DM. (2007) Helminth infection enhances disease in a murine TH2 model of colitis. Gastroenterology 132: 1320–1330.
26. Weigmann B, Tubbe I, Seidel D, Nicolaev A, Becker C, et al. (2007) Isolation and subsequent analysis of murine lamina propria mononuclear cells from colonic tissue. Nat Protoc 2: 2307–2311.
27. Badr G, Lefevre EA, Mohany M. (2011) Thymoquinone inhibits the CXCL12-induced chemotaxis of multiple myeloma cells and increases their susceptibility to Fas-mediated apoptosis. PLoS One 6: e23741.
28. Terabe M, Berzofsky JA. (2008) The role of NKT cells in tumor immunity. Adv Cancer Res 101: 277–348.
29. Yang J, Zhao J, Nakaguchi T, Gregersen H. (2009) Biomechanical changes in oxazolone-induced colitis in BALB/C mice. J Biomech 42: 811–817.
30. Wurbel MA, McIntire MG, Dwyer P, Fiebiger E. (2011) CCL25/CCR9 interactions regulate large intestinal inflammation in a murine model of acute colitis. PLoS One 6: e16442.
31. Podolsky DK. (2002) Inflammatory bowel disease. N Engl J Med 347: 417–429.
32. Nieuwenhuis EE, Matsumoto T, Exley M, Schleipman RA, Glickman J, et al. (2002) CD1d-dependent macrophage-mediated clearance of Pseudomonas aeruginosa from lung. Nat Med 8: 588–593.
33. Zlotnik A, Yoshie O. (2000) Chemokines: a new classification system and their role in immunity. Immunity 12: 121–127.
34. Mantovani A. (1999) The chemokine system: redundancy for robust outputs. Immunol Today 20: 254–257.
35. Sallusto F, Mackay CR, Lanzavecchia A. (1997) Selective expression of the eotaxin receptor CCR3 by human T helper 2 cells." Science 227: 2005–2007.
36. Papadakis KA, Prehn J, Nelson V, Cheng L, Binder SW, et al. (2000) The role of thymus-expressed chemokine and its receptor CCR9 on lymphocytes in the regional specialization of the mucosal immune system. J Immunol 165: 5069–5076.
37. Wermers JD, McNamee EN, Wurbel MA, Jedlicka P, Rivera-Nieves J. (2011) The chemokine receptor CCR9 is required for the T-cell-mediated regulation of chronic ileitis in mice. Gastroenterology 140: 1526–1535.
38. Godfrey DI, Kronenberg M. (2004) Going both ways: immune regulation via CD1d-dependent NKT cells. J Clin Invest 114: 1379–1388.
39. Smyth MJ, Godfrey DI. (2000) NKT cells and tumor immunity–a double-edged sword. Nat Immunol 1: 459–460.
40. Autschbach F, Giese T, Gassler N, Sido B, Heuschen G, et al. (2002) Cytokine/chemokine messenger-RNA expression profiles in ulcerative colitis and Crohn's disease. Virchows Arch 441: 500–513.

2

Decrease of Peripheral and Intestinal NKG2A-Positive T Cells in Patients with Ulcerative Colitis

Takehiko Katsurada[1,2]⁹, Waka Kobayashi[1,2]⁹, Utano Tomaru[1*], Tomohisa Baba[1¤], Shigeru Furukawa[2], Akihiro Ishizu[3], Kazuyoshi Takeda[4], Naoya Sakamoto[2], Masahiro Asaka[2], Hiroshi Takeda[2,5], Masanori Kasahara[1]

1 Department of Pathology, Hokkaido University Graduate School of Medicine, Sapporo, Japan, **2** Department of Gastroenterology, Hokkaido University Graduate School of Medicine, Sapporo, Japan, **3** Faculty of Health Sciences, Hokkaido University, Sapporo, Japan, **4** Department of Immunology, Juntendo University School of Medicine, Tokyo, Japan, **5** Faculty of Pharmaceutical Sciences, Hokkaido University, Sapporo, Japan

Abstract

To investigate the role of inhibitory natural killer receptors (iNKRs) in inflammatory bowel disease (IBD), we analyzed the expression of NKG2A, one of the iNKRs, on T cells in a mouse colitis model and human IBD. During the active phase of dextran sulfate sodium (DSS)-induced mouse colitis, the frequency of NKG2A+ T cells was significantly decreased in the peripheral blood, and increased in the intestine, suggesting the mobilization of this T cell subset to the sites of inflammation. Administration of anti-NKG2A antibody increased the number of inflammatory foci in DSS-induced colitis, suggesting the involvement of NKG2A+ T cells in this colitis model. In ulcerative colitis (UC) patients, the frequency of peripheral blood NKG2A+ T cells was significantly decreased, compared with Crohn's disease (CD) patients and healthy controls, regardless of clinical conditions such as treatment modalities and disease activity. Notably, in sharp contrast to the DSS-induced mouse colitis model, the frequency of NKG2A+ cells among intestinal T cells was also decreased in UC patients. These results suggest that inadequate local infiltration of NKG2A+ T cells may be involved in the pathogenesis of UC.

Editor: Sven G. Meuth, University of Muenster, Germany

Funding: This work was supported in part by Grants-in-Aid for Scientific Research from The Ministry of Education, Culture, Sports, Science and Technology of Japan. No additional external funding received for this study. The funders had no role in study design, data collection and analysis, decision to publish, or preparation of the manuscript.

Competing Interests: The authors have declared that no competing interests exist.

* E-mail: tomaruu@med.hokudai.ac.jp

⁹ These authors contributed equally to this work.

¤ Current address: Division of Molecular Bioregulation, Cancer Research Institute, Kanazawa University, Kanazawa, Japan

Introduction

The intestinal tract is home to a large number of immune cellular components that continuously encounter abundant exogenous stimuli. Normally, immune responses in the intestine remain in a state of controlled inflammation, mediated by a balance between protective immunity toward pathogens and regulatory mechanisms to circumvent host damages. Inflammatory bowel disease (IBD) is a condition characterized by chronic and refractory intestinal inflammation; there are two distinct, but sometimes overlapping clinical entities that comprise IBD: ulcerative colitis (UC) and Crohn's disease (CD). Although the pathogenesis of IBD remains poorly understood, a large body of evidence indicates that both diseases are caused by imbalances in barrier function and immune responses against pathogens, triggered by infections as well as environmental and genetic factors [1–3].

Natural killer (NK) cells are large granular lymphocytes of the innate immune system that produce many cytokines and chemokines, and exert antibody (Ab)-dependent as well as Ab-independent cytotoxicity [4]. NK-cell tolerance to self is ensured in part by the ligation of inhibitory NK receptors (iNKRs) by self-major histocompatibility complex (MHC) class I molecules [5]. These receptors include killer cell immunoglobulin-like receptors and leukocyte immunoglobulin-like receptors in humans, Ly49 molecules in mice, and CD94/NKG2 molecules in both species [6]. All of these receptors are characterized by the presence of an intracytoplasmic immunoreceptor tyrosine-based inhibition motif (ITIM) that is necessary and sufficient for the inhibitory function [7,8]. Despite being named NK receptors, iNKRs are also expressed on minor subsets of T cells [9]. There is increasing evidence that iNKRs such as NKG2A expressed on T cells are importantly involved in the regulation of immune responses by down-regulating antigen-mediated T-cell effector functions and cytokine release [9–11].

Recently, it was reported that intraepithelial CD8+ NKG2A+ $\gamma\delta$+ T cells localized in the small intestine have regulatory potential in celiac disease [12]. However, no studies have addressed the potential role of NKG2A+ T cells in the pathogenesis of IBD. In this study, we examined peripheral blood and intestinal NKG2A+ T cells in a dextran sulfate sodium (DSS)-induced mouse colitis model and UC patients.

Results

Frequency of NKG2A+ T Cells in Peripheral Blood Is Decreased in DSS-induced Colitis Mice

Mice were given 3% DSS in distilled water *ad libitum* for 7 days to induce colitis. On day 3, they started to develop clinical symptoms such as diarrhea, hematochezia, and body weight loss. After discontinuation of DSS treatment, these symptoms were improved around days 10 to 14, and their body weight returned to normal levels around day 21 (Figure 1A). Control mice, which were given distilled water, developed no clinical symptoms at all. We analyzed the frequency of NKG2A+ T cells in the peripheral blood mononuclear cells (PBMCs) of DSS-induced colitis and control mice by flow cytometry (Figure 1B). On day 7, the proportion of NKG2A+ cells among T cells (CD3+ PBMCs) decreased significantly in DSS-treated mice compared with control mice (1.77±0.60% vs 3.45±0.74%, respectively; $p=0.00002$). Thereafter, the frequency of NKG2A+ T cells in DSS-treated mice began to increase and returned to the pretreatment levels around day 14. On day 21, when colitis was cured and the body weight was restored to the level equal to that of control mice, the frequency of NKG2A+ T cells in DSS-treated mice exceeded that of control mice (7.22±1.66% vs 3.96±0.5%, respectively; $p=0.00006$). Control mice without DSS treatment showed very little change in the frequency of NKG2A+ T cells (3.51±0.71%).

Frequency of NKG2A+ T Cells Is Increased in Inflamed Intestinal Mucosa

In addition to NKG2A+ T cells in the peripheral blood, we analyzed the frequency of NKG2A+ T cells in the intestine of DSS-induced colitis mice. Mice were given 5% DSS in distilled water *ad libitum* for 7 days. There is a substantial variability in the effectiveness of different lots of DSS [13]. We therefore chose this concentration of DSS to ensure successful induction of colitis. PBMCs and lamina propria mononuclear cells (LPMCs) were obtained from identical DSS-induced colitis mice on days 0, 7, and 21, and the frequencies of NKG2A+ T cells were measured by flow cytometry. We confirmed that the frequency of NKG2A+ T cells in CD3+ PBMCs was decreased on day 7 and increased on day 21 in DSS-induced colitis mice (3.64±1.20%, 2.39±0.60%, and 7.17±3.57% on days 0, 7, and 21, respectively; Figure 2A). Conversely, the frequency of NKG2A+ T cells in CD3+ LPMCs was markedly increased on day 7 and returned to the level before DSS treatment on day 21 (4.88±1.42%, 7.84±2.12%, and 5.76±1.13% on days 0, 7, and 21, respectively; Figure 2B). These results suggest that, in addition to local expansion, some NKG2A+ T cells were recruited from the peripheral blood to the intestine during active colitis, presumably to suppress local inflammation.

Next, we performed flow cytometry analysis to examine NKG2A expression on different T cell subpopulations of LPMCs isolated from DSS-induced colitis mice (Figure 3). Although CD49b expression on T cells was generally lower in LPMCs than in PBMCs (data not shown), the frequency of CD49b+ T cells (panel C) was significantly increased on day 7 in DSS-induced colitis mice (4.49±1.66%, 9.24±2.83%, and 6.71±1.78% on days 0, 7, and 21, respectively). However, the frequency of CD8+ (panel A) or T-cell receptor (TCR) γδ+ (panel B) T cells hovered around 10% (11.22±1.64%, 9.38±2.65%, and 8.98±3.11% on days 0, 7, and 21, respectively, for CD8+ T cells; and 8.84±3.02%, 6.81±1.68%, and 9.09±3.20% on days 0, 7, and 21, respectively, for TCRγδ+ T cells). Interestingly, the frequency of NKG2A+ cells in CD8+ T cells (panel D) was significantly increased on day 7 (29.46±12.69%, 44.59±13.01%, and 39.26±9.02% on days 0, 7, and 21, respectively). There was no significant change in the frequency of NKG2A+ cells in CD3+TCRγδ+ (panel E) or CD3+CD49b+ (panel F) T cells (42.15±11.44%, 46.07±7.93%, and 48.61±5.01% on days 0, 7, and 21, respectively, for CD3+TCRγδ+ T cells; and 28.63±8.96%, 29.44±8.22%, and 25.61±5.28% on days 0, 7, and 21, respectively, for CD3+CD49b+ T cells).

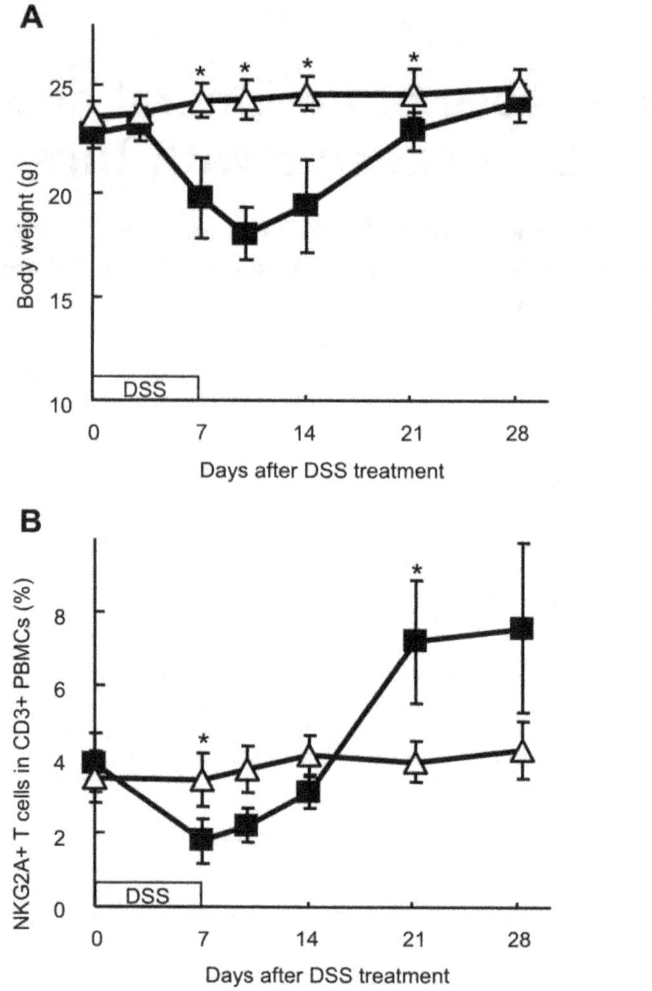

Figure 1. Frequency of NKG2A+ T cells in DSS-induced colitis mice. A) Body weight was measured chronologically. **B)** The frequency of NKG2A+ T cells in PBMCs was analyzed by flow cytometry. Data were calculated as the ratio of NKG2A+CD3+ cells to CD3+ cells. ■, DSS-induced colitis mice; △, control mice. For both DSS-induced colitis and control mice, 3 to 10 mice were subjected to analysis at each time point. *$P<0.05$.

Treatment with anti-NKG2A Ab Increases the Number of Inflammatory Foci in DSS-induced Colitis

To examine whether NKG2A+ T cells exert any immunoregulatory role in DSS-induced colitis, mice were injected intraperitoneally with control IgG or anti-NKG2A Ab and fed 5% DSS in their drinking water. On day 6, mice were sacrificed, and intestinal tissues were subjected to histological analysis. Although the difference fell slightly short of achieving statistical significance, mice injected with anti-NKG2A Ab showed an increased number of inflammatory lesions in the intestine, in comparison with mice injected with control IgG (4.58±3.15% vs 11.83±12.10%, $p=0.06$; Figure 4). When mice were fed phosphate-buffered

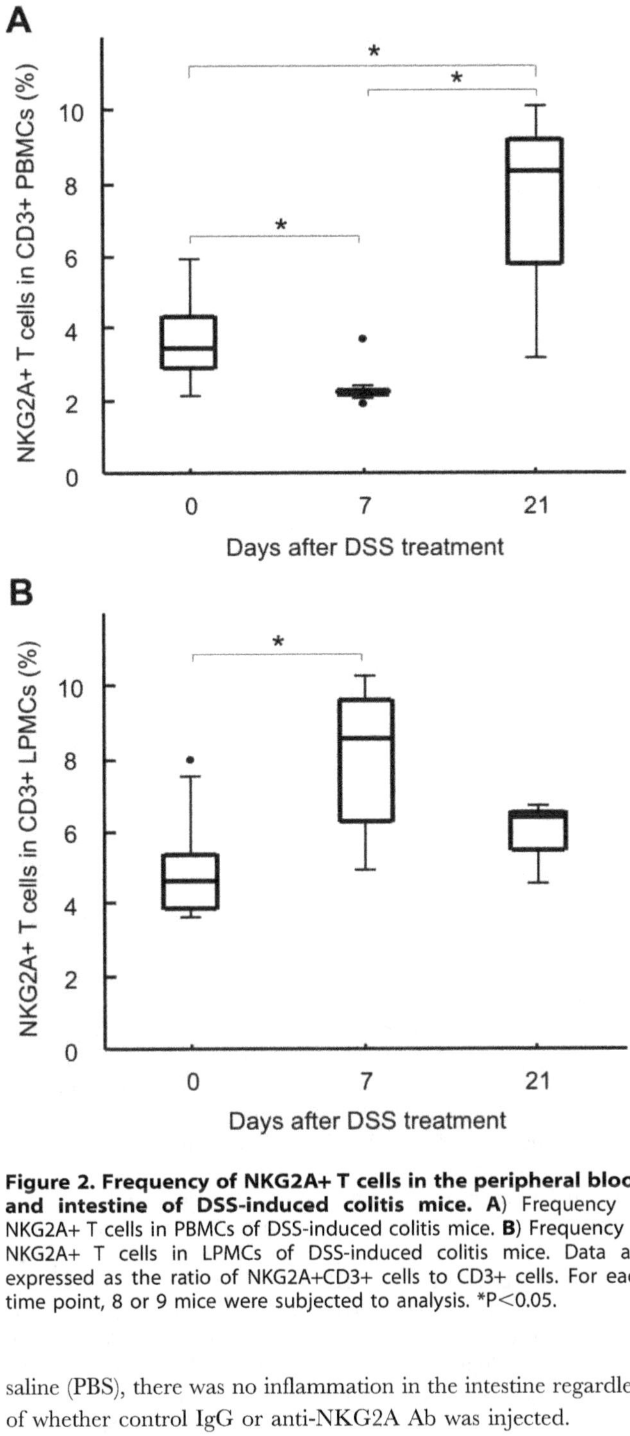

Figure 2. Frequency of NKG2A+ T cells in the peripheral blood and intestine of DSS-induced colitis mice. A) Frequency of NKG2A+ T cells in PBMCs of DSS-induced colitis mice. **B**) Frequency of NKG2A+ T cells in LPMCs of DSS-induced colitis mice. Data are expressed as the ratio of NKG2A+CD3+ cells to CD3+ cells. For each time point, 8 or 9 mice were subjected to analysis. *P<0.05.

saline (PBS), there was no inflammation in the intestine regardless of whether control IgG or anti-NKG2A Ab was injected.

Frequency of NKG2A+ T Cells Is Decreased in the PBMCs of UC Patients

Because we observed significant changes in the frequency of NKG2A+ T cells in PBMCs of DSS-induced colitis mice, we next examined the frequency of this T cell subset in PBMCs of IBD patients (Figure 5). NKG2A expression on T cells was analyzed by flow cytometry; samples from 20 patients with UC, 16 patients with CD, and 23 HCs were tested (Table 1). We observed a significant decrease of NKG2A+ T cells in the PBMCs of UC patients, compared with HC ($p = 0.004$) and CD patients ($p = 0.019$).

We then examined whether the frequency of NKG2A+ T cells in the PBMCs of UC patients correlated with clinical variables such as the methods of treatment, disease activity, and disease type (Figure 6). The frequency of NKG2A+ T cells was consistently low regardless of whether the patients were treated with steroid (panel A) or received surgical treatment (panel B). Likewise, neither disease activity (panel C) nor the extent of lesions (panel D) affected the frequency of NKG2A+ T cells. We subgrouped CD patients in a similar manner, and examined whether any specific subgroup of patients showed abnormalities in the frequency of peripheral blood NKG2A+ T cells; none of the subgroups showed a decrease in the frequency of peripheral blood NKG2A+ T cells (data not shown).

Next, to determine which T cell subsets decreased NKG2A expression in UC patients, we analyzed NKG2A expression on several T cell subsets by flow cytometry (Figure 7). Consistent with a previous observation [14], we did not detect any CD4+ T cells expressing NKG2A in patients or HCs (data not shown). In UC patients, the proportion of NKG2A+ cells was decreased in all T cell subsets including CD3+CD8+ T cells (panel A), CD3+CD56+ NKT cells (panel B), and CD3+TCRγδ+ T cells (panel C). In contrast, the proportion of NKG2A+ cells was not decreased in CD3-CD56+ NK cells (panel D), indicating that the decreased expression of NKG2A in UC patients occurs exclusively in T cells.

Number of NKG2A+ T Cells Infiltrating the Intestine Is Decreased in UC Patients, in Comparison with CD Patients and HC

In DSS-induced colitis mice, the frequency of NKG2A+ T cells was decreased in PBMCs, and increased in LPMCs on day 7. To examine whether similar alterations in the frequency of NKG2A+ T cell occurs in UC patients, we analyzed NKG2A+ T cells infiltrating into the affected intestine. Tissue sections derived from the specimens of IBD patients and HCs were double-stained using anti-CD3 and anti-NKG2A Abs. Representative immunofluorescence staining of a HC sample is shown in Figure 8A; CD3+NKG2A+ cells were scattered throughout the lamina propria. CD3+ cells and CD3+NKG2A+ cells were counted in 10 high power fields (HPF) for each section, and the frequency of NKG2A+ T cells in the lamina propria was calculated as a percentage of CD3+NKG2A+ cells among CD3+ cells.

Although massive infiltration of inflammatory cells was observed in the affected mucosa of IBD patients, the number of infiltrating T cells (CD3+ cells) did not differ significantly among UC patients, HC, and CD patients (data not shown). However, in sharp contrast to the mouse model of DSS-induced colitis, the frequency of CD3+NKG2A+ cells in the lamina propria was significantly decreased in UC patients ($4.44 \pm 1.57\%$) in comparison with HC and CD patients ($8.68 \pm 4.73\%$ and $10.49 \pm 3.33\%$, respectively; Figure 8B).

Discussion

Expression of NKG2A on T cells has been proposed as a mechanism for fine-tuning T cell responses by raising the threshold for TCR triggering, inhibiting cytokine production, and decreasing cytolytic activity [11,15,16]. In this study, we demonstrated that NKG2A+ T cells in the intestine underwent dynamic changes during DSS-induced mouse colitis; the frequency of NKG2A+ T cells was significantly increased during the active phase of DSS-induced colitis, and returned to the level before DSS treatment after the inflammation had subsided (Figure 2B). Considering the frequency of NKG2A+ cells in each subpopulation of lamina propria T cells isolated from DSS-induced colitis

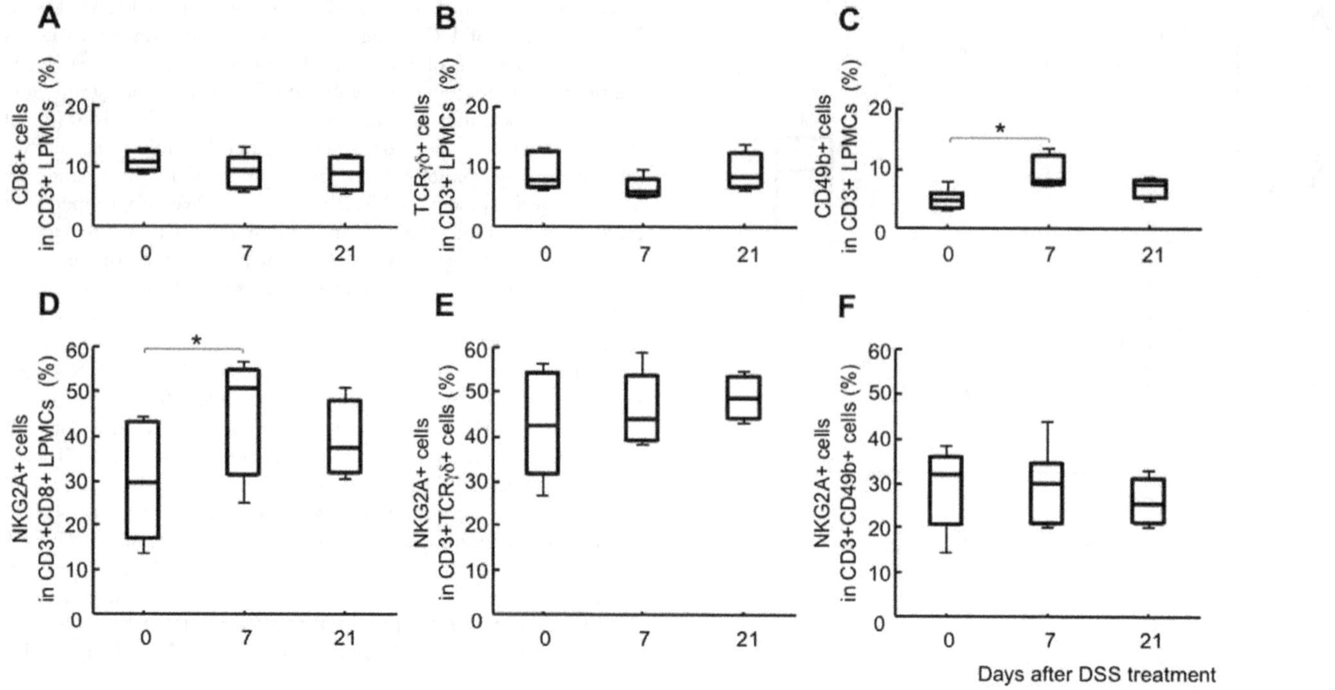

Figure 3. Frequency of NKG2A+ T cells in LPMCs isolated from the intestine of DSS-induced colitis mice. Frequencies of CD8+ T cells in CD3+ LPMCs (A), TCRγδ+ T cells in CD3+ LPMCs (B), CD49b+ T cells in CD3+ LMPCs (C), NKG2A+ cells in CD3+CD8+ LPMCs (D), NKG2A+ cells in CD3+TCRγδ+ LPMCs (E), and NKG2A+ cells in CD3+CD49b+ LPMCs (F) were analyzed by flow cytometry. For each time point, 4 to 7 mice were subjected to analysis. *$P<0.05$.

mice, it is likely that the major population of NKG2A+ T cells in the affected intestine is derived from CD8+ T cells (Figure 3). In the peripheral blood, the frequency of NKG2A+ T cells was decreased during the active phase, but gradually increased after discontinuation of DSS treatment and eventually exceeded that in DSS-untreated mice (Figures 1B and 2A). DSS-induced colitis is a simple model of acute intestinal injury [17]. Thus, the dynamic changes observed in intestinal and peripheral blood NKG2A+ T cells may reflect immune responses mounted against mucosal injuries inflicted by DSS. Although the difference fell slightly short of reaching statistical significance, DSS-fed mice injected with anti-NKG2A Ab showed an increased number of inflammatory foci in the intestine as compared with DSS-fed mice injected with control IgG (Figure 4). In view of the known immunoregulatory function of iNKRs, it seems reasonable to assume that NKG2A+ T cells were recruited to the affected intestine, and expanded there to prevent tissue damages resulting from excessive immune responses.

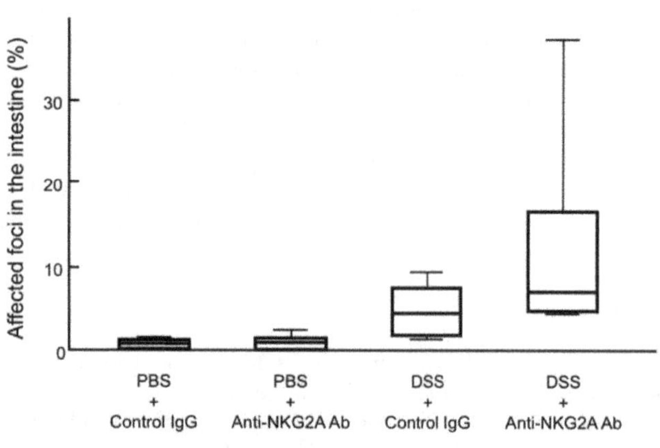

Figure 4. Frequency of inflammatory foci in the intestine of DSS-induced colitis mice treated with anti-NKG2A Ab or control IgG. For Ab blocking experiments, mice were intraperitoneally injected with 300 μg of anti-NKG2A monoclonal Ab or control IgG. The number of inflammatory foci in the intestine was counted histologically on day 6 after DSS administration. Seven mice injected with anti-NKG2D Ab and 8 mice injected with control IgG were subjected to analysis.

A growing body of evidence indicates that human NKG2A+ T cells exert immunoregulatory functions in diverse clinical conditions, including infections, autoimmune disorders, and malignant tumors [18–21]. Thus, in patients with human T-cell lymphotropic virus 1 (HTLV-1)-associated myelopathy/tropical spastic paraparesis (HAM/TSP), NKG2A+ T cells are significantly decreased, compared with asymptomatic carriers [22]. Saito *et al* [22] showed that a decrease in NKG2A+ CD8+ T cells increased the risk of developing HAM/TSP. Li *et al* [23] demonstrated that patients with systemic lupus erythematosus had lower expression of NKG2A on T cells. On the other hand, increased expression of NKG2A+ on T cells may result in impaired cytotoxic T cell activity in some diseases. In patients with malignant melanoma, increased expression of NKG2A on cytotoxic T cells was shown to impair their lytic activity against melanoma cells [16]. In chronic hepatitis C, the expression of NKG2A+ on NK and CD8+ T cells is increased, presumably acting negatively on the elimination of the virus [21]. These observations indicate that human NKG2A+ T cells have immunoregulatory, in most cases immunosuppressive functions like their mouse counterparts.

The most striking observation made in this study is that the frequency of NKG2A+ T cells was decreased not only in the peripheral blood but also in the inflamed intestine of UC patients (Figures 5 and 8). This is in sharp contrast to the observation made

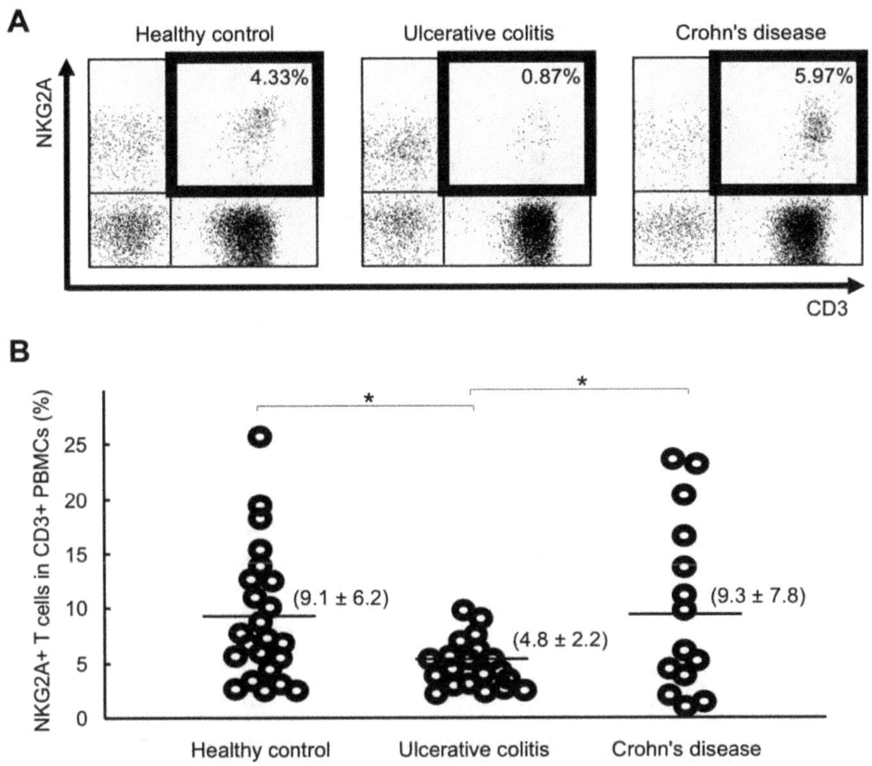

Figure 5. NKG2A+ T cells in the peripheral blood of HCs and IBD patients. A) Representative flow cytometry analysis of peripheral blood NKG2A+ T cells in HC and IBD patients. **B**) The ratio of NKG2A+CD3+ cells to CD3+ PBMCs was analyzed by flow cytometry. PBMCs from 23 HCs, 20 patients with UC, and 16 patients with CD were subjected to analysis. Numbers in parentheses represent mean ± standard deviation. *P<0.05.

in the DSS-induced mouse model of colitis, where NKG2A+ T cells accumulated in the affected intestine during the active phase of inflammation (Figure 2B). Since iNKR-expressing T cells appear to have immunosuppressive functions, the decreased presence of NKG2A+ T cells in the intestine may result in excessive local inflammation, contributing to the development and persistence of UC.

Regulatory T cells (Treg) have recently received much attention because of their involvement in the maintenance of mucosal microenvironments [24]. In both UC and CD patients, the number of Treg in LPMCs is increased during exacerbation, whereas the frequency of Treg in PBMCs is decreased during exacerbation and increased during remission [25]. In contrast, the frequency of peripheral blood NKG2A+ T cells was consistently low in UC patients regardless of disease activity, disease type, or the methods of treatment (Figure 6). These results suggest that mucosal immunosuppressive functions are predominantly mediated by Treg cells in IBD. A decrease in NKG2A+ T cells may contribute to disease amelioration through a decreased threshold for T cell activation, resulting in decreased cytotoxic activity and cytokine release rather than through decreased immunosuppression. Although the mechanism by which a decrease in NKG2A+ T cells potentially affects susceptibility to UC remains unknown, it must be emphasized that paucity of NKG2A+ T cells was seen in

Table 1. Summary of IBD patients and healthy controls.

	Healthy control	Ulcerative colitis	Crohn's disease
Number of patients	23	20	16
Age range (mean)	26–48 (32.4)	17–48 (31.8)	19–41 (28.6)
Sex:male; female	12; 11	11; 9	8; 8
Type		total colitis; left-sided colitis	small intestine; small and large intestine; large intestine
		13; 7	5; 8; 3
Steroid treatment: +; −		6; 14	NA
Activity: +; −		7; 13	5;11
Colectomy: +; −		5; 15	NA

NA: information not available.

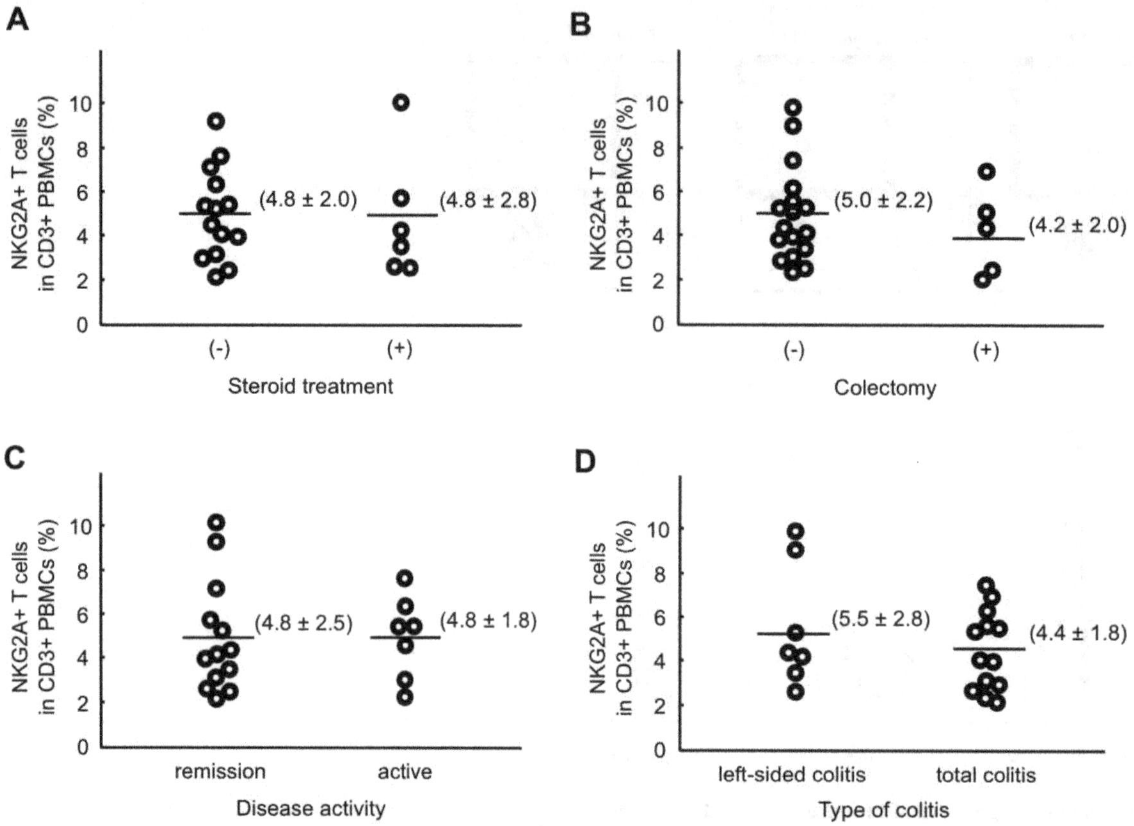

Figure 6. Frequency of NKG2A+ T cells in PBMCs of UC patients subgrouped according to clinical conditions. Data are expressed as the ratio of NKG2A+CD3+ cells to CD3+ cells. Clinical data are summarized in Table 1. Numbers in parentheses represent mean ± standard deviation.

UC, but not CD patients (Figure 5). This observation, together with generally known functions of iNKRs [26], suggests that a decrease in NKG2A+ T cells may be involved in the etiology of UC.

Why is the frequency of NKG2A+ T cells decreased in the peripheral blood and intestinal mucosa of UC patients? One explanation is that UC patients have a decreased total body pool of NKG2A+ T cells. This could happen if expansion of NKG2A+ T cells is impaired or the machinery required to express NKG2A is defective. Interestingly, decreased expression of NKG2A was observed in T, but not NK cells in UC patients (Figure 7). The GATA-3 transcription factor enhances transcription of *NKG2A* in the human NK leukemia cell line NKL, but not in Jurkat T cells [27]. Thus, UC patients might have some mutations in the promoter region of the *NKG2A* gene that affect the binding of transcription factors such as GATA-3. Alternatively, a decrease in the circulating pool of NKG2A+ T cells may occur by an accelerated recruitment of NKG2A+ T cells to the sites of inflammation within the intestine accompanied by an increased local cell death, irreversible down-regulation of NKG2A expression on mobilized T cells, and/or impaired local expansion. However, this explanation appears less likely because the frequency of peripheral blood NKG2A+ T cells remained low in UC patients who underwent a colectomy (Figure 6, panel B). Effective defense against enteric pathogens requires lymphocytes to be appropriately recruited, positioned, and expanded in the intestinal mucosa. This is mediated by a specific repertoire of adhesion molecules, chemokines, and chemokine receptors [28,29]. A third possibility is that UC patients have some defects in the recruitment of NKG2A+ T cells to the intestine. Our work does not exclude this possibility. However, impaired recruitment alone does not fully explain our observation that the peripheral blood NKG2A+ T cell frequency is consistently low in UC patients.

A significant proportion of healthy individuals have peripheral blood NKG2A+ T cells at frequencies comparable to those in UC patients (Figure 5). This observation may suggest that a decrease in NKG2A+ T cells has a relatively minor pathological role. However, it is also possible that the frequency of peripheral blood NKG2A+ T cells is low in some healthy individuals simply because their T cells are not stimulated to induce NKG2A expression. Unlike healthy individuals, UC patients have elevated serum levels of IL-15 [30–32], a cytokine that induces expression of NKG2A on T cells [9]. Nevertheless, UC patients invariably have low frequencies of peripheral blood NKG2A+ T cells (Figures 5 and 6). We therefore examined whether T cells from UC patients and HCs differ in their ability to express NKG2A after IL-15 stimulation, which, however, failed to detect any statistically significant difference between T cells derived from UC patients and HCs (unpublished observation). The possibility still remains open that the response of T cells to other NKG2A-inducing cytokines such as IL-12 [33] and TGF-β [34] is impaired in UC patients.

In summary, our study demonstrates for the first time that the frequency of NKG2A+ T cells is decreased in the peripheral blood and intestinal mucosa of UC patients, implicating this T cell subset as a potential therapeutic target for UC. Further investigation is needed to understand the molecular mechanism by which a decrease in NKG2A+ T cells potentially affects susceptibility to UC.

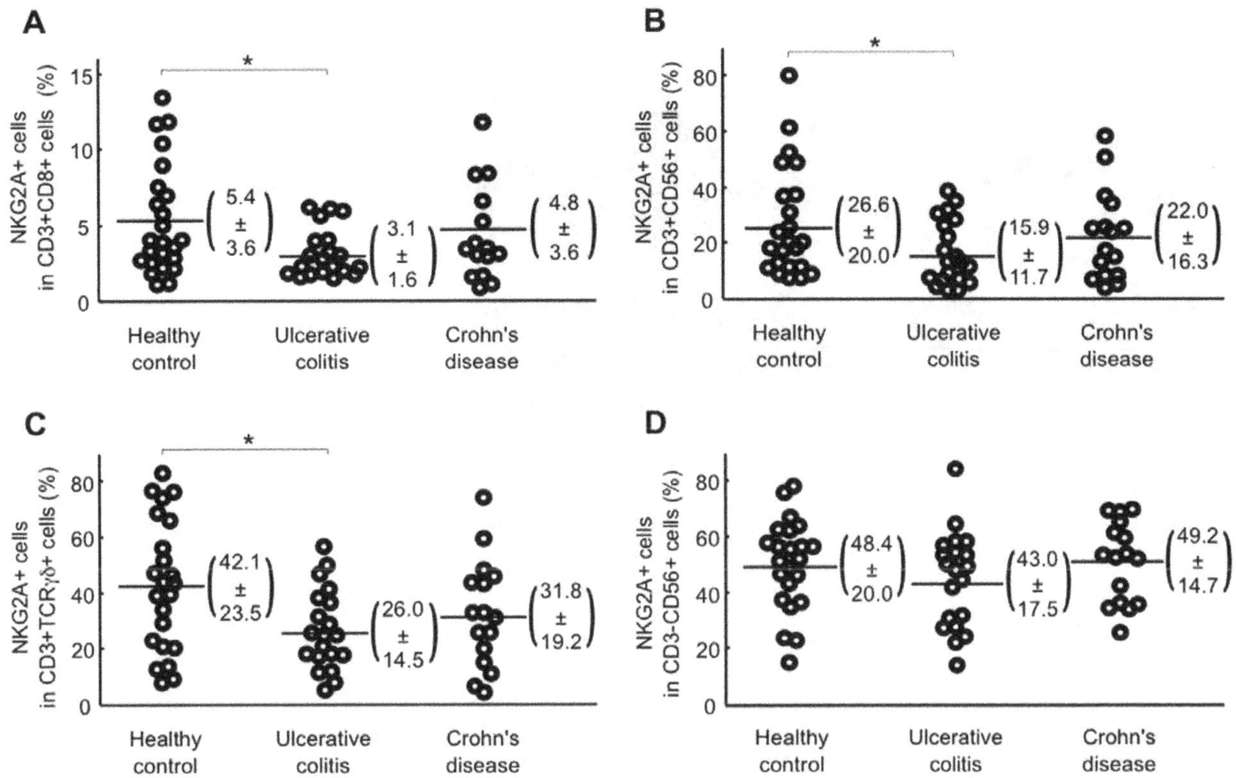

Figure 7. Frequency of NKG2A+ T cells and NKG2A+ NK cells in PBMCs from UC patients, CD patients, and healthy controls. A) Ratio of NKG2A+ cells in CD3+CD8+ T cells, **B**) Ratio of NKG2A+ cells in CD3+CD56+ NKT cells, **C**) Ratio of NKG2A+ cells in CD3+TCRγδ+ T cells, and **D**) Ratio of NKG2A+ cells in CD3-CD56+ NK cells. Numbers in parentheses represent mean ± standard deviation. PBMCs isolated from 23 HCs, 20 patients with UC, and 16 patients with CD were subjected to analysis. *$P<0.05$.

Materials and Methods

Mice

Male BALB/c mice (8–10 weeks old) were purchased from Sankyo Lab., Japan. For induction of experimental colitis, mice were orally administrated 3% or 5% DSS (molecular weight, 40 kDa, Wako) in distilled water for 7 days *ad libitum* [35]. For controls, age-matched BALB/c mice were given distilled water. For the analysis of NKG2A+ T cells in PBMCs and LPMCs, peripheral blood and intestinal tissues were obtained on days 0, 7, 10, 14, 21, and 28 (n = 3 to 10). For blocking experiments using anti-NKG2A Ab, mice were intraperiteoneally injected with 300 µg of anti-NKG2A monoclonal Ab or control IgG at three time points: 3 days before, day 0, and day 3 after oral administration of 5% DSS. The anti-NKG2A monoclonal Ab (20d5) was generated as described previously [36]. Control IgG was purchased from Sigma-Aldrich. All animal experiments were done according to the Guide for the Care and Use of Laboratory Animals, Hokkaido University Graduate School of Medicine.

Patients with IBD and HCs

PBMC samples were obtained from 20 patients with UC, 16 patients with CD, and 23 healthy volunteers. Summarized data for the patients and HCs are given in Table 1. Activity of UC was defined according to the clinical activity index (CAI); patients with index 4 or greater were considered to have active colitis [37]. Activity of CD was defined using the International Organization for the Study of Inflammatory Bowel Disease (IOIBD) score [38]. For immunohistochemical analysis, biopsies and surgical specimens were collected from patients with UC (n = 6) and CD (n = 5). Normal colonic tissues used for immunohistochemical analysis were obtained from surgical specimens of patients with colorectal cancer (n = 7). All patients and healthy volunteers provided written informed consent, and the experiments were approved by the Medical Ethics Committee of Hokkaido University Graduate School of Medicine.

Cell Isolation

PBMCs were isolated by Ficoll density gradient centrifugation. Isolation of LPMCs from mice with DSS-induced colitis was performed as previously described [39]. Briefly, freshly taken intestinal tissues were washed in PBS and incubated with 1 mmol/L EDTA/PBS for 30 minutes at 37°C. Then, the tissues were minced and digested with type IV collagenase (Sigma-Aldrich) and DNase I (TaKaRa) for 30 minutes in a shaking incubator at 37°C. Released cells were isolated by density gradient centrifugation with Lympholite M (Cedarlane).

Flow Cytometry

For the detection of NKG2A+ T cells in mouse PBMCs and LPMCs, cells were stained with phycoerythrin (PE)-conjugated rat anti-mouse NKG2A/C/E Ab (clone 20d5, Beckman Coulter) and peridinin chlorophyll-a protein (PerCP)-conjugated hamster anti-mouse CD3 Ab (clone 145-2C11, BD Bioscience). Anti-mouse NKG2A/C/E Ab is operationally monospecific for NKG2A, because CD94/NKG2A complexes, but not other CD94/NKG2 complexes, are expressed on NK cells and T cells [40]. For the analysis of T cell subpopulation, mouse PBMCs and LPMCs were stained with FITC-conjugated anti-CD8 (clone Ly-2, BD Biosci-

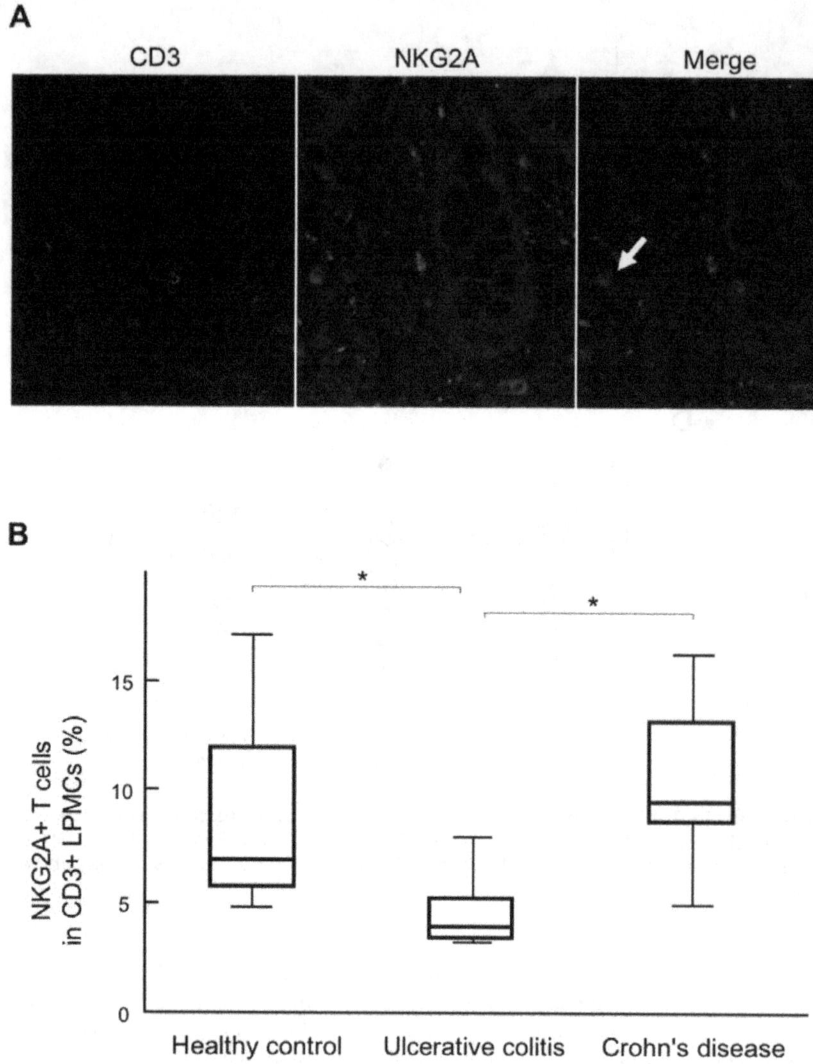

Figure 8. Frequency of NKG2A+ T cells in the intestine of UC patients. A) A representative double-stained section of normal intestinal tissues using anti-CD3 and anti-NKG2A Abs. Merged images show double positive cells (arrow). Red, CD3; green, NKG2A. **B**) The frequency of NKG2A+ T cells in the intestine was analyzed by immunohistochemistry. NKG2A+ T cells in the lamina propria were less abundant in UC patients than in HC and CD patients. Tissue sections from 7 HCs, 6 UC patients, and 5 CD patients were subjected to analysis. *$P<0.05$.

ence), FITC-conjugated anti-CD49b (clone HMa2, eBioscience), or FITC-conjugated anti-TCR-γδ (clone 3BioGL3, eBioscience) Ab. Human PBMCs were stained using PE-conjugated anti-NKG2A (clone Z199, Immunotech), FITC-conjugated anti-CD3 (clone UCHT-1, BD Bioscience), RPE-Cy5-conjugated anti-CD3 (clone UCHT-1, DAKO), FITC-conjugated anti-CD8 (clones RPA-T8, BD Bioscience), RPE-Cy5-conjugated anti-CD8 (clone DK25, DAKO), FITC-conjugated anti-CD56 (clone NCAM16.2, BD Bioscience), PE-conjugated anti-CD4 (clone RPA-T4, BD Bioscience), or FITC-conjugated anti-TCRγδ-1 Ab (clone 11F2, BD Bioscience). Isotype controls were used as negative controls. Cells were stained for 30 minutes at 4°C with optimal dilution of Abs. After washing, they were analyzed by flow cytometry (FACSCalibur and CellQuest software, BD Bioscience) by setting a gate around viable lymphocytes based on their forward and side scatter characteristics.

Histological Analysis and Immunohistochemistry

For histological analysis of DSS-induced colitis mice, formalin-fixed intestinal sections were stained with hematoxylin and eosin (H&E). The frequency of inflammatory foci in the intestine was evaluated through microscopic examination of 60 to 70 tissue sections of comparable size prepared from the whole colon of each mouse. The frequency of inflammatory foci was calculated by dividing the total number of foci by the number of tissue sections analyzed. For immunohistochemical analysis of human intestinal tissues, formalin-fixed tissue sections were deparaffinized in xylene and rehydrated in graded alcohols and distilled water. Deparaffinized and rehydrated slides were processed for antigen retrieval by a standard microwave heating technique. The slides were incubated in PBS with 10% goat serum for 1 hour at room temperature, followed by overnight incubation with goat polyclonal Ab against human NKG2A (1:100, T-20, Santa Cruz) at 4°C. After incubation, rabbit anti-human CD3 Ab (1:100, DAKO) was added on slides and incubated for 30 minutes. Negative controls were stained with normal goat serum and rabbit IgG.

Sections were labeled with chicken anti-rabbit Alexa 594 and donkey anti-goat Alexa 488 (1:400, Invitrogen), and examined by fluorescence microscopy. Positive cells in 10 HPFs were counted for each section.

Statistical Analysis

Data were evaluated using the Student's *t*-test or the Mann-Whitney U-test. P-values less than 0.05 were considered statistically significant.

Acknowledgments

We are grateful to Rika Nagashima, Chisato Sudo, and Masayo Tateyama for technical support.

Author Contributions

Conceived and designed the experiments: TK WK UT NS MA HT KT. Performed the experiments: TK WK UT. Analyzed the data: TB SF AI KT NS. Contributed reagents/materials/analysis tools: KT. Wrote the paper: TK WK UT. Supervised the entire study: MK.

References

1. Podolsky DK (2002) Inflammatory bowel disease. N Engl J Med 347: 417–429.
2. Fiocchi C (1998) Inflammatory bowel disease: etiology and pathogenesis. Gastroenterology 115: 182–205.
3. Abraham C, Cho JH (2009) Inflammatory bowel disease. N Engl J Med 361: 2066–2078.
4. Moretta A, Bottino C, Mingari MC, Biassoni R, Moretta L (2002) What is a natural killer cell? Nat Immunol 3: 6–8.
5. Ljunggren HG, Karre K (1990) In search of the 'missing self': MHC molecules and NK cell recognition. Immunol Today 11: 237–244.
6. Vivier E, Anfossi N (2004) Inhibitory NK-cell receptors on T cells: witness of the past, actors of the future. Nat Rev Immunol 4: 190–198.
7. Vivier E, Daeron M (1997) Immunoreceptor tyrosine-based inhibition motifs. Immunol Today 18: 286–291.
8. Long EO (1999) Regulation of immune responses through inhibitory receptors. Annu Rev Immunol 17: 875–904.
9. Braud VM, Aldemir H, Breart B, Ferlin WG (2003) Expression of CD94-NKG2A inhibitory receptor is restricted to a subset of CD8+ T cells. Trends Immunol 24: 162–164.
10. Jabri B, Selby JM, Negulescu H, Lee L, Roberts AI, et al. (2002) TCR specificity dictates CD94/NKG2A expression by human CTL. Immunity 17: 487–499.
11. Moser JM, Gibbs J, Jensen PE, Lukacher AE (2002) CD94-NKG2A receptors regulate antiviral CD8+ T cell responses. Nat Immunol 3: 189–195.
12. Bhagat G, Naiyer AJ, Shah JG, Harper J, Jabri B, et al. (2008) Small intestinal CD8+TCRγδ+NKG2A+ intraepithelial lymphocytes have attributes of regulatory cells in patients with celiac disease. J Clin Invest 118: 281–293.
13. Wirtz S, Neufert C, Weigmann B, Neurath MF (2007) Chemically induced mouse models of intestinal inflammation. Nat Protoc 2: 541–546.
14. Freishtat RJ, Mitchell LW, Ghimbovschi SD, Meyers SB, Hoffman EP (2005) NKG2A and CD56 are coexpressed on activated TH2 but not TH1 lymphocytes. Hum Immunol 66: 1223–1234.
15. Le Drean E, Vely F, Olcese L, Cambiaggi A, Guia S, et al. (1998) Inhibition of antigen-induced T cell response and antibody-induced NK cell cytotoxicity by NKG2A: association of NKG2A with SHP-1 and SHP-2 protein-tyrosine phosphatases. Eur J Immunol 28: 264–276.
16. Speiser DE, Pittet MJ, Valmori D, Dunbar R, Rimoldi D, et al. (1999) In vivo expression of natural killer cell inhibitory receptors by human melanoma-specific cytolytic T lymphocytes. J Exp Med 190: 775–782.
17. Kawada M, Arihiro A, Mizoguchi E (2007) Insights from advances in research of chemically induced experimental models of human inflammatory bowel disease. World J Gastroenterol 13: 5581–5593.
18. Suvas S, Azkur AK, Rouse BT (2006) Qa-1b and CD94-NKG2a interaction regulate cytolytic activity of herpes simplex virus-specific memory CD8+ T cells in the latently infected trigeminal ganglia. J Immunol 176: 1703–1711.
19. Byers AM, Andrews NP, Lukacher AE (2006) CD94/NKG2A expression is associated with proliferative potential of CD8+ T cells during persistent polyoma virus infection. J Immunol 176: 6121–6129.
20. Liao YH, Jee SH, Sheu BC, Huang YL, Tseng MP, et al. (2006) Increased expression of the natural killer cell inhibitory receptor CD94/NKG2A and CD158b on circulating and lesional T cells in patients with chronic plaque psoriasis. Br J Dermatol 155: 318–324.
21. Nattermann J, Feldmann G, Ahlenstiel G, Langhans B, Sauerbruch T, et al. (2006) Surface expression and cytolytic function of natural killer cell receptors is altered in chronic hepatitis C. Gut 55: 869–877.
22. Saito M, Braud VM, Goon P, Hanon E, Taylor GP, et al. (2003) Low frequency of CD94/NKG2A+ T lymphocytes in patients with HTLV-1-associated myelopathy/tropical spastic paraparesis, but not in asymptomatic carriers. Blood 102: 577–584.
23. Li WX, Pan HF, Hu JL, Wang CZ, Zhang N, et al. (2010) Assay of T- and NK-cell subsets and the expression of NKG2A and NKG2D in patients with new-onset systemic lupus erythematosus. Clin Rheumatol 29: 315–323.
24. Mottet C, Uhlig HH, Powrie F (2003) Cutting edge: cure of colitis by CD4+CD25+ regulatory T cells. J Immunol 170: 3939–3943.
25. Makita S, Kanai T, Oshima S, Uraushihara K, Totsuka T, et al. (2004) CD4+CD25bright T cells in human intestinal lamina propria as regulatory cells. J Immunol 173: 3119–3130.
26. Mingari MC, Pietra G, Moretta L (2005) Human cytolytic T lymphocytes expressing HLA class-I-specific inhibitory receptors. Curr Opin Immunol 17: 312–319.
27. Marusina AI, Kim DK, Lieto LD, Borrego F, Coligan JE (2005) GATA-3 is an important transcription factor for regulating human NKG2A gene expression. J Immunol 174: 2152–2159.
28. Eksteen B, Liaskou E, Adams DH (2008) Lymphocyte homing and its role in the pathogenesis of IBD. Inflamm Bowel Dis 14: 1298–1312.
29. Hart AL, Ng SC, Mann E, Al-Hassi HO, Bernardo D, et al. (2010) Homing of immune cells: role in homeostasis and intestinal inflammation. Inflamm Bowel Dis 16: 1969–1977.
30. Liu Z, Geboes K, Colpaert S, D'Haens GR, Rutgeerts P, et al. (2000) IL-15 is highly expressed in inflammatory bowel disease and regulates local T cell-dependent cytokine production. J Immunol 164: 3608–3615.
31. Sakai T, Kusugami K, Nishimura H, Ando T, Yamaguchi T, et al. (1998) Interleukin 15 activity in the rectal mucosa of inflammatory bowel disease. Gastroenterology 114: 1237–1243.
32. Kirman I, Nielsen OH (1996) Increased numbers of interleukin-15-expressing cells in active ulcerative colitis. Am J Gastroenterol 91: 1789–1794.
33. Derre L, Corvaisier M, Pandolfino MC, Diez E, Jotereau F, et al. (2002) Expression of CD94/NKG2-A on human T lymphocytes is induced by IL-12: implications for adoptive immunotherapy. J Immunol 168: 4864–4870.
34. Bertone S, Schiavetti F, Bellomo R, Vitale C, Ponte M, et al. (1999) Transforming growth factor-β-induced expression of CD94/NKG2A inhibitory receptors in human T lymphocytes. Eur J Immunol 29: 23–29.
35. Okayasu I, Hatakeyama S, Yamada M, Ohkusa T, Inagaki Y, et al. (1990) A novel method in the induction of reliable experimental acute and chronic ulcerative colitis in mice. Gastroenterology 98: 694–702.
36. Vance RE, Jamieson AM, Raulet DH (1999) Recognition of the class Ib molecule Qa-1(b) by putative activating receptors CD94/NKG2C and CD94/NKG2E on mouse natural killer cells. J Exp Med 190: 1801–1812.
37. Rachmilewitz D (1989) Coated mesalazine (5-aminosalicylic acid) versus sulphasalazine in the treatment of active ulcerative colitis: a randomised trial. BMJ 298: 82–86.
38. de Dombal FT, Softley A (1987) IOIBD report no 1: Observer variation in calculating indices of severity and activity in Crohn's disease. International Organisation for the Study of Inflammatory Bowel Disease. Gut 28: 474–481.
39. Gonzalez-Rey E, Chorny A, Delgado M (2006) Therapeutic action of ghrelin in a mouse model of colitis. Gastroenterology 130: 1707–1720.
40. Kawamura T, Takeda K, Kaneda H, Matsumoto H, Hayakawa Y, et al. (2009) NKG2A inhibits invariant NKT cell activation in hepatic injury. J Immunol 182: 250–258.

3

Enterohepatic *Helicobacter* in Ulcerative Colitis: Potential Pathogenic Entities?

John M. Thomson[1], Richard Hansen[1,2], Susan H. Berry[1], Mairi E. Hope[1], Graeme I. Murray[3], Indrani Mukhopadhya[1], Mairi H. McLean[1], Zeli Shen[4], James G. Fox[4], Emad El-Omar[1], Georgina L. Hold[1]*

1 Gastrointestinal Research Group, Division of Applied Medicine, University of Aberdeen, Foresterhill, Aberdeen, United Kingdom, **2** Child Health, University of Aberdeen, Royal Aberdeen Children's Hospital, Foresterhill, Aberdeen, United Kingdom, **3** Department of Pathology, University of Aberdeen, Foresterhill, Aberdeen, United Kingdom, **4** Division of Comparative Medicine, Massachusetts Institute of Technology, Cambridge, Massachusetts, United States of America

Abstract

Background: Changes in bacterial populations termed "dysbiosis" are thought central to ulcerative colitis (UC) pathogenesis. In particular, the possibility that novel *Helicobacter* organisms play a role in human UC has been debated but not comprehensively investigated. The aim of this study was to develop a molecular approach to investigate the presence of *Helicobacter* organisms in adults with and without UC.

Methodology/Principal Findings: A dual molecular approach to detect *Helicobacter* was developed. Oligonucleotide probes against the genus *Helicobacter* were designed and optimised alongside a validation of published *H. pylori* probes. A comprehensive evaluation of *Helicobacter* genus and *H. pylori* PCR primers was also undertaken. The combined approach was then assessed in a range of gastrointestinal samples prior to assessment of a UC cohort. Archival colonic samples were available from 106 individuals for FISH analysis (57 with UC and 49 non-IBD controls). A further 118 individuals were collected prospectively for dual FISH and PCR analysis (86 UC and 32 non-IBD controls). An additional 27 non-IBD controls were available for PCR analysis. All *Helicobacter* PCR-positive samples were sequenced. The association between *Helicobacter* and each study group was statistically analysed using the Pearson Chi Squared 2 tailed test. *Helicobacter* genus PCR positivity was significantly higher in UC than controls (32 of 77 versus 11 of 59, $p=0.004$). Sequence analysis indicated enterohepatic *Helicobacter* species prevalence was significantly higher in the UC group compared to the control group (30 of 77 versus 2 of 59, $p<0.0001$). PCR and FISH results were concordant in 74 (67.9%) of subjects. The majority of discordant results were attributable to a higher positivity rate with FISH than PCR.

Conclusions/Significance: *Helicobacter* organisms warrant consideration as potential pathogenic entities in UC. Isolation of these organisms from colonic tissue is needed to enable interrogation of pathogenicity against established criteria.

Editor: Tanya Parish, Queen Mary University of London, United Kingdom

Funding: This study was funded by the Broad Medical Research Program (Grant number IBD-0178). JMT was supported by grants from the GI Research Unit, Aberdeen Royal Infirmary; RH was supported by a Clinical Academic Training Fellowship, from the Chief Scientist Office (CAF/08/01). The funders had no role in study design, data collection and analysis, decision to publish, or preparation of the manuscript.

Competing Interests: The authors have declared that no competing interests exist.

* E-mail: g.l.hold@abdn.ac.uk

Introduction

Ulcerative colitis (UC) is a chronic condition of the human colon which affects the superficial mucosal layer from the rectum and extending proximally for variable distances [1]. This variable phenotype remains a puzzle, as does our difficulty in achieving long-term cure with current treatments. Recent developments in genetics have greatly improved our understanding of the inflammatory bowel diseases (Crohn's disease and UC), resulting in a renewed interest in the interplay between host immunology and bacteria at the mucosal surface; however genetic elements appear to be more important in Crohn's disease (CD) than UC. The possibility of infection as a trigger event for, or indeed as the cause of, inflammatory bowel disease (IBD) has long been debated with various organisms being suggested as pathogens. None of these organisms have been conclusively proven as causative agents. Studies examining the diversity of bacteria in IBD have shown increased cell counts of bacteria and reduced bacterial diversity. Changes in bacterial populations to the detriment of the host have been termed "dysbiosis" and this change is thought central to IBD pathogenesis. IBD onset following infectious episodes is well described and one possibility is that gastrointestinal infection may facilitate dysbiosis and ultimately IBD. Whether acute self-limiting infection is sufficient as a single entity, or whether chronic infection with as yet unknown agents is required to drive the chronicity of disease is unknown. UC is a stronger candidate than CD for a purely infectious aetiology because of the weaker genetic association, continuity of disease distribution and the relative limitation of disease to superficial tissue. It is likely however that a combination of host (genetic) susceptibility, a trigger event (which may be infectious) and the progression to dysbiosis are all likely required for the development of IBD.

The discovery that *Helicobacter pylori* was the causative agent underpinning gastric and duodenal ulceration and ultimately gastric cancer revolutionised our understanding of these conditions and resulted in a Nobel prize for Robin Warren and Barry Marshall. The tantalising possibility that a similar agent is responsible for IBD warrants consideration and exploration [2].

The family *Helicobacteraceae* contains the genera *Helicobacter* and *Wolinella*. The *Helicobacter* genus can be split into two groups, gastric *Helicobacter*, describing those that preferentially colonise the stomach, and enterohepatic *Helicobacter*, which preferentially colonise the intestinal or hepatobilliary system (Table 1). Enterohepatic *Helicobacter* organisms have been cultured from both Cotton-top tamarin monkeys (*Saguinus oedipus*) and rhesus monkeys (*Macaca mulatta*) with colitic disease (*Helicobacter* sp. Flexispira taxon 10, *Helicobacter macacae* and *Helicobacter* sp. Rhesus monkey 2), whilst *Helicobacter hepaticus* and *Helicobacter bilis* have been shown to be capable of causing IBD-like disease in immunodeficient rodent models [3–5]. Thus animal models demonstrating that infection with *Helicobacter* spp. on a background of host immunodeficiency can lead to colitis, and that "auto-immune" type reactions to commensal bacteria can be initiated by such organisms, would suggest the possibility of parallel mechanisms in humans resulting in IBD.

Various groups have examined human IBD for the presence of *Helicobacter* spp., from the negative studies of Bell and Grehan [6,7], through to studies by Bohr, Zhang and Laharie which have successfully demonstrated PCR evidence of non-*pylori Helicobacter* (n*pH*) in both IBD and controls [8–10]. The methodologies used, the variable rates of positivity reported between groups, and the small study numbers included in some, mean discussions at *Helicobacter* species level have been limited. Unfortunately, no-one has successfully cultured non-*pylori Helicobacter* organisms from IBD tissue (although 7 enterohepatic *Helicobacter* spp. have been cultured from the gastrointestinal tract of humans with diarrhoea or systemic disease [2]). The difficulties in isolating and culturing non-*pylori Helicobacter* from human colonic tissue highlight the importance of molecular approaches as viable alternatives to facilitate the study of the role of *Helicobacter* spp. in extra-gastric diseases. However, it is vital that these molecular methods are suitably sensitive, specific and applicable to a diverse range of samples. The purpose of the present study was to design a combined molecular approach to identify *Helicobacteraceae* organisms within a variety of gastrointestinal sample types. Our specific aim was to examine colonic tissue from IBD patients to assess the prevalence of *Helicobacteraceae* organisms against tissue from controls largely undergoing colorectal cancer screening. We elected to analyse UC cases rather than CD cases for the reasons outlined above regarding UC as a stronger candidate for an infectious aetiology.

Table 1. Classification of named *Helicobacter* spp. as Gastric or Enterohepatic.

Gastric	Enterohepatic
H. acinonychis	*H. anseris*
H. aurati	**H. bilis*
H. bizzozeroni	*H. brantae*
H. cetoreum	**H. canis*
H. felis	**H. canadensis*
H. mustelae	*H. cholecystus*
**H. pylori*	**H. cinaedi*
H. salomonis	*H. equorum*
H. suis	**H. fennelliae*
H. bovis (candidate species)	*H. ganmani*
H. suncus (candidate species)	*H. hepaticus*
H. cyanogastricus	*H. mastomyrinus*
	H. marmotae
	H. mesocricetorum
	H. magdeburgensis
	H. muridarum
	H. pametenis
	**H. pullorum*
	H. rodentium
	H. suncus
	H. trogontum
	H. typhlonicus
	H. westmeadii
	**H. winghamensis*

*Isolated from humans.

Methods

Ethics Statement

Ethical approval for the archival specimen analysis and the biopsy study was granted by North of Scotland Research Ethics Service and written informed consent was obtained from all subjects in the biopsy study.

Development of a Combined Molecular Approach for the Detection of *Helicobacteraceae* Organisms

Development of PCR Methodology. A bacterial reference panel was used to screen a series of primer combinations. The bacterial strains used in this study included: *Helicobacter bilis* (ATCC 51630), *H. canadensis* (ATCC 700968), *H. canis* (ATCC 51402), *H. cholecystus* (ATCC 700242), *H. cinaedi* (CCUG 18818), *H. felis* (ATCC 49179), *H. hepaticus* (ATCC 51449), *H. pullorum* (NCTC 12824), *H. pylori* (ATCC 700392), *Pseudomonas fluorescens* (clinical isolate), *Listeria monocytogenes* (clinical isolate), *Aeromonas caviae* (clinical isolate), *Aeromonas sobria* (clinical isolate), *Campylobacter jejuni* (clinical isolate), *Proteus mirabilis* (NCTC 3177), *Enterobacter aerogenes* (NCIMB 10102), *Yersinia enterocolitica* (NCIMB 2124), *Bifidobacterium longum* (NCIMB 8809), *Bifidobacterium infantis* (DSM 20088), *Eubacterium rectale* (NCIMB 14373), *Roseburia intestinalis* (DSM 14610), *Bacteroides vulgatus* (DSM 1447), *Bacteroides thetaiotaomicron* (NCTC 10582), *Eubacterium hallii* (DSM 17630), *Enterococcus faecalis* (NCIMB 13280), *Pseudomonas aeruginosa* (NCIMB 8626), *Enterobacter cloacae* (NCIMB 8556), *Proteus vulgaris* (NCTC 4175), *Salmonella enteritidis* (NCTC 12694), *Salmonella poona* (NCTC 4840), *Salmonella typhimurium* (NCIMB 13284), *Escherichia coli* (NCIMB 12210), *Shigella sonnei* (ATCC 25931), *Staphylococcus epidermidis* (NCIMB 8853), *Bacillus subtilis* (NCIB 8054), *Bacillus cereus* (ATCC 10876), *Klebsiella pneumoniae* (NCIMB 13281), *Staphylococcus aureus* (NCIMB 12702), *Streptococcus gordonii* (ATCC 35105), *Faecalibacterium prausnitzii* strain A2-165 (DSM 17677), *Megasphaera elsdenii* (ATCC 25940), *Bifidobacterium adolescentis* isolate L2-32, *Lactococcus lactis* strain MG1363, *Enterococcus faecalis* strain JH2-2, *Ruminococcus albus* strain SY3, *Ruminococcus flavefaciens* strain 17, *Eubacterium cylindroides* strain T2-87, *Coprococcus spp* L2-50, *Methanobrevibacter smithii* ATCC 35061, *Acinetobacter baumanii*, *Lactobacillus acidophilus* (ATCC 43561) and *Streptococcus bovis* strain *Z6*. Aerobic and microaerobic strains were grown at 37°C on Columbia agar with 10% horse blood. Anaerobic strains were grown at 37°C on M2GSC [11], MRS or M17 media (Becton Dickinson, Oxford, UK). All strains were used in fluorescent *in-situ* hybrisation (FISH) and PCR optimisation studies.

Initial assessment used a universal 16S bacterial PCR described previously [12]. To allow identification of the family *Helicobacteraceae* (genera *Helicobacter* and *Wolinella*), 8 *Helicobacteraceae* PCR primer pairs were assessed. The nested PCR combination of C05 and C97 [13] followed by a reverse complement of primer C98 [13] and1067r [14] was selected as it yielded a final product of suitable length (~400 bp) for sequence analysis. For *H. pylori* specific PCR, numerous *H. pylori* specific primer sets targeting the 16S rRNA gene were assessed with the most successful pairing being identified as 27f (5′-AGAGTTTGATCMTGGCTCAG-3′) [15] and HPY (5′-CTGGAGAGACTAAGCCCTCC-3′) [16]. Both PCRs utilised the following conditions: denaturation at 94°C for 5 min, followed by 35 cycles of 94°C for 1 min, 66°C for 1 min, 72°C for 2 min. Final extension 72°C for 10 min. To determine the sensitivity of the genus PCR, decreasing amounts of *H. pylori* and *H. hepaticus*-derived DNA were spiked into faecal samples which were previously analysed by FISH and PCR and found to be negative for *Helicobacteraceae*. Dilutions ranged from 500 pg to 0.05 pg of *Helicobacter* DNA with the detection level of 0.5 pg *Helicobacter* DNA (representing approximately 30 bacteria) consistently being achieved.

Development of FISH Methodology. Five broad-specificity probes were designed to target the small subunit rRNA of the family *Helicobacteraceae* (Table 2). The new probes were designed with the Primrose software package [17], checked against the Ribosomal Database Project (RDP) and EMBL databases, and were named according to the nomenclature suggested by the Oligonucleotide Probe Database (OPD) [18]. One of the designed *Helicobacteraceae* probe sequences S-G-Hel-1047-a-A-21 had been previously described as a *Helicobacter* genus specific PCR primer [14] but to our knowledge it has not been used as a probe. Of note, *in-silico* analysis indicated that this probe detects several bacteria of the genera *Sulfurimonas* (17 of 21), *Sulfurovum* (9 of 42) and *Wolinella* (4 of 5). The specificity of the 5 newly designed *Helicobacteraceae* probes along with four previously published *H. pylori* specific probes (Table 2) was tested by whole-cell *in situ* hybridization against a panel of 60 reference strains derived from the human and animal gastrointestinal tract (see above) including a panel of 9 *Helicobacter* type strains [19]. As a positive control for the presence of bacteria, the bacterium-specific probe S-D-Bact-0338-a-A-18 (termed Eub338) was used [20]. Following assessment of the various *Helicobacteraceae* probes, it was identified that the *Helicobacteraceae* probe S-G-Hel-1047-a-A-21 and the *H. pylori* specific probe Hp16S2 hybridized only to the respective target organisms but not to any of the other organisms tested. Both the Eub338 and Hp16S2 hybridised at 50°C and could be co-hybridised using discriminating fluorescent labels (Rhodamine red and Oregon green 488 respectively). S-G-Hel-1047-a-A-21 hybridised at 52°C.

Validation of Molecular Methods (PCR/FISH) for the Detection of *Helicobacteraceae* Organisms. In order to calculate the sensitivity and specificity of the dual molecular approach 100 gastric samples were selected on the basis of *H. pylori* status (50 positive and 50 negative). *H. pylori* status had been confirmed previously by CLO test and histology; however this was blinded to researchers until after molecular assessment. FISH was performed on archival paraffin tissue sections and PCR was performed on DNA extracted from fresh biopsies.

Biopsy blocks were cut to a thickness of 4 µm using a Leica RM2125RT rotary microtome with sections cut per block, and mounted on ChemMate capillary gap slides, 75 µm, (DakoCytomation, Cambridgeshire, UK). Following microtome sectioning and mounting of tissue, slides were dried vertically at room temperature and incubated overnight at 37°C to ensure that the tissue was adhered to the slide. Slides were then arranged by patient and block number and sections 1, 3 and 5 were used for assessing the presence of *H. pylori* coupled with the universal bacterial probe. Sections 2, 4 and 6 were used for assessing the presence of all *Helicobacteraceae*. Biopsy sections were deparaffinised

Table 2. Probes used for fluorescent *in-situ* hybridisation (FISH).

Probe	16S rDNA position [a] [b]	Probe sequence [c]	Fluorophore	Reference
Universal				
Eub A	338–355 [a]	5′ - GCT GCC TCC CGT AGG AGT - 3′	Rhodamine red	[20]
Eub B	338–355 [a]	5′ - GCT GCC ACC CGT AGG TGT - 3′	Rhodamine red	[40]
Eub C	338–355 [a]	5′ - GCA GCC ACC CGT AGG TGT - 3′	Rhodamine red	[40]
***Helicobacteraceae* family specific**				
Hgen1	218–235 [b]	5′- ARC TGA TAG GAC ATA GRC - 3′ [c]	Cy3	This study
Hgen2	666–683 [b]	5′ - TGA GTA TTC YTC TTG ATM - 3′ [c]	Oregon green 488	This study
Hgen3	657–674 [b]	5′ - CTC TTG ATC TCT ACG GAT - 3′	Oregon green 488	This study
Hgen4	630–647 [b]	5′ - ACA CCA AGA ATT CCA CCT - 3′	Oregon green 488	This study
Hgen5	1047–1067 [b]	5′ - GCC GTG CAG CAC CTG TTT TCA - 3′	Oregon green 488	This study
***Helicobacter pylori* specific**				
Hpy-1	547–567 [b]	5′- CACACCTGACTGACTATCCCG - 3′	Cy3	[21]
HP2	796–815 [b]	5′- CTG GAG AGA CTA AGC CCT CC - 3′	Oregon green 488	[16]
Hp16S-1	163–185 [b]	5′- GGAGTATCTGGTATTAATCATCG - 3′	Oregon green 488	[41]
Hp16S-2	206–227 [b]	5′- GGACATAGGCTGATCTCTTAGC -3′	Oregon green 488	[41]

[a]Indicates *E. coli* numbering.
[b]Indicates *H. pylori* numbering to strain 26695 (ATCC 700392).
[c]Indicates degeneracy of nucleotides according to IUPAC see http://www.chem.qmul.ac.uk/iubmb/misc/naseq.html.

using xylene and ethanol [21]. For glass slides carrying deparaffinised tissue sections, 50 µl of hybridisation buffer was added and coverslips were used to minimise evaporation. Hybridisation was performed for 16 hours for all tissue sections and Vectashield Hardmount (Vector Laboratories, Peterborough, UK) was used.

DNA extraction of mucosal biopsies was performed using the commercially available Qiagen QIAamp Mini kit (Qiagen Crawley UK) with the following amendments. Biopsy samples were kept frozen until the addition of ATL buffer before allowing biopsies to equilibrate to room temperature, an additional 10 µl of Proteinase K was added for an initial lysis period of 18 hours to ensure complete lysis of the biopsy material prior to DNA extraction. PCR was performed as described above with biopsy DNA initially subjected to universal bacterial PCR [12] to confirm the suitability of the DNA for further analysis.

One hundred infectious diarrhoea samples were also collected for inclusion in the validation cohort. Samples were obtained from the Department of Medical Microbiology (Aberdeen Royal Infirmary, Aberdeen) and DNA was extracted using the Nucleon phytopure DNA extraction kit. PCR was performed as described above with faecal DNA initially subjected to universal bacterial PCR [12] to confirm the suitability of the DNA for further analysis.

Assessment of *Helicobacteraceae* Prevalence in Human Colonic Tissue Using the Combined Molecular Approach

Archival colonic tissue specimens. Paraffin embedded colonic specimens from a total of 106 patients were obtained from the Department of Pathology (Aberdeen Royal Infirmary). Fifty-seven ulcerative colitis (UC) patients and forty-nine healthy controls (HC) were included. All UC patients were assessed during active disease and analysis was performed on all available colonic sites that were biopsied at the time of colonoscopy. The HC subjects comprised individuals who had undergone a colonoscopy in which colonic tissue was macroscopically normal, and subsequently confirmed as microscopically normal by histology. This cohort was examined exclusively by the FISH method outlined above. This sample cohort was not amenable to PCR methodologies.

Fresh colonic biopsy specimens. A total of 145 individuals were recruited for the prospective fresh biopsy study, 86 formed the ulcerative colitis (UC) cohort and were analysed alongside a cohort of 59 healthy controls (HC). Of the UC cohort 9 individuals were excluded, 3 could not undergo colonoscopy for clinical reasons and 6 had an alternative final diagnosis. The HC cohort comprised two groups. The first group (N = 32) were recruited specifically for this study and had biopsies collected for both FISH and PCR studies (as outlined above). The second group (N = 27) had been recruited previously and all 27 had biopsies collected from normal colon whilst undergoing polypectomy.

Biopsies were collected during colonoscopy using standard endoscopic forceps (Boston Scientific Nanterre Cedex France). The colonic mucosa was rinsed with sterile water via the colonoscope to remove residual faecal material. Biopsies were immediately snap frozen in liquid nitrogen and then transferred to a −80°C freezer until used for DNA analysis. Additional biopsies were also sent for histopathology assessment and FISH analysis.

Biopsies were only collected for PCR based studies and so FISH analysis was not studied in this cohort. Therefore mucosal biopsies were obtained from 136 individuals, 77 with a clinical and histological diagnosis of UC (55 established disease – three had antibiotic therapy in the 6 months prior to study recruitment, 22 *de-novo*) and 59 healthy controls. The entire UC group had biopsies collected for both fluorescent *in-situ* hybridisation (FISH) and PCR studies. Samples that generated positive PCR results with *Helicobacteraceae* or *H. pylori* PCR primers were sequenced to confirm identity. Based on sequence analysis results, samples that were suspected of containing multiple *Helicobacter* sequences were cloned [12] and 5 clones per sample were sent for sequence analysis (400 bp).

Ethical approval for the archival specimen analysis and the biopsy study was granted by North East of Scotland Research Ethics Service and written informed consent was obtained from all subjects in the biopsy study.

Statistical analysis

Statistical analysis with the Pearson Chi Squared 2 tailed test, was performed using SPSS statistics software version 17.0.1 (December 1 2008).

Results

Validation of Molecular Methods (PCR/FISH) for the Detection of *Helicobacteraceae* Organisms

Fifty of the gastric biopsy samples demonstrated FISH positivity using both *Helicobacteraceae* and *H. pylori* specific probes along with the universal Eub338 probe. The same 50 samples tested positive by PCR for *Helicobacteraceae, H. pylori* specific and universal bacterial primer sets with a subset of results (N = 10) subjected to sequence analysis which confirmed the presence of *H. pylori* (sequence identities >99%). The molecular results were 100% concordant with the findings of clinical investigation indicating that the combined approach had a high diagnostic sensitivity and specificity.

The combined molecular approach was then applied to 100 infectious diarrhoea samples. All infectious diarrhoea samples showed positivity with the universal bacterial FISH probe (Eub338) and the universal bacterial PCR. One diarrhoea sample was positive for *Helicobacter* by FISH and both *Helicobacteraceae* and *H. pylori* specific PCR with sequencing confirming the presence of *H. pylori*. As non-*pylori Helicobacter* organisms have been isolated from diarrheal samples previously, we performed a series of spiking experiments to confirm that the diarrheal samples were not inhibiting PCR amplification. Ten samples which were negative for *Helicobacteraceae* by both FISH and PCR were spiked with *H. pylori* DNA (500 pg to 0.5 pg) prior to PCR amplification. All spiked samples yielded positive PCR and subsequent sequencing results (>99% sequence similarity, over 360 bp, to the spiked *H. pylori* 16S rDNA gene sequence) confirming that if present these organisms would have been detected.

Helicobacteraceae Prevalence in Human Colonic Tissue

Archival study. The UC archival cohort (n = 57, 44% Male) had a median age of 40 (range 15–82) at the time of colonoscopy and were classified as extensive (40%), left sided (37%) and proctitis (23%) according to the Montreal criteria [22]. A total of 284 biopsies were analysed with 46% of subjects having biopsies from inflamed and un-involved mucosa available (E1 n = 8, E2 n = 9, E3 n = 9) and the remainder having biopsies only from inflamed mucosa. The HC archival cohort (n = 49, 35% Male) had a median age of 42 (range 14–80) at the time of colonoscopy. A total of 127 biopsies were processed in triplicate to assess the presence of *Helicobacteraceae* from the available pathology blocks of the right and left colon including rectum. Subjects were considered to be positive if appropriate fluorescent organisms were observed in at least 1 slide. All fluorescent *in-situ* hybridisations were assessed alongside *H. pylori* positive gastric biopsy reference slides and a selection of *Helicobacter* reference strains. All of the 106 subjects had bacteria detected with the universal bacterial probe. Of the 55 subjects positive for *Helicobacteraceae*, 29 were from the UC cohort and 26 were from the HC cohort. In both groups there was no statistically significant correlation with gender or age of the subjects and in the UC cohort the extent of disease did not correlate with the rate of positivity either as detailed in Table 3. Interestingly there was a statistically significant difference in the presence of *Helicobacter pylori* with 13 of the *Helicobacteraceae* positive subjects from the HC cohort also having a positive result for *Helicobacter pylori* compared with only 3 of the UC cohort ($p = 0.002$). Assuming that these *Helicobacter pylori* positive results represent transported gastric *Helicobacter pylori* we consequently removed these from the *Helicobacteraceae* positive results, thus creating a new category of non-pylori *Helicobacter* positive organisms. By this approach there was also a statistically significant difference in the presence of non-*pylori Helicobacter* organisms between the UC and HC cohorts ($p = 0.04$). There was no correlation with age, gender or severity of disease as detailed in Table 3. Because of limitations of the archival FISH technique it was not possible to ascertain if the *H. pylori* organisms were entirely responsible for the genus positivity or if the *H. pylori* were cohabiting with other non-*pylori Helicobacter*. Indeed, it was also not possible to ascertain if more than one *Helicobacteraceae* species was present within a sample. Attempts were made to extract microbial DNA from the archival tissue but these were unsuccessful and therefore a prospectively collected cohort was established with samples taken for PCR based analyses and FISH analysis.

Prospective study. The prospective UC cohort ($n = 77$, 46% Male) had a median age of 42 (range 16–84) at the time of index colonoscopy and were classified as extensive (25%), left sided (62%), proctitis (13.0%). A total of 137 biopsy sites were analysed. Twenty one (27%) subjects had a single site analysed, all of which represented inflamed mucosa and 56 (73%) had more than one biopsy site assessed, of which 42 both had inflamed and uninvolved mucosa. The prospective HC cohort ($n = 59$, 59% Male) had a median age of 63 (range 30–75) at the time of index colonoscopy. There was a statistically significant median age difference between the UC cohort and the control groups (Mann Whitney U test $p < 0.001$). A single biopsy site ($n = 59$) was analysed from each control subject. All 136 subjects (77 UC and 59 controls) had colonic biopsies available for PCR analysis and all were positive for universal bacterial PCR indicating the presence of bacterial DNA within all samples. Of the 136 subjects, 43 (32%) were PCR positive for *Helicobacteraceae* and 3 (2%) were PCR positive for both *Helicobacter pylori* and *Helicobacter* genus (Table 4). Subsequent sequence analysis of the *Helicobacteraceae* PCR products confirmed the presence of only *Helicobacter pylori* in these 3 samples. Thus 40 subjects were PCR positive for *Helicobacteraceae* but not *H. pylori*. Sequence analysis revealed a further 4 subjects (3 controls and 1 UC) with only *Helicobacter pylori* identified.

In the remaining 36 subjects sequence analysis identified the presence of a further 8 *Helicobacter* species and a *Wollinella succinogenes* with 6 subjects having more than one species identified (Table 5). Of these subjects, 3 had multiple *Helicobacter* species present within the same biopsy sample and 3 had different *Helicobacter* species spread between the samples analysed (Table S1). *Helicobacter pylori* were not found to co-exist with any other *Helicobacteraceae* species. The species identified and the number of samples they were identified in is detailed in Table S1.

Helicobacteraceae PCR positivity was significantly higher in UC than controls 32 of 77 (42%) versus 11 of 59 (19%), $p = 0.004$). By analysing the sequences obtained and including only those *Helicobacter* species classified as "enterohepatic," the prevalence was 29 of 77 (38%) in the UC group versus 2 of 59 (3%) in the controls ($p < 0.0001$). There was also a negative association between the identification of gastric *Helicobacter* species in UC (2 of 77) versus controls (9 of 59, $p = 0.007$) (Table 4). There was no correlation between the age, gender or extent of disease.

The effect of bowel preparation on *Helicobacteraceae* PCR positivity was also considered. Of the 77 UC subjects, 32 had full bowel preparation prior to colonoscopy along with all 59 control subjects. *Helicobacteraceae* PCR positivity in subjects with bowel preparation was significantly higher in UC than controls [20 of 32 (63%) versus 11 of 59 (19%), (Pearson Chi squared test $p < 0.0001$)]. There was also a significant difference in *Helicobacteraceae* PCR positivity within the UC cohort based on bowel preparation 20 of 32 (63% full bowel preparation), 1 of 5 (20% phosphate enema preparation) vs 11 of 40 (28% no bowel preparation), Pearson Chi squared test $p = 0.007$). There was also no statistically significant association with antibiotic usage.

Table 3. Archival Study FISH results.

	Gender	Montreal Extent of Disease	Median Age	Eub 338 +ve (%)	HFam +ve (%)	HP +ve (%)	NpH +ve (%)
UC	Male	1	29	8 (100)	3 (38)	0 (0)	3 (38)
		2	45	8 (100)	6 (75)	1 (13)	5 (63)
		3	40	9 (100)	6 (67)	1 (11)	5 (56)
		Total	32	25 (100)	15 (60)	2 (8)	13 (52)
	Female	1	37	5 (100)	3 (60)	0 (0)	3 (60)
		2	49	13 (100)	4 (31)	0 (0)	4 (31)
		3	39	14 (100)	7 (50)	1 (7)	6 (43)
		Total	42	32 (100)	14 (44)	1 (3)	13 (41)
	Combined Total		**40**	**57 (100)**	**29 (51)**	**3 (5)***	**26 (46) ****
Control	Male		39	17 (100)	10 (59)	6 (35)	4 (24)
	Female		47	32 (100)	16 (50)	7 (22)	9 (28)
	Combined Total		**42**	**49 (100)**	**26 (53)**	**13 (27)***	**13 (27)****

*$p = 0.002$ (Pearson Chi Squared 2 tailed test).
**$p = 0.04$ (Pearson Chi Squared 2 tailed test).

Table 4. Prospective Study PCR results

	Gender	Montreal Extent of Disease	Median Age	Universal Bacteria +ve (%)	HFam +ve (%)	Gastric Species (%)	EHH species (%)
UC	Male	1	53	2 (100)	1 (50)	0 (0)	1 (50)
		2	44	21 (100)	10 (48)	1 (5)	9 (43)
		3	53	12 (100)	7 (58)	0 (0)	7 (58)
		Total	45	35 (100)	18 (51)	1 (3)	17 (49)
	Female	1	52	8 (100)	2 (25)	1 (13)	1 (13)
		2	42	27 (100)	9 (33)	0 (0)	9 (33)
		3	28	7 (100)	3 (43)	0 (0)	3 (43)
		Total	41	42 (100)	14 (33)	1 (2)	13 (31)
	Combined Total		**42**	**77 (100)**	**32 (42)***	**2 (3)****	**30 (39)*****
Control	Male		61	35 (100)	6 (17)	4 (11)	2 (6)
	Female		64	24 (100)	5 (21)	5 (21)	0 (0)
	Combined Total		**63**	**59 (100)**	**11 (19)***	**9 (15)****	**2 (3)*****

*p = 0.004 (Pearson Chi Squared 2 tailed test).
**p = 0.007 (Pearson Chi Squared 2 tailed test).
***p<0.0001 (Pearson Chi Squared 2 tailed test).

For 109 (77 UC, 32 HC) of the 136 subjects, samples were available for both FISH and PCR based analyses. All samples analysed by FISH were Eub338 positive indicating the presence of bacteria. 62 of 77 (81%) UC were *Helicobacteraceae* positive whilst 1 was also *H. pylori* positive. In the 32 controls, 12 (38%) were *Helicobacteraceae* positive whilst 2 were also *H. pylori* positive (Table 6). The *Helicobacteraceae* positivity was significantly higher in the UC cohort ($p<0.0001$) but no negative association with *Helicobacter pylori* as seen in the archival FISH and prospective PCR studies. As in the other studies there was no correlation between the age, gender or extent of disease. Correlation between PCR and FISH results for these 109 subjects were examined which demonstrated concordance in 74 (68%) of subjects. The majority of discordant results were attributable to a higher positivity rate for *Helicobacteraceae* with FISH than PCR (Table 7).

Discussion

During the development of our combined molecular approach, both the PCR and FISH techniques were highly sensitive and specific (100% each) when interrogating gastric biopsies with known *H. pylori* status. A further validation cohort utilising

Table 5. *Helicobacteraceae* species identified by sequencing.

Helicobacteraceae **Species Identified**	**Number of Subjects Combination of Species identified in**	
	UC	**Control**
Single species identified		
Helicobacter cinaedi	1	0
Helicobacter canadensis	1	0
Helicobacter cholecystus	9	0
Helicobacter hepaticus	5	1
Helicobacter mustelae	0	4
Helicobacter pullorum	5	1
Helicobacter pylori	2	5
Wolinella succinogenes	1	0
Two species co-existing within Subject		
Helicobacter brantae *Helicobacter pullorum*	1	0
Helicobacter cholecystus *Helicobacter bilis*	1	0
Helicobacter cholecystus *Helicobacter canadensis*	1	0
Helicobacter cholecystus *Helicobacter hepaticus*	3	0

Table 6. Prospective Study FISH results.

	Gender	Montreal Extent of Disease	Median Age	Eub 338 +ve (%)	HFam +ve (%)	HP +ve (%)	NpH +ve (%)
UC	**Male**	1	53	2 (100)	2 (100)	0	2 (100)
		2	44	21 (100)	16 (76.2)	1 (4.8)	15 (71.4)
		3	53	12 (100)	12 (100)	0	12 (100)
		Total	45	35 (100)	30 (85.7)	1	29 (64.4)
	Female	1	53	8 (100)	8 (100)	0	8 (100)
		2	42	27 (100)	20 (74.1)	0	20 (74.1)
		3	28	7 (100)	4 (57.4)	0	4 (57.4)
		Total	41	42 (100)	32 (76.2)	0	32 (76.2)
	Combined Total		**42**	**77** (100)	**62 (85.7)***	**1 (1.3)**	**61 (79.2) ****
Control	**Male**		64	15 (100)	5 (33.3)	0	5 (33.3)
	Female		64	17 (100)	7 (41.2)	2 (11.7)	5 (29.4)
	Combined Total		**64**	**32** (100)	**12 (37.5)***	**2 (6.3)**	**10 (31.1)****

*p<0.0001 (Pearson Chi Squared 2 tailed test).
**p<0.0001 (Pearson Chi Squared 2 tailed test).

diarrhoeal samples demonstrated limited *Helicobacteraceae* positivity. However spiking experiments on this cohort indicate that organisms would have been identified had they been present. These findings suggest that *Helicobacteraceae* are not a prominent causative agent in infectious diarrhoea in our setting although they have been isolated from diarrhoeal samples by other investigators [23–33]. Part of the rationale behind our developing a combined approach to identify *Helicobacteraceae*, rather than one based solely on either PCR or FISH, was that the combination of techniques allows visualisation of organisms *in-situ* and species-level identification from sequencing. PCR-only studies can be criticised based on the possibility that contaminant environmental DNA could bias results. In the gastrointestinal tract for instance, DNA could be transited to the colon in the faecal stream from foodstuffs. FISH addresses these concerns by allowing direct visualisation and localisation of organisms to the colonic mucosa. FISH-only studies however are limited by the constraints of designing species-specific probes and therefore they lack species-level sensitivity at times. By utilising both approaches *Helicobacteraceae* species present could be visualised and also identified. Based on the strength of these validation studies, we considered that this combined methodology was suitable for investigating *Helicobacteraceae* prevalence in UC colonic biopsies. A combined FISH/PCR approach has also been utilised to examine *Helicobacteraceae* prevalence in a small cohort of children with IBD (n = 12) (Crohn's disease n = 11), irritable bowel syndrome (IBS; n = 5) and controls (n = 4) [9]. This small study identified a strikingly high prevalence in both IBD (11/12) and IBS (5/5) versus controls (1/4). Through sequence analysis of DGGE bands several *Helicobacteraceae* were identified including *Helicobacter ganmani*, *Wolinella succinogenes*, *H. hepaticus* and *H. pylori*. Two further bands were identified as *Helicobacter* although equal sequence similarity was attributed to multiple species.

The results of our study show that rates of *Helicobacteraceae* positivity are significantly higher in the colonic tissue of UC patients than in controls. When sequencing data is analysed and species identities attributed, in control patients, the species identified are almost exclusively gastric (namely *H. pylori* and *H. mustelae* (99–100% sequence similarity); comprising 9 of 11). This finding is in stark contrast to the *Helicobacter* sequences from the UC cohort where 32 patients had *Helicobacteraceae* species identified, although only 2 of these were attributed to *H. pylori* and curiously, *H. mustelae* was absent. Our study was not designed to obtain gastric *Helicobacter* species. As such it was not possible to confirm or refute the notion that *Helicobacter* species detected in the colon are truly colonising the mucus or merely transiting from the stomach. For the former, *Helicobacter* grown from both sites (stomach and colon) would be necessary in order to undertake a detailed strain comparison, which was not feasible within this study. As indicated in the results section there was also a statistically significant difference in age between the UC and control groups. The difference in age between the two groups is a result of the control group predominantly being recruited from a colorectal cancer screening programme whose lower age limit is 50 years.

Interestingly, bowel preparation appeared to increase the detection of *Helicobacter* species. It might be anticipated that the wash-out effect of bowel preparation might reduce the positivity.

Table 7. Correlation of PCR and FISH results.

	FISH *Helicobacter* negative (%)	FISH *Helicobacteraceae* positive (%)	FISH *H. pylori* positive (%)
PCR *Helicobacter* Negative	35 (32%)	35 (32%)	0
PCR *Helicobacteraceae* positive	0	39 (36%)	2 (2%)
PCR *H. pylori* positive	0	0	1 (1)

This surprising result may be the result of an unidentified confounding factor or could be a surrogate disease severity marker. This was due to it being a clinical decision whether subjects received bowel preparation or not. As no bowel preparation was given when there was the clinical impression of severe disease. This suggests that *Helicobacteraceae* positivity is associated with less severe disease. However no association between *Helicobacteraceae* positivity and the Montreal classification of disease extent and severity was observed.

Six of the UC patients appear to have multiple *Helicobacter* species present within their colonic tissue. Two of the six had different *Helicobacter* sequences identified from the same biopsy whereas the other four had single *Helicobacter* species identified from biopsies taken from different regions of the colon. Mixed species were not identified in the control cohort although it should be acknowledged that only single colonic sites were investigated by biopsy. Nevertheless our findings suggest that more than one enterohepatic *Helicobacter* species can be present in the same human host although this does not appear to be the case for gastric species.

It should be noted that allocation of species should not rely solely on 16S rRNA sequencing as comparison of these sequences can be misleading and does not always provide conclusive evidence for species level identification. *Helicobacter* species identity cannot be firmly established by 16S sequencing and the 400 bp product of the nested PCR further compounded this by only allowing sequencing over this short segment. However there is confidence that the sequence belonged to the genus *Helicobacter* based on the sequenced product. For example, although our nested PCR technique amplified a hyper-variable region of the 16S rRNA *Helicobacter* genome which equated to an estimated average evolutionary diversity of 14 base pairs within the 9 species identified [34], it is not possible to be certain of the *Helicobacter* species without additional genotypic or phenotypic characterisation [35]. There is always the possibility that mixed *Helicobacter* organisms were present that had identical sequences over the 400 bp 16S rDNA region analysed. It is possible that alternative identification approaches including denaturing gradient gel electrophoresis (DGGE) could have been used to address this potential issue. Where sequence analysis indicated that mixed species were present, the additional cloning and sequencing approach was undertaken which demonstrated the presence of multiple *Helicobacter* sequences within a few samples.

The use of nested PCR is known to increase the sensitivity of the PCR test; however it is also known that without strict use of appropriate control strategies including sequencing of positive results, it can lead to false positives. In the current study, all positive nested PCR findings were sequenced in order to eliminate the query of false positives due to nested PCR. Extensive attempts were made to isolate *Helicobacter* species from the prospective cohort, however this was not successful. *Helicobacter* species are notoriously fastidious and although novel *Helicobacter* species have been isolated from human faeces, to date none have been isolated from colonic tissue. Examining both FISH and PCR analyses on a large number of samples (n = 109) revealed a correlation rate of ~68%. In the majority of cases, discordant results showed that FISH was more likely to yield a positive result than PCR. This was not seen in our gastric validation cohort. The most likely explanation is that the number of *H. pylori* strains present in infected gastric tissue is higher than the corresponding number of *Helicobacter* species in the colon. These results suggest that the FISH technique is more sensitive but lacks the specificity to identify the *Helicobacteraceae* species. Regardless of these technical issues, both techniques demonstrate a statistically significant correlation between the presence of *Helicobacteraceae* species, particularly the enterohepatic *Helicobacter* species and the UC cohort.

The PCR methodology that we developed used a nested PCR approach for *Helicobacteraceae* but a single PCR was used for *H. pylori*. It is likely that a nested PCR for *H. pylori* would have been more sensitive in the colonic samples and would have increased the detection rate. This is a plausible explanation for at least 3 of the four samples which were shown by sequence analysis of the *Helicobacteraceae* PCR product to contain *H. pylori* despite *H. pylori* PCR results being negative. Nevertheless, in order to identify every *Helicobacter* that was detected, we chose to sequence every positive PCR reaction including those that were *H. pylori* positive in order to determine whether multiple species were present.

Attributing causation to putative pathogens has always been a difficult endeavour with the gold standard remaining fulfilment of Koch's postulates [36]. In an era of molecular biology and an increasing awareness of the "unculturable" microbiota of the human colon however, these postulates are perhaps outdated. Swidsinski and colleagues recently proposed alternative postulates for a modern era [37]:

- There must be a clear link between a pathogen and a disease,
- The pathogenic organism should be identified and characterised (by traditional culture and phenotyping or by "reliable" modern methods such as PCR, DNA sequencing and FISH),
- There should be positive evidence of the chain of infection (this can be from individual transfections or from epidemiological observation)
- Knowledge of a specific pathogen should assist the development of new diagnostic methods and treatment

We would add that host factors, in particular genetic or immunological susceptibility should be considered, particularly in the context of IBD. We believe that our data adds considerable weight to fulfilling Swidsinski's second postulate and that the first has already been firmly established in animal models. Further work is required to address the third postulate which would clearly be aided by successful culture of these organisms from the colonic tissue of UC patients.

Finally, the presence of *H. mustelae* in the colonic tissue of controls but not UC patients warrants further consideration. Since *H. mustelae* is a gastric organism (previously only identified in ferrets [38]), it would be interesting to see if this species is co-colonising the human stomach and colon, the colon alone or simply being transited to the colon from the stomach. *H. mustelae* has a similar morphology to *H. pylori* and is also a urease positive organism so it could easily be mistaken with current clinical testing (CLO test) for *H. pylori* in human gastric disease. It may be that *H. mustelae* represents a less pathogenic organism in the human host which nonetheless confers the IBD protective benefits of *H. pylori* [39]. In terms of the extra-gastric *Helicobacters* our findings clearly demonstrate compelling molecular evidence for their presence in the human colon. Their presence in the human host is not well established compared to animal models however; there is no reason to suggest that they do not reside in the human intestinal tract. Clearly these hypotheses require further exploration.

Acknowledgments

We are grateful to Dr Sylvia Duncan (Rowett Institute for Nutrition and Health, Aberdeen) for supplying many of the bacterial isolates used in this work. We gratefully acknowledge technical assistance from Mrs Nicky Fyfe.

Author Contributions

Conceived and designed the experiments: JMT RH GIM JGF EEO GLH. Performed the experiments: JMT RH SHB MEH IM MHM ZS. Analyzed the data: JMT RH GLH. Contributed reagents/materials/analysis tools: JMT RH ZS JGF EEO GLH. Wrote the paper: JMT RH GLH.

References

1. Lennard-Jones JE (1989) Classification of inflammatory bowel disease. Scand J Gastroenterol 24(S170): 2–6.
2. Hansen R, Thomson JM, Fox JG, El-Omar EM, Hold GL (2011) Could *Helicobacter* organisms cause inflammatory bowel disease? FEMS Imm Med Micro 61(1): 1–14.
3. Cahill RJ, Foltz CJ, Fox JG, Dangler CA, Powrie F, et al. (1997) Inflammatory bowel disease: An immunity-mediated condition triggered by bacterial infection with *Helicobacter hepaticus*. Infect Immun 65(8): 3126–3131.
4. Kullberg MC, Ward JM, Gorelick PL, Caspar P, Hieny S, et al. (1998) *Helicobacter hepaticus* triggers colitis in specific-pathogen-free interleukin-10 (IL-10)-deficient mice through an IL-12-and gamma interferon-dependent mechanism. Infect Immun 66(11): 5157–5166.
5. Jergens AE, Wilson-Welder JH, Dorn A, Henderson A, Liu Z, et al. (2007) *Helicobacter bilis* triggers persistent immune reactivity to antigens derived from the commensal bacteria in gnotobiotic C3H/HeN mice. Gut 56(7): 934–940.
6. Bell SJ, Chisholm SA, Owen RJ, Borriello SP, Kamm MA (2003) Evaluation of *helicobacter* species in inflammatory bowel disease. Aliment Pharmacol Ther 18(5): 481–486.
7. Grehan M, Danon S, Lee A, Daskalopoulos G, Mitchell H (2004) Absence of mucosa-associated colonic *helicobacters* in an australian urban population. J Clin Microbiol 42(2): 874–876.
8. Bohr URM, Glasbrenner B, Primus A, Zagoura A, Wex T, et al. (2004) Identification of enterohepatic *helicobacter* species in patients suffering from inflammatory bowel disease. J Clin Microbiol 42(6): 2766–2768.
9. Zhang L, Day A, McKenzie G, Mitchell H (2006) Nongastric *helicobacter* species detected in the intestinal tract of children. J Clin Microbiol 44(6): 2276–2279.
10. Laharie D, Asencio C, Asselineau J, Bulois P, Bourreille A, et al. (2009) Association between entero-hepatic *helicobacter* species and crohn's disease: A prospective cross-sectional study. Aliment Pharmacol Ther 30(3): 283–293.
11. Miyazaki K, Martin JC, Marinsek-Logar R, Flint HJ (1997) Degradation and utilization of xylans by the rumen anaerobe prevotella bryantii (formerly P. ruminicola subsp. brevis) B14. Anaerobe 3(6): 373–381.
12. Hold GL, Pryde SE, Russell VJ, Furrie E, Flint HJ (2002) Assessment of microbial diversity in human colonic samples by 16S rDNA sequence analysis. FEMS Microbiol Ecol 39(1): 33–39.
13. Fox JG, Dewhirst FE, Shen Z, Feng Y, Taylor NS, et al. (1998) Hepatic *helicobacter* species identified in bile and gallbladder tissue from chileans with chronic cholecystitis. Gastroenterology 114(4): 755–763.
14. Grehan M, Tamotia G, Robertson B, Mitchell H (2002) Detection of *Helicobacter* colonization of the murine lower bowel by genus-specific PCR-denaturing gradient gel electrophoresis. Appl Environ Microbiol 68(10): 5164–5166.
15. Weisburg WG, Barns SM, Pelletier DA, Lane DJ (1991) 16S ribosomal DNA amplification for phylogenetic study. J Bacteriol 173(2): 697–703.
16. Moreno Y, Ferrus MA, Alonso JL, Jimenez A, Hernandez J (2003) Use of fluorescent in situ hybridization to evidence the presence of *helicobacter pylori* in water. Water Res 37(9): 2251–2256.
17. Ashelford KE, Weightman AJ, Fry JC (2002) PRIMROSE: A computer program for generating and estimating the phylogenetic range of 16S rRNA oligonucleotide probes and primers in conjunction with the RDP-II database. Nucleic Acids Res 30(15): 3481–3489.
18. Loy A, Maixner F, Wagner M, Horn M (2007) probeBase–an online resource for rRNA-targeted oligonucleotide probes: New features 2007. Nucleic Acids Res 35(Database issue): D800–D804.
19. Schwiertz A, Le Blay G, Blaut M (2000) Quantification of different eubacterium spp. in human fecal samples with species-specific 16S rRNA-targeted oligonucleotide probes. Appl Environ Microbiol 66(1): 375–382.
20. Amann RI, Binder BJ, Olson RJ, Chisholm SW, Devereux R, et al. (1990) Combination of 16S rRNA-targeted oligonucleotide probes with flow cytometry for analyzing mixed microbial populations. Appl Environ Microbiol 56(6): 1919–1925.
21. Trebesius K, Panthel K, Strobel S, Vogt K, Faller G, et al. (2000) Rapid and specific detection of *Helicobacter pylori* macrolide resistance in gastric tissue by fluorescent in situ hybridisation. Br Med J 46(5): 608–614.
22. Silverberg MS, Satsangi J, Ahmad T, Arnott IDR, Bernstein CN, et al. (2005) Towards an integrated clinical, molecular and serological classification of inflammatory bowel disease: Report of a working party of the 2005 montreal world congress of gastroenterology. Can J Gastroenterol 19(Suppl A): 5A–36A.
23. Tee W, Anderson BN, Ross BC, Dwyer B (1987) Atypical *campylobacters* associated with gastroenteritis. J Clin Microbiol 25(7): 1248–1252.
24. Vandamme P, Falsen E, Pot B, Kersters K, De Ley J (1990) Identification of *Campylobacter cinaedi* isolated from blood and feces of children and adult females. J Clin Microbiol 28(5): 1016–1020.
25. Burnens AP, Stanley J, Schaad UB, Nicolet J (1993) Novel *campylobacter*-like organism resembling helicobacter fennelliae isolated from a boy with gastroenteritis and from dogs. J Clin Microbiol 31(7): 1916–1917.
26. Stanley J, Linton D, Burnens AP, Dewhirst FE, Owen RJ, et al. (1993) *Helicobacter canis* sp. nov., a new species from dogs: An integrated study of phenotype and genotype. Microbiology 139(10): 2495–2504.
27. Romero S, Archer JR, Hamacher ME, Bologna SM, Schell RF (1988) Case report of an unclassified microaerophilic bacterium associated with gastroenteritis. J Clin Microbiol 26(1): 142–143.
28. Stanley J, Linton D, Burnens AP, Dewhirst FE, On SLW, et al. (1994) *Helicobacter pullorum* sp. nov.-genotype and phenotype of a new species isolated from poultry and from human patients with gastroenteritis. Microbiology 140(12): 3441–3449.
29. Burnens AP, Stanley J, Morgenstern R, Nicolet J (1994) Gastroenteritis associated with *Helicobacter pullorum*. Lancet 344(8936): 1569–1570.
30. Steinbrueckner B, Haerter G, Pelz K, Weiner S, Rump JA, et al. (1997) Isolation of *Helicobacter pullorum* from patients with enteritis. Scand J Infect Dis 29(3): 315–318.
31. Melito PL, Munro C, Chipman PR, Woodward DL, Booth TF, et al. (2001) *Helicobacter winghamensis* sp. nov., a novel helicobacter sp. isolated from patients with gastroenteritis. J Clin Microbiol 39(7): 2412–2417.
32. Lastovica AJ (2000) Efficient isolation of campylobacteria from stools. J Clin Microbiol 38(7): 2798–2799.
33. Fox JG, Chien CC, Dewhirst FE, Paster BJ, Shen Z, et al. (2000) *Helicobacter canadensis* sp. nov. isolated from humans with diarrhea as an example of an emerging pathogen. J Clin Microbiol 38(7): 2546–2549.
34. Tamura K, Dudley J, Nei M, Kumar S (2007) MEGA4: Molecular evolutionary genetics analysis (MEGA) software version 4.0. Mol Biol Evol 24(8): 1596–1599.
35. Whary MT, Fox JG (2004) Natural and experimental *helicobacter* infections. Comp Med 36: 139–177.
36. Koch R (1884) Die aetiologie der tuberkulose. Mittbeilungen Kaiserlichen Gesundbeitsamte 2: 1–88.
37. Swidsinski A, Doerffel Y, Loening-Baucke V, Theissig F, Ruckert JC, et al. (2010) Acute appendicitis is characterized by local invasion with *Fusobacterium nucleatum/necrophorum*. Gut:doi:10.1136/gut.2009.191320.
38. Fox JG, Correa P, Taylor NS, Lee A, Otto G, et al. (1990) *Helicobacter mustelae*-associated gastritis in ferrets. An animal model of *Helicobacter pylori* gastritis in humans. Gastroenterology 99(2): 352–361.
39. Luther J, Dave M, Higgins PDR, Kao JY (2009) Association between *Helicobacter pylori* infection and inflammatory bowel disease: A meta-analysis and systematic review of the literature. Inflamm Bowel Dis 16(6): 1077–1084.
40. Daims H, Brühl A, Amann R, Schleifer KH, Wagner M (1999) The domain-specific probe EUB 338 is insufficient for the detection of all bacteria: Development and evaluation of a more comprehensive probe set. Syst Appl Microbiol 22(3): 434–444.
41. Morotomi M, Hoshina S, Green P, Neu HC, LoGerfo P, et al. (1989) Oligonucleotide probe for detection and identification of *Campylobacter pylori*. J Clin Microbiol 27(12): 2652–2655.

4

Ulcerative Colitis Impairs the Acylethanolamide-Based Anti-Inflammatory System Reversal by 5-Aminosalicylic Acid and Glucocorticoids

Juan Suárez[1,3], Yanina Romero-Zerbo[1], Lucia Márquez[2], Patricia Rivera[1], Mar Iglesias[4], Francisco J. Bermúdez-Silva[1,3], Montserrat Andreu[2]*, Fernando Rodríguez de Fonseca[1,3]*

1 Laboratorio de Medicina Regenerativa, Hospital Carlos Haya, Mediterranean Institute for the Advance of Biotechnology and Health Research Fundación, Málaga, Spain, **2** Department of Gastroenterology, Parc de Salut Mar, Universidad Autónoma, Barcelona, Spain, **3** El Centro de Investigación Biomédica en Red de Fisiopatología de Obesidad y Nutrición, Instituto de Salud Carlos III, Ministerio de Ciencia e Innovación, Madrid, Spain, **4** Department of Pathology, Parc de Salut Mar, Universidad Autónoma, Barcelona, Spain

Abstract

Studies in animal models and humans suggest anti-inflammatory roles on the N-acylethanolamide (NAE)-peroxisome proliferators activated receptor alpha (PPARα) system in inflammatory bowel diseases. However, the presence and function of NAE-PPARα signaling system in the ulcerative colitis (UC) of humans remain unknown as well as its response to active anti-inflammatory therapies such as 5-aminosalicylic acid (5-ASA) and glucocorticoids. Expression of PPARα receptor and PPARα ligands-biosynthetic (NAPE-PLD) and -degrading (FAAH and NAAA) enzymes were analyzed in untreated active and 5-ASA/glucocorticoids/immunomodulators-treated quiescent UC patients compared to healthy human colonic tissue by RT-PCR and immunohistochemical analyses. PPARα, NAAA, NAPE-PLD and FAAH showed differential distributions in the colonic epithelium, lamina propria, smooth muscle and enteric plexus. Gene expression analysis indicated a decrease of PPARα, PPARγ and NAAA, and an increase of FAAH and iNOS in the active colitis mucosa. Immunohistochemical expression in active colitis epithelium confirmed a PPARα decrease, but showed a sharp NAAA increase and a NAPE-PLD decrease, which were partially restored to control levels after treatment. We also characterized the immune cells of the UC mucosa infiltrate. We detected a decreased number of NAAA-positive and an increased number of FAAH-positive immune cells in active UC, which were partially restored to control levels after treatment. NAE-PPARα signaling system is impaired during active UC and 5-ASA/glucocorticoids treatment restored its normal expression. Since 5-ASA actions may work through PPARα and glucocorticoids through NAE-producing/degrading enzymes, the use of PPARα agonists or FAAH/NAAA blockers that increases endogenous PPARα ligands may yield similar therapeutics advantages.

Editor: Jörn Karhausen, Duke University Medical Center, United States of America

Funding: This study was supported by grants to FRdF from the European Union's 7th Framework Programme (Health-F2-2008-223713, REPROBESITY); the following grants from the Spanish Ministry of Science and Innovation (SAF2010-20521); National Institute of Health "Carlos III" (PI07/1226, PI07/0880 and PI 07/0953), Red de Trastornos Adictivos-UE-ERDF (RD06/0001/0000) and El Centro de Investigación Biomédica en Red de Fisiopatología de Obesidad y Nutrición; grants from the Consejería de Economía, Innovación y Ciencia de la Junta de Andalucía, UE/ERDF (CTS-433 and PI45403); and a grant from the Consejería de Salud de la Junta de Andalucía (PI0232/2008), Spain. FJBS holds a Miguel Servet research contracts CD07/00283, and JS holds a Sara Borrell postdoctoral contract CD08/00203, both from the National Institute of Health "Carlos III", Madrid, Spain. The funders had no role in study design, data collection and analysis, decision to publish, or preparation of the manuscript.

Competing Interests: The authors have declared that no competing interests exist.

* E-mail: fernando.rodriguez@fundacionimabis.org (FRdF); MAndreu@parcdesalutmar.cat (MA)

Introduction

Ulcerative colitis (UC) is a chronic relapsing inflammation of the colonic tissue caused by the influence of complex genetic and environmental interactions [1]. Different pro-inflammatory factors, including reactive oxygen and nitrogen metabolites, eicosanoids, platelet-activating factors and cytokines, are upregulated and actively contribute to an exacerbated intestinal immune response to otherwise innocuous stimuli [2,3]. For the management of human UC, several drugs are currently used as 5-aminosalicylic acid (5-ASA), glucocorticoids, anti-TNFα and immunomodulators as thiopurines, which interfere with pro-inflammatory cascades and effectively down-regulate the overstated inflammatory response [4–6]. Evidences suggested that the anti-inflammatory effect of 5-ASA can be mediated by the activation of peroxisome proliferator-activated receptors (PPARs), such as PPARα and PPARγ [7–11], which are highly expressed in the intestinal and colonic mucosa by both epithelial cells and macrophages [12–14]. UC patients seem to have reduced levels of PPARγ in their colonic epithelium and similar deficiencies were observed in colitis mouse models, but only in macrophages of the lamina propria [15,16]; confirming the beneficial effects of PPARγ agonists on the attenuation of colon inflammation [17,18]. Less information is available on PPARα and β/δ receptors.

Recent studies in experimental colitis suggested that PPARα ligands also have anti-inflammatory properties, which was enhanced after glucocorticoid treatment, but was weakened in PPARα-null mice [19–23]. Moreover, 5-ASA is able to induce PPARα expression and promote its translocation to the nucleus in

Table 1. Characteristics of UC patients.

Case	Gender	Age	Smoking habits	Alcohol intake gr/day	BMI kg/m^2	Year at diagnosis	CRP$^{\$}$	UC Extension*	Mayo score at diagnosis	MTWSI$^{\&}$	Extraintestinal manifestations	Treatment: Induction of remission	Treatment: Maintenance
1	Female	35	No	No	24,97	2006	1.4	E3	2	Moderate	No	5-ASA+ glucocorticoids	5-ASA
2	Female	29	No	No	26,10	2006	4.4	E3	2	Moderate	Aphthous stomatitis	5-ASA+ glucocorticoids+ azathioprine	5-ASA+ azathioprine
3	Male	29	Yes	No	21,88	2006	7.4	E3	3	Severe	No	glucorticoids+ cyclosporine	5-ASA+ azathioprine
4	Female	28	Yes	No	30,86	2006	1.2	E3	2	Moderate	No	5-ASA+ glucocorticoids	5-ASA
5	Female	46	Yes	No	28.00	2006	1.2	E3	3	Moderate	No	5-ASA+ glucocorticoids	5-ASA
6	Female	38	No	No	23,87	2006	0.5	E3	1	Mild	No	5-ASA	5-ASA
7	Male	69	No	40	22.00	2006	0.8	E3	1	Mild	No	5-ASA+ glucocorticoids	5-ASA
8	Male	20	No	No	22,98	2006	0.2	E3	3	Severe	No	glucocorticoids+ cyclosporine	5-ASA+ azathioprine
9	Male	23	No	No	25,01	2007	8.8	E3	2	Moderate	Arthritis	5-ASA+ glucocorticoids	5-ASA+ azathioprine
10	Female	26	Yes	No	23,42	2006	2	E3	3	Severe	Erythema nodosum	5-ASA+ glucocorticoids	5-ASA
11	Male	37	No	No	22.00	2006	0.2	E3	1	Mild	No	5-ASA	5-ASA
12	Male	48	No	100	21.24	2006	0.4	E2	2	Moderate	No	5-ASA+ glucocorticoids	5-ASA
13	Male	34	No	No	22,86	2006	33.9	E3	3	Severe	No	5-ASA+ glucocorticoids	Azathioprine+ Infliximab
14	Male	61	No	No	23,26	2006	8.9	E3	2	Severe	No	5-ASA+ glucocorticoids	5-ASA
15	Female	28	No	No	23,05	2007	1.4	E3	2	Mild	Arthritis	5-ASA	infliximab
16	Male	26	No	No	24,30	2008	0.4	E3	2	Moderate	No	5-ASA+ glucocorticoids	5-ASA
17	Male	39	No	No	22,52	2007	0.6	E2	2	Moderate	No	5-ASA+ glucocorticoids	5-ASA
18	Male	17	Yes	No	22,53	2006	3	E3	2	Moderate	No	5-ASA+ glucocorticoids	5-ASA
19	Male	62	Yes	No	25,27	2006	1.2	E3	3	Moderate	No	5-ASA+ glucocorticoids	5-ASA
20	Male	30	No	No	22,86	2006	14.9	E3	2	Moderate	Arthritis	glucocorticoids+ azathioprine	azathioprine

Table 1. Cont.

Case	Gender	Age	Smoking habits	Alcohol intake gr/day	BMI kg/m^2	Year at diagnosis	CRP$	UC Extension*	Mayo score at diagnosis	MTWSI&	Extraintestinal manifestations	Treatment: Induction of remission	Treatment: Maintenance
21	Female	42	No	No	27,34	2007	0.9	E3	2	Mild	No	5-ASA+ glucocorticoids	5-ASA+ azathioprine
22	Male	73	Yes	No	26,95	2007	8.5	E2	2	Moderate	No	5-ASA+ glucocorticoids	5-ASA
23	Male	44	No	No	23,98	2006	2.9	E2	2	Moderate	No	5-ASA+ glucocorticoids+ cyclosporine	5-ASA+ azathioprine
24	Female	62	No	No	24.00	2006	0.6	E3	1	Moderate	No	5-ASA	5-ASA

$C-reactive protein at diagnosis (mg/L);
*Ulcerative colitis extension by Montreal criteria;
&Modified Truelove-Witts Severity index (MTWSI): Mild 11–15 points, Moderate 16–20 points, Severe 21–27 points.

an animal model of irradiation-induced intestinal inflammation [11]. PPARα is specifically expressed in the more differentiated colonic epithelial cells facing the intestinal lumen of the small intestine and colon [12–14]. Thus, PPARα has been proposed to participate in the intestinal epithelial barrier system; absence of PPARα expression resulted in an increase of tight junction permeability associated with apoptosis in an animal model of experimental colitis [20]. PPARα signaling system is an anti-inflammatory system composed of the PPARα receptor and its endogenous ligands, the N-acylethanolamides oleoylethanolamide (OEA) and palmitoylethanolamide (PEA). It also includes the enzymes involved in their biosynthesis and release, such as N-acyl phosphatidylethanolamide-specific phospholipase D (NAPE-PLD), as well as mechanisms for cellular uptake and hydrolysis, such as fatty acid amide hydrolase (FAAH) and N-acylethanolamide-hydrolyzing acid amidase (NAAA) [24–26]. Increased PPARα expression or enhanced PPARα ligand production can attenuate inflammatory process observed in current animal models of experimental colitis. For instance, treatment with FAAH antagonists or genetic ablation of FAAH protected against colitis inflammation [27–29]. Thus, PPARα system is positioned to exert a putative role in many of the points where homeostasis breaks in UC, although the anti-inflammatory role of PPARα remains to be determined in humans.

The aim of the present study is to analyze the expression and distribution of components of the acylethanolamide-PPARα anti-inflammatory system such as PPARα receptor and the enzymes involved in endogenous ligand degradation (FAAH and NAAA) and biosynthesis (NAPE-PLD) in the normal human colonic tissue compared to untreated active UC at disease onset and after achieving remission, according to clinical and endoscopic criteria, and depending on treatment received (5-ASA, glucocorticoids and/or immunomodulators).

Methods

Ethics statement

Biopsies and colonic resection samples used for the present study were obtained after a written inform consent from all the patients, as requested by the clinical guides of Hospital del Mar. Research procedures were approved by the Hospital del Mar and Hospital Carlos Haya Clinical Research and Ethics Committee and were conducted according to the principles expressed in the Declaration of Helsinki.

Subjects

We selected retrospectively 24 consecutive patients diagnosed from January 2006 to December 2007 of a first flare of UC, with extensive or left-side extension according to the Montreal classification (E2 and E3) [30]. UC was defined by the criteria of Lennard-Jones [31]. All patients had to achieve clinical and endoscopic remission after medical treatment according to Truelove-Witts index (<6 points) [32] and endoscopic Mayo score (score = 0) [33] during 12 months of diagnosis. We excluded patients with distal UC according to Montreal classification (E1) and patients without clinical and endoscopic remission criteria after treatment. Thus, we obtained several endoscopic samples of UC mucosa from each patient collected before any treatment (active group), and after medical treatment and endoscopic remission (quiescent group).

Colonic samples were retrieved from tissue bank of Pathology Service at the Hospital del Mar. Data from each patients were collected retrospectively from medical records including age, sex, smoking habits and alcohol history, body mass index and

Table 2. Clinical characteristics of control group.

Case	Age at diagnosis	Gender	Smoking habit	Alcohol	*BMI kg/m^2	Co-morbidity	Medical treatment	Colon cancer location	Year at diagnosis
1	74	Male	No	No	23.20	Diabetes mellitus; dislipemia; hypertension	Torvastatine Metformine	Sigmoid colon	2006
2	76	Female	No	No	20.80	Diabetes mellitus; hypertension	Glibenclamide Enalapril	Rectal	2006
3	68	Male	No	No	28.10	Diabetes mellitus; hypertension	Enalapril Atenolol	Rectal	2006
4	78	Male	No	No	31.98	Diabetes mellitus; hypertension	Glibenclamide Enalapril	Right colon	2006
5	80	Male	No	No	27.30	Diabetes mellitus; dislipemia; hypertension	Metformine Insulin Bisoprolol	Cecum	2006
6	74	Female	No	No	28.23	Hypertension	Enalapril	Sigmoid colon	2006
7	56	Male	No	No	19.81	No	No	Sigmoid colon	2006
8	61	Female	No	No	24.25	No	No	Rectal	2006
9	68	Female	No	No	28.98	No	No	Sigmoid colon	2006
10	74	Male	No	No	29.09	Diabetes mellitus; hypertension	Metformine Enalapril	Sigmoid colon	2006
11	79	Female	No	No	26.40	Hypertension	Enalapril	Right colon	2006
12	56	Male	Yes	No	30.91	Dislipemia	Simvastatine	Sigmoid colon	2006
13	62	Female	No	No	26.75	Hypertension Atrial fibrillation	Digoxine; Warfarine	Rectal	2006
14	80	Male	No	No	21.64	No	No	Right colon	2006
15	69	Female	No	No	21.50	No	No	Rectal	2006
16	79	Male	No	No	34.41	No	No	Cecal	2006
17	68	Female	No	No	26.74	No	No	Sigmoid colon	2006
18	76	Male	No	No	26.12	Diabetes mellitus;hypertension	Metformine Enalapril;	Right colon	2006
19	67	Female	No	No	22.00	No	No	Descending colon	2006
20	67	Male	No	No	22.00	No	No	Sigmoid colon	2006
21	78	Male	No	No	23.80	Diabetes mellitus	No	Right colon	2006
22	75	Female	No	No	20.60	Hypertension	Enalapril	Sigmoid colon	2006

*BMI: body mass index Kg/m^2; Medical treatment at the time to take samples of colon mucosa.

Table 3. Primers sequences used for RT-PCR.

Gene symbol (name)	Oligosense (5'→3') Oligoantisense (5'→3')	GenBank® accession no.	Product size (bp)	Annealing temperature (C°)
SP1	AGCAGGATGGTTCTGGTCAA AGGTGATGTTCCCATTCAGG	NM_138473.2	210	54.0
NAPE-PLD	CACGGTAATGGTGGAAATGG GTCCAGATGGTCATAGTGGTTG	NM_001122838.1	178	57.0
FAAH	CCCAGATGGAACATTACAGG CAGGATGACTGGTTTTCAGG	NM_001441.2	187	57.6
NAAA	ATGGCGCAAGTCATCGGGGA TGAAGTCACACATGCCGCGGA	NM_014435.3	127	59.0
PPARα	ATCACGGACACGCTTTCAC GGTCGCACTTGTCATACACC	NM_001001928.2	220	58,9
PPARγ	TGCCATCAGGTTTGGGCGGA AATGTTTTGCCAGGGCCCGGA	NM_138712.3	118	61.4
iNOS	TCAGCAAGCAGCAGAATGAG ATAATGGACCCCAGGCAAGA	NM_000625.4	210	63.3

extraintestinal manifestations, date of diagnosis, disease location (Montreal classification), endoscopic lesions (Mayo clinic score) and clinical score according Truelove and Witts index at onset, and medical treatment received to induce remission after diagnosis: 5-aminosalicilates (3 cases), glucocorticoids (15 cases), and/or the immunomodulators cyclosporine A and azathioprine (6 cases) (Table 1).

For the control group, we selected retrospectively 22 patients who were pathohistologically given a definite diagnosis of colorectal cancer and who had not received preoperative radiotherapy or chemotherapy treatment and underwent colonic resections for colorectal cancer. Several colonic resections were obtained from each patient at least 10 cm from the tumour (control group). We confirmed histopathologically the absence of microscopic alterations (Table 2).

Colonic samples were frozen at $-80°C$ for molecular analysis (N = 7–8) or fixated with 4% paraformadehyde in 0.1 M phosphate buffered saline (PBS) by immersion and included in paraffin until immunohistochemical analysis (N = 22–24). The analysis of the immunostaining patterns was carried out at transmural planes of the normal and pathological colonic tissue by comparing it with hematoxylin-eosin staining.

mRNA isolation and quantitative RT-PCR analysis

In order to evaluate the mRNA expression we collected prospectively 7 colonic endoscopic biopsies from patients with a first flare of active UC and 8 colonic resections, at least 10 cm from the tumour, of patients with colorectal cancer (control group). Colonic resections were divided into mucosa, containing both epithelium and lamina propria, and submucosa layers, containing smooth muscle and enteric plexi. Reverse transcript reaction was carried out from 4 µg of mRNA using the Transcriptor Reverse Transcriptase kit and random hexamer primers (Transcriptor RT, Roche Diagnostic GmbH, Manheim, Germany). Quantitative real-time reverse transcription polymerase chain reaction (quantitative RT-PCR) was performed using a CFX96TM Real-Time PCR Detection System (Bio-Rad Laboratories, Hercules, CA, USA), and the SYBR Green detection format (FastStart Universal Master Kit, Roche, Mannheim, Germany). Each reaction was run in duplicate and contained 5 µl of cDNA. Quantification was carried out with the classic standard curve method run at the same time. We analyzed the housekeeping genes SP1 transcription factor and βACTIN, selecting the most suitable according to their homogeneity (Figure S1). Absolute values from each sample were normalized with regard to the housekeeping gene SP1. Primers for PCR reaction were designed based on NCBI database sequences of human reference mRNA (Table 3), checked for specificity with BLAST software from NCBI website (http://blast.ncbi.nlm.nih.gov/Blast.cgi) and synthesized by Invitrogen.

Western blotting

In order to evaluate the presence of PPARα, NAAA, NAPE-PLD and FAAH in the colon mucosa we collected prospectively 8 colonic resection of control patients processed as previously described [34,35]. Each blotted membrane lane was incubated separately with the specific rabbit anti-PPARα (1:100; Fitzgerald, cat. no. RDI-PPARAabrx), rabbit anti-NAAA (1:1000; R&D Systems, cat. no. AF4494), rabbit anti-NAPE-PLD (1:100) and rabbit anti-FAAH (1:100) antibodies [35], overnight at 4°C. Western blots showed that each primary antibody detects a protein of the expected molecular weight (see Methods S1).

Immunohistochemistry

We analyzed the distribution of PPARα, NAAA, NAPE-PLD and FAAH in the normal colonic tissue and in the active and quiescent UC mucosa by immunohistochemistry, following methods previously described in Marquez et al [35]. Sections were incubated overnight at room temperature with rabbit anti-PPARα antibody (diluted 1:75; Fitzgerald), rabbit anti-NAAA (diluted 1:200; R&D Systems), rabbit anti-NAPE-PLD antibody (diluted 1:100) and rabbit anti-FAAH (diluted 1:100). Then, sections were incubated in a biotin-conjugated donkey anti-rabbit immunoglobulin (Amersham) diluted 1:500 for 1 hour, and incubated in ExtrAvidin peroxidase (Sigma) diluted 1:2000 for 1 hour. We revealed immunolabeling with 0.05% diaminobenzidine (DAB; Sigma), 0.05% nickel ammonium sulphate, and 0.03% H_2O_2 in 0.1 M phosphate-buffered saline (pH 7.4). Sections were dehydrated in ethanol, cleared in xylene, and coverslipped with Eukitt mounting medium (Kindler GmbH and Co., Freiburg, Germany).

Double immunofluorescence

Paraffin-embedded sections of colonic tissue were analyzed for the presence of NAAA, NAPE-PLD and FAAH in plasma cells (CD38+), B lymphocytes (CD19+), T lymphocytes (CD3+) and macrophages (CD14+) of the lamina propria of control and UC colitis groups. Sections were incubated overnight at room temperature in a cocktail containing rabbit anti-NAAA, NAPE-PLD or FAAH antibody (see above) and mouse monoclonal anti-human CD14-IgG1 conjugated to R-phycoerythrin-Cy7 (eBioscience, San Diego, CA, USA, cat. no. 25-0149), anti-human CD3-IgG1 conjugated to R-phycoerythrin-Cy7 (eBioscience, cat. no. 25-0038) or conjugated to eFluor® 450 (eBioscience, cat.

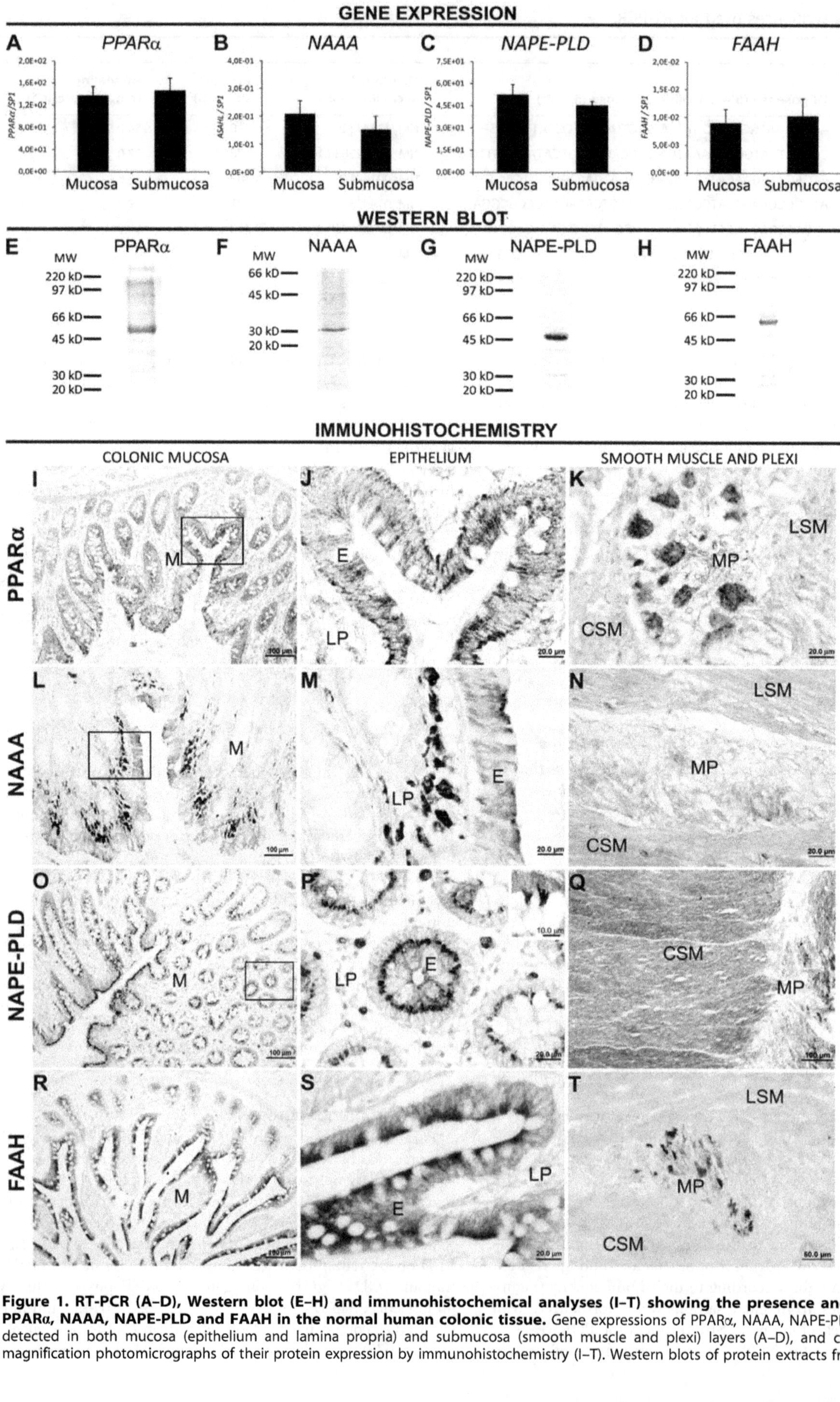

Figure 1. RT-PCR (A–D), Western blot (E–H) and immunohistochemical analyses (I–T) showing the presence and distribution of PPARα, NAAA, NAPE-PLD and FAAH in the normal human colonic tissue. Gene expressions of PPARα, NAAA, NAPE-PLD and FAAH were detected in both mucosa (epithelium and lamina propria) and submucosa (smooth muscle and plexi) layers (A–D), and confirmed by high-magnification photomicrographs of their protein expression by immunohistochemistry (I–T). Western blots of protein extracts from human colonic

tissue showed prominent immunoreactive bands of the expected size for PPARα (52 kDa), NAAA (31 kDa), NAPE-PLD (46 kDa) and FAAH (62 kDa). Positions of molecular markers (MW) are indicated at the left (E–H). Abbreviations: CSM, circular smooth muscle; E, epithelium; LSM, longitudinal smooth muscle; LP, lamina propria; M, mucosa; MP, myenteric plexus.

Table 4. Rating scale that summarizes the immunohistochemical distribution in the normal human colonic tissue (n = 24)[1].

	Epithelium	Lamina propria	Smooth muscle	Myenteric plexus
PPARα	+++	–	–	++
NAAA	+	+++	+	–
NAPE-PLD	++	+	+++	–
FAAH	++	+	–	++

[1]Gray-scale values measured in single epithelium, lamina propria, muscular layers and plexi are represented on an arbitrary rating scale of the immunoreactivity of each structure. Symbols are as follows: high (+++), moderate (++), low (+) and without immunoreactivity (–).

no. 48-0038), anti-human CD19-IgG2a conjugated to R-Phycoerythrin (Immunostep, Salamanca, Spain, cat. no. 19PE1-100T) or anti-human 38-IgG1 conjugated to fluorescein isothiocyanate (Immunostep, cat. no. 38F-100T). Then, the sections were incubated for 2 hours at room temperature in secondary donkey anti-rabbit IgG-Cy3 antibody (dilution 1:300; Jackson Immunoresearch Laboratories, West Grove, PA, USA, cat. no. 711-165-152) or goat anti-rabbit IgG-FITC antibody (dilution 1:300; Jackson Immunoresearch Laboratories, cat. no. 111-095-003).

Quantification of mucosa immunostaining

For epithelium, we carried out a densitometrical quantification for each protein. For lamina propria, we evaluated the type and the number of immunostained immune cells per area (μm^2) analyzed. In addition, quantification was segregated depending on UC severity and treatment received: 5-ASA, glucocorticoids, and/

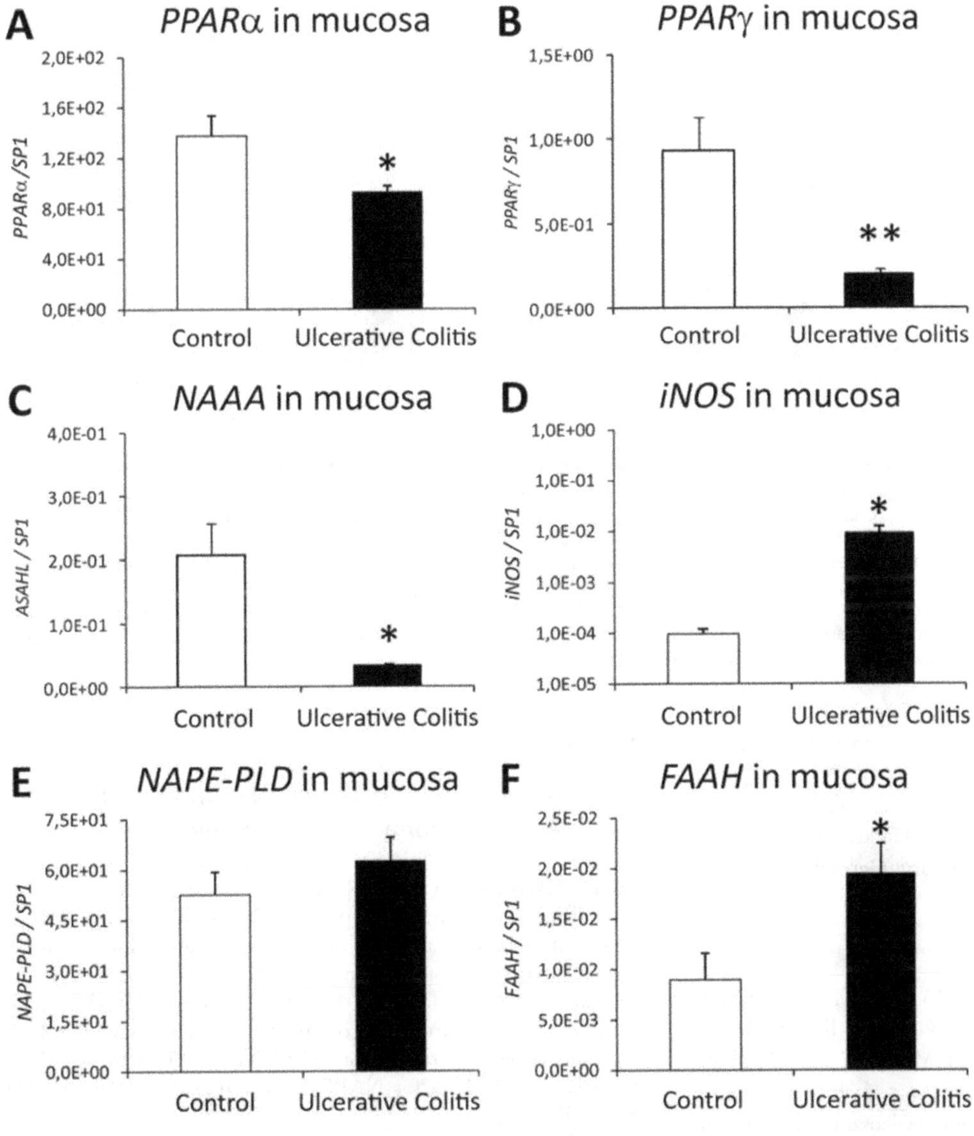

Figure 2. Relative quantification of PPARα (A), PPARγ (B), NAAA (C), iNOS (D), NAPE-PLD (E) and FAAH (F) gene expression in the colonic mucosa of active UC patients compared to human healthy colonic tissue (control). Absolute values were normalized with regard to the housekeeping gene SP1. Active UC at disease onset showed lower PPARα, PPARγ and NAAA gene expression, but higher iNOS and FAAH gene expression compared to control. No change was detected for NAPE-PLD gene expression. Student *t* test (N = 8): *$P<0.05$, **$P<0.01$ *versus* control group.

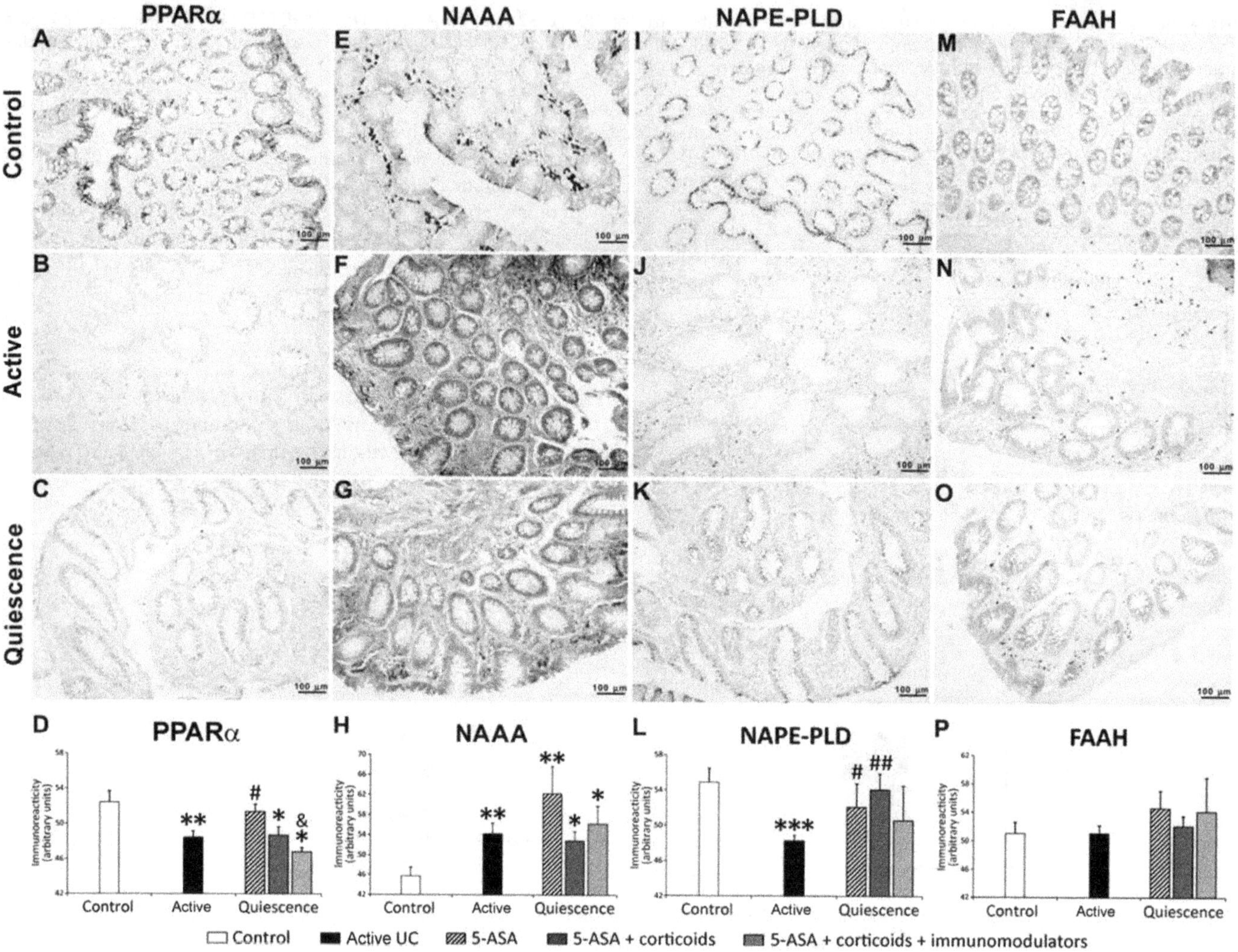

Figure 3. Representative photomicrographs and densitometrical quantification of PPARα (A–D), NAAA (E–H), NAPE-PLD (I–L) and FAAH (M–P) immunoreactivity in human healthy (control; A, E, I, M), active UC (B, F, J, N) and quiescent UC (C, G, K, O) colonic epithelium depending on treatment. Active UC at disease onset showed a decrease in PPARα and NAPE-PLD immunoreactivity, but an increase in NAAA immunoreactivity. PPARα immunoreactivity showed significant differences depending on treatment. Treatment with 5-ASA in UC patients restored completely PPARα and NAPE-PLD protein levels to control ones. However, PPARα expression dropped again in UC patients treated with 5-ASA and glucocorticoids, and 5-ASA, glucocorticoids and immunomodulators compared to control group. In contrasts, treatment with 5-ASA and glucocorticoids increased NAPE-PLD immunoreactivity. No changes were observed in FAAH immunoreactivity in the epithelium of control, active (untreated) UC and quiescent (treated) UC patients. Mann-Whitney U and Wilcoxon tests (N = 22–24): *$P<0.05$, **$P<0.01$, ***$P<0.001$ versus control group; $^{\#}P<0.05$, $^{\#\#}P<0.01$ *versus* UC group; $^{\&}P<0.05$ *versus* 5-ASA-treated quiescent UC group.

or immunomodulators. Digital high-resolution microphotographs were taken under the same conditions of light and brightness/contrast by an Olympus BX41 microscope equipped with an Olympus DP70 digital camera and a Metal Halide epifluorescence system (Olympus Europa GmbH, Hamburg, Germany).

Statistical analysis

Data were analyzed using SPSS 15.0 software (Statistical Package for the Social Sciences Inc., Chicago, Illinois, USA). Results are expressed as mean ± S.E.M. Differences between groups were evaluated using Student *t* test for parametric observation and Mann-Whitney U and Wilcoxon tests for non parametric observations. A *P* value of $P<0.05$ was considered statistically significant.

Results

Presence and distribution of PPARα, NAAA, NAPE-PLD and FAAH in the normal human colonic tissue

The normal colonic tissue showed gene expression of PPARα, NAAA, NAPE-PLD and FAAH in the mucosa, including epithelium and lamina propria, and the submucosa layers, containing smooth muscle and enteric plexi (Figs. 1A–D). Protein extracts from normal colonic tissue confirmed the presence of protein levels of PPARα, NAAA, NAPE-PLD and FAAH. They appeared as prominent immunoreactive bands of expected molecular masses at ~52 kDa for PPARα, ~31 kDa for NAAA, ~46 kDa for NAPE-PLD and ~62 kDa for FAAH (Figs. 1E–H).

Results of the immunohistochemical distribution were summarized in a rating scale (Table 4). PPARα immunoreactivity was observed in the colonic epithelium of both absorptive and goblet

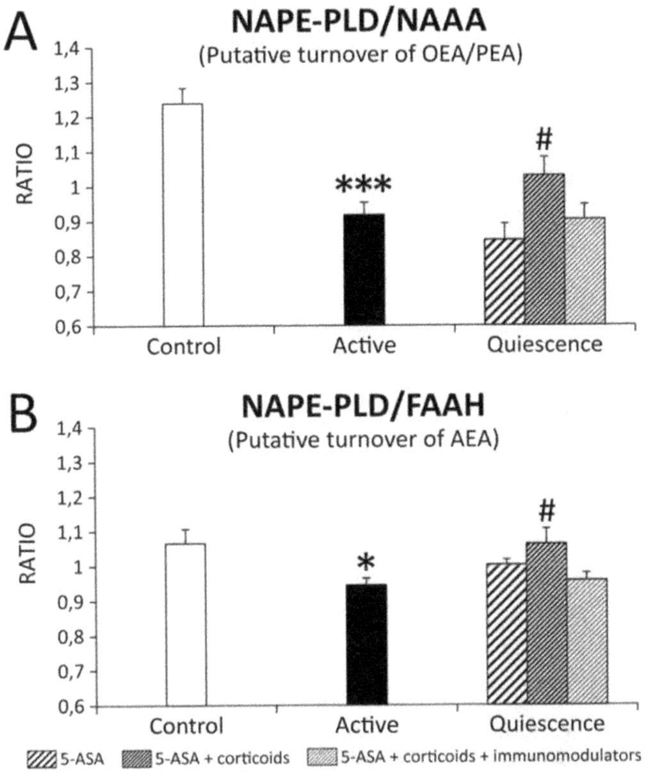

Figure 4. Estimation of acylethanolamide turnover by analyzing the NAPE-PLD/NAAA (A) and NAPE-PLD/FAAH (B) ratios in the epithelium of the untreated active and treated quiescent UC patients in comparison with control patients. Active UC produced a significant decrease in NAPE-PLD/NAAA and NAPE-PLD/FAAH ratios, which were restored to control levels only after the treatment with 5-ASA and glucocorticoids. Mann-Whitney U and Wilcoxon tests (N = 22–24): *$P<0.05$, ***$P<0.001$ *versus* control group; #$P<0.05$ *versus* active UC group.

cells (Figs. 1I, J). The immunoreactivity filled the epithelial cells, showing prominent staining in the apical and basal portions. We did not detected PPARα immunoreactivity in immune cells of the lamina propria, the muscularis mucosae, the muscularis externa (circular and longitudinal smooth muscle) and the serosa (Figs. 1I, J). Numerous PPARα-immunopositive ganglion cells were evident only in the myenteric plexi (Figure 1K). Moderate to low intensity of NAAA immunostaining was observed in the colonic epithelium (Figs. 1L, M). Interestingly, we detected numerous NAAA immune cells in the lamina propria, which showed a variety of shapes and sizes (Fig. 1M). Muscularis mucosae, muscularis externa, plexi and serosa showed very weak staining for NAAA (Fig. 1N). Intense NAPE-PLD immunoreactivity was widely distributed in the colonic epithelium, being prominent in the perinuclear portion of the absorptive cells (Figs. 1O, P, inset). Some positive plasma cells were also observed in the lamina propria (Fig. 1P). Strong NAPE-PLD immunostaining defined both layers of muscularis externa, but low immunostaining was detected in fibers of the myenteric plexi (Fig. 1Q). FAAH immunoreactivity was mainly detected in the colonic epithelium, which shows higher expression in the apical portion of the epithelial cells (Figs. 1R, S). A low number of immunoreactive immune plasma cells were observed in the lamina propria and no staining was detected in the muscularis mucosae, the muscularis externa and the serosa. However, we can observe a specific FAAH immunoreactivity in nervous cells of the myenteric plexi (Fig. 1T).

Quantification of PPARα, PPARγ, NAAA, iNOS, NAPE-PLD and FAAH gene expression in the mucosa of UC patients

In order to evaluate any changes on the expression of PPARα signaling system in the colonic mucosa (epithelium and lamina propria) of UC patients, we analyzed the relative differences in the mRNA levels of selected genes such as PPARα, PPARγ, NAAA, iNOS, NAPE-PLD and FAAH in the UC mucosa, containing epithelium and lamina propria, by quantitative RT-PCR. We detected significantly lower levels of PPARα ($P<0.05$), PPARγ ($P<0.01$) and NAAA ($P<0.05$) mRNA in the mucosa of UC patients compared to that of control ones (Figs. 2A–C). In contrast, iNOS and FAAH gene expression was significantly higher in the mucosa of UC patients ($P<0.05$) (Figs. 2D, F). We observed no change in the levels of NAPE-PLD mRNA between both groups (Fig. 2E).

Densitometrical quantification of PPARα, NAAA, NAPE-PLD and FAAH immunoreactivity in the epithelium of UC patients depending on treatment

Figure 3 shows representative microphotographs showing qualitative differences of the immunohistochemical expression of PPARα, NAAA, NAPE-PLD and FAAH in the colonic epithelium of control, active and quiescent groups. Results corresponding to the quantification of immunoreactivity are shown in Figures 3D, H, L, P respectively. We detected a decrease of PPARα and NAPE-PLD immunoreactivity in the epithelium of UC patients compared to that of control ones ($P<0.01$ and $P<0.001$ respectively) (Figs. 3D, L). In contrast, NAAA immunoreactivity was more prominent in the epithelium of active UC patients ($P<0.01$) (Fig. 3H). No change was detected in FAAH immunoreactivity in the epithelium between active UC and control groups (Fig. 3P). In order to address the disease severity, we analyzed the NAE-PPARα signaling system depending on the clinical score (mild, moderate and severe) in active UC patients (Figure S2). UC patients with moderate clinical score showed a significant reduction ($P<0.05$) of PPARα immunohistochemical expression (Figure S2A). When NAPE-PLD immunoreactivity was analyzed, we detected significant decreases in UC patients with mild ($P<0.01$), moderate ($P<0.01$) and severe ($P<0.001$) clinical score (Figure S2B). However, FAAH immunoreactivity was no affected (Figure S2C). Finally, UC patients with moderate ($P<0.05$) and severe ($P<0.01$) clinical score showed significant increases in NAAA immunoreactivity (Figure S2D). We also analyzed the possible effect of gender and smoking habits on the NAE-PPARα signaling system in active UC patients. We did not detect differences between females and males or between smokers and non-smokers in the immunohistochemical expression in the epithelium of active UC patients (Figures S3 and S4).

We also quantified the immunoreactivity in the colonic epithelium of quiescent UC patients depending on the treatment received: 5-ASA (3 cases), 5-ASA and glucocorticoids (15 cases), or 5-ASA, glucocorticoids and immunomodulators (6 cases). 5-ASA treatment produced an increase of PPARα immunoreactivity in the colonic epithelium of active UC patients ($P<0.05$), but not when UC patients were treated with 5-ASA in combination with other drugs (Fig. 3D). Thus, no difference in PPARα immunoreactivity was observed in UC patients treated with 5-ASA plus glucocorticoids only or 5-ASA, glucocorticoids and immunomodulators with respect untreated active UC ones. Interestingly, the decrease in PPARα immunoreactivity observed in the epithelium

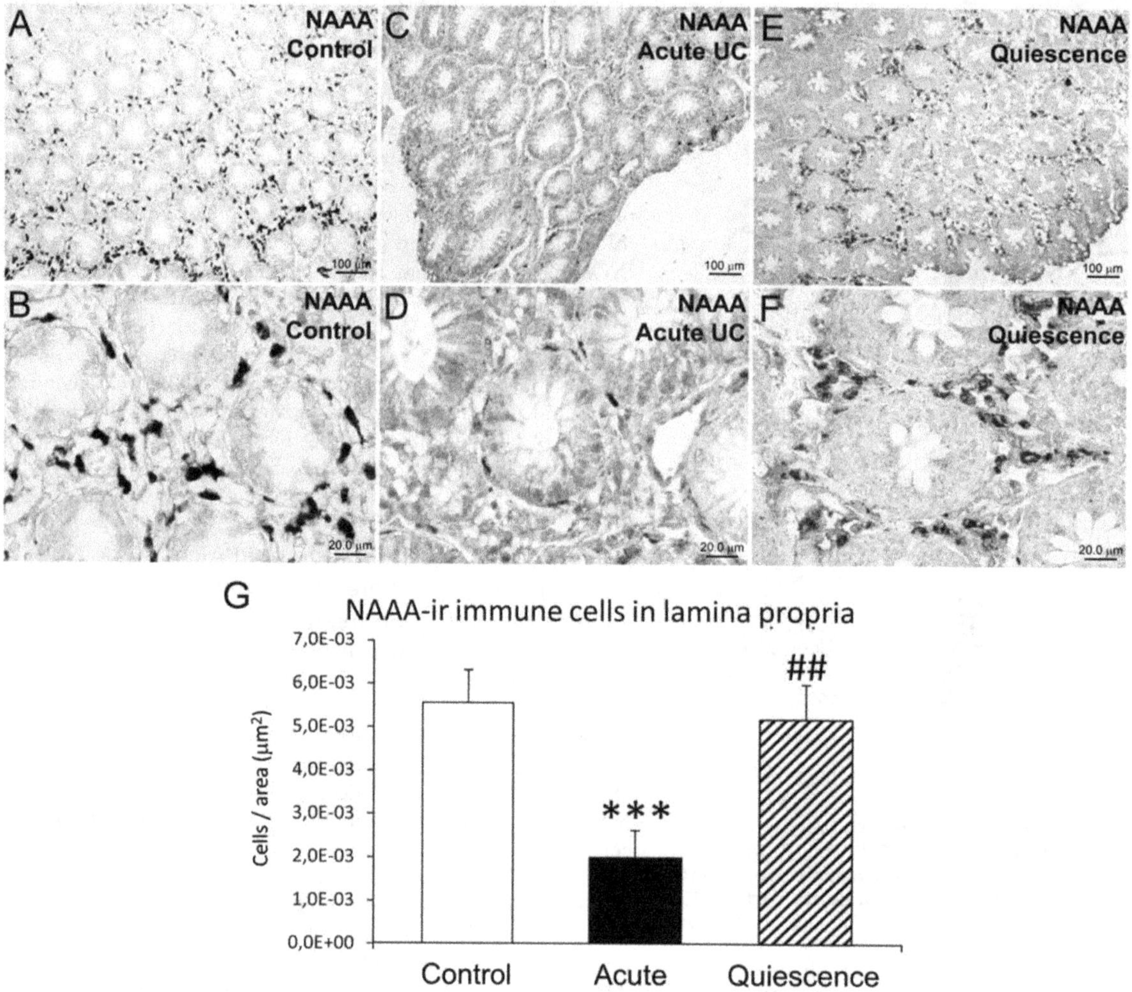

Figure 5. Analysis of the number of NAAA-ir cells per area (μm^2) in the lamina propria of control group compared to acute UC patients and after 5-ASA and corticosteroid treatment (quiescent group). A–F: Representative high-magnification photomicrographs showing NAAA immunostaining in the lamina propria. G: Acute UC at disease onset was associated with a significant decrease in the number of NAAA-ir cells in the infiltrate of the lamina propria. The number of NAAA-ir cells was increased to control levels after treatment (5-ASA and corticoids). Mann-Whitney U and Wilcoxon tests (N = 15–22): ***$P<0.001$ *versus* control group; ##$P<0.01$ *versus* acute UC group.

of UC patients treated with 5-ASA, glucocorticoids and immunomodulators was significant compared to that of UC patients treated with 5-ASA only ($P<0.05$). However, we cannot detect significant changes in NAAA immunoreactivity in the epithelium of quiescent UC patients treated with any of the drugs, being similar to that of active UC patients (Fig. 3H). Regarding NAPE-PLD immunoreactive levels, there was a significant increase to control levels in UC patients treated with 5-ASA ($P<0.05$) or 5-ASA and glucocorticoids ($P<0.01$) compared to the active UC patients (Fig. 3L). However, a wide variability in the intensity of NAPE-PLD immunoreactivity was detected in UC patients treated with 5-ASA, glucocorticoids and immunomodulators. Finally, we cannot observe any difference in FAAH immunoreactivity in the UC epithelium after treatment (Fig. 3P).

Acylethanolamide producing/degrading enzyme ratio in the colonic epithelium

In order to analyze whether the differential immunohistochemical expression of either acylethanolamide producing or degrading enzymes may have resulted in an altered PPARα endogenous ligand tone in the untreated active and treated quiescent UC epithelium, we calculated the ratios between NAPE-PLD and NAAA expressions, and between NAPE-PLD and FAAH expressions. These ratios can suggest possible changes of OEA/PEA levels (Fig. 4). The main result of these analysis was that there was a significant decrease of both NAPE-PLD/NAAA ($P<0.001$) and NAPE-PLD/FAAH ($P<0.05$) ratios in the epithelium of untreated active UC patients. Interestingly, we detected an increase of NAPE-PLD/NAAA and NAPE-PLD/FAAH ratios (both at $P<0.05$) only in the epithelium of quiescent UC patients treated with 5-ASA and glucocorticoids, but not with 5-ASA or 5-ASA, glucocorticoids and immunomodulators (Fig. 4).

NAAA, NAPE-PLD and FAAH immunoreactive cells in the lamina propria of UC patients and after treatment

The number of NAAA and FAAH immunoreactive cells in the lamina propria showed significant changes in active UC patients and after treatment (quiescent group). We found a significant low number of NAAA-ir cells (2.75-fold; $P<0.001$) in the infiltrate of active UC patients, but was completely restored, similar to control level, after treatment (Fig. 5). Performing double immunofluorescence, NAAA expression was found in CD19-positive (+) B

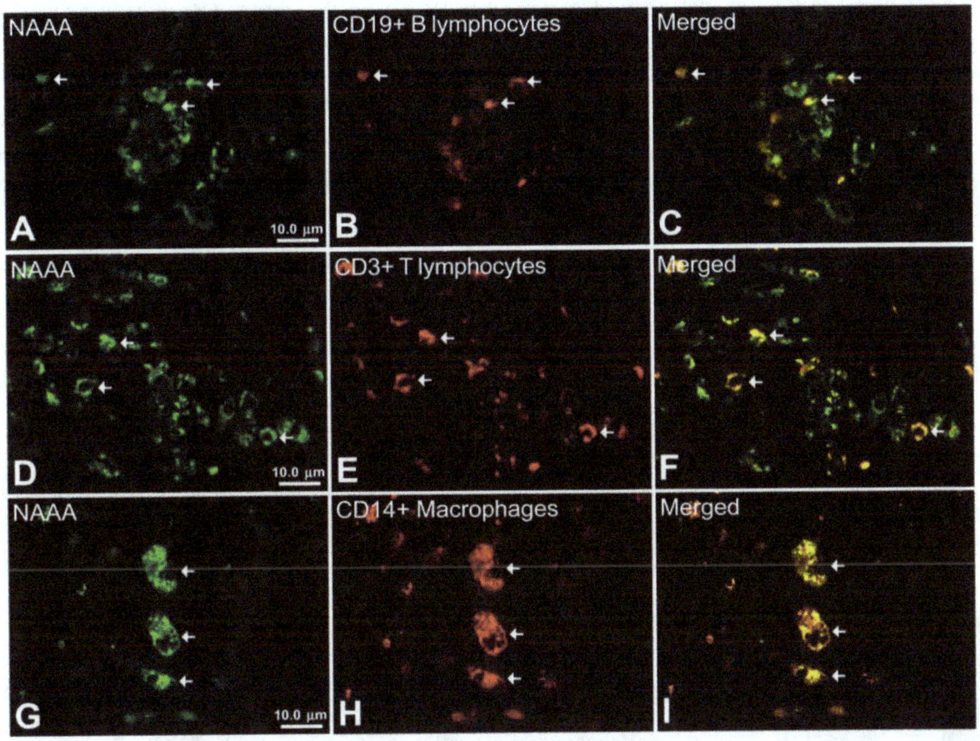

Figure 6. Representative high-magnification photomicrographs showing double immunofluorescence for NAAA, CD19, CD3 and CD14 in order to characterize the immune cells in the mucosa infiltrate of UC patients. NAAA immunofluorescence was observed in CD19+ B lymphocytes (A–C), CD3+ T lymphocytes (D–F) and CD14+ macrophages (G–I).

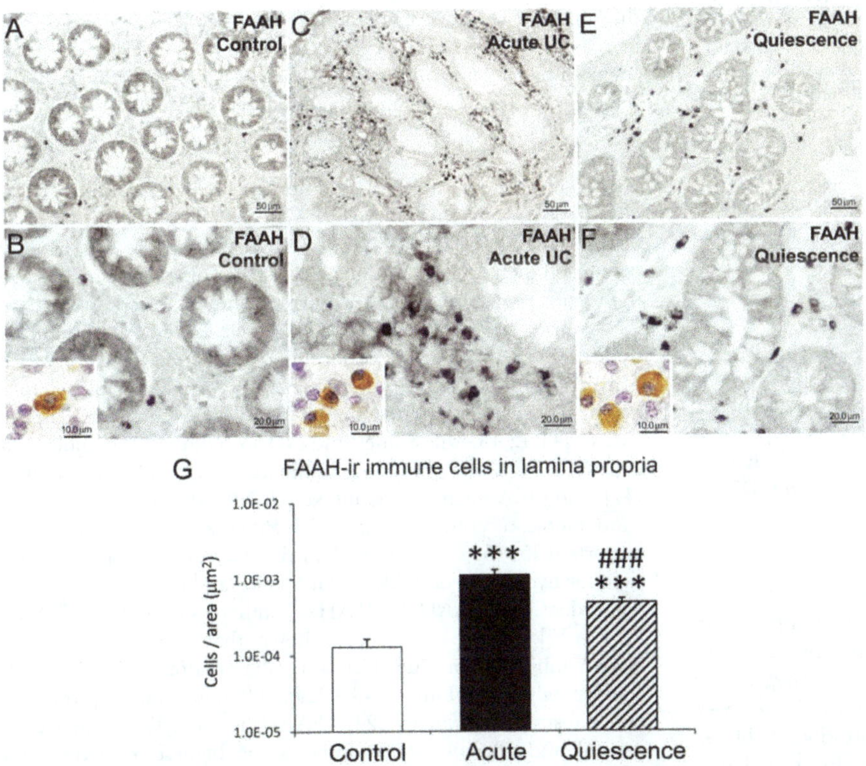

Figure 7. Analysis of the number of FAAH-ir cells per area (μm^2) in the lamina propria of acute and quiescent (5-ASA and corticoid-treated) UC patients compared to control ones. A–F: Representative high-magnification photomicrographs showing FAAH immunostaining in the lamina propria. G: Acute UC at disease onset was associated with a dramatic increase in the number of FAAH-ir cells in the infiltrate of the lamina propria. The number of FAAH-ir cells was significantly dropped after treatment, but do not reach control levels. Mann-Whitney U and Wilcoxon tests (N = 15–22): ***$P<0.001$ *versus* control group; ###$P<0.001$ *versus* acute UC group.

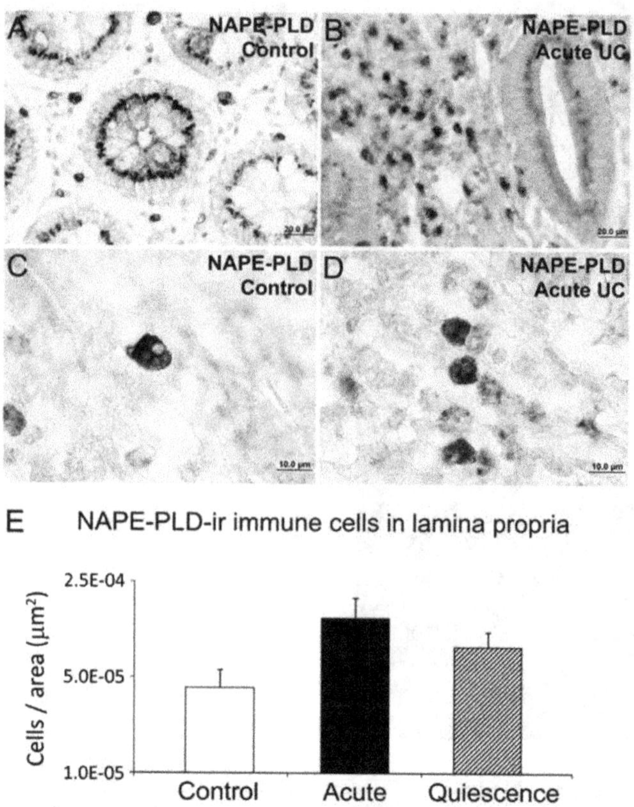

Figure 8. Analysis of the number of NAPE-PLD-ir cells per area (μm²) in the lamina propria of acute and quiescent (5-ASA and corticoid-treated) UC patients compared to control ones. A–D: Representative high-magnification photomicrographs showing NAPE-PLD immunostaining in the lamina propria. E: No significant change in the number of NAPE-PLD-ir cells was observed in the infiltrate of the lamina propria of acute UC patients and after treatment (5-ASA and corticoids). Mann-Whitney U and Wilcoxon tests (N = 15–22).

lymphocytes, CD3+ T lymphocytes and CD14+ macrophages (Fig. 6). In contrast, the number of FAAH-ir cells of the lamina propria increased dramatically (10-fold; $P<0.001$) in active UC patient (Fig. 7). After treatment, the number of FAAH-ir cells decreased significantly in quiescent UC patients ($P<0.001$), but did not reach control level. We did not find change in the number of NAPE-PLD-ir cells in the lamina propria of active UC patients and after treatment (Fig. 8). Nearly all the FAAH-ir cells in the infiltrate expressed the plasma cell-specific CD38, which include B lymphocytes and natural killer cells (Figs. 9A–C). NAPE-PLD expression was mainly found in CD38+ plasma cells and CD3+ T lymphocytes (Figs. 9 D–I).

Discussion

The key findings of this study are to demonstrate that profound changes in the acylethanolamide-PPARα anti-inflammatory system are produced in human UC. Overall the findings suggest that active UC deactivate this anti-inflammatory system while 5-ASA/glucocorticoids treatment restores its normal expression (Table 5). The process involves both receptors and enzymes for acylethanolamides.

Considering PPARα receptor we found that it is mainly expressed in the human colonic epithelium, but not in immune cells of the lamina propria [14]. Interestingly, colonic mucosa (epithelium and lamina propria) in active UC patients at disease onset showed a significant down-regulation of both PPARα and PPARγ mRNA expression in colonic mucosa of active UC patients. These data indicate that, not only PPARγ, but also PPARα, are implicated in the pathophysiology of the human colonic inflammation. We also detected an over-expression of iNOS mRNA, a pro-inflammatory mediator that produces nitric oxide species and leads oxidative stress and cell death [11,36,37]. This enzyme is under the active control of PPARα receptor since PPARα agonists enhance its degradation [38]. Immunohistochemical results demonstrated that PPARα mRNA down-expression in the UC mucosa correlated with PPARα protein down-expression in the UC epithelium. Moreover, only 5-ASA treatment increased immunohistochemical expression of PPARα to control expression level, but not when UC patients were treated with 5-ASA in combination with glucocorticoids and/or immunomodulators.

5-ASA is structurally related to nonsteroidal anti-inflammatory drugs that shares molecular targets including inflammation, proliferation and/or apoptosis [39–41]. 5-ASA inhibits inflammation by scavenging free radicals and thus interfering with the arachidonic acid metabolism [42]. Recent studies indicated that the anti-inflammatory effect of 5-ASA is mediated by the activation of PPARγ [9–11], a nuclear receptor whose agonists can suppress or delay inflammation effectively by inhibiting multiple steps in NF-κB and AP-1 signaling pathways [7,8] and attenuating the production of nitric oxide (iNOS) and macrophage-derived cytokines such as TNFα, IL-1 and IL-6 in mouse models of colitis [16,43,44]. Moreover, Linard et al. [11] showed that 5-ASA is able to induce PPARα, PPARγ and RXRα co-expression and promote their translocation to the nucleus in an animal model of irradiation-induced intestinal inflammation. In the present study, we demonstrated that 5-ASA specifically increased the expression of PPARα in the human UC epithelium suggesting that, not only PPARγ, but also PPARα can be a key receptor for the potent anti-inflammatory effect of 5-ASA in the human UC [9,10]. At this time, nothing at all is known about the regulation of PPARα expression and much more studies are needed to elucidate the anti-inflammatory mechanisms of 5-ASA.

Others components of the PPARα signaling system, such as NAPE-PLD, FAAH and NAAA, are expressed in the healthy colonic epithelium and immune cells of the colonic lamina propria in humans [35]. NAPE-PLD is one of several N-acylethanolamide-biosynthesis enzymes that catalyze the release of N-acylethanolamide (NAE) from N-acyl-phosphatidylethanolamine (NAPE), converting endogenous lipids into chemical signals like oleoylethanolamine (OEA), palmitoylethanolamine (PEA) and anandamide (AEA) [41,42,45,46]. Some studies showed that the biological activity of PEA, such as anti-inflammatory and analgesic activities [47], and OEA, such as food intake [48–50], are mediated by non-cannabinoid receptors among which PPARα is probably the most important [51–53]. In mammalian tissues, three enzymes responsible for hydrolyses of NAEs to fatty acids and ethanolamine have been identified: FAAH-1, FAAH-2 (human isozyme) and NAAA [24,54–57]. Thus, it has been shown that selective FAAH or NAAA inhibitors produced an anti-inflammatory effect [26–29]. Interestingly, FAAH and NAAA have different catalytic properties and substrate specificity [24]. FAAH is catalytically active at neutral and alkaline pH and shows the highest reactivity with anandamide, followed by OEA and PEA [58]. In contrast, NAAA activity is optimum at pH 4.5–5, being inactive at alkaline pH, and hydrolyzes PEA much faster than others NAEs [24,55]. Therefore, alterations of FAAH and NAAA activity can be as a result of variations of luminal pH in colonic inflammation, and it is

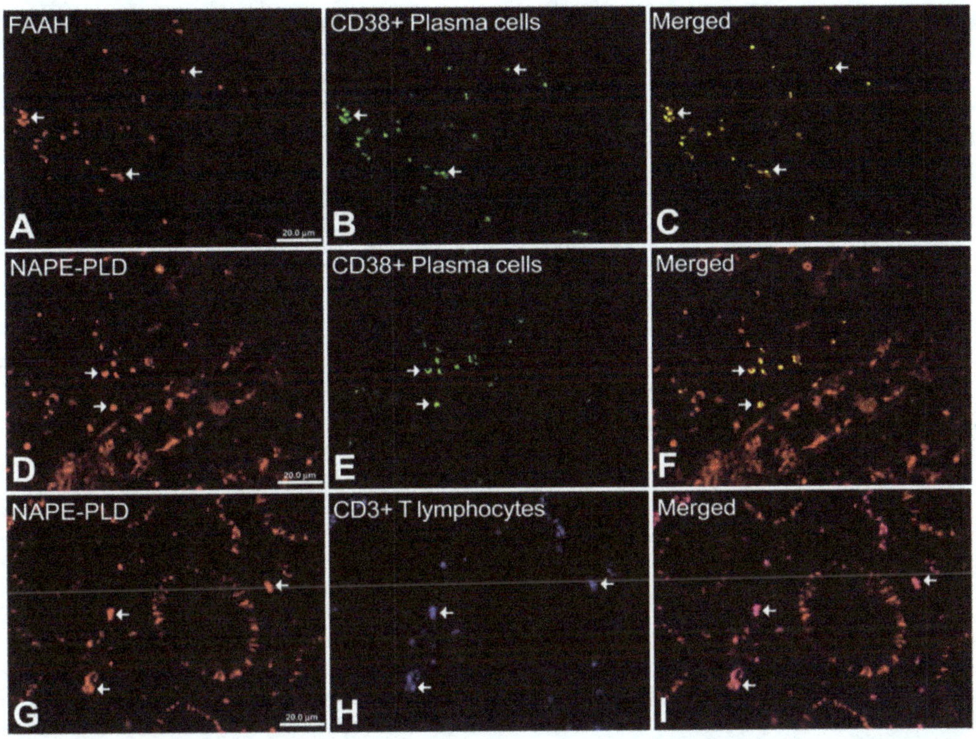

Figure 9. Representative high-magnification photomicrographs showing double immunofluorescence for FAAH, NAPE-PLD, CD38 and CD3 in order to characterize the immune cells in the mucosa infiltrate of UC patients. Nearly all FAAH immunofluorescent cells are plasma cell-specific CD38 (A–C). NAPE-PLD immunofluorescence was observed in both CD38+ plasma cells (D–F) and CD3+ T lymphocytes (G–I).

conceivable that reduced intracolonic pH in active UC impairs the anti-inflammatory effects of PPAR endogenous agonists [59].

In the present study, we demonstrated that mRNA and protein expression of NAPE-PLD, FAAH and NAAA was partially altered in active colitis, and immunohistochemical expression of these enzymes was partially restored after treatment (quiescent colitis) in a tissue-dependent manner (epithelium and immune cells of the lamina propria). Overall, the present data suggested that both increase of NAAA expression and lack of change in FAAH expression in the UC epithelium agree with a substantial reduction of luminal pH in the colon of UC patients [59]. Therefore, NAPE-PLD down-expression and NAAA over-expression in UC epithelium might let to a net reduction in NAEs turnover (specifically PEA) in the epithelium, leading the attenuation of the anti-inflammatory response via the activation of PPAR receptors (Fig. 10). Interestingly, inflammation associated with osteoarthritis and rheumatoid arthritis showed a lower concentration of PEA in the synovial fluid compared to non-inflamed normal volunteers [60]. Changes observed in NAPE-PLD, FAAH and NAAA mRNA expression in the mucosa (epithelium and lamina propria) correlated completely with changes observed in the number of immunoreactive cells in the lamina propria of UC patients, but not with their immunohistochemical expression in the UC epithelium (see Table 5). These discrepancies can be explained by a higher expression of these enzymes in the immune cells during UC

Table 5. Summary of the changes detected in PPARα signaling system (PPARα, NAPE-PLD, FAAH and NAAA) in the colonic epithelium and lamina propria of active UC patients and after treatment (quiescent UC patients)[1].

	Gene expression	Immunohistochemical expression in epithelium		Number of immunoreactive cells in lamina propria	
	Active untreated-UC	Active untreated-UC	Quiescent treated-UC	Active untreated-UC	Quiescent treated-UC
PPARα	↓ (*)	↓ (**)	↑ (*) (5-ASA)	nc	nc
NAPE-PLD	nc	↓ (***)	↑ (**) (5-ASA+ glucocortic.)	nc	nc
FAAH	↑ (*)	nc	nc	↑ (***)	↓ (***)
NAAA	↓ (*)	↑ (**)	nc	↓ (***)	↑ (**)

[1]Symbols are as follows: increased expression (↑), decreased expression (↓), no change (nc). Statistical significance was represented by.
*$P<0.05$,
**$P<0.01$ and
***$P<0.001$.

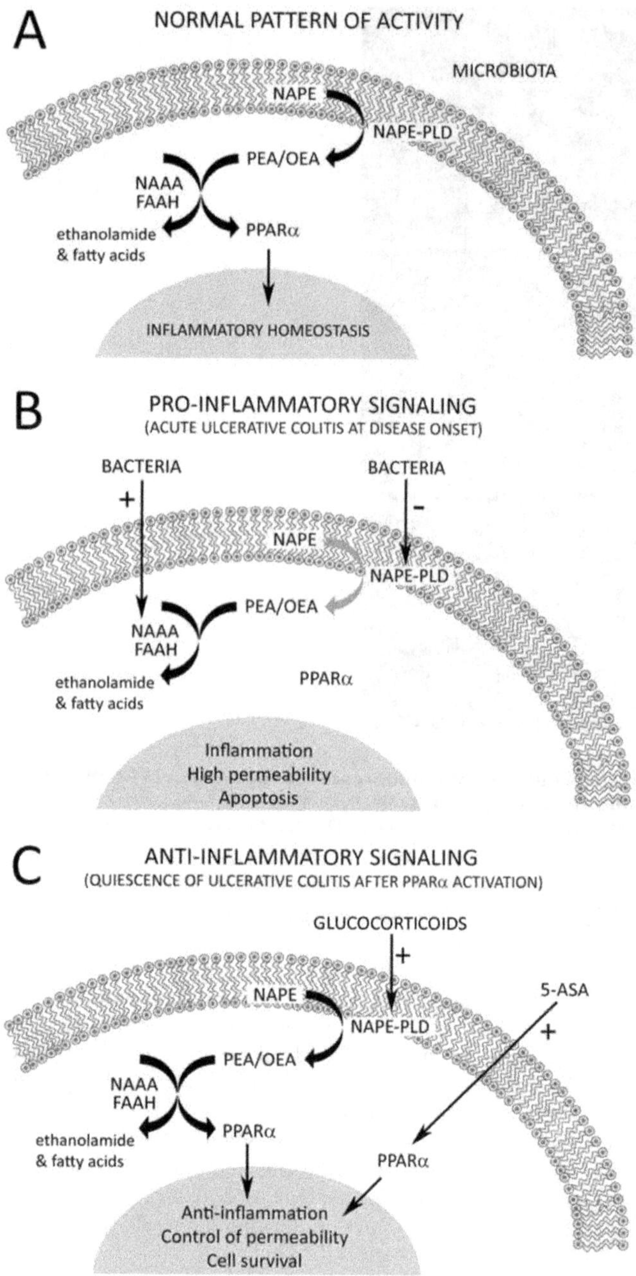

Figure 10. Schematic drawings that hypothesize the normal pattern of NAE-PPARα activity (A), and the pro- and anti-inflammatory NAE-PPARα signaling that may occur in the colonic epithelial cells of active UC at disease onset (B) and after a putative treatment with 5-ASA and/or glucocorticoids (C).

infiltration, but also the different roles of the NAE-PPARα signaling system in colonic epithelium and lamina propria.

In the lamina propria of healthy human colon, we found that the number of NAAA-ir immune cells was 50-fold higher than the number of FAAH-ir immune cells. These data can suggest a higher rate of PEA hydrolysis in comparison with AEA hydrolysis. In the lamina propria of active UC, we found that the number of FAAH-ir immune cells increased up to 10-fold, whereas the number of NAAA-ir immune cells decreased up to 2.75-fold, suggesting a concomitant increase of AEA hydrolysis as well as decrease of PEA hydrolysis. These results can be related with the fact that AEA activates cannabinoid (CB1 and CB2) receptors, whereas PEA is inactive on these receptors, but activates PPARα [51], playing different roles in inflammatory activation. Previous biochemical and immunochemical analysis demonstrated NAAA expression in macrophage cells of the rat lung and brain [25]. Here, we showed that NAAA is predominantly expressed in macrophages and B and T lymphocytes in the lamina propria of UC patients. Most FAAH-ir cells in the lamina propria of UC patients expressed CD38, a surface glycoprotein found in plasma B and natural killer cells, and this result agrees with previous studies showing FAAH activity in lymphocytes [61]. NAPE-PLD-ir cells in the lamina propria of UC patients were CD38+ plasma cells and CD3+ T lymphocytes, but not CD14+ macrophages, contrary to expectation after pro-inflammatory stimuli [62].

UC-specific treatments produced tissue-dependent impairments in the expression of PPARα signaling system. NAPE-PLD, but not NAAA or FAAH, responded to treatment in the epithelium, while NAAA and FAAH, but not NAPE-PLD, responded to treatment in the immune cells of the lamina propria of UC patients. 5-ASA produced an increase of NAPE-PLD immunohistochemical expression (similar to control levels) in the quiescent UC epithelium, which was enhanced after corticosteroid treatment. Interestingly, the analysis of the NAPE-PLD/NAAA and NAPE-PLD/FAAH ratios suggested an increase of NAEs production in the UC epithelium after 5-ASA/corticosteroid treatment, but not when patients were treated exclusively with 5-ASA. It is clear that 5-ASA treatment leads to an increase of NAPE-PLD and PPARα expression, so probably both 5-ASA and the concomitant over-production of NAEs via glucocorticoids can enhance an anti-inflammatory response in the epithelium of UC patients by the activation of PPARα (Fig. 10). This hypothesis agrees with previous data indicating that glucocorticoids generate anti-inflammatory regulatory responses by promoting arachidonic acid-containing lipid biosynthesis [63]. Treatment also increases the number of NAAA-ir immune cells, reaching control levels and, probably, normalizing PEA hydrolysis. However, the significant decrease of FAAH-ir immune cells after treatment did not reach control levels, so there may be still an over-degradation of AEA in the lamina propria of UC patients.

We must pay attention on two limitations related with the cohort of patients used in the present study. As a result of prioritizing clinical, endoscopical and histopathological considerations to obtain a homogeneous cohort, control and UC groups were not-age matched. Additionally, smoker patients and patients and controls from both genders were included in the study. However, these factors cannot be included in additional analysis because of the size of the cohort, designed to be a within-subject design (patients were they own control for quiescence status).

In conclusion, our results indicated that PPARα, NAPE-PLD, FAAH and NAAA form part of a key lipid signaling system that regulates UC-activated inflammatory response in human. 5-ASA, through PPARα receptor, and glucocorticoids, through acylethenolamide producing/degrading enzymes, reduces colitis-associated inflammation suggesting PPARα agonists or FAAH/NAAA inhibitors as potential drugs for the treatment of inflammatory bowel diseases in human.

Supporting Information

Figure S1 Housekeeping gene expressions of SP1 transcription factor (A) and βACTIN (B) represented by the threshold cycles (C(t)). We cannot detect differences in gene expression between control and active UC patients. Student *t*-test

(N = 7–8): SP1, F = 0.291, P = 0.734; βACTIN, F = 0.388, P = 0.597).

Figure S2 Densitometrical quantification of PPARα (A), NAPE-PLD (B), FAAH (C) and NAAA (D) immunoreactivity in human healthy (control) and active UC colonic epithelium depending on severity (mild, moderate and severe). Mann-Whitney U and Wilcoxon tests (N = 22–24): *P<0.05, **P<0.01, ***P<0.001 versus control group.

Figure S3 Densitometrical quantification of PPARα (A), NAPE-PLD (B), FAAH (C) and NAAA (D) immunoreactivity in active UC colonic epithelium depending on gender. No statistical difference was observed. Student t-test (N = 22–24).

Figure S4 Densitometrical quantification of PPARα (A), NAPE-PLD (B), FAAH (C) and NAAA (D) immunoreactivity in active UC colonic epithelium depending on smoking habits. No statistical difference was observed. Student t-test (N = 22–24).

Methods S1 mRNA isolation and quantitative RT-PCR analysis.

Author Contributions

Conceived and designed the experiments: JS MA FRdF. Performed the experiments: JS YRZ LM. Analyzed the data: JS YRZ MI PR FJBS. Contributed reagents/materials/analysis tools: FJBS MA FRdF. Wrote the paper: JS FRdF.

References

1. Strober W, Fuss I, Mannon P (2007) The fundamental basis of inflammatory bowel disease. J Clin Invest 117: 514–521.
2. Sartor RB (1997) Pathogenesis and immune mechanisms of chronic inflammatory bowel diseases. Am J Gastroenterol 92(suppl): 5S–11S.
3. Fiocchi C (1998) Inflammatory bowel disease: aetiology and pathogenesis. Gastroenterology 115: 182–205.
4. Travis SPL, Jewel DP (1994) Salicylates for ulcerative colitis–their mode of action. Pharmacol Ther 63: 135–161.
5. Bratts R, Linden M (1996) Cytokine modulation by glucocorticoids: mechanisms and actions in cellular studies. Aliment Pharmacol Ther 10: 81–90.
6. Kho YH, Pool MO, Jansman FG, Harting JW (2001) Pharmacotherapeutic options in inflammatory bowel disease: an update. Pharm World Sci 23: 17–21.
7. Ricote M, Li AC, Willson TM, Kelly CJ, Glass CK (1998) The peroxisome proliferator-activated receptor g is a negative regulator of macrophage activation. Nature 391: 79–82.
8. Delerive P, Fruchart JC, Staels B (2001) Peroxisome proliferator-activated receptors in inflammation control. J Endocrinol 169: 453–459.
9. Rousseaux C, Lefebvre B, Dubuquoy L, Lefebvre P, Romano O, et al. (2005) Intestinal antiinflammatory effect of 5-aminosalicylic acid is dependent on peroxisome proliferator-activated receptor-gamma. J Exp Med 201: 1205–15.
10. Dubuquoy L, Rousseaux C, Thuru X, Peyrin-Biroulet L, Romano O, et al. (2006) PPARgamma as a new therapeutic target in inflammatory bowel diseases. Gut 55: 1341–9.
11. Linard C, Grémy O, Benderitter M (2008) Reduction of peroxisome proliferation-activated receptor gamma expression by gamma-irradiation as a mechanism contributing to inflammatory response in rat colon: modulation by the 5-aminosalicylic acid agonist. J Pharmacol Exp Ther 324: 911–20.
12. Braissant O, Foufelle F, Scotto C, Dauca M, Wahli W (1996) Differential expression of peroxisome proliferatoractivated receptors (PPARs): tissue distribution of PPAR-alpha, -beta, and -gamma in the adult rat. Endocrinology 137: 354–66.
13. Mansen A, Guardiola-Diaz H, Rafter J, Branting C (1996) Expression of the peroxisome proliferator-activated receptor (PPAR) in the mouse colonic mucosa. Biochem Biophys Res Commun 222: 844–851.
14. Huin C, Corriveau L, Bianchi A, Keller JM, Collet P, et al. (2000) Differential expression of peroxisome proliferator-activated receptors (PPARs) in the developing human fetal digestive tract. J Histochem Cytochem 48: 603–611.
15. Dubuquoy L, Jansson EA, Deeb S, Rakotobe S, Karoui M, et al. (2003) Impaired expression of peroxisome proliferator-activated receptor g in ulcerative colitis. Gastroenterology 124: 1265–1276.
16. Katayama K, Wada K, Nakajima A, Mizuguchi H, Hayakawa T, et al. (2003) A novel PPAR gamma gene therapy to control inflammation associated with inflammatory bowel disease in a murine model. Gastroenterology 124: 1315–1324.
17. Dworzanski T, Celinski K, Korolczuk A, Slomka M, Radej S, et al. (2010) Influence of the peroxisome proliferator-activated receptor gamma (PPAR-γ) agonist, rosiglitazone and antagonist, biphenol-A-diglicydyl ether (BADGE) on the course of inflammation in the experimental model of colitis in rats. J Physiol Pharmacol 61: 683–93.
18. Celinski K, Dworzanski T, Korolczuk A, Piasecki R, Slomka M, et al. (2011) Effects of peroxisome proliferator-activated receptors-gamma ligands on dextran sodium sulphate-induced colitis in rats. J Physiol Pharmacol 62: 347–56.
19. Cuzzocrea S, Di Paola R, Mazzon E, Genovese T, Muià C, et al. (2004) Role of endogenous and exogenous ligands for the peroxisome proliferators activated receptors alpha (PPAR-alpha) in the development of inflammatory bowel disease in mice. Lab Invest 84: 1643–54.
20. Mazzon E, Cuzzocrea S (2007) Absence of functional peroxisome proliferator-activated receptor-alpha enhanced ileum permeability during experimental colitis. Shock 28: 192–201.
21. Esposito E, Mazzon E, Paterniti I, Dal Toso R, Pressi G, et al. (2010) PPAR-alpha contributes to the anti-inflammatory activity of verbascoside in a model of inflammatory bowel disease in mice. PPAR Res 2010: 917312.
22. Cuzzocrea S, Bruscoli S, Mazzon E, Crisafulli C, Donato V, et al. (2008) Peroxisome proliferator-activated receptor-alpha contributes to the anti-inflammatory activity of glucocorticoids. Mol Pharmacol 73: 323–37.
23. Riccardi L, Mazzon E, Bruscoli S, Esposito E, Crisafulli C, et al. (2009) Peroxisome proliferator-activated receptor-alpha modulates the anti-inflammatory effect of glucocorticoids in a model of inflammatory bowel disease in mice. Shock 31: 308–16.
24. Tsuboi K, Takezaki N, Ueda N (2007) The N-acylethanolamine-hydrolyzing acid amidase (NAAA). Chem Biodivers 4: 1914–25.
25. Tsuboi K, Zhao LY, Okamoto Y, Araki N, Ueno M, et al. (2007) Predominant expression of lysosomal N-acylethanolamine-hydrolyzing acid amidase in macrophages revealed by immunochemical studies. Biochim Biophys Acta 1771: 623–32.
26. Solorzano C, Zhu C, Battista N, Astarita G, Lodola A, et al. (2009) Selective N-acylethanolamine-hydrolyzing acid amidase inhibition reveals a key role for endogenous palmitoylethanolamide in inflammation. Proc Natl Acad Sci U S A 106: 20966–20971.
27. Massa F, Marsicano G, Hermann H, Cannich A, Monory K, et al. (2004) The endogenous cannabinoid system protects against colonic inflammation. J Clin Invest 113: 1202–1209.
28. D'Argenio G, Valenti M, Scaglione G, Cosenza V, Sorrentini I, et al. (2006) Upregulation of anandamide levels as an endogenous mechanism and a pharmacological strategy to limit colon inflammation. FASEB J 20: 568–570.
29. Storr MA, Keenan CM, Emmerdinger D, Zhang H, Yuce B, et al. (2008) Targeting endocannabinoid degradation protects against experimental colitis in mice: involvement of CB1 and CB2 receptors. J Mol Med 86: 925–936.
30. Silverberg MS, Satsangi J, Ahmad T, Arnott ID, Bernstein CN, et al. (2005) Toward an integrated clinical, molecular and serological classification of inflammatory bowel disease: Report of a Working Party of the 2005 Montreal World Congress of Gastroenterology. Can J Gastroenterol 19 Suppl A: 5–36.
31. Lennard-Jones JE, Shivananda S (1997) Clinical uniformity of inflammatory bowel disease a presentation and during the first year of disease in the north and south of Europe. EC-IBD Study Group. Eur J Gastroenterol Hepatol 9: 353–9.
32. Truelove SC, Witts LJ (1955) Cortisone in ulcerative colitis; final report on a therapeutic trial. Br Med J 2: 1041–8.
33. D'Haens G, Sandborn WJ, Feagan BG, Geboes K, Hanauer SB, et al. (2007) A review of activity indices and efficacy end points for clinical trials of medical therapy in adults with ulcerative colitis. Gastroenterology 132: 763–86.
34. Suárez J, Bermúdez-Silva FJ, Mackie K, Ledent C, Zimmer A, et al. (2008) Immunohistochemical description of the endogenous cannabinoid system in the rat cerebellum and functionally related nuclei. J Comp Neurol 509: 400–21.
35. Marquéz L, Suárez J, Iglesias M, Bermudez-Silva FJ, Rodríguez de Fonseca F, et al. (2009) Ulcerative colitis induces changes on the expression of the endocannabinoid system in the human colonic tissue. PLoS ONE 4: e6893.
36. Cross RK, Wilson KT (2003) Nitric oxide in inflammatory bowel disease. Inflamm Bowel Dis 9: 179–89.
37. Sklyarov AY, Panasyuk NB, Fomenko IS (2011) Role of nitric oxide-synthase and cyclooxygenase/lipooxygenase systems in development of experimental ulcerative colitis. J Physiol Pharmacol 62: 65–73.
38. Paukkeri EL, Leppänen T, Sareila O, Vuolteenaho K, Kankaanranta H, et al. (2007) PPARalpha agonists inhibit nitric oxide production by enhancing iNOS degradation in LPS-treated macrophages. Br J Pharmacol 152: 1081–91.
39. Brown WA, Farmer KC, Skinner SA, Malcontenti-Wilson C, Misajon A, et al. (2000) 5-aminosalicyclic acid and olsalazine inhibit tumor growth in a rodent model of colorectal cancer. Dig Dis Sci 45: 1578–84.

40. Reinacher-Schick A, Schoeneck A, Graeven U, Schwarte-Waldhoff I, Schmiegel W (2003) Mesalazine causes a mitotic arrest and induces caspase-dependent apoptosis in colon carcinoma cells. Carcinogenesis 24: 443–51.
41. Clapper ML, Gary MA, Coudry RA, Litwin S, Chang WC, et al. (2008) 5-aminosalicylic acid inhibits colitis-associated colorectal dysplasias in the mouse model of azoxymethane/dextran sulfate sodium-induced colitis. Inflamm Bowel Dis 14: 1341–7.
42. Tromm A, Griga T, May B (1999) Oral mesalazine for the treatment of Crohn's disease: clinical efficacy with respect to pharmacokinetic properties. Hepatogastroenterology 46: 3124–35.
43. Desreumaux P, Dubuquoy L, Nutten S, Peuchmaur M, Englaro W, et al. (2001) Attenuation of colon inflammation through activators of the retinoid X receptor (RXR)/peroxisome proliferator-activated receptor gamma (PPARgamma) heterodimer: a basis for new therapeutic strategies. J Exp Med 193: 827–838.
44. Saubermann LJ, Nakajima A, Wada K, Zhao S, Terauchi Y, et al. (2002) Peroxisome proliferatoractivated receptor gamma agonist ligands stimulate a Th2 cytokine response and prevent acute colitis. Inflamm Bowel Dis 8: 330–339.
45. Okamoto Y, Morishita J, Tsuboi K, Tonai T, Ueda N (2004) Molecular characterization of a phospholipase D generating anandamide and its congeners. J Biol Chem 279: 5298–305.
46. Ueda N, Tsuboi K, Uyama T (2010) Enzymological studies on the biosynthesis of N-acylethanolamines. Biochim Biophys Acta 1801: 1274–85.
47. Lambert DM, Vandevoorde S, Jonsson KO, Fowler CJ (2002) The palmitoylethanolamide family: a new class of anti-inflammatory agents? Curr Med Chem 9: 663–674.
48. Rodríguez de Fonseca F, Navarro M, Gómez R, Escuredo L, Nava F, et al. (2001) An anorexic lipid mediator regulated by feeding. Nature 414: 209–212.
49. Nielsen MJ, Petersen G, Astrup A, Hansen HS (2004) Food intake is inhibited by oral oleoylethanolamide. J Lipid Res 45: 1027–1029.
50. Fu J, Astarita G, Gaetani S, Kim J, Cravatt BF, et al. (2007) Food intake regulates oleoylethanolamide formation and degradation in the proximal small intestine. J Biol Chem 282: 1518–28.
51. Fu J, Gaetani S, Oveisi F, Lo Verme J, Serrano A, et al. (2003) Oleylethanolamide regulates feeding and body weight through activation of the nuclear receptor PPAR-alpha. Nature 425: 90–93.
52. Lo Verme J, La Rana G, Russo R, Calignano A, Piomelli D (2005) The search for the palmitoylethanolamide receptor. Life Sci 77: 1685–1698.
53. Lo Verme J, Fu J, Astarita G, La Rana G, Russo R, et al. (2005) The nuclear receptor peroxisome proliferator-activated receptor-alpha mediates the anti-inflammatory actions of palmitoylethanolamide. Mol Pharmacol 67: 15–19.
54. McKinney MK, Cravatt BF (2005) Structure and function of fatty acid amide hydrolase. Annu Rev Biochem 74: 411–432.
55. Tsuboi K, Sun YX, Okamoto Y, Araki N, Tonai T, et al. (2005) Molecular characterization of N-acylethanolamine-hydrolyzing acid amidase, a novel member of the choloylglycine hydrolase family with structural and functional similarity to acid ceramidase. J Biol Chem 280: 11082–11092.
56. Wei BQ, Mikkelsen TS, McKinney MK, Lander ES, Cravatt BF (2006) A second fatty acid amide hydrolase with variable distribution among placental mammals, J Biol Chem 281: 36569–36578.
57. Ueda N, Tsuboi K, Uyama T (2010) N-acylethanolamine metabolism with special reference to N-acylethanolamine-hydrolyzing acid amidase (NAAA). Prog Lipid Res 49: 299–315.
58. Ueda N, Puffenbarger RA, Yamamoto S, Deutsch DG (2000) The fatty acid amide hydrolase (FAAH). Chem Phys Lipids 108: 107–21.
59. Nugent SG, Kumar D, Rampton DS, Evans DF (2001) Intestinal luminal pH in inflammatory bowel disease: possible determinants and implications for therapy with aminosalicylates and other drugs. Gut 48: 571–7.
60. Richardson D, Pearson RG, Kurian N, Latif ML, Garle MJ, et al. (2008) Characterisation of the cannabinoid receptor system in synovial tissue and fluid in patients with osteoarthritis and rheumatoid arthritis. Arthritis Res Ther 10: R43.
61. Battista N, Bari M, Tarditi A, Mariotti C, Bachoud-Lévi AC, et al. (2007) Severe deficiency of the fatty acid amide hydrolase (FAAH) activity segregates with the Huntington's disease mutation in peripheral lymphocytes. Neurobiol Dis 27: 108–16.
62. Zhu C, Solorzano C, Sahar S, Realini N, Fung E, et al. (2011) Proinflammatory stimuli control N-acylphosphatidylethanolamine-specific phospholipase D expression in macrophages. Mol Pharmacol 79: 786–92.
63. Malcher-Lopes R, Franco A, Tasker JG (2008) Glucocorticoids shift arachidonic acid metabolism toward endocannabinoid synthesis: a non-genomic anti-inflammatory switch. Eur J Pharmacol 583: 322–39.

5

Up-Regulation of Annexin-A1 and Lipoxin A4 in Individuals with Ulcerative Colitis may Promote Mucosal Homeostasis

Linda Vong[1]*, Jose G. P. Ferraz[3], Neil Dufton[2], Remo Panaccione[3], Paul L. Beck[3], Philip M. Sherman[1], Mauro Perretti[4], John L. Wallace[2]

1 Hospital for Sick Children, Research Institute, Toronto, Ontario, Canada, **2** Farncombe Family Digestive Health Research Institute, McMaster University, Hamilton, Ontario, Canada, **3** Division of Gastroenterology, University of Calgary, Calgary, Alberta, Canada, **4** Centre for Biochemical Pharmacology, William Harvey Research Institute, London, United Kingdom

Abstract

Background: One of the characteristics of an active episode of ulcerative colitis (UC) is the intense mucosal infiltration of leukocytes. The pro-resolution mediators Annexin-A1 (AnxA1) and lipoxin A_4 (LXA_4) exert counter-regulatory effects on leukocyte recruitment, however to date, the dual/cumulative effects of these formyl peptide receptor-2 (FPR2/ALX) agonists in the context of human intestinal diseases are unclear. To define the contribution of these mediators, we measured their expression in biopsies from individuals with UC.

Methods: Colonic mucosal biopsies were collected from two broad patient groups: healthy volunteers without ('Ctrl' n = 20) or with a prior history of UC ('hx of UC' n = 5); individuals with UC experiencing active disease ('active' n = 8), or in medically-induced remission ('remission' n = 16). We assessed the mucosal expression of LXA_4, AnxA1, and the FPR2/ALX receptor in each patient group using a combination of fluorescence microscopy, biochemical and molecular analyses.

Results: Mucosal expression of LXA_4 was elevated exclusively in biopsies from individuals in remission (3-fold, $P<0.05$ vs. Ctrl). Moreover, in this same group we observed an upregulation of AnxA1 protein expression (2.5-fold increase vs. Ctrl, $P<.01$), concurrent with an increased level of macrophage infiltration, and an elevation in FPR2/ALX mRNA (7-fold increase vs. Ctrl, $P<.05$). Importantly, AnxA1 expression was not limited to cells infiltrating the lamina propria but was also detected in epithelial cells lining the intestinal crypts.

Conclusions: Our results demonstrate a specific up-regulation of this pro-resolution circuit in individuals in remission from UC, and suggest a significant role for LXA_4 and AnxA1 in promoting mucosal homeostasis.

Editor: Jörn Karhause, Duke University Medical Center, United States of America

Funding: This research was supported by a grant-in-aid from the Crohn's and Colitis Foundation of Canada (to J.G.P.F. and J.L.W.; http://www.ccfc.ca/site/c.ajIRK4NLLhJ0E/b.6319851/k.BDBF/Home.htm) and a grant from the Canadian Institutes of Health Research (to J.L.W; http://www.cihr-irsc.gc.ca/e/193.html). P.M.S is the recipient of a Canada Research Chair in Gastrointestinal Disease. The funders had no role in study design, data collection and analysis, decision to publish, or preparation of the manuscript.

Competing Interests: The authors have declared that no competing interests exist.

* E-mail: linda.vong@sickkids.ca

Introduction

Ulcerative colitis (UC) is a relapsing disease characterized by periods of exacerbation and remission. One of the hallmarks of an active episode is the intense mucosal infiltration of lymphocytes, macrophages and polymorphonuclear leukocytes (PMN) [1]. These cells release an array of injurious mediators including proteases, cytokines and free radicals, resulting in edema, goblet cell depletion and extensive mucosal ulceration [2,3]. Although recruited to extinguish a pro-inflammatory stimulus, there is emerging evidence that infiltrating leukocytes also release anti-inflammatory mediators to trigger resolution [4,5]. Central to this paradigm is the existence of distinct pro-resolution circuits which modulate both the duration and intensity of the inflammatory response [6]. Their effectiveness is governed by the timely introduction and removal of various leukocyte subsets; for example, during an acute inflammatory response, resolution of inflammation is preceded by the replacement of PMNs with macrophages. At each step these cells act as a source, or contain the enzymatic machinery, for the synthesis of pro-resolution mediators. A deficiency of these 'stop-signals', exemplified in rodent models where such mediators are absent, results in a persistent and dysregulated inflammatory response [7,8].

Annexin-A1 (AnxA1) is a calcium- and phospholipid-binding protein with potent anti-inflammatory activities. It is particularly abundant in cells of the host immune system, including monocytes, macrophages, and PMNs [9]. Functionally, AnxA1 attenuates leukocyte recruitment by inhibiting cell adhesion and trans-migration [10,11]. AnxA1-deficient mice display an increased susceptibility to dextran sodium-sulfate (DSS)-induced colitis, and an impaired recovery following withdrawal of DSS [12]. Important roles for AnxA1 in the regulation of mucosal regeneration and healing have also been reported [13].

Lipoxin A_4 (LXA_4) is a lipoxygenase (LO)-derived eicosanoid generated *in situ* by the sequential lipoxygenation of arachidonic acid during cell-cell interaction [14,15]. LXA_4 inhibits eosinophil and PMN trafficking, adhesion and transmigration [16,17], and is strongly chemotactic for monocytes and macrophages [18,19]; in the latter case the ability of LXA_4 to stimulate the non-phlogistic phagocytosis of apoptotic PMNs [20,21] defines its role as an innate modulator of resolution. Native LXA_4, LXA_4 analogues and aspirin-triggered lipoxins (ATL) inhibit PMN adhesion to intestinal epithelial cells [22,23], as well as attenuate the secretion of chemokines from intestinal epithelia *in vitro* [24,25].

Both AnxA1 and LXA_4 activate and signal via a common receptor, the formyl peptide receptor 2/LXA_4 receptor (FPR2/ALX) [26]. Individually, the counter-regulatory effects of AnxA1 and LXA_4 on leukocyte recruitment are abolished following administration of FPR2/ALX antagonists [27–30], indicating the central role of this receptor in immune-regulatory responses. However, little is known regarding the dual or cumulative effects of these pro-resolution mediators in human pathological settings.

In this study, we examined the possibility that AnxA1 and LXA_4 exert protective and/or reparative roles in human intestinal inflammation. Given that resolution is an active process, we hypothesized that a microenvironment which favors a resolution phenotype would drive an increase in levels of both these mediators. We demonstrate that LXA_4 biosynthesis is elevated in mucosal biopsies from UC patients in medically-induced remission. Moreover, we observed in these same patients a concurrent up-regulation of AnxA1 in the mucosal lamina propria and intestinal epithelia, suggesting a reparative role for AnxA1 in healing of the intestinal mucosa. Together, these results are consistent with a significant role, and possibly concerted actions, for LXA_4 and AnxA1 in promoting mucosal homeostasis.

Results

Proinflammatory cytokine and enzyme expression

The expression of mRNA for cytokines TNF-α, IFN-γ, and IL-1β, as well as COX-2 (Table 1), was significantly elevated in biopsies from individuals with active disease. These findings were consistent with the level of macroscopic inflammation described at the time of colonoscopy. In contrast, in biopsies from individuals in medically-induced remission the expression of all genes, but COX-2, was not significantly different from that in the healthy group.

Mucosal infiltration by granulocytes and macrophages

Given the divergent roles of PMN and macrophages in the inflammatory response, we next assessed the infiltration of these cells into the colonic mucosa. PMN infiltration was significantly elevated in biopsies from patients with active disease, as assessed by HNE staining (Fig.1*A Upper* and Fig. 1*B*). The number of $CD68^+$ cells, a pan macrophage marker, was increased in biopsies from patients with active disease, those in medically induced remission, as well as those with a prior history of colitis (Fig. 1*A Lower* and Fig. 1*C*). Dual-labeling of macrophages with CD68 and CD206 revealed a significant reduction in the percentage of alternatively activated macrophages in biopsies of those with active disease (Fig. 1D).

Colonic LXA_4 biosynthesis

LXA_4 levels were significantly elevated (~3-fold) in biopsies from patients in medically-induced remission (Fig. 2*A*) but not in any of the other groups. To assess for alterations in enzymes responsible for LXA_4 biosynthesis, we first examined the mRNA expression of LO enzymes. 5-lipoxygenase (5-LO) mRNA expression was increased only in patients with active disease (Fig. 2*B*), with no significant changes in 12-lipoxygenase (12-LO) or 15-LO mRNA being identified (Fig. 2*C and 2D*, respectively). The increase in 5-LO mRNA expression was confirmed by immunohistochemistry (i.e., there was an increase in 5-LO^+ cells in biopsies of patients with active disease) (Fig. 2*E*).

AnxA1 expression in colonic mucosa

We used fluorescence microscopy to assess the expression and localization of AnxA1 in colonic mucosal biopsies. In healthy volunteers, a basal low level of AnxA1 expression was observed in cells of the intestinal lamina propria (Fig. 3*A*, 3*B*). In contrast, there was a significant increase in AnxA1 expression in biopsies from patients with active UC or those in medically-induced remission. Double-staining experiments revealed marked AnxA1 staining in neutrophils (co-localisation with HNE, a neutrophil granule protease) in biopsies of patients with active disease (Fig. 3*C*). In patients who were in medically-induced remission, AnxA1 expression was associated with macrophages, as evident from the paralleled expression with CD68 (Fig. 3*D*). Interestingly, AnxA1 immunostaining in biopsies from patients with UC (active or remission) was not limited to cells of the lamina propria, but appeared also in some of the epithelial cells lining the intestinal crypts (Fig. 3*E*). Such staining of epithelial cells was absent in biopsies from healthy volunteers.

Many of the biological effects of AnxA1 are mediated by the NH_2-terminal domain [31,32]. It is thought that proteolytic cleavage of the native 37 kDa protein results in termination of

Table 1. Pro-inflammatory cytokine expression.

	Healthy		UC	
mRNA expression (fold change)	**Ctrl**	**Hx of UC**	**Active**	**Rem**
TNF-α	1.00±0.46	1.09±0.26	4.77±1.67 *	1.19±0.21
IL-1β	1.00±0.47	3.57±0.66	7.87±1.41 *	1.36±1.36
IFN-γ	1.00±0.43	0.91±0.37	5.61±1.64 Ψ*	1.19±0.28
COX-2	1.00±0.23	0.65±0.16	3.91±0.84 Ψ	3.03±0.77 *

Quantitative RT-PCR analysis of pro-inflammatory cytokine and COX-2 expression in human colon biopsies. Assessment of TNF-α, IFN-γ, IL-1β and COX-2 mRNA levels in healthy subjects without (Ctrl) or with a prior history (Hx) of UC, UC patients with active disease (active), or UC patients in medically-induced remission. Data were normalized to β-actin gene expression (n = 5–20; *P<.05 vs. Ctrl, ΨP<.05 vs. Hx of UC).

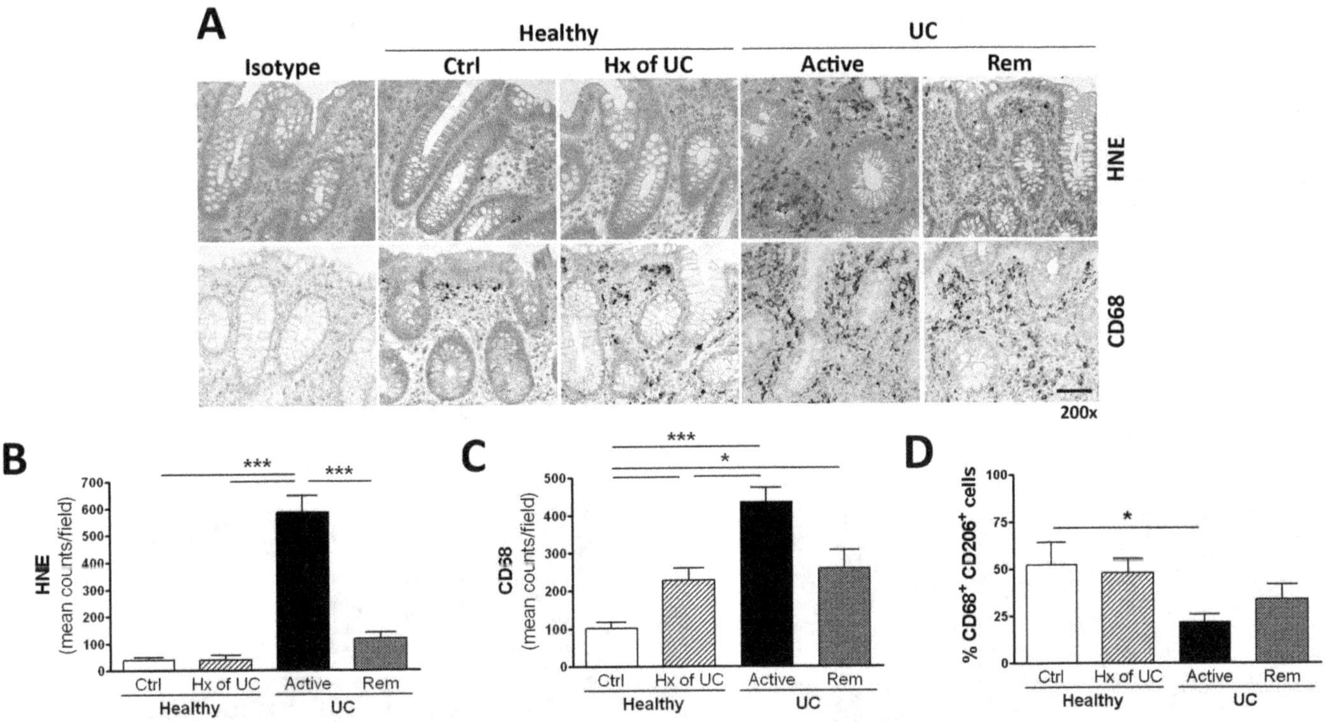

Figure 1. Expression of HNE and CD68 in colonic mucosal biopsies from healthy subjects without (Ctrl) or with a prior history (Hx) of UC, or UC patients with active disease (Active) or medically-induced remission (Rem) (**A**). HNE expression (Upper), used to detect PMNs was elevated in UC patients with active disease. CD68 expression (Lower), a pan macrophage marker, was elevated in active disease as well as in medically-induced remission. Cumulative analysis (mean counts/field) of HNE (**B**) and CD68 expression (**C**). Dual-staining of macrophage populations with CD68 and CD206, markers for alternatively activated (M2) macrophages (**D**), Data are expressed as mean ± SEM (**P*<.05, ****P*<.001, n = 4). Magnification bar = 100μm.

bioactivity, and cleavage-resistant AnxA1 mutants exhibit increased and prolonged anti-inflammatory activities [33]. Given the pro-inflammatory milieu in patients with active UC, we next assessed whether the expression of AnxA1 isoforms were altered among the patient groups. Biopsies from patients with active disease displayed a significant increase in AnxA1 protein

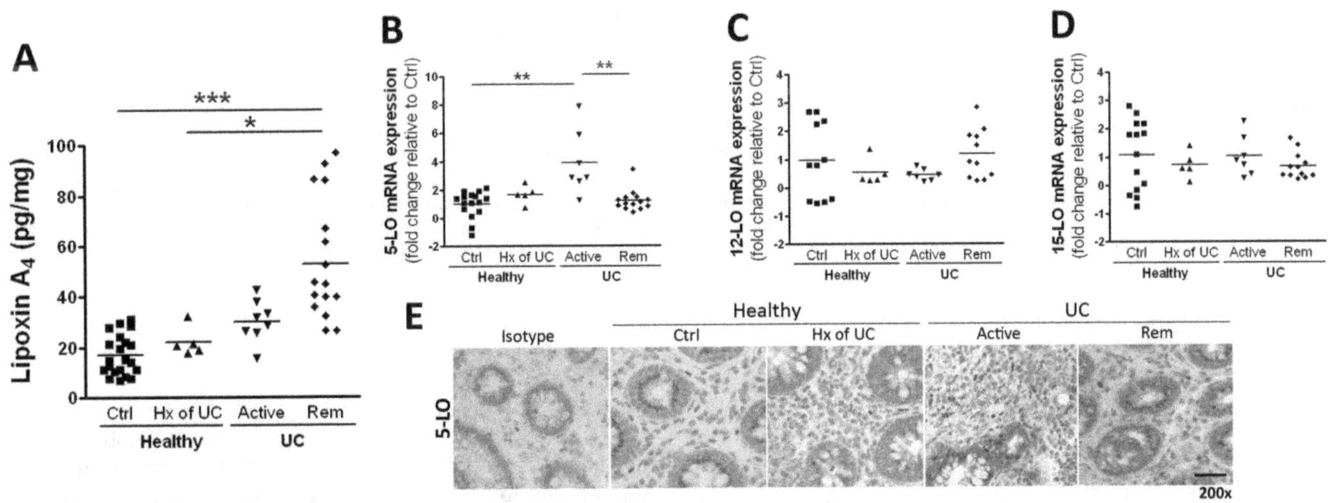

Figure 2. Colonic mucosal lipoxin A_4 levels (**A**) in biopsies from healthy subjects without (Ctrl) or with a prior history (Hx) of UC, or UC patients with active disease (Active) or medically-induced remission (Rem). Lipoxin A_4 levels were significantly elevated in the samples from patients who were in medically-induced remission compared with healthy subjects and those with a prior history of UC (>4 years disease-free). Quantitative RT-PCR analysis of 5-LO (**B**), 12-LO (**C**) and 15-LO (**D**) expression revealed an increase of 5-LO expression in patients with active disease. This correlated with an increase in the number of 5-LO-positive cells as assessed by immunohistochemistry (**E**). Data are expressed as fold change relative to Ctrl (**P*<.05, ***P*<.01 ****P*<.001, n = 5–20). Magnification bar = 100 μm.

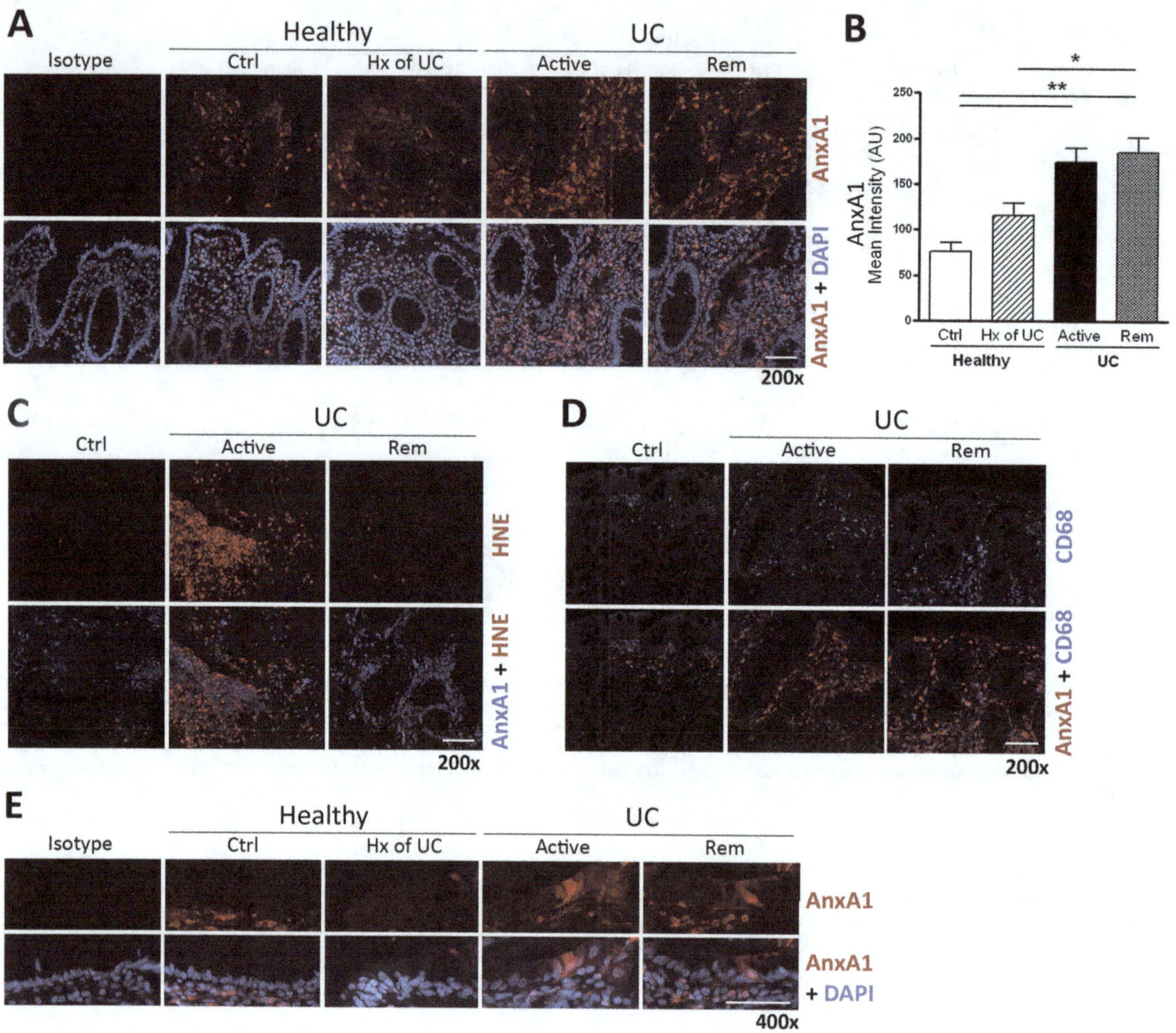

Figure 3. Expression of Annexin-A1 in colonic mucosal biopsies from healthy subjects without (Ctrl) or with a prior history (Hx) of UC, or UC patients with active disease (Active) or medically-induced remission (Rem) (**A**). Immunofluorescence detection of Annexin-A1 (red) demonstrates expression is increased in patients with UC, whether active or in medically-induced remission. Integrated pixel intensity revealed ~3-fold increase in these groups, compared to healthy subjects (**B**). In biopsies from patients with active UC, Annexin-A1 (blue) staining could be localized to infiltrating PMNs (red; stained with anti-HNE) (**C**), however in biopsies from patients in medically-induced remission, Annexin-A1 staining (red) closely paralleled tissue infiltration by CD68$^+$ macrophages (blue; stained with anti-CD68) (**D**). Annexin-A1 expression was also detected in crypt epithelial cells in subjects with UC, but not healthy subjects without/with a prior history of UC (**E**). Data are expressed as mean $\pm$ SEM (*$P<.05$, ***$P<.001$, n = 4). Magnification bar = 100 μm.

expression, present as a characteristic NH_2-terminal-cleaved 37/33kDa doublet (Fig. 4*A*, 4*B*). A similar increase was observed in patients in medically-induced remission, relative to healthy controls.

Expression of FPR2/ALX receptor

In line with colonic mucosal levels of AnxA1, analysis of FPR2/ALX mRNA expression revealed an increase in expression in biopsies from patients with active disease (10.7$\pm$3.6-fold, $P<.05$) as well as in those in medically-induced remission (7.3$\pm$2.9-fold, $P<.05$), relative to healthy controls (Fig. 5).

Discussion

Much evidence supports the capacity of infiltrating leukocytes to synthesize, either individually or cooperatively, a number of anti-inflammatory and pro-resolving factors [34]. In the present study, we set out to document the contribution of a distinct pro-resolution circuit, namely the liberation and actions of AnxA1 and LXA_4, in individuals with active or remittent UC.

Transepithelial migration of PMN from the microcirculation to the mucosa results in impaired barrier function and destruction of tissues [35,36]. Consistent with the literature, we observed PMN infiltration in colonic biopsies taken from individuals with active UC, but not in the other patient groups. Alongside the elevation in

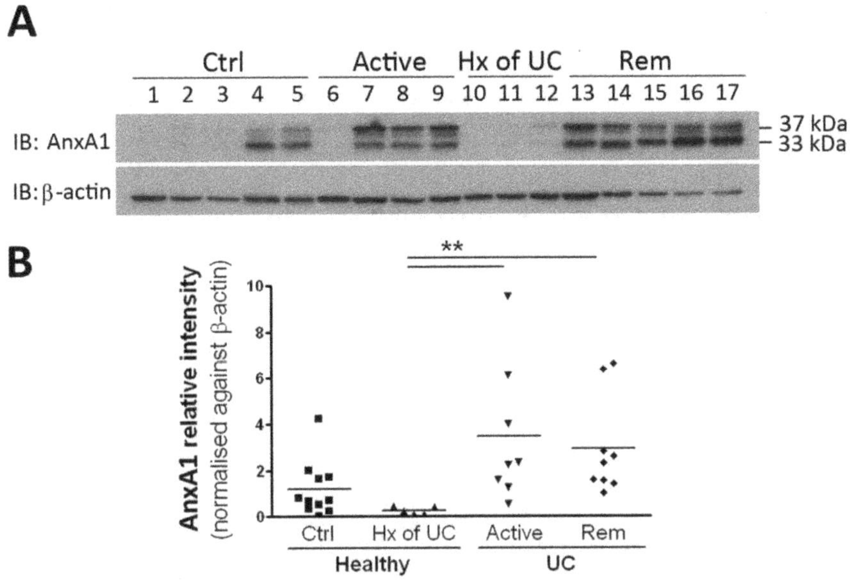

Figure 4. Detection of annexin-A1 NH_2-terminal-intact and -cleaved fragments in biopsies from healthy subjects without (Ctrl) or with a prior history (Hx) of UC, or UC patients with active disease (Active) or medically-induced remission (Rem). Annexin-1 was overexpressed in colonic mucosal biopsies of patients with UC compared to healthy patients with a prior history of UC (**A**). Alongside the native 37 kDa fragment, a NH_2-terminal cleaved isoform (33 kDa) could also be visualized, indicating specific degradation in response to externalization from activated cells. Analysis of relative intensity, where annexin-A1 immunoreactivity was normalized against β-actin (**B**). Data are expressed as mean ± SEM (***P*<.01, n = 5–11).

pro-inflammatory cytokine transcript levels (TNF-α, IFN-γ and IL-1β) and COX-2 mRNA expression, the local infiltration by cell types such as monocytes and macrophages likely contributes to this inflammatory milieu [37]. Intestinal macrophages play a fundamental role in host defense, including the phagocytosis and killing of microorganisms. Blood monocytes recruited to the inflamed mucosa do not display the same level of tolerogenicity as their resident counterparts; instead, these cells retain or have increased inflammatory capabilities [38]. Consistent with the high numbers of PMN in biopsies from individuals with active UC, we also observed an increase in infiltration of $CD68^+$ macrophages. Only a small proportion of these cells were of the M2 phenotype, as demonstrated by dual-labeling of macrophages with CD68 and CD206. However, the abundance of macrophages in biopsies from individuals in medically-induced remission, where there was an absence of PMN infiltration and an increase in COX-2 transcript levels, likely denoting an environment that is more conducive to the resolution of mucosal inflammation.

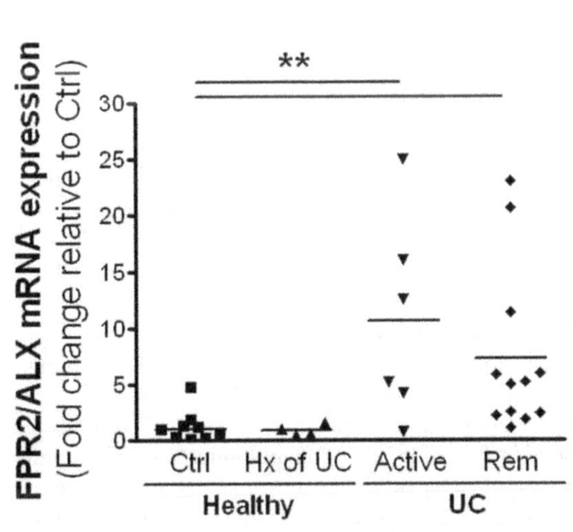

Figure 5. mRNA expression of FPR2/ALX in colonic mucosal biopsies from healthy subjects without (Ctrl) or with a prior history (Hx) of UC, or UC patients with active disease (Active) or medically-induced remission (Rem). Increased expression of FPR2/ALX was detected in biopsies from individuals with UC. Data are expressed as fold change relative to Ctrl (***P*<.01, n = 5–12).

In a rodent model of self-resolving peritonitis, analysis of macrophage phenotypes, specifically during the resolution phase, revealed a new class of resolution-phase macrophages that share markers of both classically activated and alternatively activated cells [39]. These resolution-phase macrophages synthesize high levels of COX-2 as well as the anti-inflammatory mediator PGD_2. We noted an increase in the number of infiltrating macrophages in biopsies from individuals in long-term remission, previously reported to be high producers of PGD_2 [40].

Given their roles in host defense, invading leukocytes are often viewed as pro-inflammatory. However, there is accumulating evidence that such cells synthesize distinct counter-regulatory mediators that promote the resolution of mucosal inflammation. Previous studies have documented the inhibitory effects of LXA_4 on leukocyte adhesion and transmigration [41,42], and LXA_4 analogues have also been shown to accelerate resolution in rodent models of colitis [43,44].

The results from our study identify a significant increase in LXA_4 synthesis exclusively in biopsies from patients in medically-induced remission. This further supports the hypothesis that there exists a pro-resolution microenvironment in the intestinal mucosa of individuals in remission from UC, and may be a means through which recruited macrophages coordinate the clearance of PMN. LXA_4 synthesis has been reported in pulmonary disease [45], periodontitis [46] and nasal polyps [47]. We observed an increase in 5-LO expression, at the transcript and protein levels, in biopsies taken from individuals with active UC. This is consistent with known increases of leukotriene-dependent enzymes in active IBD [48]. However, we found no changes in LO expression in biopsies obtained from individuals in medically-induced remission. Thus, the observed increase in mucosal LXA_4 synthesis likely stems from an augmentation of LO enzyme activity, rather than enzyme expression.

A new view regarding mechanisms of inflammatory resolution emerged when the short-lived lipid LXA_4 and the glucocorticoid-regulated protein AnxA1 were shown to share the same receptor target (FPR2/ALX) [49]. This indicates the existence of a convergence between specific effectors for theresolution of inflammation. Of interest, both LXA_4 and AnxA1 mediate IL-10-dependent inflammatory hyporesponsiveness in a model of intestinal ischemia/reperfusion injury [50]. Blockade of FPR2/ALX, LXA_4 production, and the use of neutralizing AnxA1 antibodies result in an increase in tissue injury, TNF-α production and lethality. A direct functional association between LXA_4 and endogenous AnxA1 has recently been described in human resting PMN *in vitro* [51]. However, the association between LXA_4 and AnxA1 has not been studied in man and, more importantly, in human pathological settings. Thus, alongside LXA_4 synthesis, we determined the expression and proteolysis of the AnxA1 in intestinal human samples.

Examination of colonic perfusates from UC patients indicates that AnxA1 secretion may be dependent on the severity of inflammation [52]. In the present study, we observed AnxA1-expression in the colonic mucosa of healthy individuals and those with UC, although expression was significantly elevated in the latter group. Whereas AnxA1 was localized predominately to PMN in biopsies of individuals with active disease, during disease remission AnxA1 expression switched to CD68+ macrophages. We speculate that high AnxA1 levels may be a characteristic of the recently described pro-resolving macrophages, at least in pre-clinical and clinical models of IBD, though future studies will be needed to specifically address this hypothesis. It is of interest to note that an increased susceptibility, mucosal injury, and clinical morbidity is observed in AnxA1-deficient mice administered dextran sodium sulfate (DSS) [53]. This dysregulated inflammatory response is compounded by an abated recovery following withdrawal of DSS administration, thereby providing strong proof-of-concept to the pro-resolving nature of AnxA1 in gut inflammation.

There is accumulating evidence that AnxA1 may also enhance mucosal healing. Peptides based on the NH_2-terminal region of AnxA1 stimulate epithelial cell migration [54], which is an important step in the restitution and wound healing process. Gastric mucosal repair of acetic acid-induced ulcers is significantly impaired in AnxA1-deficient mice, whereas in wild-type littermates healing of the ulcer region is accompanied by an increase of AnxA1 at the ulcer margin [55]. Rodents administered DSS also display an increase of AnxA1 in both surface and crypt epithelial cells [56]. When assessing colonic biopsies for the formation of cleaved AnxA1 products by western blotting, we observed a similar elevation of AnxA1 expression in biopsies from individuals with UC, relative to those in the healthy group. In each case, AnxA1 was present as a 37/33kDa doublet, corresponding to the NH_2-terminal-intact and -cleaved species, respectively [57].

Another interesting observation was the up-regulation of AnxA1 in intestinal epithelial cells of biopsies from individuals with active UC or in medically-induced remission. The increase of AnxA1 was diffuse, and not present in all crypt epithelial cells, which we speculate is likely reflective of the degree of mucosal inflammation and rate of cell turnover at any one point in time. This finding may be further evidence of the reparative roles of AnxA1 in the context of intestinal mucosa, independent of infiltrating leukocytes. It is noteworthy though that stimulation of epithelial cell motility, while important for mucosal healing, may also have pathophysiological consequences if dysregulated. In line with this view, an increase of AnxA1 expression has been associated with the development of tumor metastasis and colonic adenocarcinoma [58–60].

As mentioned above, the effects of AnxA1 and LXA_4 are mediated via a common G_i-protein-coupled receptor, namely FPR2/ALX [61]. FPR2/ALX is one of a family of pertussis toxin-sensitive FPR receptors [62] that interact with structurally diverse pro-and anti-inflammatory ligands [63]. The actions of AnxA1 and LXA_4 are abolished with the use of FPR2/ALX antagonists [64–70] as well as in FPR2/ALX-deficient mice [71], highlighting the fundamental role of this receptor in transducing non-redundant anti-inflammatory signals. We demonstrate herein the up-regulation of FPR2/ALX mRNA in biopsies of UC patients in medically-induced remission. The concurrent up-regulation of this receptor, alongside the observed increase in synthesis of the pro-resolution mediators AnxA1 and LXA_4 is consistent with a microenvironment that favors mucosal homeostasis. LXA_4-dependent ligation of FPR2/ALX down-regulates epithelial secretion of the chemokine CXCL-8 [72], which likely contributes to the reduced inflammation observed in biopsies obtained from patients in medically-induced remission, compared to those with active disease. No changes in FPR2/ALX expression were observed in biopsies taken from patients with a prior history of UC (long-term, medication-free remission for >4 years), perhaps indicating other pro-homeostatic mechanisms are in effect [73].

In summary, this study has documented an increase in mucosal synthesis of two pro-resolution mediators, AnxA1 and LXA_4, in individuals in medically-induced remission from UC. The concerted up-regulation of both ligand and receptor, in a previously pro-inflammatory setting, indicates a switch to a microenvironment that is conducive to the resolution of inflammation. Moreover, in the same individuals there was an up-regulation of AnxA1 synthesis by intestinal epithelial cells, consistent with its role in mucosal repair. We propose that this short-lived lipid and protein/peptide pair act in concert to safeguard effective inflammatory resolution. It is likely that parallel or converging pro-resolution networks, exemplified by the LXA_4/AnxA1 pair, are activated in multiple inflammatory settings, and is a scenario that could become paradigmatic for other mediators of inflammation.

Materials and Methods

Ethics Statement

This study was approved by the Ethics Committee at the University of Calgary. Each patient gave their written consent prior to participation in this study and all experiments were conducted according to the principles expressed in the Declaration of Helsinki.

Patients and tissue samples

Colonic mucosal biopsies were obtained from two broad patient groups: healthy individuals undergoing colonoscopy for routine colon cancer screening, and individuals with UC. These groups were subdivided; for healthy individuals, samples were obtained from those with no history of UC ('control' group; n = 8 male and 12 female; mean age 51±9 years), or those diagnosed previously with UC but had not experienced any bout of disease nor required any medication for UC for at least 4 years ('prior history of UC' group; n = 5 female; mean age 47±11 years). Patients with UC were divided into two groups: those with active disease ('active' group; n = 5 male and 3 female; mean age 43±16 years), and those in clinical and endoscopic remission while on maintenance therapy with either oral/topical 5-aminosalicylic acid or immunosuppressive/ biological therapy ('remission' group; n = 9 male and 7 female; mean age 44±13 years). Details regarding patient characteristics, such as gender, age, and clinical activity were obtained from medical records. Mucosal biopsies were taken from the left colon in close proximity to biopsies used for histological assessment. Samples intended for quantitative PCR, LXA_4 measurement, or western blotting were stored at −80°C until ready for processing. Samples for immunohistochemistry were fixed in 10% neutral-buffered formalin.

Quantitative PCR

Total RNA from colonic biopsies was extracted using the RNeasy Mini Kit (Qiagen, Valencia, CA) and two-step quantitative PCR was performed, as described [74]. Bioinformatic-validated high efficiency primer assays for human TNF-α (NM_000594), IL-1β (NM_000576), IFN-γ (NM_000619), COX-2 (NM_000963), 5-LO (NM_000698), 12-LO (NM_000697), 15-LO (NM_001140), FPR2/ALX (NM_001462) and β-actin (NM_001101) were obtained from Qiagen (Valencia, CA). All data were analyzed using Ct values obtained from Realplex software (Eppendorf, Ontario, CA), and amplification and relative quantification of gene products determined using the $\Delta\Delta C_t$ method, where target genes were normalized against the housekeeping gene β-actin.

Western blotting

Tissue samples were processed and proteins separated by 12% SDS-PAGE, as described previously [75]. Primary polyclonal rabbit anti-AnxA1 (Invitrogen) and monoclonal mouse anti-β-actin (Sigma Aldrich) antibodies were used. Secondary anti-rabbit and anti-mouse IgG antibodies were conjugated to horseradish peroxidase (GE Healthcare), and visualized using enhanced chemiluminescence (ECL) detection kit (GE Healthcare) on a Chemi-doc gel imaging system (Bio-Rad). Densitometric analysis was performed using ImageLab 2.0 software (Bio-Rad, Ontario, CA), with AnxA1 protein normalized against β-actin expression.

Histology and immunohistochemical analysis

Colonic biopsies from four patients per group were used for immunohistochemistry. For analysis of HNE and CD68 (markers of PMNs and macrophages, respectively), or 5-LO expression, sections were incubated in 3% H_2O_2 for 15min and then steamed for 30min in 10mM citrate buffer (pH 6.0)/0.05% Triton X-100. Sections were blocked in 10% normal serum, and incubated with mouse anti-human HNE (clone NP57, DAKO Cytomation), mouse anti-human CD68 (clone PG-M1, DAKO), mouse anti-human CD206 (ABCAM) or rabbit anti-5-LO (Cayman Chemical) overnight at 4°C. Sections were washed in PBS, incubated with anti-mouse or anti-rabbit biotinylated secondary antibodies (Vector Laboratories), and visualized by avidin-biotin-peroxidase detection using the Vectastain Elite ABC kit (Vector Laboratories). 3–3′ diaminobenzidine (DAB; Vector Laboratories) was used as the chromagen, and sections counterstained with Mayer's hematoxylin (Sigma Aldrich). For immunofluorescence detection of AnxA1, sections were blocked with 3% BSA and incubated with a monoclonal antibody raised against full-length human AnxA1 (mAb1B [76]) overnight, 4°C. To examine co-localization of AnxA1 with HNE or CD68, rabbit anti-AnxA1 antibody (Invitrogen) was incubated alongside anti-HNE or anti-CD68 antibodies. Sections were washed and incubated with AlexaFluor®568 goat anti-mouse IgG, AlexaFluor®350 goat anti-mouse IgG, AlexaFluor®568 goat anti-rabbit IgG, or AlexaFluor®350 goat anti-rabbit IgG (Invitrogen). To examine co-localization of CD68 with CD206, sections were incubated with AlexaFlour®568 goat anti-mouse and AlexaFluor®488 goat anti-mouse, respectively. Sections were then mounted with ProLong Gold containing DAPI (Invitrogen) or Vectashield fluorescence mounting medium (Vector Laboratories). Fluorescence was visualized on a Nikon Eclipse 80i microscope (Nikon) equipped with a DS-QiMc monochromatic camera (Nikon) and X-Cite® Series 120Q Xenon lamp. NIS-Elements BR3.1 software (Nikon) was used for all analyses. Images were recorded at identical gain settings, and mean intensity calculated per image field. Four image fields were taken of each section.

Lipoxin A_4 measurement

Measurement of LXA_4 was performed, as previously described [77], using a commercially available LXA_4 ELISA kit (Oxford Biomedical Research, Canada). Briefly, colonic biopsies were homogenized in extraction buffer (isopropranol/ethanol/0.1N HCl; 3:3:1), and diluted 1:1 with deionized water. The sample was centrifuged at 1,500*g* for 10min at 4°C, the organic phase transferred to a new tube, acidified to pH 3.5 and purified on pre-conditioned C18 Sep-Pak light columns (Millipore). The eluate was evaporated to dryness under a gentle stream of nitrogen gas and levels of LXA_4 determined using a commercially available LXA_4 ELISA kit (Oxford Biomedical Research, Canada).

Statistical analysis

Data are presented as mean±SEM. Comparisons among groups of data were made using a one-way ANOVA followed by the Kruskal-Wallis test. An associated probability ($P<.05$) was considered significant.

Acknowledgments

We thank Ida Rabbani-Nejad of the Intestinal Tissue Bank at the University of Calgary for her assistance with these studies.

Author Contributions

Conceived and designed the experiments: LV JGPF JLW. Performed the experiments: LV ND JGPF RP PLB. Analyzed the data: LV JGPF PLB MP JLW. Contributed reagents/materials/analysis tools: LV PLB JLW. Wrote the paper: LV JGPF PMS MP JLW.

References

1. Xavier RJ, Podolsky DK (2007) Unravelling the pathogenesis of inflammatory bowel disease. Nature 448: 427–434.
2. Grisham MB (1994) Oxidants and free radicals in inflammatory bowel disease. Lancet 344: 859–861.
3. Nusrat A, Parkos CA, Liang TW, Carnes DK, Madara JL (1997) Neutrophil migration across model intestinal epithelia: monolayer disruption and subsequent events in epithelial repair. Gastroenterology 113: 1489–1500.
4. Levy BD, Clish CB, Schmidt B, Gronert K, Serhan CN (2001) Lipid mediator class switching during acute inflammation: signals in resolution. Nat Immunol 2: 612–619.
5. Spite M, Norling LV, Summers L, Yang R, Cooper D, et al. (2009) Resolvin D2 is a potent regulator of leukocytes and controls microbial sepsis. Nature 461: 1287–1291.
6. Serhan CN, Savill J (2005) Resolution of inflammation: the beginning programs the end. Nat Immunol 6: 1191–1197.
7. Babbin BA, Laukoetter MG, Nava P, Koch S, Lee WY, et al. (2008) Annexin A1 regulates intestinal mucosal injury, inflammation, and repair. J Immunol 181: 5035–5044.
8. Rajakariar R, Hilliard M, Lawrence T, Trivedi S, Colville-Nash P, et al. (2007) Hematopoietic prostaglandin D2 synthase controls the onset and resolution of acute inflammation through PGD2 and 15-deoxyDelta12 14 PGJ2. Proc Natl Acad Sci U S A 104: 20979–20984.

9. Flower RJ, Rothwell NJ (1994) Lipocortin-1: cellular mechanisms and clinical relevance. Trends Pharmacol Sci 15: 71–76.
10. Chatterjee BE, Yona S, Rosignoli G, Young RE, Nourshargh S, et al. (2005) Annexin 1-deficient neutrophils exhibit enhanced transmigration in vivo and increased responsiveness in vitro. J Leukoc Biol 78: 639–646.
11. Mancuso F, Flower RJ, Perretti M (1995) Leukocyte transmigration, but not rolling or adhesion, is selectively inhibited by dexamethasone in the hamster post-capillary venule. Involvement of endogenous lipocortin 1. J Immunol 155: 377–386.
12. Babbin BA, Laukoetter MG, Nava P, Koch S, Lee WY, et al. (2008) Annexin A1 regulates intestinal mucosal injury, inflammation, and repair. J Immunol 181: 5035–5044.
13. Babbin BA, Lee WY, Parkos CA, Winfree LM, Akyildiz A, et al. (2006) Annexin I regulates SKCO-15 cell invasion by signaling through formyl peptide receptors. J Biol Chem 281: 19588–19599.
14. Fiore S, Serhan CN (1990) Formation of lipoxins and leukotrienes during receptor-mediated interactions of human platelets and recombinant human granulocyte/macrophage colony-stimulating factor-primed neutrophils. J Exp Med 172: 1451–1457.
15. Serhan CN, Sheppard KA (1990) Lipoxin formation during human neutrophil-platelet interactions. Evidence for the transformation of leukotriene A4 by platelet 12-lipoxygenase in vitro. J Clin Invest 85: 772–780.
16. Bandeira-Melo C, Bozza PT, Diaz BL, Cordeiro RS, Jose PJ, et al. (2000) Cutting edge: lipoxin (LX) A4 and aspirin-triggered 15-epi-LXA4 block allergen-induced eosinophil trafficking. J Immunol 164: 2267–2271.
17. Clish CB, Gronert K, Serhan CN (2000) Local and systemic delivery of an aspirin-triggered lipoxin stable analog inhibits neutrophil trafficking. Ann N Y Acad Sci 905: 274–278.
18. Godson C, Mitchell S, Harvey K, Petasis NA, Hogg N, et al. (2000) Cutting edge: lipoxins rapidly stimulate nonphlogistic phagocytosis of apoptotic neutrophils by monocyte-derived macrophages. J Immunol 164: 1663–1667.
19. Maddox JF, Serhan CN (1996) Lipoxin A4 and B4 are potent stimuli for human monocyte migration and adhesion: selective inactivation by dehydrogenation and reduction. J Exp Med 183: 137–146.
20. Maddox JF, Serhan CN (1996) Lipoxin A4 and B4 are potent stimuli for human monocyte migration and adhesion: selective inactivation by dehydrogenation and reduction. J Exp Med 183: 137–146.
21. Mitchell S, Thomas G, Harvey K, Cottell D, Reville K, et al. (2002) Lipoxins, aspirin-triggered epi-lipoxins, lipoxin stable analogues, and the resolution of inflammation: stimulation of macrophage phagocytosis of apoptotic neutrophils in vivo. J Am Soc Nephrol 13: 2497–2507.
22. Colgan SP, Serhan CN, Parkos CA, Delp-Archer C, Madara JL (1993) Lipoxin A4 modulates transmigration of human neutrophils across intestinal epithelial monolayers. J Clin Invest 92: 75–82.
23. Goh J, Baird AW, O'Keane C, Watson RW, Cottell D, et al. (2001) Lipoxin A(4) and aspirin-triggered 15-epi-lipoxin A(4) antagonize TNF-alpha-stimulated neutrophil-enterocyte interactions in vitro and attenuate TNF-alpha-induced chemokine release and colonocyte apoptosis in human intestinal mucosa ex vivo. J Immunol 167: 2772–2780.
24. Gewirtz AT, McCormick B, Neish AS, Petasis NA, Gronert K, et al. (1998) Pathogen-induced chemokine secretion from model intestinal epithelium is inhibited by lipoxin A4 analogs. J Clin Invest 101: 1860–1869.
25. Gronert K, Gewirtz A, Madara JL, Serhan CN (1998) Identification of a human enterocyte lipoxin A4 receptor that is regulated by interleukin (IL)-13 and interferon gamma and inhibits tumor necrosis factor alpha-induced IL-8 release. J Exp Med 187: 1285–1294.
26. Perretti M, Chiang N, La M, Fierro IM, Marullo S, et al. (2002) Endogenous lipid- and peptide-derived anti-inflammatory pathways generated with glucocorticoid and aspirin treatment activate the lipoxin A4 receptor. Nat Med 8: 1296–1302.
27. Babbin BA, Laukoetter MG, Nava P, Koch S, Lee WY, et al. (2008) Annexin A1 regulates intestinal mucosal injury, inflammation, and repair. J Immunol 181: 5035–5044.
28. Gastardelo TS, Damazo AS, Dalli J, Flower RJ, Perretti M, et al. (2009) Functional and ultrastructural analysis of annexin A1 and its receptor in extravasating neutrophils during acute inflammation. Am J Pathol 174: 177–183.
29. Gavins FN, Yona S, Kamal AM, Flower RJ, Perretti M (2003) Leukocyte antiadhesive actions of annexin 1. Blood 101: 4140–4147.
30. Martin GR, Perretti M, Flower RJ, Wallace JL (2008) Annexin-1 modulates repair of gastric mucosal injury. Am J Physiol Gastrointest Liver Physiol 294: G764–G769.
31. Croxtall JD, Waheed S, Choudhury Q, Anand R, Flower RJ (1993) N-terminal peptide fragments of lipocortin-1 inhibit A549 cell growth and block EGF-induced stimulation of proliferation. Int J Cancer 54: 153–158.
32. Croxtall JD, Choudhury Q, Flower RJ (1998) Inhibitory effect of peptides derived from the N-terminus of lipocortin 1 on arachidonic acid release and proliferation in the A549 cell line: identification of E-Q-E-Y-V as a crucial component. Br J Pharmacol 123: 975–983.
33. Pederzoli-Ribeil M, Maione F, Cooper D, Al Kashi A, Dalli J, et al. (2010) Design and characterization of a cleavage-resistant Annexin A1 mutant to control inflammation in the microvasculature. Blood 116: 4288–4296.
34. Serhan CN, Savill J (2005) Resolution of inflammation: the beginning programs the end. Nat Immunol 6: 1191–1197.
35. Grisham MB (1994) Oxidants and free radicals in inflammatory bowel disease. Lancet 344: 859–861.
36. Nusrat A, Parkos CA, Liang TW, Carnes DK, Madara JL (1997) Neutrophil migration across model intestinal epithelia: monolayer disruption and subsequent events in epithelial repair. Gastroenterology 113: 1489–1500.
37. Rugtveit J, Nilsen EM, Bakka A, Carlsen H, Brandtzaeg P, et al. (1997) Cytokine profiles differ in newly recruited and resident subsets of mucosal macrophages from inflammatory bowel disease. Gastroenterology 112: 1493–1505.
38. Rugtveit J, Haraldsen G, Hogasen AK, Bakka A, Brandtzaeg P, et al. (1995) Respiratory burst of intestinal macrophages in inflammatory bowel disease is mainly caused by CD14+L1+ monocyte derived cells. Gut 37: 367–373.
39. Bystrom J, Evans I, Newson J, Stables M, Toor I, et al. (2008) Resolution-phase macrophages possess a unique inflammatory phenotype that is controlled by cAMP. Blood 112: 4117–4127.
40. Vong L, Ferraz JG, Panaccione R, Beck PL, Wallace JL (2010) A pro-resolution mediator, prostaglandin D(2), is specifically up-regulated in individuals in long-term remission from ulcerative colitis. Proc Natl Acad Sci U S A 107: 12023–12027.
41. Colgan SP, Serhan CN, Parkos CA, Delp-Archer C, Madara JL (1993) Lipoxin A4 modulates transmigration of human neutrophils across intestinal epithelial monolayers. J Clin Invest 92: 75–82.
42. Goh J, Baird AW, O'Keane C, Watson RW, Cottell D, et al. (2001) Lipoxin A(4) and aspirin-triggered 15-epi-lipoxin A(4) antagonize TNF-alpha-stimulated neutrophil-enterocyte interactions in vitro and attenuate TNF-alpha-induced chemokine release and colonocyte apoptosis in human intestinal mucosa ex vivo. J Immunol 167: 2772–2780.
43. Fiorucci S, Wallace JL, Mencarelli A, Distrutti E, Rizzo G, et al. (2004) A beta-oxidation-resistant lipoxin A4 analog treats hapten-induced colitis by attenuating inflammation and immune dysfunction. Proc Natl Acad Sci U S A 101: 15736–15741.
44. Gewirtz AT, Collier-Hyams LS, Young AN, Kucharzik T, Guilford WJ, et al. (2002) Lipoxin a4 analogs attenuate induction of intestinal epithelial proinflammatory gene expression and reduce the severity of dextran sodium sulfate-induced colitis. J Immunol 168: 5260–5267.
45. Lee TH, Crea AE, Gant V, Spur BW, Marron BE, et al. (1990) Identification of lipoxin A4 and its relationship to the sulfidopeptide leukotrienes C4, D4, and E4 in the bronchoalveolar lavage fluids obtained from patients with selected pulmonary diseases. Am Rev Respir Dis 141: 1453–1458.
46. Pouliot M, Clish CB, Petasis NA, Van Dyke TE, Serhan CN (2000) Lipoxin A(4) analogues inhibit leukocyte recruitment to Porphyromonas gingivalis: a role for cyclooxygenase-2 and lipoxins in periodontal disease. Biochemistry 39: 4761–4768.
47. Edenius C, Kumlin M, Bjork T, Anggard A, Lindgren JA (1990) Lipoxin formation in human nasal polyps and bronchial tissue. FEBS Lett 272: 25–28.
48. Jupp J, Hillier K, Elliott DH, Fine DR, Bateman AC, et al. (2007) Colonic expression of leukotriene-pathway enzymes in inflammatory bowel diseases. Inflamm Bowel Dis 13: 537–546.
49. Perretti M, Chiang N, La M, Fierro IM, Marullo S, et al. (2002) Endogenous lipid- and peptide-derived anti-inflammatory pathways generated with glucocorticoid and aspirin treatment activate the lipoxin A4 receptor. Nat Med 8: 1296–1302.
50. Souza DG, Fagundes CT, Amaral FA, Cisalpino D, Sousa LP, et al. (2007) The required role of endogenously produced lipoxin A4 and annexin-1 for the production of IL-10 and inflammatory hyporesponsiveness in mice. J Immunol 179: 8533–8543.
51. Brancaleone V, Dalli J, Bena S, Flower RJ, Cirino G, et al. (2011) Evidence for an Anti-Inflammatory Loop Centered on Polymorphonuclear Leukocyte Formyl Peptide Receptor 2/Lipoxin A4 Receptor and Operative in the Inflamed Microvasculature. J Immunol.
52. Vergnolle N, Pages P, Guimbaud R, Chaussade S, Bueno L, et al. (2004) Annexin 1 is secreted in situ during ulcerative colitis in humans. Inflamm Bowel Dis 10: 584–592.
53. Babbin BA, Laukoetter MG, Nava P, Koch S, Lee WY, et al. (2008) Annexin A1 regulates intestinal mucosal injury, inflammation, and repair. J Immunol 181: 5035–5044.
54. Babbin BA, Lee WY, Parkos CA, Winfree LM, Akyildiz A, et al. (2006) Annexin I regulates SKCO-15 cell invasion by signaling through formyl peptide receptors. J Biol Chem 281: 19588–19599.
55. Martin GR, Perretti M, Flower RJ, Wallace JL (2008) Annexin-1 modulates repair of gastric mucosal injury. Am J Physiol Gastrointest Liver Physiol 294: G764–G769.
56. Babbin BA, Laukoetter MG, Nava P, Koch S, Lee WY, et al. (2008) Annexin A1 regulates intestinal mucosal injury, inflammation, and repair. J Immunol 181: 5035–5044.
57. Vong L, D'Acquisto F, Pederzoli-Ribeil M, Lavagno L, Flower RJ, et al. (2007) Annexin 1 cleavage in activated neutrophils: a pivotal role for proteinase 3. J Biol Chem 282: 29998–30004.
58. Duncan R, Carpenter B, Main LC, Telfer C, Murray GI (2008) Characterisation and protein expression profiling of annexins in colorectal cancer. Br J Cancer 98: 426–433.
59. Jiang D, Ying W, Lu Y, Wan J, Zhai Y, et al. (2003) Identification of metastasis-associated proteins by proteomic analysis and functional exploration of interleukin-18 in metastasis. Proteomics 3: 724–737.

60. Xin W, Rhodes DR, Ingold C, Chinnaiyan AM, Rubin MA (2003) Dysregulation of the annexin family protein family is associated with prostate cancer progression. Am J Pathol 162: 255–261.
61. Perretti M, Chiang N, La M, Fierro IM, Marullo S, et al. (2002) Endogenous lipid- and peptide-derived anti-inflammatory pathways generated with glucocorticoid and aspirin treatment activate the lipoxin A4 receptor. Nat Med 8: 1296–1302.
62. Ye RD, Boulay F, Wang JM, Dahlgren C, Gerard C, et al. (2009) International Union of Basic and Clinical Pharmacology. LXXIII. Nomenclature for the formyl peptide receptor (FPR) family. Pharmacol Rev 61: 119–161.
63. Le Y, Murphy PM, Wang JM (2002) Formyl-peptide receptors revisited. Trends Immunol 23: 541–548.
64. Babbin BA, Lee WY, Parkos CA, Winfree LM, Akyildiz A, et al. (2006) Annexin I regulates SKCO-15 cell invasion by signaling through formyl peptide receptors. J Biol Chem 281: 19588–19599.
65. der Weid PY, Hollenberg MD, Fiorucci S, Wallace JL (2004) Aspirin-triggered, cyclooxygenase-2-dependent lipoxin synthesis modulates vascular tone. Circulation 110: 1320–1325.
66. Gastardelo TS, Damazo AS, Dalli J, Flower RJ, Perretti M, et al. (2009) Functional and ultrastructural analysis of annexin A1 and its receptor in extravasating neutrophils during acute inflammation. Am J Pathol 174: 177–183.
67. Gavins FN, Yona S, Kamal AM, Flower RJ, Perretti M (2003) Leukocyte antiadhesive actions of annexin 1. Blood 101: 4140–4147.
68. Martin GR, Perretti M, Flower RJ, Wallace JL (2008) Annexin-1 modulates repair of gastric mucosal injury. Am J Physiol Gastrointest Liver Physiol 294: G764–G769.
69. Scannell M, Flanagan MB, deStefani A, Wynne KJ, Cagney G, et al. (2007) Annexin-1 and peptide derivatives are released by apoptotic cells and stimulate phagocytosis of apoptotic neutrophils by macrophages. J Immunol 178: 4595–4605.
70. Souza DG, Fagundes CT, Amaral FA, Cisalpino D, Sousa LP, et al. (2007) The required role of endogenously produced lipoxin A4 and annexin-1 for the production of IL-10 and inflammatory hyporesponsiveness in mice. J Immunol 179: 8533–8543.
71. Dufton N, Hannon R, Brancaleone V, Dalli J, Patel HB, et al. (2010) Anti-inflammatory role of the murine formyl-peptide receptor 2: ligand-specific effects on leukocyte responses and experimental inflammation. J Immunol 184: 2611–2619.
72. Gronert K, Gewirtz A, Madara JL, Serhan CN (1998) Identification of a human enterocyte lipoxin A4 receptor that is regulated by interleukin (IL)-13 and interferon gamma and inhibits tumor necrosis factor alpha-induced IL-8 release. J Exp Med 187: 1285–1294.
73. Vong L, Ferraz JG, Panaccione R, Beck PL, Wallace JL (2010) A pro-resolution mediator, prostaglandin D(2), is specifically up-regulated in individuals in long-term remission from ulcerative colitis. Proc Natl Acad Sci U S A 107: 12023–12027.
74. Chavez-Pina AE, Vong L, McKnight W, Dicay M, Zanardo RC, et al. (2008) Lack of effects of acemetacin on signalling pathways for leukocyte adherence may explain its gastrointestinal safety. Br J Pharmacol 155: 857–864.
75. Vong L, Ferraz JG, Panaccione R, Beck PL, Wallace JL (2010) A pro-resolution mediator, prostaglandin D(2), is specifically up-regulated in individuals in long-term remission from ulcerative colitis. Proc Natl Acad Sci U S A 107: 12023–12027.
76. Perretti M, Chiang N, La M, Fierro IM, Marullo S, et al. (2002) Endogenous lipid- and peptide-derived anti-inflammatory pathways generated with glucocorticoid and aspirin treatment activate the lipoxin A4 receptor. Nat Med 8: 1296–1302.
77. Souza MH, de Lima OM Jr, Zamuner SR, Fiorucci S, Wallace JL (2003) Gastritis increases resistance to aspirin-induced mucosal injury via COX-2-mediated lipoxin synthesis. Am J Physiol Gastrointest Liver Physiol 285: G54–G61.

6

The *Mutyh* Base Excision Repair Gene Influences the Inflammatory Response in a Mouse Model of Ulcerative Colitis

Ida Casorelli[1]*, Tania Pannellini[2], Gabriele De Luca[1], Paolo Degan[3], Federica Chiera[1], Ivano Iavarone[1], Alessandro Giuliani[1], Alessia Butera[4], Monica Boirivant[4], Piero Musiani[2], Margherita Bignami[1]*

1 Department of Environment and Primary Prevention, Istituto Superiore di Sanità, Rome, Italy, 2 Aging Research Center, Gabriele D'Annunzio University of Chieti, Chieti, Italy, 3 Istituto Tumori di Genova, Genova, Italy, 4 Department of Infectious Parasitic and Immuno-mediated Diseases, Istituto Superiore di Sanità, Rome, Italy

Abstract

Background: The *Mutyh* DNA glycosylase is involved in the repair of oxidized DNA bases. Mutations in the human *MUTYH* gene are responsible for colorectal cancer in familial adenomatous polyposis. Since defective DNA repair genes might contribute to the increased cancer risk associated with inflammatory bowel diseases, we compared the inflammatory response of wild-type and *Mutyh*$^{-/-}$ mice to oxidative stress.

Methodology/Principal Findings: The severity of colitis, changes in expression of genes involved in DNA repair and inflammation, DNA 8-oxoguanine levels and microsatellite instability were analysed in colon of mice treated with dextran sulfate sodium (DSS). The *Mutyh*$^{-/-}$ phenotpe was associated with a significant accumulation of 8-oxoguanine in colon DNA of treated mice. A single DSS cycle induced severe acute ulcerative colitis in wild-type mice, whereas lesions were modest in *Mutyh*$^{-/-}$ mice, and this was associated with moderate variations in the expression of several cytokines. Eight DSS cycles caused chronic colitis in both wild-type and *Mutyh*$^{-/-}$ mice. Lymphoid hyperplasia and a significant reduction in Foxp3^{+} regulatory T cells were observed only in *Mutyh*$^{-/-}$ mice.

Conclusions: The findings indicate that, in this model of ulcerative colitis, Mutyh plays a major role in maintaining intestinal integrity by affecting the inflammatory response.

Editor: Guillaume Dalmasso, Emory Unviersity, United States of America

Funding: This work was supported by grants from Association for International Cancer Research, Associazione Italiana Ricerca sul Cancro, Alleanza Contro il Cancro and Fondo per gli Investimenti della Ricerca di Base to MB. The funders had no role in study design, data collection and analysis, decision to publish, or preparation of the manuscript.

Competing Interests: The authors have declared that no competing interests exist.

* E-mail: ida.casorelli@ospedalesantandrea.it (IC); margherita.bignami@iss.it (MB)

These authors contributed equally to this work.

Introduction

Inflammatory processes induce oxidative/nitrosative stress and lipid peroxidation by generating an excess of radical reactive species. Experimental and epidemiological evidences suggested a link between oxidative stress and cancer. Persistent inflammation is considered an important risk factor for colorectal cancer development in Ulcerative colitis (UC) and Crohn's disease, two major Inflammatory Bowel Diseases (IBDs) [1].

Oxidative stress causes different kinds of DNA damage, including single and double strand breaks and base modifications. One of the predominant products, 8-oxoguanine (8-oxoG), is potentially mutagenic and is implicated in carcinogenesis. DNA 8-oxoG codes ambiguously during replication and directs incorporation of C and A with almost equal efficiencies. The mutagenic consequence of 8-oxoG:A mismatches, G:C->T:A transversions, are regarded as the signature mutations of DNA 8-oxoG. Base Excision Repair (BER) initiated by the MUTYH DNA glycosylase provides protection against 8-oxoG:A mispairs [2,3]. This enzyme removes A incorrectly inserted opposite 8-oxoG. The APE/REF1 endonuclease incises the resulting apurinic site and insertion of a C across the 8-oxoG creates a substrate for enzymes which remove this oxidized purine [4]. In addition, Mutyh can remove other sources of potentially mutagenic lesions such as oxidized adenines [5]. The absence of this repair pathway in *Mutyh*$^{-/-}$ cells is associated with accumulation of DNA 8-oxoG and a mutator phenotype [6,7]. In addition, *Mutyh*-null mice show enhanced susceptibility to spontaneous and $KBrO_3$-induced intestinal carcinogenesis [8] and Mutyh deficiency enhances intestinal tumorigenesis in *Apc*$^{min/+}$ mice [9]. Biallelic germ-line mutations in human *MUTYH* have been identified in patients affected by colorectal adenomatous polyposis [10]. Accumulation of somatic GC->TA transversions in *APC* and *KRAS*, most likely because of defective repair of 8-oxoG:A mismatches, characterize this autosomal recessive syndrome [11,12].

Oxidative stress in IBDs is associated with increased levels of oxidized DNA bases [1]. Furthermore the accumulation of 8-oxoG in the mucosa of UC-associated neoplasia accompanied by functional inactivation human MUTYH have been proposed as early events in UC-associated carcinogenesis [13]. Since DNA repair genes might play a role in cancer risk associated with chronic inflammation occurring in IBDs [1,14], in this study we compared the response of *Mutyh*$^{-/-}$ and wild-type (wt) mice to single or multiple cycles of dextran sulfate sodium (DSS) in drinking water. DSS induces colonic oxidative stress and colitis that mimics human IBDs [15]. In the acute phase, exposure of the mucosa to bacterial antigens generates an acute inflammatory response and damage to the epithelium. In the chronic phase, the mucosa is still inflamed although the epithelium is restored, albeit with an irregular structure. Long-term DSS exposure can be associated with the induction of colonic tumors. Indeed DSS has been shown to enhance 8-oxoG levels in rat and mouse colonic mucosa [16,17].

Following a DSS-induced oxidative stress we investigated the role of Mutyh in modulating levels of DNA oxidation and patterns of expression of 40 genes involved in the inflammatory response or in DNA repair. Our findings indicate that the inflammatory response elicited by acute DSS exposure is diminished in *Mutyh*$^{-/-}$ mice in comparison to their wt counterparts. In contrast, a chronic exposure to DSS induces an inflammatory response in both wt and *Mutyh*$^{-/-}$ mice, although a more florid lymphoid hyperplasia with a significant reduction of Foxp3^{+} regulatory T cells (Tregs) is apparent in the latter animals.

Results

Acute colitis

A single cycle of 3% DSS for 7 days followed by a 10-day period with water (1 cycle) induced acute colitis. In wt animals, colitis was associated with decrease of body weight in comparison to controls ($P<0.01$ from day 4 of DSS exposure)(Figure 1A). Weight loss was less pronounced in *Mutyh*$^{-/-}$ animals ($P<0.05$, days 14th and 16th) and their weights differed significantly from untreated mice only at the end of the DSS treatment ($P<0.05$, day 16)(Figure 1A).

Histopathological analyses of colonic sections from wt mice, revealed signs of frank inflammation and confirmed the presence of severe acute UC in most animals (10/11, >90%). Colitis was characterized by the presence of mucosal ulcerations, infiltration of the lamina propria by inflammatory cells, oedema, crypt erosion and abscesses, gland loss, goblet cell reduction and signs of epithelial regeneration (Figure 1B). These features were signifi-

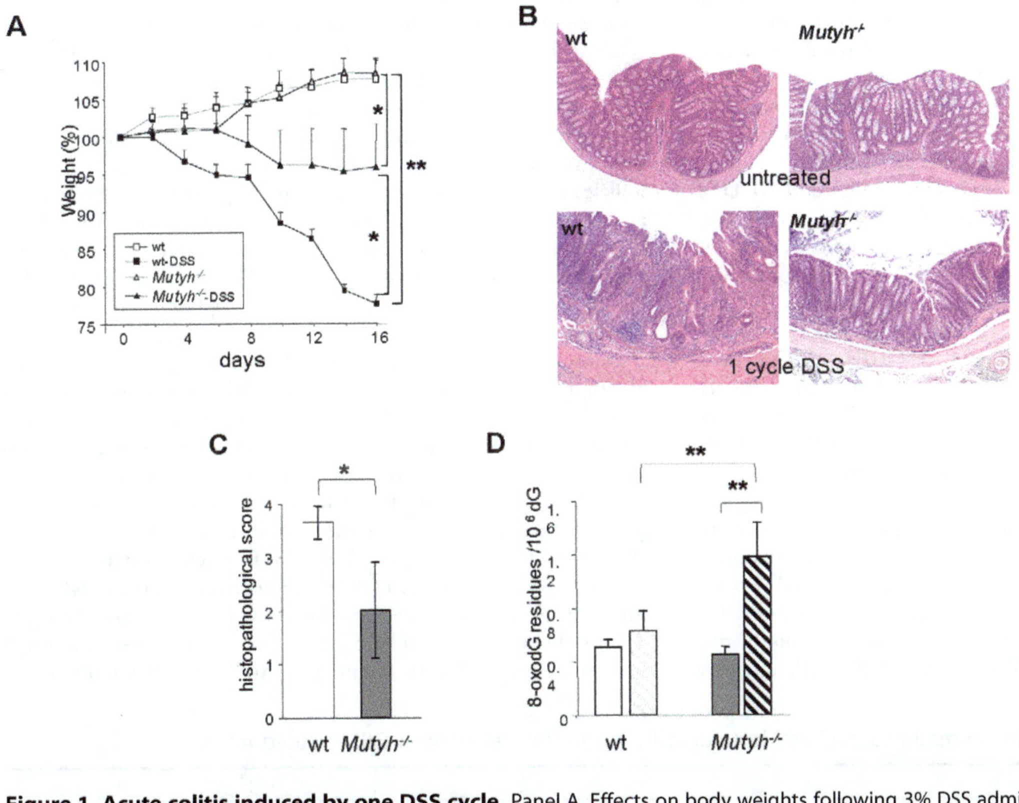

Figure 1. Acute colitis induced by one DSS cycle. Panel A. Effects on body weights following 3% DSS administration in 10 wt and 7 *Mutyh*$^{-/-}$ mice. Body weight variations are shown as percentage of weights at the beginning of the analysis in the control or DSS-treated groups. Data are mean ± SE. *P* values were calculated by comparing wt and *Mutyh*$^{-/-}$ mice at the same days of DSS treatment. Untreated wt (open circles), DSS-treated wt (closed circles); untreated *Mutyh*$^{-/-}$ (open triangles), DSS-treated *Mutyh*$^{-/-}$ (closed triangles). Panel B. Photomicrographs of colon from wt (left) and *Mutyh−/−* (right) mice exposed (lower row) or not (upper row) to one DSS cycle. Severe colitis in wt animals is indicated by ulcerations of the mucosa, crypt erosion and abscesses, goblet cell reduction, oedema and marked presence of inflammatory cells in the lamina propria. A reduction in the number of epithelial lesions and infiltrating inflammatory cells is observed in Mutyh−/− mice. Lesions correspond to an average histopathological score of 3 and 1 in wt and Mutyh−/− mice, respectively. Scale bars: 100 mm. Panel C. The extent of inflammation was calculated at the end of treatment as histopathological score according to indicated criteria (Table 1 and ref. [15]). Data are mean + SE of 11 wt and 6 *Mutyh−/−* mice. Panel D. Levels of DNA 8-oxoG in colonic mucosa of untreated and DSS-treated mice. Data are the mean + SE from 20 untreated (open bars) and 10 DSS-treated wt (dashed bars) and 8 untreated (grey bars) and 5 DSS-treated *Mutyh−/−* mice (dashed bars). DSS-treated groups are compared to untreated controls by t-tests and two-way P-values (*P = 0.05; ** P<0.05).

cantly attenuated in *Mutyh*$^{-/-}$ mice and only 50% showed signs of inflammation. Lesions were either absent or modest and we observed few ulcers (Figure 1B). Table 1 details the severity of colitis quantified from histological scores [15], with minor modifications. The mean histopathological scores for colitis in wt animals were significantly higher than those of *Mutyh*$^{-/-}$ mice ($P = 0.05$)(Figure 1C).

Since DSS is known to induce oxidative stress we investigated whether this treatment resulted in the accumulation of 8-oxoG in colon DNA (Figure 1D). Acute DSS treatment increased the amount of DNA 8-oxoG in *Mutyh*$^{-/-}$ mice >2.5-fold compared to untreated controls. The levels of this oxidized base remained unchanged in wt mice (Figure 1D). As previously reported [18], basal levels of 8-oxoG in colon DNA were unaffected by Mutyh inactivation.

These findings indicate that the inflammatory response to DSS exposure in *Mutyh*$^{-/-}$ mice is attenuated in comparison to that in wt animals. This is accompanied by the accumulation of significantly higher levels of DSS-induced DNA 8-oxoG in the colon of *Mutyh*$^{-/-}$ animals.

Gene expression in DSS–induced acute colitis

Gene expression in colon samples from 20 wt and 19 *Mutyh*$^{-/-}$ animals was analysed using low-density arrays containing 40 genes involved in DNA repair and inflammatory responses (Table 2). Samples were classified on the basis of genotypes and treatment. In untreated animals, only a few genes differed in basal expression between the two genotypes. In *Mutyh*$^{-/-}$ mice, expression of hMOX1, IL-17A and NOX1 was 2-fold lower ($P<0.05$) and IL-6 ($P = 0.02$) was 2-fold higher than in wt mice (Figure 2). Significant differences in steady-state levels of DNA repair gene mRNA were also observed. LIG1 and PARP1 levels were higher and NUDT1 expression was lower in *Mutyh*$^{-/-}$ mice ($P\leq0.05$) (Figure 2).

Acute DSS treatment induced widespread changes in gene expression in the colon of wt mice (Figure 3A–B). Acute colitis was associated with up-regulation of several genes involved in pro-inflammatory pathways (IFNγ, IL-17a, IL-1b, IL-6, NOS2, PTGS2, hMOX1, TNFα and IL-12a) ($P<0.01$). hMOX1 was induced to a similar degree in *Mutyh*$^{-/-}$ mice but changes in IL-17a, IL-1b and NOS2 were less pronounced ($P\leq0.01$) (Figure 3A) and there was no significant increase in expression of IL-12a, IL-6, PTGS2, or TNFα (data not shown). Strikingly, there was no up-regulation of IFNγ in *Mutyh*$^{-/-}$ mice.

Another set of genes, the majority of which encode DNA repair factors, was significantly down-regulated by acute DSS treatment (Figure 3B). The extent of these changes was less marked (2-fold). In *Mutyh*$^{-/-}$ mice the down-regulation was restricted to a subset of these genes, although the degree of variation was similar in the two genotypes. The only down-regulated gene of the inflammatory panel, IL-13, was affected more significantly in *Mutyh*$^{-/-}$ than in wt mice (10- versus 3-fold change).

In conclusion following an acute DSS treatment, *Mutyh*$^{-/-}$ mice display a lower number of modulated genes as compared to wt animals, when either up-regulated (4 *versus* 9 genes) or down-regulated genes (7 *versus* 13) are taken into consideration. Overall, the limited modulation of pro- or anti-inflammatory cytokines in *Mutyh*$^{-/-}$ mice nicely parallels the moderate degree of inflammation observed histologically in these animals.

Chronic colitis

After three 1.5% DSS cycles, severe lesions of the glandular epithelium and ulcers coupled with a decrease in the number of mucus-secreting cells and a marked increase in the number of reactive cells in the lamina propria and submucosa similar to those of acute UC were observed in wt mice (mean histopathological score 3.7±0.5 and Figure 4B). In contrast, colitis in *Mutyh*$^{-/-}$ mice was less aggressive with few ulcers, the lesions of the glandular epithelium were focally distributed and the lamina propria and submucosa were moderately infiltrated by reactive cells (mean histopathological score 2.7±0.4 and Figure 4B).

Eight DSS courses resulted in chronic colitis in wt mice with residual glands coated with an epithelium containing few mucus-secreting cells (Figure 4C). Numerous reactive cells with lymphoid cells, sometimes arranged in follicles, occupied the lamina propria and the submucosa. Often granulation tissue filled in the ulcer craters, followed by regeneration of the mucosal epithelium. In some areas submucosal fibrosis and mucosal architectural disarray and atrophy remained as residual of healed disease. The same treatment induced chronic UC in *Mutyh*$^{-/-}$ mice, although this was less severe. *Mutyh*$^{-/-}$ mice had numerous ample lymphoid follicles at the level of the colonic lamina propria or between this and the submucosa. A hyperplastic mantle zone and florid Germinal Centers (GCs) characterized these follicles, with a large number of leukocytes located in inter-follicular zones (Figure 4C). Neither wt nor *Mutyh*$^{-/-}$ mice showed neoplastic transformation of mucosal glands.

Immunohistochemical analysis of lymphoid aggregates revealed an impressive lymphoid hyperplasia of B220+ B lymphocytes in *Mutyh*$^{-/-}$ mice (Figure 4D). These were organized in PNA+ GCs and were more pronounced and larger than in wt mice. Numerous CD4+ T lymphocytes were present in the inter-follicular zones and at the borders of the follicles, again in larger numbers in *Mutyh*$^{-/-}$ mice (Figure 4D), although the architecture of these lymphoid structures did not show gross deviations from the normal structure.

In comparison to wt mice, the lymphoid hyperplasia in *Mutyh*$^{-/-}$ mice was always associated with very low levels of CD4+/Foxp3^{+} T regs (Figure 5A–B). These cells were significantly diminished both in follicles without (Figure 5A) and with GCs (continuous

Table 1. Scoring system for inflammation-associated histological changes in the colon of DSS -treated mice.

Colitis Grade	Histological Parameters
0	No evidence of inflammation
1	Slight colitis: low level of inflammation with scattered infiltrating granulocytes, monocytes and plasmacells (1–2 foci).
2	Moderate colitis: moderate inflammation with multiple foci, oedema of lamina propria, scattered granulocytes.
3	Severe colitis: high level of inflammation with marked wall thickening, oedema of the lamina propria, glands distortion, gland erosion and abscesses, ulcerations of superficial epithelial cells.
4	Maximal severity of inflammation with transmural leukocyte infiltration, almost complete loss of goblet cells, large ulcerations involving all mucosal wall and deep suppuration foci.

Table 2. List of genes involved in the inflammatory response and in DNA repair and analyzed for expression.

CODE	GENE	CODE	GENE
INFLAMMATORY RESPONSE		*RECOMBINATIONAL REPAIR*	
Mm00443258_m1	*TNFα*	Mm00450600_m1	*Mre11a*
Mm00484741_m1	*SMAD7*	Mm00487905_m1	*RAD51*
Mm00489637_m1	*SMAD3*	Mm00550147_m1	*XRCC5 (KU70)*
Mm00478374_m1	*PTGS2*	Mm00487458_m1	*XRCC6 (KU80)*
Mm00477214_m1	*PTGS1*	Mm00465092_m1	*PRKDC (DNA-PK)*
Mm00500821_m1	*NQO1*		
Mm00549170_m1	*NOX1*	*MISMATCH REPAIR*	
Mm00440485_m1	*NOS2*	Mm00500563_m1	*MSH2*
Mm00479807_m1	*NFKB2*	Mm00487756_m1	*MSH3*
Mm00446190_m1	*IL6*	Mm00487761_m1	*MSH6*
Mm00518984_m1	*IL23a*	Mm00503449_m1	*MLH1*
Mm00434228_m1	*IL1b*	Mm00476986_m1	*PMS2*
Mm00444686_m1	*IL17b*		
Mm00439619_m1	*IL17a*	*BASE EXCISION REPAIR*	
Mm00434204_m1	*IL13*	Mm00521933_m1	*LIG3*
Mm00434165_m1	*IL12a*	Mm00495331_m1	*LIG1*
Mm00439616_m1	*IL10*	Mm00494229_m1	*XRCC1*
Mm00801778_m1	*IFNΓ*	Mm00448234_m1	*POLB*
Mm00516004_m1	*HMOX1*	Mm00507805_g1	*APEX1*
Mm00599683_m1	*CD3E*	Mm00449156_m1	*UNG*
		Mm00500154_m1	*PARP1*
		Mm00447872_m1	*MPG*
DNA DAMAGE RESPONSE		DAMAGE AVOIDANCE	
Mm00458141_m1	*TRP53inp1*	Mm00599710_m1	*NUDT1*

line, Figure 5B) as well as in the mantle zone (dotted line, Figure 5B). No difference was observed between the two genotypes in the relatively low number of Foxp3$^+$ cells scattered in the lamina propria and intraepithelia (Figure 5C).

In summary, the extent of inflammation associated with chronic DSS exposure differs quantitatively and qualitatively between wt and *Mutyh*$^{-/-}$ mice. In particular, the marked lymphoid hyperplasia in *Mutyh*$^{-/-}$ mice is associated with very low levels of CD4+/Foxp3$^+$ Tregs.

Gene expression in chronic colitis

The progression from acute to chronic colitis was associated with more limited changes in inflammatory response genes. In wt mice there were fewer genes with significantly altered expression (3 *versus* 9). Only IFNγ, NOS2 and NQO1 ($P \leq 0.01$) were up-regulated after chronic DSS treatment (Figure 6A). The extent of induction was also lower compared to acute colitis. Examples include IFNγ (7- *versus* 24-fold) and NOS2 (3- *versus* 10-fold)(Figure 3A and Figure 6A). None of these genes showed a statistically significant change in *Mutyh*$^{-/-}$ mice, although a trend towards up-regulation of IFNγ, IL-12a, IL-6 was observed (data not shown).

In wt mice with chronic colitis, IL-23a, IL-13, NF-kB2, PTGS1, SMAD3 and SMAD7 ($P \leq 0.05$) were significantly down-regulated, with the largest variations affecting the expression of IL-23a and IL-13 (100- and 10-fold) (Figure 6A).

A smaller subset of genes was down-regulated in the colon of *Mutyh*$^{-/-}$ mice (7 *versus* 20 in wt mice), and these included SMAD3, SMAD7, APEX1, LIG3, MLH1, LIG1 and MRE11 ($P \leq 0.05$) (Figure 6B).

Overall, the differences in inflammation between acute and chronic colitis are paralleled by differences in the expression of pro-inflammatory cytokines. In contrast the down-regulation of DNA repair genes is largely unaffected by the shift from acute to chronic colitis. The response of *Mutyh*$^{-/-}$ mice to a chronic DSS exposure is more restricted with altered expression of fewer genes in both categories.

Gene expression data were also analyzed by another statistical method, Principal Component Analysis (PCA). This unsupervised learning approach investigates natural co-expression structures (components) of the analysed genes. A significant *a posteriori* discrimination between samples from treated and untreated mice was accomplished by the first five components as shown by the analysis of variance on the component scores (Figure S1). The global concordance of analyses gene-by-gene and by a multi-dimensional perspective is a robust proof-of-concept of the existence of strict links between DNA repair and the inflammatory response in terms of gene expression.

DNA oxidation and microsatellite instability

The levels of DNA 8-oxoG in the colon of wt mice increased 1.7-fold after chronic DSS treatment (Figure 7A). The increased

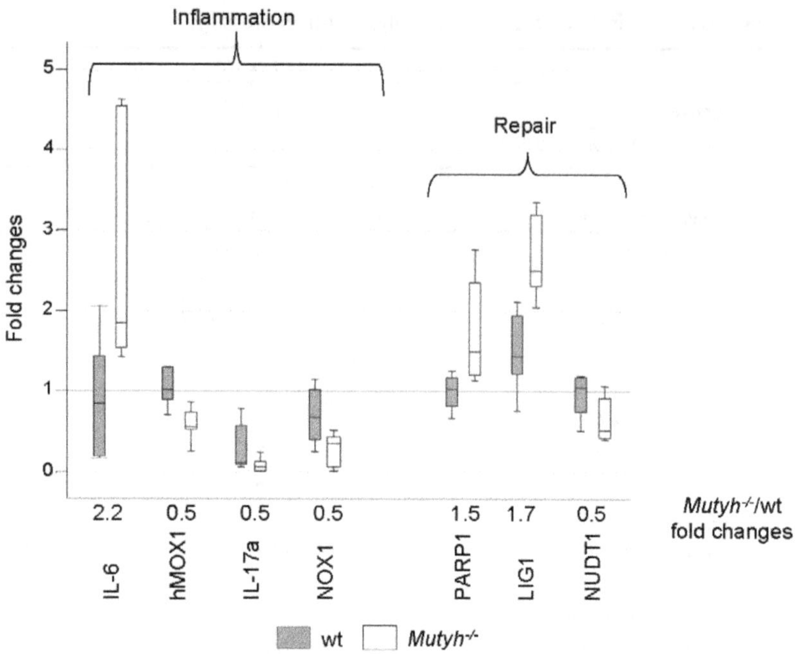

Figure 2. Expression levels of selected genes in untreated wt and *Mutyh−/−* mice. Box Plots of fold-changes in the expression of genes are shown for untreated wt and *Mutyh−/−* mice (8 and 7 animals, respectively). For each gene, fold-change ratios between *Mutyh−/−* and wt groups are also displayed. A representative untreated wt colon sample was chosen as calibrator. Only genes with statistically significant variations in the expression levels are shown. wt (closed symbol), *Mutyh−/−* mice (open symbols).

accumulation in the DNA of *Mutyh*$^{-/-}$ mice was 2-fold higher (Figure 7A).

MSI in colon DNA was investigated using four microsatellite probes (*Aa006036, L24372, D1Mit62, D6Mit59*) (Figure 7B). A very limited MSI was identified in DSS-treated animals at two loci (*Aa006036* and *D1Mit62*). There were no apparent difference between wt and *Mutyh*$^{-/-}$ mice in this regard.

These findings indicate that chronic DSS treatment results in a more pronounced accumulation of 8-oxoG in colon DNA of *Mutyh*$^{-/-}$ mice than in their wt counterparts. This increased amount of oxidized DNA bases is not accompanied by widespread MSI in both genetic backgrounds.

Discussion

In this study of the effect of Mutyh deficiency on the inflammatory response, we used the DSS mouse model for IBDs. In view of the known substrate specificity of Mutyh [3] and the association between DSS treatment and increased levels of DNA 8-oxoG [16,17], we measured this lesion in colon DNA of wt and *Mutyh*$^{-/-}$ mice. Several cycles of DSS were required to significantly increase 8-oxoG levels in wt animals whereas the accumulation of the lesion was evident in *Mutyh*$^{-/-}$ mice after a single DSS cycle and the levels increased further with chronic exposures. These results indicate that Mutyh is an important barrier against accumulation of DNA damage during oxidative stress associated with UC. High levels of oxidative DNA damage have also been reported in UC-inflamed human colonic mucosa [19] accompanied by altered expression of MUTYH [13].

Accumulation of DNA 8-oxoG was not accompanied by high levels of MSI in either wt or Mutyh-defective mice, even after prolonged periods (6 months). These findings are in agreement with reports that chronic oxidative stress being associated with low-MSI [1].

DSS treatment caused down-regulation of DNA repair genes involved in different DNA repair pathways. We did not observe any DNA repair gene up-regulation. This contrasts to the up-regulation of some BER genes (*APE1, AAG*) in human IBDs [14]. Whether this is due to differences between the mouse model and human IBDs remains to be clarified.

The most striking observation of our study is the significant and unexpected role of Mutyh in modulating the inflammatory response occurring in DSS-induced colitis [20]. Histopathological examination and gene expression analyses concur that *Mutyh*$^{-/-}$ mice are less prone to the induction of acute colitis by DSS. Mutyh modulates DSS-mediated inflammation both quantitatively and qualitatively. Thus, the reduced inflammation in *Mutyh*$^{-/-}$ mice is reflected in fewer changes in gene expression as well as in reduced induction of the pro-inflammatory cytokines IL-17a, IL-1b, IL-6 and no variation in IFNγ. The expression of inducible nitric oxide synthase NOS*2* - an important mediator of intestinal inflammation in this colitis model [21] - is also reduced. The qualitative difference in the inflammatory response is exemplified by the prevalence of Th17 *vs* Th-1/Th-17 response [22] and suggests that Mutyh might act as an inflammatory/immune system modulator affecting DSS-mediated inflammation both quantitatively and qualitatively. The anti-inflammatory IL-13 cytokine was significantly down-regulated in both wt and *Mutyh*$^{-/-}$ mice. This indicates that Mutyh deficiency, while contributing significantly to the induction of the pro-inflammatory response to DSS, does not significantly affect anti-inflammatory mechanisms.

Chronic inflammatory stimuli underlined the involvement of Mutyh in the inflammatory response. Chronic colitis in *Mutyh*$^{-/-}$ mice was accompanied by an obvious lymphoid hyperplasia, with lymphocytes organized in follicles often characterized by the presence of large GCs. Similarly to previous reports [23], progression from acute to chronic colitis in wt mice was associated with a reduced expression of IFNγ and IL-6, accompanied by an

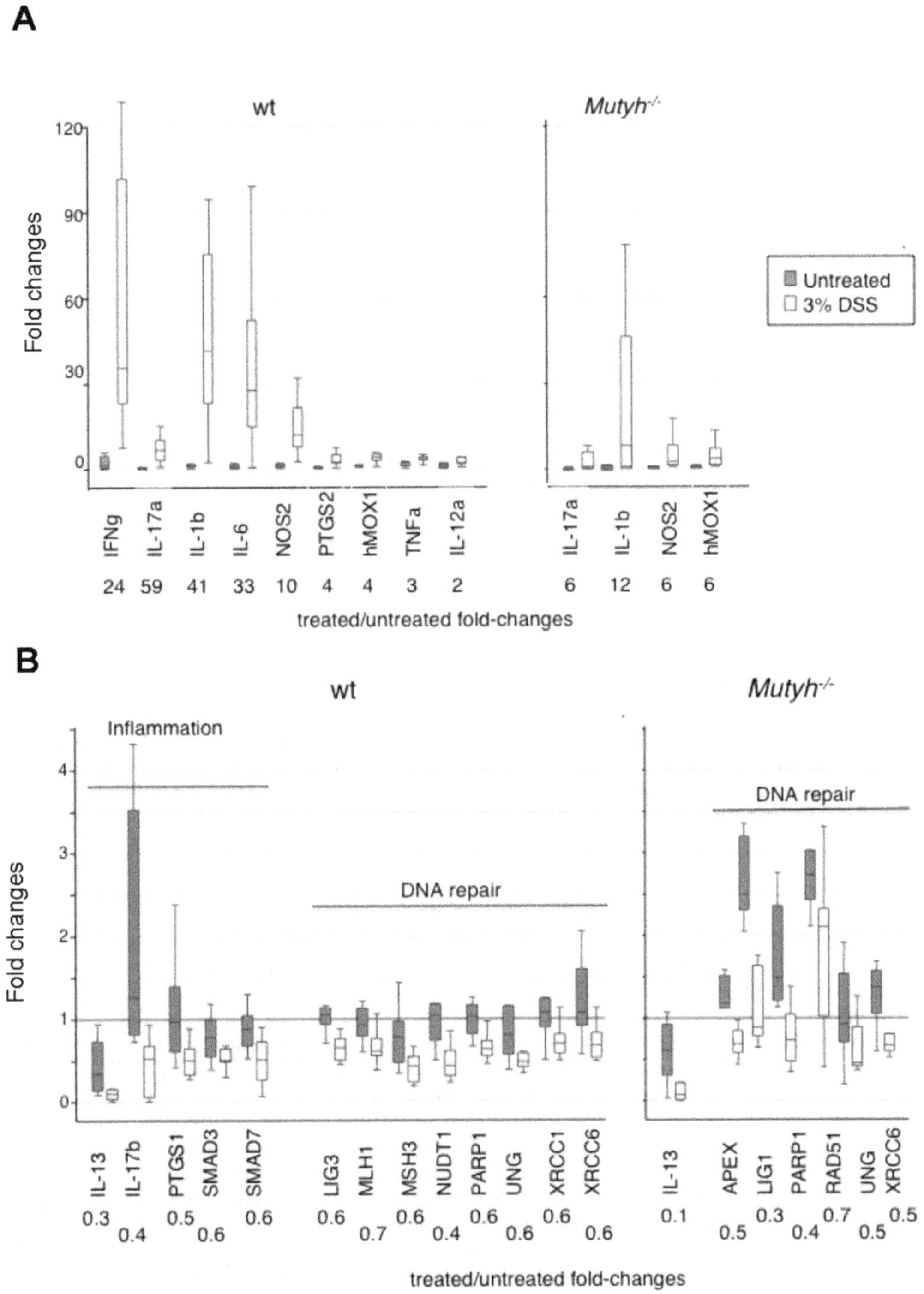

Figure 3. Changes in gene expression induced by one DSS cycle. Box Plots of fold-changes in the expression of up-regulated (Panel A) or down-regulated genes (Panel B) for untreated and DSS-treated wt (left) (8 and 12 animals, respectively) and *Mutyh−/−* mice (right)(7 and 12 animals, respectively). For each gene fold-change ratios between treated and untreated groups are also displayed. A representative untreated wt colon sample was chosen as calibrator. Only genes with statistically significant variations in the expression levels are shown.

increased (albeit not significant) IL-10 levels. In contrast chronically-treated *Mutyh*$^{-/-}$ mice show a trend towards up-regulation of IFNγ, IL12a and IL-6 suggesting that the chronic inflammation occurring in these mice is characterized by the persistence of cytokines dominating the acute phase. Taken together these data suggest that Mutyh somehow contributes to the cellular adaptation towards chronic inflammatory stimuli.

This view is supported by the striking decrease in CD4+/ Foxp3$^+$ Tregs in chronically treated *Mutyh*$^{-/-}$ mice. Tregs control the bacteria-driven inflammatory response in the gastrointestinal tract [24,25]. In experimental models of colitis, the appearance of increased numbers of Foxp3$^+$ cells precedes the spontaneous resolution of inflammation, whereas a low number is associated with persistence of inflammation [26]. Thus intense lymphoid

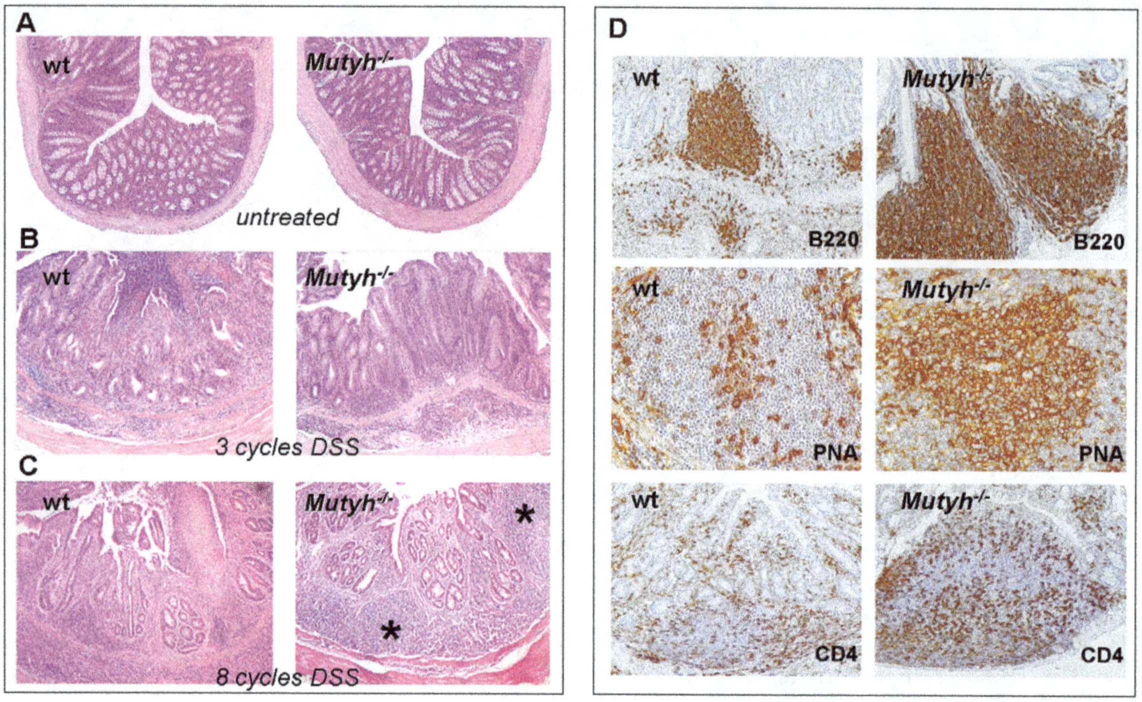

Figure 4. Histological analysis of colon from untreated or DSS-treated wt and *Mutyh−/−* mice. After three DSS cycles (Panel B), wt mice show a severe acute UC with several lesions of the glandular epithelium, ulcers and a marked increase of reactive cells. The colitis in *Mutyh−/−* mice is less aggressive with few ulcers and a moderate increase of reactive cells (100× magnification). After eight DSS cycles (Panel C), chronic UC in *Mutyh−/−* is less severe than in wt mice. In *Mutyh−/−* mice numerous and ample lymphoid follicles (asterisks) are present in the lamina propria or between this and submucosa (100× magnification). After eight DSS cycles (Panel D), lymphoid hyperplasia occurring in Mutyh−/− mice is formed by B220+ cells, PNA+ GCs filled with centroblasts and centrocytes and CD4+ T lymphocytes, mostly located around follicles and in the interfollicular zones. In wt animals the number of B220+ cells, PNA+ GCs and CD4+ T lymphocyte is lower than in Mutyh−/− (B220 and CD4: 200× magnification; PNA: 400× magnification).

hyperplasia observed in the colon of in *Mutyh*$^{-/-}$ mice is consistent with the observed reduction in the number of Tregs. Of interest, the reduction of CD4+/Foxp3^{+} cells in the follicles might be the conversion of Foxp3^{+} T cells into follicular (CD4+/Foxp3^{-}) helper T cells, as recently described in mouse Peyer's patches [27]. These follicular CD4+/Foxp3^{-} helper T cells might cooperate with B cells in inducing the formation of GCs in colon mucosa and contribute to establishing and chronically-maintaining the observed lymphoid hyperplasia.

A limited set of genes was also affected by Mutyh inactivation in untreated animals. The decreased IL-17a level together with an increased IL-6 observed in *Mutyh*$^{-/-}$ in comparison to wt animals suggest that Mutyh germline inactivation might modify both the immune response to external stimuli and baseline protective immunity.

The limited inflammatory response induced by various inflammatory stimuli (LPS-induced endotoxic shock, streptozotocin-induced Type I diabetes, oxazolone-induced contact hypersensitivity and *Helicobacter pylori*-induced gastritis) in mice in which Ogg1, the DNA glycosylase involved in the removal of 8-oxoG [28], is inactive is also consistent with the involvement of oxidized DNA guanine in inflammation [29,30]. In addition long exposures to DSS (15 cycles) significantly increased adenocarcinoma development in the colon of *Ogg1*$^{-/-}$ in comparison to wt mice, even in the absence of carcinogen treatment [31]. This appears to be a specific response to oxidative DNA damage and other DNA repair-defective animals (*Aag*$^{-/-}$, *Msh2*$^{-/-}$ and *Mlh1*$^{-/-}$ mice) are more susceptible to colorectal carcingenesis with no apparent changes in the inflammatory response [17,32,33].

The anti-inflammatory activity exerted *in vivo* by 8-oxoGTP or 7,8-dihydro-8-oxo-deoxyguanosine (but not by 8-oxoG) indicates that some oxidation by-products can modulate immune functions [34,35]. The mechanism by which Mutyh influences the inflammatory response remains however to be ascertained. It is possible that repair intermediates (apurinic sites and/or single strand breaks) generated by the removal of A incorporated opposite DNA 8-oxoG might act as a signal triggering/amplifying the cascade of inflammation processes. Supporting evidence of a major role of repair intermediates in mediating several biological processes is the block in cell proliferation and activation of cell death induced by accumulation of abasic DNA damage in APE/REF1-defective human cells [36]. Alternatively Mutyh might act as a fine tuner of the redox function of the APE/REF1 endonuclease. This enzyme displays a powerful redox activity [37] that regulates the expression of multiple transcription factors involved in the regulation of the immune and pro-inflammatory responses [38,39]. Finally Mutyh might play a role in cellular functions needed for an efficient native and adaptive immunity and its inactivation might result in an impairment of correct cellular maturation and ability to respond to inflammatory stimuli. These functions might not be necessarily mutually exclusive and could be the link between processing of DNA damage and inflammation processes.

In conclusion we show here that Mutyh activity is needed for eliciting the intense inflammatory response following an acute oxidative stress and is also involved in its attenuation during the chronic phase, probably by affecting the local occurrence of regulatory T cells. In view of the cancer prone phenotype

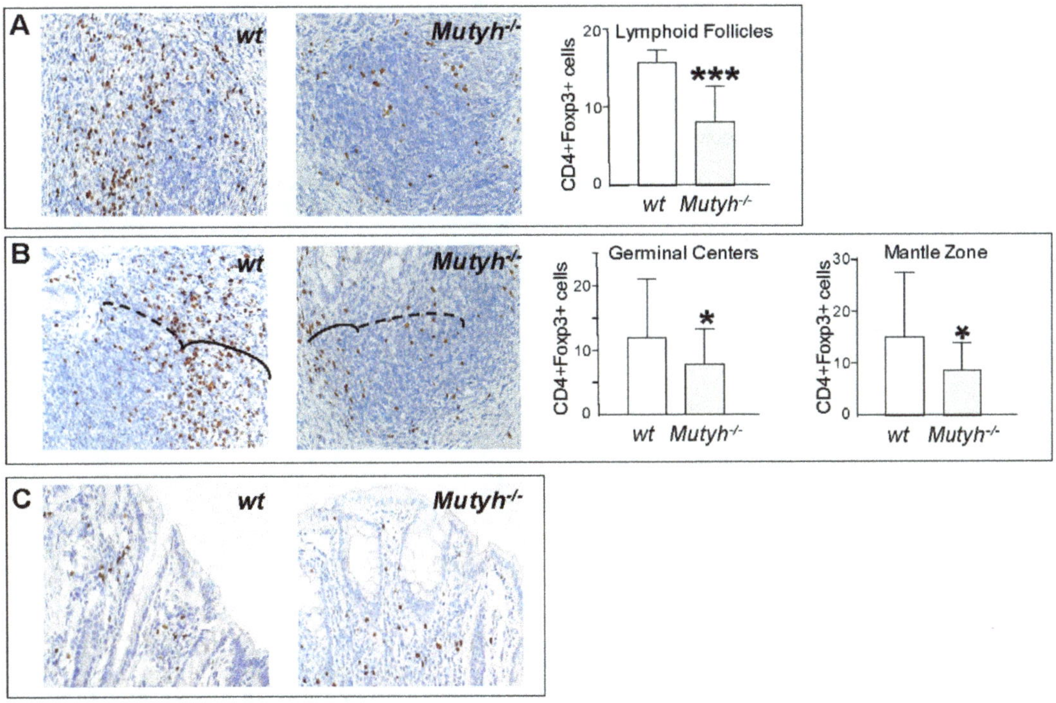

Figure 5. CD4+ Foxp3^{+} cells quantisation in colon samples from mice exposed to eight DSS cycles. Following eight DSS cycles, *Mutyh*$^{-/-}$ mice animals show a reduction in the number of Foxp3^{+} cells in lymphoid follicles without active GCs (A), in GCs (solid line in B) or in the Mantle Zone (dotted line in B) in comparison to wt mice. No differences were found in the Foxp3^{+} cells scattered in the lamina propria (C). The number of CD4+ Foxp3^{+} cells is reported as the number of CD4+ Foxp3^{+} cells/number of Mantle Zone, or GCs, or Lymphoid Follicles (400× magnification). Unpaired t test. * $p < 0.05$, *** $p < 0.005$.

associated with inactivation of the human *MUTYH* gene, it is tempting to speculate that the inability of *Mutyh* - defective mice to properly resolve the acute cellular response to external inflammatory stimuli and the consequent chronic persistence of the response might also plays a role in colorectal carcinogenesis in humans.

Materials and Methods

Animals

Animal care followed the directives of the EC Council (86/609/EEC). The experimental protocol was approved by the National Committee of the Italian Ministry of Health (authorization No. 162/2008-B). Mice were housed under pathogen-free conditions in the Laboratory Animal Services of Istituto Superiore di Sanità. *Mutyh*$^{-/-}$ mice were kindly provided by J.H. Miller [40]. Genotypes were confirmed by polymerase chain reaction of tail DNA using specific oligonucleotide primers [7]. The experimental protocol was approved by the Italian Ministry of Health. Acute colitis was induced in 10 week-old mice by treatment with 3%DSS (MW: ~36,000–50,000, ICN Pharmaceuticals, Costa Mesa, CA, USA) in drinking water for 1 week followed by 2 weeks of tap water (1 cycle). The control groups were given ordinary tap water during the whole period. Body weights were recorded daily. Chronic colitis was induced by 8 cycles of 1.5%DSS treatment. For histology and immunohistochemistry, cross-sections of colon were dipped in Tissue Freezing Medium (Electron Microscopy Sciences, Hatfield, PA, USA) and kept at −80°C or fixed in periodate-lysine-paraformaldehyde (PLP) [41]. For DNA and RNA isolation, tissue sections were minced and snap frozen in liquid nitrogen within a few minutes after euthanasia (cervical dislocation).

Histology and immunohistochemistry

Cryostatic sections were stained with hematoxylin/eosin or processed for immunohistochemistry. Sections were incubated with anti-mouse antibodies against CD4 (Abcam, Cambridge UK), CD8 (Oxford Biotechnology, Cambridge, UK), CD45R/B220 (a subset of mouse CD45 isoforms predominantly expressed on B lymphocytes; BD Pharmingen, San Diego, CA, USA), CD11b (a marker of monocyte/macrophage lineage; BD Pharmingen), PAX-5 (a marker for B lineage-committed cells; BD Biosciences, San Jose, CA, USA), Foxp3 (e-Bioscience, San Diego CA, USA). To immunostain Germinal Centers (GC), the sections were incubated with biotinylated peanut agglutinin lectin (PNA), whose binding to a common carbohydrate sequence distinguishes monocytes, macrophages and particularly centroblasts (Vector Laboratories, Burlingame, CA, USA). In CD4/Foxp3 double immunostaining experiments, binding of the primary Ab (anti CD4) in the first label was detected using avidin-biotin alkaline phosphatase (Thermo Scientific, Rockford, IL, USA) and Ferangi Blu (Biocare, Concord, CA, USA) as chromogen. Before the second staining with anti-Foxp3, frozen tissues were subjected to Ag retrieval by heat treatment in citrate (pH 6) buffer. The second label was detected using an indirect avidin-biotin phosphatase (Thermo Scientific) and Vulcan fast Red (Biocare) as a chromogen.

Nucleic Acids extraction

DNA and RNA were extracted from colon tissues using the Puregene DNA Purification Kit (Gentra Systems, MN, USA) and QIAGEN RNeasy Midi Kit (QIAGEN, Valencia, CA, USA) according to the manufacturer's protocol. Briefly, colon sections were placed in 1.5 ml tubes of QIAGEN RLT® buffer

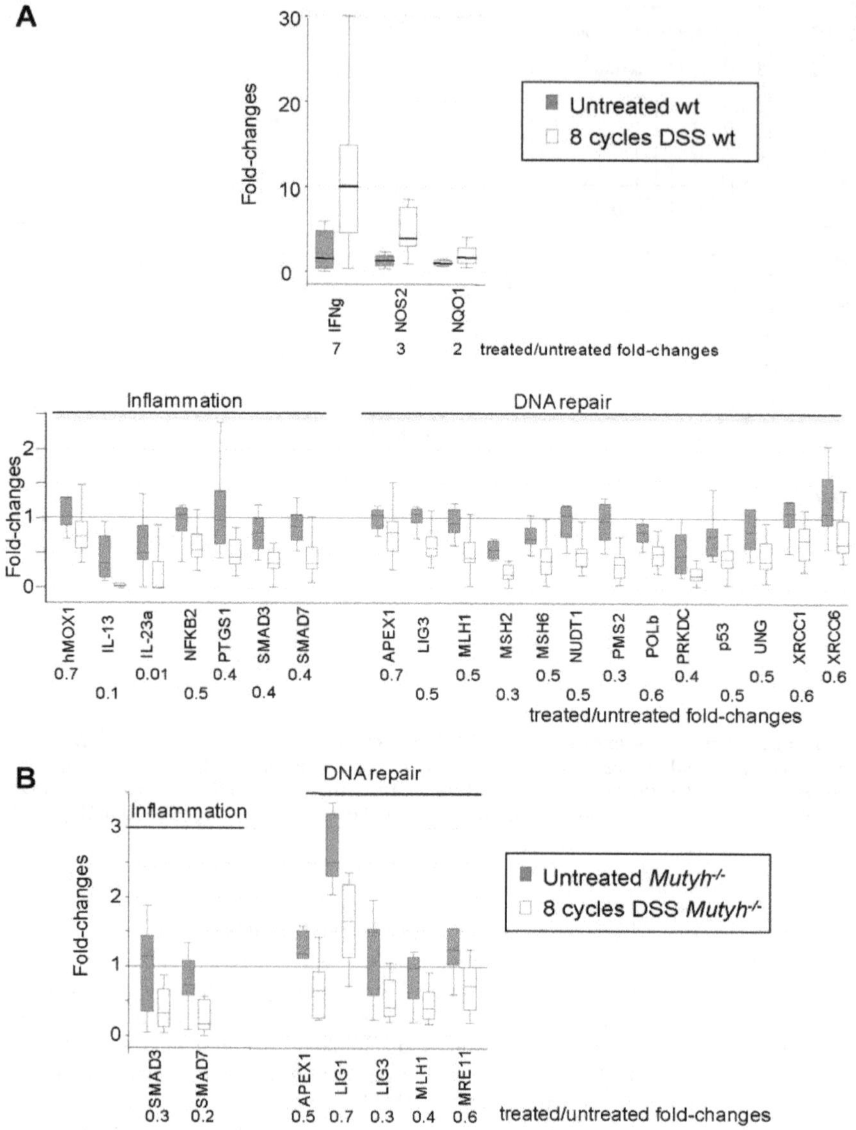

Figure 6. Changes in gene expression induced by eight DSS cycles. Panel A. Box Plots of fold-changes in the expression of up-regulated (top) and down-regulated (bottom) genes are shown for 8 untreated and 16 DSS-treated wt mice. Panel B. Box Plots of fold-changes in the expression of down-regulated genes are shown for 7 untreated and 8 DSS-treated *Mutyh*$^{-/-}$ mice.

and homogenized using the QIAGEN homogenizer. Homogenates were further processed according to the standard protocol for animal tissues. To determine purity, concentration and total yield of RNA samples, absorbance was determined spectrophotometrically at 260 and 280 nm and verified by the Agilent Bioanalyzer (Santa Clara, CA, USA) according to manufacturer's instructions.

8-oxoG determinations

8-oxodG was measured by HPLC/EC as previously described [42]. Following DNA extraction, RNase treatment and enzymatic hydrolysis, DNA hydrolysate was analysed by HPLC/EC (Coulochem I, Esa, Chelmsford, MA, USA) using a C18 250×46 mm 5 µm Uptishere column (Interchim, San Pedro, CA, USA) equipped with a C18 guard column. The eluent was 50 mM ammonium acetate, pH 5.5, containing 9% methanol, at a flow rate of 0.7 ml/min. Deoxyguanosine was measured in the same run of corresponding 8-oxodG with a UV detector (model SPD-2A; Shimadzu, Kyoto, Japan) at 256 nm.

Microsatellite instability

For analysis of microsatellite instability (MSI), genomic DNA, isolated from the colon mucosa and the tail of the same mice, was analysed at mononucleotide *L24372*, *Aa006036* and dinucleotide *D1Mit62* and *D6Mit59* microsatellites. Primers, labelled with the fluorescent compound FAM were previously described [43,44]. PCR reactions were carried out in a reaction buffer containing DNA (100 ng), primers (2 pmol/µl), dNTPs (200 mM), 0,5 U/µlTaq polimerase (Applied Biosystems, Foster City, CA, USA). After denaturation (95°C for 2 min), DNA was amplified by 25 cycles (30 s at 95°C, 30 s at 55°C, 30 s at 72°C). Amplification products (10 µl) were digested with 0,4 U/µl T4 DNA polymerase (Roche Diagnostic, Indianapolis, IN, USA)(30 min, 37°C) denatured in deionized formamide (2 min, 95°C) and analyzed with an

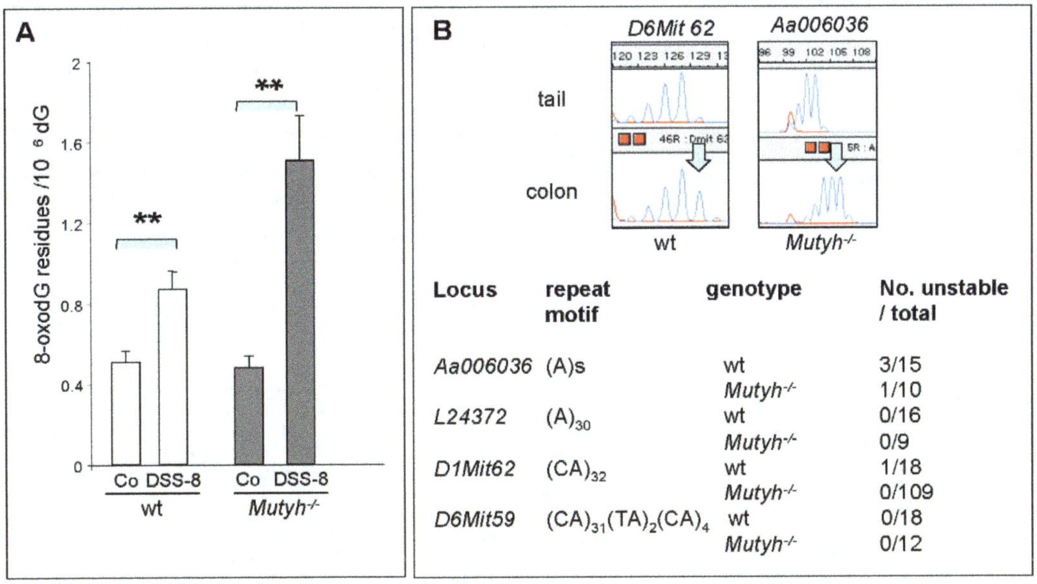

Figure 7. DNA 8-oxoG and MSI levels in colonic mucosa of mice exposed to eight DSS cycles. Panel A. Data are the mean ± SE of measurements from wt (open bars) and *Mutyh*$^{-/-}$ mice (closed bars) (20 animals per genotype) ** P<0.05.Panel B. The numbers of mice with MSI are shown together with examples of unstable *D6Mit62* and *Aa006036* loci. The arrows indicate the shift in the highest peak.

ABI Prism 310 automatic sequencer by the GeneScan software (Applied Biosystems).

Gene Expression Analysis

Gene expression was analysed using low-density arrays. Briefly, total RNA was converted to single stranded cDNA by reverse transcriptase and High-Capacity cDNA Archive Kit (Applied Biosystems, Foster City, CA, USA). cDNA was used for determination of gene expression level using TaqMan Low Density Arrays (Applied Biosystems). Relative quantification values have been normalized to the hypoxanthine phosphoribosyltransferase 1 housekeeping gene and then normalized to a calibrator sample (untreated wild-type colon sample) according to the $2^{-\Delta\Delta Ct}$ comparative threshold cycle (C_t) method. Amplification was performed with ABI-Prism-7900 Sequence Detection System (Applied Biosystems) and mRNA was quantified using the CT method of relative quantification using SDS software version 2.2.1 (Applied Biosystems).

Computational analyses

To analyse differences between experimental groups at single-gene expression level, the STATA statistical package was used [45]. To verify the independence of samples, non-parametric two-sample Wilcoxon rank-sum (Mann-Whitney) test for unmatched data was adopted. Genes were ranked on the basis of the discriminative ability of their *P*-values and data are shown as fold-change ratios between different subgroups with box-whisker plots graphically showing variations in gene expression levels among experimental groups. To perform PCA, SAS/STAT (http://www.sas.com/technologies/analytics/statistics/stat/index.html) was used. The effect of genotype, treatment and the mutual interaction of these two variation sources on the component scores were assessed by Analysis of Variance (General Linear Model, SAS).

Author Contributions

Conceived and designed the experiments: IC TP M. Boirivant PM M. Bignami. Performed the experiments: IC TP GDL PD FC II AB. Analyzed the data: IC TP GDL PD FC II AG AB M. Boirivant PM M. Bignami. Wrote the paper: IC PM M. Bignami.

References

1. Risques RA, Rabinovitch PS, Brentnall TA (2006) Cancer surveillance in inflammatory bowel disease: new molecular approaches. Curr Opin Gastroenterol 22: 382–390.
2. Slupska MM, Luther WM, Chiang JH, Yang H, Miller JH (1999) Functional expression of hMYH, a human homolog of the Escherichia coli MutY protein. J Bacteriol 181: 6210–6213.
3. David SS, O'Shea VL, Kundu S (2007) Base-excision repair of oxidative DNA damage. Nature 447: 941–950.
4. D'Errico M, Parlanti E, Dogliotti E (2008) Mechanism of oxidative DNA damage repair and relevance to human pathology. Mutat Res 659: 4–14.
5. Ohtsubo T, Nishioka K, Imaiso Y, Iwai S, Shimokawa H, et al. (2000) Identification of human MutY homolog (hMYH) as a repair enzyme for 2-hydroxyadenine in DNA and detection of multiple forms of hMYH located in nuclei and mitochondria. Nucleic Acids Res 28: 1355–1364.
6. Hirano S, Tominaga Y, Ichinoe A, Ushijima Y, Tsuchimoto D, et al. (2003) Mutator phenotyper of MUTYH-null Mouse embryonic stem cells. J Biol Chem 278: 38121–38124.
7. Russo MT, De Luca G, Casorelli I, Degan P, Molatore S, et al. (2009) Role of MUTYH and MSH2 in the control of oxidative DNA damage, genetic instability, and tumorigenesis. Cancer Res 69: 4372–4379.
8. Sakamoto K, Tominaga Y, Yamauchi K, Nakatsu Y, Sakumi K, et al. (2007) MUTYH-null mice are susceptible to spontaneous and oxidative stress induced intestinal tumorigenesis. Cancer Res 67: 6599–6604.
9. Sieber OM, Howarth KM, Thirlwell C, Rowan A, Mandir N, et al. (2004) Myh deficiency enhances intestinal tumorigenesis in multiple intestinal neoplasia (ApcMin/+) mice. Cancer Res 64: 8876–8881.
10. Al-Tassan N, Chmiel NH, Maynard J, Fleming N, Livingston AL, et al. (2002) Inherited variants of MYH associated with somatic G:C>T:A mutations in colorectal tumors. Nat Genet 30: 227–232.

11. Jones S, Emmerson P, Maynard J, Best JM, Jordan S, et al. (2002) Biallelic germline mutations in MYH predispose to multiple colorectal adenoma and somatic G:C>T:A mutations. Hum Mol Genet 11: 2961–2967.
12. Lipton L, Halford SE, Johnson V, Novelli MR, Jones A, et al. (2003) Carcinogenesis in MYH-associated polyposis follows a distinct genetic pathway. Cancer Res 63: 7595–7599.
13. Gushima M, Hirahashi M, Matsumoto T, Fujita K, Fujisawa R, et al. (2009) Altered expression of MUTYH and an increase in 8-hydroxydeoxyguanosine are early events in ulcerative colitis-associated carcinogenesis. J Pathol 219: 77–86.
14. Hofseth LJ, Khan MA, Ambrose M, Nikolayeva O, Xu-Welliver M, et al. (2003) The adaptive imbalance in base excision-repair enzymes generates microsatellite instability in chronic inflammation. J Clin Invest 112: 1887–1894.
15. Wirtz S, Neufert C, Weigmann B, Neurath MF (2007) Chemically induced mouse models of intestinal inflammation. Nat Protoc 2: 541–546.
16. Tardieu D, Jaeg JP, Cadet J, Embvani E, Corpet DE, et al. (1998) Dextran sulfate enhances the level of an oxidative DNA damage biomarker, 8-oxo-7,8-dihydro-2′-deoxyguanosine, in rat colonic mucosa. Cancer Lett 134: 1–5.
17. Meira LB, Bugni JM, Green SL, Lee CW, Pang B, et al. (2008) DNA damage induced by chronic inflammation contributes to colon carcinogenesis in mice. J Clin Invest 118: 2516–2525.
18. Russo MT, De Luca G, Degan P, Parlanti E, Dogliotti E, et al. (2004) Accumulation of the oxidative base lesion 8-hydroxyguanine in DNA of tumor-prone mice defective in both the Myh and Ogg1 DNA glycosylases. Cancer Res 64: 4411–4414.
19. D'Incà R, Cardin R, Benazzato L, Angriman I, Martines D, et al. (2004) Oxidative DNA damage in the mucosa of ulcerative colitis increases with disease duration and dysplasia. Inflamm Bowel Dis 10: 23–27.
20. Egger B, Bajaj-Elliott M, MacDonald TT, Inglin R, Eysselein VE, et al. (2000) Characterisation of acute murine dextran sodium sulphate colitis: cytokine profile and dose dependency. Digestion 62: 240–248.
21. Beck PL, Li Y, Wong J, Chen CW, Keenan CM, et al. (2007) Inducible nitric oxide synthase from bone marrow-derived cells plays a critical role in regulating colonic inflammation. Gastroenterology 132: 1778–1790.
22. Ito R, Kita M, Shin-Ya M, Kishida T, Urano A, et al. (2008) Involvement of IL-17A in the pathogenesis of DSS-induced colitis in mice. Biochemical and Biophysical Research Communications 377: 12–16.
23. Eijkelkamp N, Heijnen CJ, Lucas A, Premont RT, Elsenbruch S, et al. (2007) G protein-coupled receptor kinase 6 controls chronicity and severity of dextran sodium sulphate-induced colitis in mice. Gut 56: 847–854.
24. de Zoeten EF, Hancock WW (2008) Strategies to cure experimental autoimmune colitis using antigen-specific Foxp3+ regulatory T cells. Gastroenterology 134: 2171–2174.
25. Singh B, Read S, Asseman C, Malmström V, Mottet C, et al. (2001) Control of intestinal inflammation by regulatory T cells. Immunol Rev 182: 190–200.
26. Alex P, Zachos NC, Nguyen T, Gonzales L, Chen TE, et al. (2009) Distinct cytokine patterns identified from multiplex profiles of murine DSS and TNBS-induced colitis. Inflamm Bowel Dis 15: 341–352.
27. Tsuji M, Komatsu N, Kawamoto S, Suzuki K, Kanagawa O, et al. (2009) Preferential generation of follicular B helper T cells from Foxp3+ T cells in gut Peyer's patches. Science 323: 1488–1492.
28. Klungland A, Rosewell I, Hollenbach S, Larsen E, Daly G, et al. (1999) Accumulation of premutagenic DNA lesions in mice defective in removal of oxidative base damage. Proc Natl Acad Sci U S A 96: 13300–13305.
29. Mabley J, Pacher P, Deb A, Wallace R, Elder R, et al. (2005) Potential role for 8-oxoguanine DNA glycosylase in regulating inflammation. FASEB J 19: 290–292.
30. Touati E, Michel V, Thiberge JM, Avé P, Huerre M, et al. (2006) Deficiency in OGG1 protects against inflammation and mutagenic effects associated with H. pylori infection in mouse. Helicobacter 11: 494–505.
31. Liao J, Seril DN, Lu GG, Zhang M, Toyokuni S, et al. (2008) Increased susceptibility of chronic ulcerative colitis-induced carcinoma development in DNA repair enzyme Ogg1 deficient mice. Mol Carcinog 47: 638–46.
32. Kohonen-Corish MR, Daniel JJ, te Riele H, Buffinton GD, Dahlstrom JE (2002) Susceptibility of Msh2-deficient mice to inflammation-associated colorectal tumors. Cancer Res 62: 2092–2097.
33. Taniguchi K, Kakinuma S, Tokairin Y, Arai M, Kohno H, et al. (2006) Mild inflammation accelerates colon carcinogenesis in Mlh1-deficient mice. Oncology 71: 124–130.
34. Choi S, Choi HH, Lee SH, Ko SH, You HJ, et al. (2007) Anti-inflammatory effects of 8-hydroxy-2′-deoxyguanosine on lipopolysaccharide-induced inflammation via Rac suppression in Balb/c mice. Free Radic Biol Med 43: 1594–603.
35. Kim HJ, Yoon SH, Ryu HO, Yoon BH, Choi S, et al. (2007) 8-oxo-7,8-dihydroguanosine triphosphate(8-oxoGTP) down-regulates respiratory burst of neutrophils by antagonizing GTP toward Rac, a small GTP binding protein. Free Radic Res 41: 655–62.
36. Fung H, Demple B (2005) A Vital Role for Ape1/Ref1 Protein Short Article in Repairing Spontaneous DNA Damage in Human Cells. Mol Cell 17: 463–470.
37. Xanthoudakis S, Smeyne RJ, Wallace JD, Curran T (1996) The redox/DNA repair protein, Ref-1, is essential for early embryonic development in mice. Proc Natl Acad Sci U S A 93: 8919–8923.
38. Luo M, He H, Kelley MR, Georgiadis M (2009) Redox Regulation of DNA Repair: Implications for Human Health and Cancer Therapeutic Development. Antioxid Redox Signal. [Epub ahead of print].
39. Ando K, Hirao S, Kabe Y, Ogura Y, Sato I, et al. (2008) A new APE1/Ref-1-dependent pathway leading to reduction of NF-kappaB and AP-1, and activation of their DNA-binding activity. Nucleic Acids Res 36: 4327–4336.
40. Xie Y, Yang H, Cunanan C, Okamoto K, Shibata D, et al. (2004) Deficiencies in mouse Myh and Ogg1 result in tumor predisposition and G to T mutations in codon 12 of the K-ras oncogene in lung tumors. Cancer Res 64: 3096–3102.
41. McLean IW, Nakane PK (1974) Periodate-lysine-paraformaldehyde fixative. A new fixation for immunoelectron microscopy. J Histochem Cytochem 12: 1077–1083.
42. Chiera F, Meccia E, Degan P, Aquilina G, Pietraforte D, et al. (2008) Overexpression of human NOX1 complex induces genome instability in mammalian cells. Free Radic Biol Med 44: 332–342.
43. Oda S, Maehara Y, Ikeda Y, Oki E, Egashira A, et al. (2005) Two modes of microsatellite instability in human cancer: differential connection of defective DNA mismatch repair to dinucleotide repeat instability. Nucleic Acids Research 33: 1628–1636.
44. Yao X, Buermeyer AB, Narayanan L, Tran D, Baker SM, et al. (1999) Different mutator phenotypes in Mlh1- versus Pms2-deficient mice. Pro. Natl. Acad. Sci. USA 96: 6850–6855.
45. StataCorp (2003) Stata Statistical Software: release 8.1. College StationTX: Stata Corporation, Cary, Illinois, USA.

Association of Single Nucleotide Polymorphisms of IL23R and IL17 with Ulcerative Colitis Risk in a Chinese Han Population

Pengli Yu[1], Fangcheng Shen[1], Xiaofei Zhang[1], Risheng Cao[1], Xiaodan Zhao[1], Pengfei Liu[2], Huiming Tu[3], Xiaozhong Yang[4], Ruihua Shi[1*], Hongjie Zhang[1*]

1 Department of Gastroenterology, the First Affiliated Hospital of Nanjing Medical University, Nanjing, China, 2 Department of Gastroenterology, the People's Hospital of Jiangyin, Jiangyin, China, 3 Department of Gastroenterology, the Fourth People's Hospital of Wuxi, Wuxi, China, 4 Department of Gastroenterology, the First Hospital of Huaian, Huaian, China

Abstract

Background: Previous studies implicated that IL23R and IL17 genes play an important role in autoimmune inflammation. Genome-wide association studies have also identified multiple single nucleotide polymorphisms (SNPs) in the IL23R gene region associated with inflammatory bowel diseases. This study examined the association of IL23R and IL17A gene SNPs with ulcerative colitis susceptibility in a population in China.

Methodology: A total of 270 ulcerative colitis and 268 healthy controls were recruited for the analyses of 23 SNPs in the IL23R and IL17A regions. Genomic DNA was extracted and analysis of these 23 SNPs using ligase detection reaction allelic (LDR) technology. Genotype and allele associations were calculated using SPSS 13.0 software package.

Principal Findings: Compared to the healthy controls, the variant alleles IL23R rs7530511, and rs11805303 showed a statistically significant difference for ulcerative colitis susceptibility (0.7% *vs* 3.3%, $P = 0.002$; 60.4% *vs* 53.2%, $P = 0.0017$, respectively). The linkage disequilibrium (LD) patterns of these SNPs were measured and three LD blocks from the SNPs of IL23R and one block from those of IL17A were identified. A novel association with ulcerative colitis susceptibility occurred in haplotypes of IL23R (Block1 H3 $P = 0.02$; Block2 H2 $P = 0.019$; Block3 H4 $P = 0.029$) and IL17A (H4 $P = 0.034$). Pair-wise analyses showed an interaction between the risk haplotypes in IL23R and IL17A ($P = 0.014$).

Conclusions: Our study demonstrated that rs7530511, and rs11805303 of IL23R were significantly associated with ulcerative colitis susceptibility in the Chinese population. The most noticeable finding was the linkage of IL23R and IL17A gene region to ulcerative colitis risk due to the gene-gene interaction.

Editor: Robert Lafrenie, Sudbury Regional Hospital, Canada

Funding: This work was supported by the National Natural Science Foundation of China (no.30771039) (http://www.nsfc.gov.cn/Portal0/default152.htm) and the Key Medical Personnel of Jiangsu Province (no. RC2011063) (http://www.jswst.gov.cn/gb/jsswst/index.html). The funders had no role in study design, data collection and analysis, decision to publish, or preparation of the manuscript.

Competing Interests: The authors have declared that no competing interests exist.

* E-mail: ruihuashi@126.com (RS); hjzhang06@163.com (HZ)

These authors contributed equally to this work.

Introduction

Ulcerative colitis (UC) is characterized by chronic and relapsing inflammation in the gastrointestinal tract, and mostly affects the colorectal region of the gastrointestinal tract [1]. As one of two major phenotypes of inflammatory bowel disease (IBD), UC still remains of unknown etiology. Several studies have indicated that UC is caused by complex interactions of environmental, genetic, and immunoregulatory factors. Of these, immune dysregulation and genetic factors are thought to play important roles in the pathogenesis of UC [2–3]. Genome-wide association studies and linkage analyses have uncovered some susceptibility genes related to IBD, such as nucleotide-binding oligomerization domains 2 (NOD2), autophagy-related gene 16 like 1 (ATG16L1), and IL-23 receptors (IL23R) [3–7]. Furthermore, several meta-analyses of genome-wide association scanning studies showed some susceptibility genes related to IBD [8–9]. However, the genetic polymorphisms located within these genes did not thoroughly explain the pathogenesis of IBD or the variations in disease phenotypes.

Recently, it is shown that the IL-23/IL-17 axis plays an important role in IBD development [10]. IL-23 is essential for expansion and maintenance of Th17 response [11–12]. Moreover, IL-23R was expressed on a variety of cells and can directly activate a subset of macrophages, monocytes, natural killer cells, and dendritic cells which secrete IL-17[13–14]. As for IL23R polymorphisms, a study by Lappalainen *et al.* [15] demonstrated that IL23R polymorphisms (rs1004819, 10889677, rs2201841, rs11465804, and rs11209026) increased Crohn's disease (CD) susceptibility in a Finnish population, while another study revealed that an association of IL23R with UC, but not with CD in Swedish patients [16]. A study from Magyaril *et al.* [17] indicated that the IL23R gene variants rs10889677 C/A and rs2201841 T/C appeared to increase the susceptibility of CD but not of UC in a Hungarian population. These results showed that functional variants in the IL23R gene were identified as susceptibility loci in Caucasian IBD patients; however, literature on genetic associations of IBD in Asian populations is currently limited [18]. Therefore, further study on the association of IL23R polymorphisms with UC definitely needs to be performed to identify functional variations in IL23R in Asian patients with UC. In addition, accumulated evidence has demonstrated that IL-17 as the downstream cytokines of IL-23 plays an important role in IBD development. Others have shown that IL17A or IL17F gene polymorphisms play a role in Rheumatoid Arthritis (RA) and asthma [19–22], but there are fewer reports on associations of the IL17A gene polymorphisms with UC; particularly, there are no reports about IL17A gene polymorphism in Chinese UC patients.

Thus, in this study, we examined the distribution of 16 SNPs in the IL23R gene and 7 SNPs in the IL17A gene for analysis of the allele/genotype–phenotype association and gene-gene interaction, which could provide insightful information for their role in UC development in a Chinese Han population.

Methods

Study Population

In this study, we recruited 270 cases of UC and 268 healthy controls from four different hospitals (The First Affiliated Hospital of Nanjing Medical University, the First Hospital of Huaian, the Fourth People's Hospital of Wuxi, and the People's Hospital of Jiangyin) between 2008 and 2011. The diagnosis of UC was based on standard clinical, endoscopic, radiological, and histological criteria [23]. Cases were determined according to Montreal classification system, and cases with indeterminate colitis were excluded. The UC lesions were classified according to the Montreal classification [24], and severity was assessed by the Mayo disease activity index [25]. Healthy controls consisted of a randomly selected and ethnically matched healthy individuals without tumors, autoimmune diseases, and IBD family history. The main clinical characteristics of the study population are summarized in Table 1. In addition, the SNP positions of IL23R and IL17A in genomic DNA are listed in Table S1.

Table 1. The basic characteristics of the UC patients.

Clinical Characteristics	UC (n = 270)
Mean age ± SD (range)	44.49±14.24
(age of onset)	(14–77)
Male	48.1%
Female	51.9%
Lesion localization	
ulcerative proctitis	17.8%
left sided UC	43.0%
extensive UC	39.2%
Perianal lesions	
anal fistula	1.9%
anal fissure	3.7%
perianal abscess	1.5%
Extraintestinal manifestations	
Aphthous ulcer	2.9%
Arthritis/Arthragia	9.6%
IBD-related skin diseases	1.5%
Hepatopathy	1.9%
Oculopathy	0
Clinical severity	
Mild	39.3%
Moderate	51.9%
Severe	7.4%
Remission	1.4%
Endoscopic severity	REI 4.52±2.279
Family history	0.7%
Smoking	
Never smoking	80.0%
Quit smoking	5.9%
On smoking	14.1%
Appendectomy	2.2%

Note: REI Rachmilewitz endoscopic index. UC lesions were classified according to the Montreal classification. UC disease severity was assessed by the Mayo disease activity index. The control group included 136 males and 132 females, and the average age was 47.1±12.9.

Ethical Approvals

This study was approved by the ethics committees of all four hospitals (Ethics Committee of the First Affiliated Hospital of Nanjing Medical University, Ethics Committee of Jiangyin People's Hospital, Ethics Committee of the Fourth People's Hospital of Wuxi, and Ethics Committee of the First Hospital of Huaian) involved in this study, and all patients signed informed consent forms for participation in this study. Clinical data were collected from the patients' medical history and from questionnaires.

Genomic DNA Extraction and Genotyping Analysis

Approximately 2 ml of blood from the cases and controls was collected and stored in tubes containing EDTA. Blood cells and serum were separated in conditions of 4°C at 3000 rpm/min for 10 min within 4 h of blood collection. Genomic DNA was then extracted from peripheral blood lymphocytes using the RelaxGene Blood DNA System (TianGen Biotech, Beijing, China). The single nucleotide polymorphisms were genotyped by a predesigned ligase detection reaction allelic (LDR) technology (Shanghai Jierui Bio Co., Ltd., Shanghai, China). The PCR amplification was carried out in a volume of 15 μl, including 1 μl of genomic DNA, 1.5 μl 10× buffer, 1.5 μl $MgCl_2$, 0.3 μl dNTP (10 mM), 0.5 μl of each primer and H_2O for an initial DNA denature at 94°C for 2 min and then 35 cycles of 94°C for 20 s, 56°C for 20 s, and 72°C for 40 s and a final extension at 72°C for 3 min. Then, 3 μl of the PCR product was mixed with 1 μl of 10× Taq DNA ligase buffer, 0.125 μl of 40 U/μl Taq DNA ligase, 0.01 μl of probe (10 p)/Article and then PCR amplified for 30 cycles of 94°C for 30 s and 56°C for 3 min. After that, 1 μl of PCR product was added to 10 μl of sample loading buffer containing a molecular weight marker, and then denatured at 95°C for 3 min and immediately put into an ice bath for DNA sequence analysis using an ABI 3730 system.

Table 2. Allele frequency variants in IL23R and IL17A genes.

SNP		Variant allele	Controls n (%)	UC n (%)	OR⁺	95% CI⁺
IL23R	rs1004819	T	306 (57.1)	334 (61.9)	1.219	(0.955–1.555)
	rs1495965	A	270 (50.4)	264 (48.9)	0.942	(0.742–1.197)
	rs1884444	T	190 (35.4)	160 (29.6)	0.767	(0.594–0.990)
	rs2201841	C	382 (71.3)	408 (75.6)	1.246	(0.950–1.634)
	rs6677188	A	114 (21.3)	96 (17.8)	0.800	(0.591–1.083)
	rs7517847	G	226 (42.2)	204 (37.8)	0.833	(0.652–1.063)
	rs7530511	T	18 (3.3)	4 (0.7)	0.215	**(0.072–0.639)***
	rs10489629	A	400 (74.6)	412 (76.3)	1.094	(0.829–1.445)
	rs10889677	A	390 (72.8)	414 (76.7)	1.230	(0.934–1.620)
	rs1343151	C	524 (97.8)	528 (97.8)	1.008	(0.449–2.263)
	rs11209032	A	244 (45.5)	270 (50.0)	1.197	(0.974–1.470)
	rs11805303	T	285 (53.2)	326 (60.4)	1.342	**(1.053–1.709)****
	rs17375018	A	172 (32.1)	136 (28.2)	0.712	(0.489–1.037)
	rs11209026	A	0	0	-	-
IL17A	rs2275913	A	246 (45.9)	238 (44.1)	0.929	(0.731–1.181)
	rs8193036	T	148 (27.6)	148 (27.4)	0.990	(0.757–1.293)
	rs3804513	T	76 (14.2)	60 (11.1)	0.757	(0.527–1.086)
	rs1974226	T	32 (5.9)	38 (7.0)	1.192	(0.599–2.371)
	rs8193037	A	78 (14.6)	68 (12.6)	0.846	(0.516–1.387)
	rs8193038	C	78 (14.6)	72 (13.3)	0.903	(0.554–1.472)
	rs3748067	A	80 (14.9)	94 (17.4)	1.201	(0.758–1.904)

*$P = 0.002$,
**$P = 0.017$.
⁺Patients with UC versus healthy controls.
Note: There were 270 UC patients and 268 healthy controls in this study, so the total number of alleles in one SNP was 270×2 in UC and 268×2 in controls.

Statistical Analysis

Allele frequencies were first calculated for the Hardy-Weinberg balance test. Genotype, haplotype, and allele frequencies were compared between cases and controls using the chi-square (χ^2) test, Fisher's exact test or Student's t-test, when each was appropriate. Odds radios (OR) and 95% confidence intervals (95% CIs) were applied for 2×2 tables. Bonferroni correction was used for multiple comparisons. Bivariate correlate analysis and binary classification Logistic regression analysis were used to search risk factors associated with SNPs loci mutations. Subgroups were based on clinical and endoscopic severity, disease location, extra-intestinal manifestations, and tobacco smoke history. Subgroups dependent on the relative risk factors were used to find the different distribution of alleles and genotypes.

Haplotype frequencies and linkage disequilibrium (LD) were estimated and visualized by Haploview 4.2 (http://www.broadinstitute.org//haploview/haploview-downloads). SNPs with minor allele frequencies (MAF) below 5% were excluded. Tagger SNPs were picked up as $r^2>0.8$, of which adjacent SNPs with 95% CI = (0.70–0.98) of D' value were considered the haplotype. Mantel-Haenszel and logistic regression methods were used to determine the interaction between haplotypes in different genes. For all the analyses, differences were considered statistically significant when the P value was less than or equal to 0.05.

Table 3. The association between IL23R rs17375018/IL17A rs2275913 and Clinical severity of UC.

Variables (n)	OR (95%CI)⁺			
	IL23R rs17375018		IL17A rs2275913	
	Allele A⁺	AA+AGvsGG	Allele A⁺	AA+AGvsGG
Clinical severity				
Mild (106)	0.49*	0.34*	1.05	1.7
	(0.33–0.72)	(0.21–0.54)	(0.77–1.45)	(0.98–2.96)
Moderate (140)	0.88	0.68	0.88	0.71
	(0.64–1.20)	(0.45–1.01)	(0.66–1.18)	(0.46–1.10)
Severe (20)	1.06	0.71	0.45**	0.21***
	(0.49–2.31)	(0.29–1.77)	(0.22–0.91)	(0.82–0.55)

*$P<0.001$,
**$P = 0.024$,
***$P = 0.001$.
There was 266 subjects included in this comparison, 4 patients with Mayo disease activity index ≤2 were not included.
⁺UC Patients versus healthy controls.

Results

Allele frequency of IL23R and IL17A in ulcerative colitis and healthy controls.

Allele frequency data are shown in Table 2 and the allele frequencies met Hardy-Weinberg equilibrium in both UC cases and controls ($P>0.05$; data not shown). The data showed that one disease risk and two protective mutations in the IL23R polymorphisms were found (Table 2). The frequency of the mutant allele T of IL23R rs1884444 and rs7530511 was significantly lower than that of controls (29.6% *vs* 35.4%, $P = 0.042$; 0.7% *vs* 3.3%, $P = 0.002$, respectively). Compared to the controls, the mutant allele T for IL23R rs11805303 was significantly higher in UC patients (60.4% *vs* 53.2%, $P = 0.0017$). Only two (rs7530511 and rs11805303) genome-wide significant SNPs passed the Bonferroni correction threshold (0.05/16 = 0.0031). Our study only showed wild type alleles in IL23R rs11209026 and rs11465804, and heterozygous alleles in IL23R rs11465788 of all the participants. However, we did not find any association between IL17A variant alleles and UC risk.

Allele or Genotype Frequency of IL23R and IL17A in Subgroups of Ulcerative Colitis

Next, we performed Logistic regression analysis to examine the association of the relative risk factors of these two gene polymorphisms with UC development, and found several significant associations. For example, the IL23R rs17375018 and IL17A rs2275913 variant alleles were associated with UC severity. Allele frequency of IL23R rs17375018 in mild UC was significantly lower than the control subjects (18.9% *vs* 32.1%, $P<0.001$, OR = 0.49, 95%CI = 0.33–0.76, Table 3). The IL17A rs2275913 variant allele frequency distribution in patients with severe UC was significantly different from that in the controls ($P = 0.024$, OR = 0.45, 95% CI = 0.21–0.91, Table 3). Next, we combined the mutant homozygous AA and mutant heterozygous AG compared to the wild homozygous GG, and there were also significant differences for the IL23R rs17375018 in the mild patients ($P<0.001$) and IL7A rs2275913 in the severe patients ($P = 0.001$). From Table 3, we found that the OR value of IL23R rs17375018 was increasing from mild UC to severe UC, but the OR value of IL17A rs2275913 was decreasing. We also compared the average disease activity index in patients who took the variant allele and the wild homozygous patients (Table S2), and the results demonstrated that the IL23R rs17375018 was positively correlated to UC disease severity (AA+AG: $\overline{X}=6.92$; GG: $\overline{X}=5.97$; $P=0.028$), while the IL17A rs2275913 was negatively correlated to UC disease severity (AA+AG: $\overline{X}=6.02$; GG: $\overline{X}=6.91$; $P=0.035$). The IL23R rs6677188 genotype distribution between UC endoscopic remission and activity was significantly different ($P=0.010$). The heterozygous type AT frequency distribution was significantly higher in the endoscopic inactivity group than that in the endoscopic activity group (33.8% *vs* 17.2%, $P=0.019$, OR = 1.958, 95% CI = 1.108–3.460, Table 4). However, no genotype-phenotype association was found between UC disease lesion location or extra-intestinal manifestations and these two (IL23R, IL17A) gene polymorphisms.

Haplotypes of IL23R and IL17A and Gene-gene Interaction

Then, we measured the linkage disequilibrium (LD) patterns of the SNPs and identified three LD blocks from the SNPs of IL23R and one LD block in the SNPs of IL17A (Figure 1). To determine whether any specific haplotype would confer a higher risk or protection for UC, we performed specific and global-haplotype tests of association. Analysis of the haplotype structure revealed 15 distinct haplotypes, and 4 of them were associated with UC (Table 5). The most common haplotype (TT) of IL23R, formed with rs11805303 and rs7517847, was observed to be a risk haplotype, with a frequency of 60% in UC patients and 50% in controls ($P=0.020$). The rare haplotype (GGTT) of IL17A, formed with four SNPs (rs2275913, rs8193037, rs8193038, and rs3804513), was also a risk haplotype with a frequency of 3.3% in UC patients and 0.7% in controls ($P=0.034$). Another two haplotypes of IL23R were both protective factors, one was tagged by the rs10489629-A and rs2201841-T alleles, and the frequency of this haplotype was 0.7% in UC patients and 3.7% in controls ($P=0.019$). Another rare haplotype formed with three wild type alleles (GTG) of rs11209032, rs6677188 and rs1495965, the frequency of which was 1.1% in UC patients and 4.1% in controls ($P=0.029$).

In the analysis of gene-gene interactions of the IL23/IL17 genes, we combined the two risk haplotypes of IL23R and IL17A together, and found a significant increase in UC risk in IL23R block1 Haplotyp3, when the risk haplotype of IL17A, Haplotyp4, was also present ($P=0.004$ by Mantel-Haenszel test, Table 6). The interaction between these two risk haplotypes was statistically significant ($P=0.014$). Furthermore, the "risk" haplotypes of IL23R and IL17A synergistically increased UC risk (Figure 2), suggesting that there was a gene-gene interaction between the IL23R and IL17A haplotypes in the IL-23/IL-17 pathway that affected the pathogenesis of UC.

Table 4. Frequency of IL23R rs6677188 genotypes in UC patients with endoscopic remission and activity.

		Endoscopic staging		
SNP	**Genotype**	**Remission No (%)**	**Activity No (%)**	***P* value[+]**
rs6677188	AT	52 (33.8)	20 (17.2)	**0.019**
	AA	6 (3.9)	6 (5.17)	0.630
	TT	96 (62.3)	90 (77.6)	0.253

Endoscopic stage was assessed by Rachmilewitz endoscopic index, Endoscopic remission: 0–4, Endoscopic activity: 5–12.
[+]Endoscopic remission group versus Endoscopic activity group.

Discussion

To date, there is emerging evidence showing that the IL-23/IL-17 axis plays an important role in UC development [10,26]. In this regard, recent studies have suggested that Th17 cells mediated intestinal inflammation [27–28]. IL-23 was reported to promote production of IL-17 and to be required for Th17 differentiation in a pro-inflammatory context [29–31], especially in the presence of TGF-β and IL-6 for production of IL-17A, IL-17F, IL-6, IL-22, IL-26, TNF-α and GM-CSF [30,32]. IL-23 and Th17 cytokines act coordinately to influence the balance between tolerance and immunity in the intestine [33]. Moreover, a study on linking genetic susceptibility to CD with Th17 cell function demonstrated that IL23R genotypes influence Th17 cytokine IL-22 serum expression [5]. IL-22 is considered to have protective functions in IBD in many studies [34–35]. Genetic studies showed that IL23R variants were associated with both CD and UC [36]. Recently, an accumulating body of evidence indicated that the IL23R genotype might affect the response to anti-TNF therapy in UC [37].

In our study, the data were the first findings to show that the IL23R rs7530511 and rs11805303 variants were associated with UC susceptibility in a Chinese Han population. IL23R rs7530511 variant allele was protective factor for UC, while rs11805303 was significantly associated with an increased risk for UC development. We also demonstrated that patients with the IL23R haplotypes who also carry the IL17A risk haplotypes had higher susceptibility to UC. This indicates that gene-gene interaction between IL23R and IL17A might occur.

A study from Magyaril *et al.* [17] showed that the IL23R gene variants, rs10889677 C/A and rs2201841 T/C appeared to increase susceptibility to CD. However, the rs10889677 and rs2201841 in our study had no significant relationship with UC susceptibility. Ferguson *et al.* [38] detected five common SNPs in IL23R gene (rs11805303, rs7517847, rs1343151, rs11209026, and rs10889677) in CD patients from a New Zealand population and found that rs1343151 and/or rs7517847 variants strongly reduced the risk of developing CD at both allelic and genotype levels. Nevertheless, we did not find the apparent association between these SNPs in IL23R with UC susceptibility, but the rs11805303 and rs7517847 could form three haplotypes with TT to increase UC susceptibility. The IL23R rs11209026 was reported to be associated with IBD and many other immune-related diseases [39–44]. Several studies reported that the rs11209026 variant allele A was significant lower in CD patients than the controls; this indicated that the IL23R rs11209026 variant confers a protective effect against CD [39–41,45]. However, the association between rs11209026 variant and UC susceptibility has some controversy. Some studies revealed that there was no relationship between rs11209026 and UC [39–40], but other studies have demonstrated that the IL23R rs11209026 variant also conferred a protective effect against UC [44–47]. Glas *et al.* [47] analyzed 10 IL23R SNPs (including 9 SNPs in our study) in a large German IBD cohort, and found that the rs1004819 was the major IL23R variant associated with CD in the German population, while the rs11209026 IL23R variant was a protective marker for CD and UC. Furthermore, all IL23R gene variants in this study showed highly significant associations with CD, and 7 IL23R SNPs variants were significantly associated with UC except rs11465804 and rs11209032. However, in our study, there was only wild type allele G on IL23R rs11209026 in UC and controls. We did not find any association of these IL23R gene polymorphisms with UC.

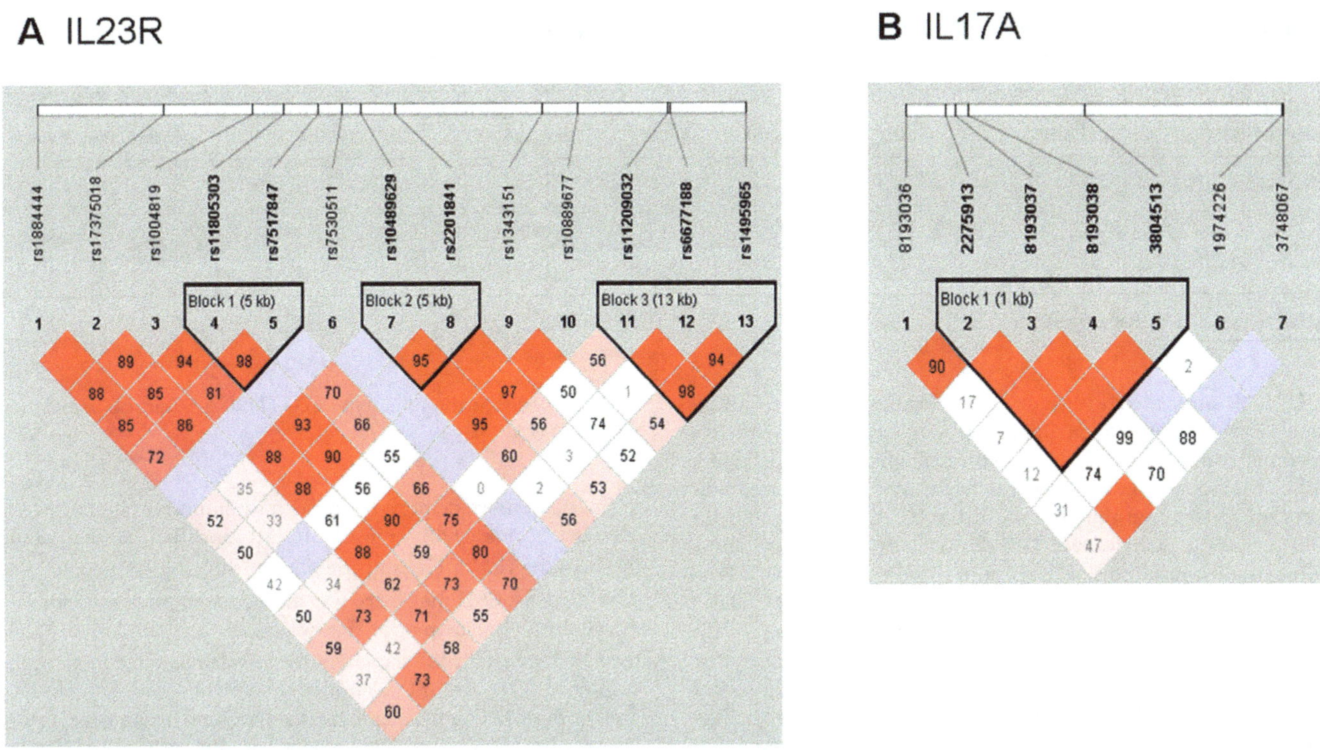

Figure 1. Linkage disequilibrium patterns of the region around the IL23R and 17A gene in the Chinese Han population. Numbers indicate the extent of D′ between 2 SNPs and in the dark area which have no digital respective D′ = 1. Dark color indicates strong connection. Three linkage disequilibrium blocks were found in IL23R, and one LD block was in IL17A. A, LD patterns of IL23R. B, LD patterns of IL17A.

Table 5. Frequency of IL23R and IL17A haplotypes in UC patients and healthy controls.

Gene							Frequency UC with Haplotype Present	Frequency Controls with Haplotype Present	*P* value[+]
IL23R			rs11805303	rs7517847					
		H1	C	G			0.356	0.418	0.138
		H2	C	T			0.041	0.078	0.062
	risk	H3	T	T			0.600	0.500	**0.020**
			rs10489629	rs2201841					
		H1	A	C			0.756	0.709	0.222
	protective	H2	A	T			0.070	0.370	**0.019**
		H3	G	T			0.226	0.250	0.624
		H4	G	C			0.011	0.004	0.521
			rs11209032	rs6677188	rs1495965				
		H1	A	T	G		0.496	0.455	0.340
		H2	G	A	A		0.170	0.213	0.257
		H3	G	T	A		0.315	0.291	0.612
	protective	H4	G	T	G		0.110	0.410	**0.029**
IL17A			rs2275913	rs8193037	rs8193038	rs3804513			
		H1	A	G	T	A	0.443	0.457	0.744
		H2	G	G	T	A	0.397	0.391	0.883
		H3	G	A	C	T	0.126	0.137	0.717
	risk	H4	G	G	T	T	0.033	0.007	**0.034**

[+]Patients with UC versus healthy controls.

Table 6. Interaction between IL23R risk haplotype and IL17A risk haplotype in all UC patients.

Presence of IL23R Block1 H3	Presence of IL17A H4	UC	Control	OR	0.95% Confidence Interval	Mantel-Haenszel *P* value	Interaction *P* value
–	–	216	268	1			
–	+	2	0	2.24	2.03–2.48		
+	–	306	264	1.44	1.13–1.83	**0.004**	**0.014**
+	+	16	4	4.96	1.64–15.06		

H3: Haplotype 3; H4: Haplotype 4.

IL-17 is associated with host defense against infectious agents and chronic inflammation [28]. IL17A is located on 6p12.1, a genomic region containing putative susceptibility loci (IBD3) for IBD. Moreover, a few studies have recently reported the associations between the G-197A in the IL7A promoter and the UC phenotype. Arisawa *et al.* [48] showed a significant association between polymorphisms of IL17A and IL17F genes and UC. Both IL17A (rs2275913, G-197A) and IL17F (rs763780, 7488T) alleles were significantly associated with the increased risk in the development of UC. However, our data did not support this. The IL17A (rs2275913, G-197A) variant allele did not associate with UC susceptibility in our patients. But in a subgroup analysis, we found that the IL17A (rs2275913, G-197A) variant was associated with disease severity; patients with mutant allele gene A tended towards mild disease severity.

From the LD analysis, we found that three haplotypes of IL23R and one haplotype of IL17A were significant associated with UC in the Chinese Han population. The haplotypes AT and GTG from the IL23R block2 H2 and block3 H4 were two protective haplotypes that reduced UC susceptibility. In contrast, the haplotypes TT and GGTT from IL23R and IL17A, respectively, were two risk haplotypes that increased UC susceptibility. These data are novel and have not been reported before. Einarsdottir *et al.* [16] showed that two haplotypes TTCTGAAA and CTCTGCAA (rs1004819, rs10489629, rs2201841, rs11465804, rs11209026, rs1343151, rs10889677, and rs11209032) were associated with UC risk, but a report from Lappalainen *et al.* [15] showed that the haplotype CTCTGCAA had no association with UC risk.

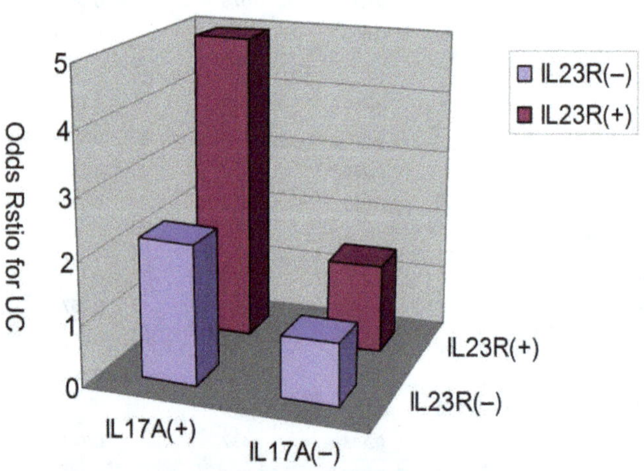

Figure 2. Increase of ulcerative colitis risk with the haplotypes of IL23R and IL17A. Relative risk haplotypes were plotted and demonstrate association between IL23R block1 haplotype3 and IL17A haplotype4 (p = 0.014 for interaction).

In addition, we demonstrated the most important finding of the gene-gene interaction between IL23R and IL17A that could increase the risk of UC susceptibility in the Chinese people. The data demonstrated that there was an increased odds ratio for UC as the "risk" haplotypes for the two genes were combined. While the OR for each "risk" haplotype alone was relatively modest, the combined OR for the identified haplotypes was substantially greater than 4. This finding suggested that there was a gene dosage effect of the IL23R and other genetic variants within IL17A in the IL-23/IL-17 pathway in increased UC risk. McGovern *et al.* [49] found some "risk" and "protective" haplotypes of IL23R and IL17A in CD patients. Another study from Kim *et al.* [18] showed significant increases of UC risk when decreasing protective or increasing risk alleles. Consequently, cumulative risk alleles of IL17A diminished the protective OR of IL23R in IBD patients, demonstrating an additive risk of UC along with an increase in the number of risk alleles in IL17A. These results provide insights into the genetic interactions in the IL23/IL17 pathway.

Finally, in our study, we also found an association of these two gene SNPs with disease severity and other clinical characteristics in UC. The variant allele A for the IL23R rs17375018 was positively correlated to UC disease severity, but the IL17A rs2275913 variant allele A had a negative relationship with UC disease severity. In IL23R rs6677188 patients with heterozygous type AT had a higher endoscopic remission rate. However, Tremelling *et al.* [50] analyzed eight IL23R SNPs including rs1343151 and found that there was no significant genotype-phenotype correlation based on sub-groups of UC. No genotype-phenotype association was found in the lesion localizations and extra intestinal manifestations of UC in our study.

In summary, our study investigated the association of SNPs of IL23R and IL17A with UC risk in Chinese Han population. The most novel finding was the linkage of the IL23R and IL17A gene regions to UC and the gene-gene interactions in the IL-23/IL-17 pathway that could increase the risk of UC susceptibility in this Chinese population. However, our study also has some limitations, such as no extensive coverage of both genes, and small size of the cohort. Thus, future study will confirm our current data using a more diverse and larger UC population.

Author Contributions

Conceived and designed the experiments: HZ RS PY FS. Performed the experiments: PY FS XFZ XDZ RC. Analyzed the data: PY FS XFZ RC HZ. Contributed reagents/materials/analysis tools: HZ RS. Wrote the paper: PY FS HZ RS. Provided material and collected the clinical data: PY FS XDZ PL HT XY.

References

1. Head KA, Jurenka JS (2003) Inflammatory bowel disease Part 1: ulcerative colitis–pathophysiology and conventional and alternative treatment options. Altern Med Rev 8: 247–83.
2. Cho JH (2008) The genetics and immunopathogenesis of inflammatory bowel disease. Nat Rev Immunol 8: 458–66.
3. Bouma G, Strober W (2003) The immunological and genetic basis of inflammatory bowel disease. Nat Rev Immunol 3: 521–33.
4. Lees CW, Barrett JC, Parkes M, Satsangi J (2011) New IBD genetics: common pathways with other diseases. Gut 60: 1739–53
5. Schmechel S, Konrad A, Diegelmann J, Glas J, Wetzke M, et al. (2008) Linking genetic susceptibility to Crohn's disease with Th17 cell function: IL-22 serum levels are increased in Crohn's disease and correlate with disease activity and IL23R genotype status. Inflamm Bowel Dis. 14: 204–12.
6. Hampe J, Franke A, Rosenstiel P, Till A, Teuber M, et al. (2007) A genome-wide association scan of nonsynonymous SNPs identifies a susceptibility variant for Crohn disease in ATG16L1. Nat Genet 39: 207–11.
7. Silverberg MS, Cho JH, Rioux JD, McGovern DP, Wu J, et al. (2009) Ulcerative colitis-risk loci on chromosomes 1p36 and 12q15 found by genome-wide association study. Nat Genet 41: 216–20.
8. Anderson CA, Boucher G, Lees CW, Franke A, D'Amato M, et al. (2011) Meta-analysis identifies 29 additional ulcerative colitis risk loci, increasing the number of confirmed associations to 47. Nat Genet 43: 246–52.
9. Franke A, McGovern DP, Barrett JC, Wang K, Radford-Smith GL, et al. (2010) Genome-wide meta-analysis increases to 71 the number of confirmed Crohn's disease susceptibility loci. Nat Genet 42:1118–25.
10. Abraham C, Cho J (2009) Interleukin-23/Th17 pathways and inflammatory bowel disease. Inflamm Bowel Dis 15: 1090–100.
11. Murphy CA, Langrish CL, Chen Y, Blumenschein W, McClanahan T, et al. (2003) Divergent pro- and antiinflammatory roles for IL-23 and IL-12 in joint autoimmune inflammation. J Exp Med 198: 1951–7.
12. Langrish CL, Chen Y, Blumenschein WM, Mattson J, Basham B, et al.(2005) IL-23 drives a pathogenic T cell population that induces autoimmune inflammation. J Exp Med 201: 233–40.
13. Bailey SL, Schreiner B, McMahon EJ, Miller SD (2007) CNS myeloid DCs presenting endogenous myelin peptides' preferentially' polarize CD4+ T(H)-17 cells in relapsing EAE. Nat Immunol 8: 172e80.
14. Schmidt-Weber CB, Akdis M, Akdis CA (2007) TH17 cells in the big picture of immunology. J Allergy Clin Immunol 120: 247e54.
15. Lappalainen M, Halme L, Turunen U, Saavalainen P, Einarsdottir E, et al. (2008) Association of IL23R, TNFRSF1A, and HLA-DRB1*0103 allele variants with inflammatory bowel disease phenotypes in the Finnish population. Inflamm Bowel Dis 14 : 1118–24.
16. Einarsdottir E, Koskinen LL, Dukes E, Kainu K, Suomela S, et al. (2009) IL23R in the Swedish, Finnish, Hungarian and Italian populations: association with IBD and psoriasis, and linkage to celiac disease. BMC Med Genet 10:8.
17. Magyaril L, Melegh B (2009) Susceptibility genetic variants in Hungarian morbus Crohn and ulcerative colitis patients. Orv Hetil 150: 81–8.
18. Kim SW, Kim ES, Moon CM, Park JJ, Kim TI, et al. (2011) Genetic polymorphisms of IL-23R and IL-17A and novel insights into their associations with inflammatory bowel disease. Gut 60:1527–36.
19. Wang JY, Shyur SD, Wang WH, Liou YH, Lin CG, et al. (2009) The polymorphisms of interleukin 17A (IL17A) gene and its association with pediatric asthma in Taiwanese population. Allergy 64: 1056–60.
20. Ramsey CD, Lazarus R, Camargo CA Jr, Weiss ST, Celedón JC (2005) Polymorphisms in the interleukin 17F gene (IL17F) and asthma. Genes Immun 6: 236–41.
21. Nordang GB, Viken MK, Hollis-Moffatt JE, Merriman TR, Førre ØT, et al. (2009) Association analysis of the interleukin 17A gene in Caucasian rheumatoid arthritis patients from Norway and New Zealand. Rheumatology (Oxford) 48: 367–70.
22. Furuya T, Hakoda M, Ichikawa N, Higami K, Nanke Y, et al. (2007) Associations between HLA-DRB1, RANK, RANKL, OPG, and IL-17 genotypes and disease severity phenotypes in Japanese patients with early rheumatoid arthritis. Clin Rheumatol 26: 2137–41.
23. Sakamoto J, Munakata A (2005) The concept, criteria for diagnosis, and disease classification of ulcerative coliti. Nihon Rinsho 63: 744–9.
24. Satsangi J, Silverberg MS, Vermeire S, Colombel JF (2006) The Montreal classification of inflammatory bowel disease: controversies, consensus, and implications. Gut 55: 749–53.
25. Lewis JD, Chuai S, Nessel L, Lichtenstein GR, Aberra FN, et al. (2008) Use of the noninvasive components of the Mayo score to assess clinical response in ulcerative colitis. Inflamm Bowel Dis 14: 1660–6.
26. Sarra M, Pallone F, Macdonald TT, Monteleone G (2010) IL-23/IL-17 axis in IBD. Inflamm Bowel Dis 16: 1808–13.
27. Liu ZJ, Yadav PK, Su JL, Wang JS, Fei K (2009) Potential role of Th17 cells in the pathogenesis of inflammatory bowel disease. World J Gastroenterol 14;15: 5784–8.
28. Hundorfean G, Neurath MF, Mudter J (2012) Functional relevance of T helper 17 (Th17) cells and the IL-17 cytokine family in inflammatory bowel disease. Inflamm Bowel Dis 18: 180–6.
29. Zelante T, De Luca A, Bonifazi P, Montagnoli C, Bozza S, et al. (2007) IL-23 and the Th17 pathway promote inflammation and impair antifungal immune resistance. Eur J Immunol 37: 2695–706.
30. Yen D, Cheung J, Scheerens H, Poulet F, McClanahan T, et al. (2006) IL-23 is essential for T cell-mediated colitis and promotes inflammation via IL-17 and IL-6. J Clin Invest 116: 1310–6.
31. Duvallet E, Semerano L, Assier E, Falgarone G, Boissier MC (2011) Interleukin-23: A key cytokine in inflammatory diseases. Ann Med 43: 503–511.
32. Dambacher J, Beigel F, Zitzmann K, De Toni EN, Göke B, et al. (2009) The role of the novel Th17 cytokine IL-26 in intestinal inflammation. Gut 58: 1207–17.
33. Shen W, Durum SK (2010) Synergy of IL-23 and Th17 cytokines: new light on inflammatory bowel disease. Neurochem Res 35: 940–6.
34. Sugimoto K, Ogawa A, Mizoguchi E, Shimomura Y, Andoh A, et al. (2008) IL-22 ameliorates intestinal inflammation in a mouse model of ulcerative colitis. J Clin Invest 118:534–44.
35. Brand S, Beigel F, Olszak T, Zitzmann K, Eichhorst ST, et al. (2006) IL-22 is increased in active Crohn's disease and promotes proinflammatory gene expression and intestinal epithelial cell migration. Am J Physiol Gastrointest Liver Physiol 290:G827–38.
36. Duerr RH, Taylor KD, Brant SR, Rioux JD, Silverberg MS (2006) A genome-wide association study identifies IL23R as an inflammatory bowel disease gene. Science 314: 1461–3.
37. Jürgens M, Laubender RP, Hartl F, Weidinger M, Seiderer J, et al. (2010) Disease activity, ANCA, and IL23R genotype status determine early response to infliximab in patients with ulcerative colitis. Am J Gastroenterol 105: 1811–9.
38. Ferguson LR, Han DY, Fraser AG, Huebner C, Lam WJ, et al. (2010) IL23R and IL12B SNPs and Haplotypes Strongly Associate with Crohn's Disease Risk in a New Zealand Population. Gastroenterol Res Pract 2010: 539461.
39. Lacher M, Schroepf S, Helmbrecht J, von Schweinitz D, Ballauff A, et al. (2010) Association of the interleukin-23 receptor gene variant rs11209026 with Crohn's disease in German children. Acta Paediatr 99: 727–33.
40. Lakatos PL, Szamosi T, Szilvasi A, Molnar E, Lakatos L, et al. (2008) ATG16L1 and IL23 receptor (IL23R) genes are associated with disease susceptibility in Hungarian CD patients. Dig Liver Dis 40: 867–73.
41. Pidasheva S, Trifari S, Phillips A, Hackney JA, Ma Y, et al. (2011) Functional Studies on the IBD Susceptibility Gene IL23R Implicate Reduced Receptor Function in the Protective Genetic Variant R381Q. PLoS One 6: e25038.
42. Huber AK, Jacobson EM, Jazdzewski K, Concepcion ES, Tomer Y (2008) Interleukin (IL)-23 receptor is a major susceptibility gene for Graves' ophthalmopathy: the IL-23/T-helper 17 axis extends to thyroid autoimmunity. J Clin Endocrinol Metab 93: 1077–81.
43. Hazlett J, Stamp LK, Merriman T, Highton J, Hessian PA (2011) IL-23R rs11209026 polymorphism modulates IL-17A expression in patients with rheumatoid arthritis. Genes Immun [Epub ahead of print].
44. Roberts RL, Gearry RB, Hollis-Moffatt JE, Miller AL, et al. (2007) IL23R R381Q and ATG16L1 T300A are strongly associated with Crohn's disease in a study of New Zealand Caucasians with inflammatory bowel disease. Am J Gastroenterol 102: 2754–61.
45. Oliver J, Rueda B, López-Nevot MA, Gómez-García M, Martín J (2007) Replication of an association between IL23R gene polymorphism with inflammatory bowel disease. Clin Gastroenterol Hepatol 5: 977–81, 981.e1–2.
46. Büning C, Schmidt HH, Molnar T, De Jong DJ, Fiedler T, et al. (2007) Heterozygosity for IL23R p.Arg381Gln confers a protective effect not only against Crohn's disease but also ulcerative colitis. Aliment Pharmacol Ther 26: 1025–33.
47. Glas J, Seiderer J, Wetzke M, Konrad A, Török HP, et al. (2007) rs1004819 is the Main Disease-Associated IL23R Variant in German Crohn's Disease Patients: Combined Analysis of IL23R, CARD15, and OCTN1/2 Variants. PLoS One 2: e819.
48. Arisawa T, Tahara T, Shibata T, Nagasaka M, Nakamura M, et al. (2008) The influence of polymorphisms of interleukin-17A and interleukin-17F genes on the susceptibility to ulcerative colitis. J Clin Immunol 28: 44–9.
49. McGovern DP, Rotter JI, Mei L, Haritunians T, Landers C, et al. (2009) Genetic epistasis of IL23/IL17 pathway genes in Crohn's disease. Inflamm Bowel Dis 15: 883–9.
50. Tremelling M, Cummings F, Fisher SA, Mansfield J, Gwilliam R, et al. (2007) IL23R variation determines susceptibility but not disease phenotype in inflammatory bowel disease. Gastroenterology 132: 1657–64.

Interleukin-6 Induces S100A9 Expression in Colonic Epithelial Cells through STAT3 Activation in Experimental Ulcerative Colitis

Min Jeoung Lee[1,2,9], Jin-Ku Lee[1,2,9], Ji Won Choi[1,2], Chang-Seok Lee[1,2], Ji Hyun Sim[3], Chung-Hyun Cho[1,2], Kwang-Ho Lee[4], Ik-Hyun Cho[5,6], Myung-Hee Chung[1,2], Hang-Rae Kim[3]*, Sang-Kyu Ye[1,2]*

1 Department of Pharmacology, Seoul National University College of Medicine, Seoul, Republic of Korea, **2** Ischemic/Hypoxic Disease Institute, Seoul National University College of Medicine, Seoul, Republic of Korea, **3** Department of Anatomy, Seoul National University College of Medicine, Seoul, Republic of Korea, **4** Department of Biotechnology, College of Biomedical & Health Science, Konkuk University, Chungju, Republic of Korea, **5** Department of Anatomy, College of Oriental Medicine, Kyung Hee University, Seoul, Republic of Korea, **6** Institute of Oriental Medicine, Kyung Hee University, Seoul, Republic of Korea

Abstract

Background: Intestinal epithelium is essential for maintaining normal intestinal homeostasis; its breakdown leads to chronic inflammatory pathologies, such as inflammatory bowel diseases (IBDs). Although high concentrations of S100A9 protein and interleukin-6 (IL-6) are found in patients with IBD, the expression mechanism of S100A9 in colonic epithelial cells (CECs) remains elusive. We investigated the role of IL-6 in S100A9 expression in CECs using a colitis model.

Methods: IL-6 and S100A9 expression, signal transducer and activator of transcription 3 (STAT3) phosphorylation, and infiltration of immune cells were analyzed in mice with dextran sulfate sodium (DSS)-induced colitis. The effects of soluble gp130-Fc protein (sgp130Fc) and S100A9 small interfering (si) RNA (si-S100A9) on DSS-induced colitis were evaluated. The molecular mechanism of S100A9 expression was investigated in an IL-6-treated Caco-2 cell line using chromatin immunoprecipitation assays.

Results: IL-6 concentrations increased significantly in the colon tissues of DSS-treated mice. sgp130Fc or si-S100A9 administration to DSS-treated mice reduced granulocyte infiltration in CECs and induced the down-regulation of S100A9 and colitis disease activity. Treatment with STAT3 inhibitors upon IL-6 stimulation in the Caco-2 cell line demonstrated that IL-6 mediated S100A9 expression through STAT3 activation. Moreover, we found that phospho-STAT3 binds directly to the *S100A9* promoter. S100A9 may recruit immune cells into inflamed colon tissues.

Conclusions: Elevated S100A9 expression in CECs mediated by an IL-6/STAT3 signaling cascade may play an important role in the development of colitis.

Editor: David L. Boone, University of Chicago, United States of America

Funding: This work was supported in part by grants from the National Research & Development (R&D) Program for Cancer Control, Ministry of Health & Welfare, Republic of Korea (1020160 and 0720540 to SK Ye) and from National Research Foundation (NRF), Ministry of Education, Science and Technology (2010-0027827 and 2011-0010571 to SK Ye). The funders had no role in study design, data collection and analysis, decision to publish, or preparation of the manuscript.

Competing Interests: The authors have declared that no competing interests exist.

* E-mail: sangkyu@snu.ac.kr (SKY); hangrae2@snu.ac.kr (HK)

9 These authors contributed equally to this work.

Introduction

Crohn's disease (CD) and ulcerative colitis (UC), which develop as the result of chronic inflammatory reactions in the gastrointestinal tract and are defined collectively as inflammatory bowel disease (IBD), are among the most common autoimmune diseases worldwide [1–4]. IBD results from the unregulated response of the mucosal immune system in the gut [5]. It is involved in autoimmune diseases and increases the risk of developing colorectal cancer, one of the most common fatal malignancies [6]. Despite recent advances in our understanding of IBD, important questions about the molecular mechanisms of its immunopathology remain unanswered.

Immune cells, which infiltrate the inflamed guts of patients with IBD, produce various cytokines and chemokines that trigger inflammatory responses [5]. Among the cytokines, interleukin-6 (IL-6) has a positive correlation with the disease activities of IBD, and its production returns to normal levels when gut inflammation becomes inactive [7–11]. Of important, IL-6 production was also increased in DSS-induced colitis [11–14].

IL-6 plays an important role in enhancing T-cell survival and apoptosis resistance in the lamina propria at the inflamed site [13,15]. It is also involved in the immune deviation of regulatory T cells toward inflammatory cells (e.g., Th17) [16] and promotes the survival of intestinal epithelial cells [14,17]. In general, IL-6 binds to soluble or membrane-bound IL-6 receptors (e.g., sIL-6Rα or

IL-6Rα), resulting in the activation of janus kinase 2 (JAK2) and the downstream effectors signal transducer and activator of transcription 3 (STAT3) and phosphatidyl inositol 3′ kinase [11,18]. In particular, genome-wide association studies have found a significant association between polymorphisms in the *STAT3* region and clinical phenotypes of CD and UC, as well as those of multiple sclerosis (MS) [19].

S100A8 (also called myeloid-related protein 8 [MRP8]) and S100A9 (MRP14) are members of the S100 family of calcium-binding proteins and exist mainly as a S100A8/S100A9 heterodimer (i.e., calprotectin) in the extracellular milieu [20–22]. They are expressed constitutively in granulocytes, monocytes, and activated macrophages [21–27], as well as in epithelial cells under inflammatory conditions [28,29]. Of important, it has been known that STAT3 regulate the expression of S100A9 in breast cancer cells and myeloid-derived suppressor cells in cancer [30,31].

The S100A8/S100A9 heterodimer as well as S100A9 induce neutrophil adhesion to fibrinogen by activating the β2 integrin Mac-1 and adhesion molecules (e.g., VCAM-1 and ICAM-1), as well as proinflammatory chemokines [32–34]. In addition, this complex functions as an endogenous activator of Toll-like receptor 4 (TLR4), promoting lethal, endotoxin-induced shock [35]. In vascular inflammation, S100A8/S100A9 characteristically damages endothelial integrity and prompts caspase-dependent and -independent cell death [34,36,37]. Due to their functions in monocyte activation and leukocyte recruitment, S100A8/S100A9 have been considered hallmarks of many pathologic conditions characterized by chronic inflammation and autoimmunity, such as rheumatoid arthritis, systemic lupus erythematosus, MS, and IBD [29,38–40].

Apart from their known functions under inflammatory conditions, little has been proven about the expression mechanism of S100A9 in intestinal epithelial cells (IECs), which are important in intestinal homeostasis [2,3]. Because IECs are able to express IL-6Rα on the basal surface, and the ligation of IL-6Rαactivates nuclear factor kappa B (NF-κB) [41,42], we investigated whether IL-6, which is abundantly expressed in the inflamed colon, modulates the expression of S100A9 in colonic epithelial cells (CECs) using an experimental colitis model. We generated a mouse model of experimental colitis induced by dextran sulfate sodium (DSS) and showed that IL-6 triggered S100A9 production in CECs, which was mediated through STAT3 activation. In addition, we suggest that the increased expression of S100A9 might give rise to the recruitment of immune cells into the colonic epithelial area in this model, resulting in the progression of inflammation.

Results

IL-6 is Up-Regulated in the Colon Tissue in DSS-Induced Colitis

We established DSS-induced colitis shown a loss of approximately 20% body weight on day 11(Fig. S1A, left). Notably, the DSS-treated mice scored up to 13 points at the end of the cycle and their DAI scores increased gradually during the course of DSS treatment (Fig. S1A, right). We histologically examined the colon tissues of normal mice and those exposed to DSS for 6 and 12 days. Both groups of DSS-exposed mice showed prominent changes in colon tissues, with mucosal ulceration and degeneration, a decreased number of goblet cells, inflammatory cellular infiltration, and submucosal edema compared to normal mice (Fig. S1B). Histological changes were more severe on day 12, with mucosal ulceration and degeneration as well as inflammatory cellular infiltration into the mucosa and submucosa, indicating that the murine colitis model was well established in our system.

To characterize the expression of the effector cytokine IL-6 during DSS-induced colitis, the mRNA expression of IL-6 was evaluated by conventional PCR. We found that IL-6 concentrations increased significantly in the colon tissue of DSS-treated mice (Fig. 1A), although the type of cells contributing to this IL-6 production remained unclear.

STAT3 Activation and S100A9 Expression in the Colonic Epithelial Cells in DSS-Induced Colitis

To investigate whether STAT3 is activated in CECs, where IL-6 was increased, from DSS-treated mice, we measured $STAT3^{PY705}$ by immunofluorescence and immunoblotting. STAT3 was highly activated in the CEC regions of colon tissues after DSS exposure for 6 days, whereas it was not expressed in control mice (Fig. 1B). To further confirm the activation of STAT3, we isolated CECs from control or DSS-treated mice. The purity of the isolated CECs was confirmed that they express E-cadherin and villin, but not CD45, common leukocyte antigen (Fig S2 A–B). Indeed, STAT3 activation was markedly elevated in the CECs from mice with DSS-induced colitis (Fig. 1C). Since the secretion of S100A9 was correlated with STAT3 [30,31], we further investigated the expression levels of S100A9 in the CECs. The mRNA expression of S100A9 was strongly elevated in CECs from DSS-treated mice, with the highest expression observed after the longest DSS exposure (Fig. 1D). These data indicate that STAT3 activation may be related to the expression of S100A9 in CECs during DSS-induced colitis.

IL-6 Blockade or STAT3 Knockdown Suppresses S100A9 Expression in CECs from DSS-Treated Mice

Based on these findings, the possibility that IL-6 acts as a regulator of S100A9 expression through STAT3 activation in CECs was examined using an IL-6 blockade method. In brief, IL-6 was abrogated by the intraperitoneal injection of 0.5 mg/kg sgp130Fc into a group of mice after 2 days of 3% DSS treatment, as described previously [43]. This method was used because signaling in response to IL-6 involves binding of the cytokine to its receptor (IL-6Rα) and subsequent homodimerization of the signal transducer gp130. Disease severity was significantly reduced in the sgp130Fc-injected group compared to the group receiving DSS alone (Fig. 2A). Then we investigated whether STAT3 phosphorylation could be inhibited by sgp130Fc treatment using immunofluorescence staining. While the expression of $STAT3^{PY705}$ was highly up-regulated in the colon tissues of the 3% DSS-treated group, it was notably repressed in the group of mice treated with 3% DSS and a subsequent injection of sgp130Fc (Fig. 2B). Remarkably, a significant reduction in the expression of *S100A9* mRNA (Fig. 2C) and protein (Fig. 2D) was observed in CECs from the 3% DSS + sgp130Fc group compared to mice receiving DSS alone, and was associated with $STAT3^{PY705}$ expression (Fig. 2B).

Next, to provide direct evidence that the increased S100A9 expression by IL-6 was mediated through STAT3 activation, we introduced a delivery system of si-STAT3 using CH-NPs [44]. si-negative/CH-NPs or si-STAT3/CH-NPs were injected intravenously twice on days 2 and 3 into the 3% DSS-treated group. Then we also investigated whether STAT3 knockdown could affect disease development using si-STAT injection. Disease activities were significantly decreased on day 6 of DSS exposure in the STAT3 suppression group compared to the negative si-RNA-treated mice (Fig. 3A). The expression levels of *S100A9* mRNA (Fig. 3B) were notably suppressed in the group of mice

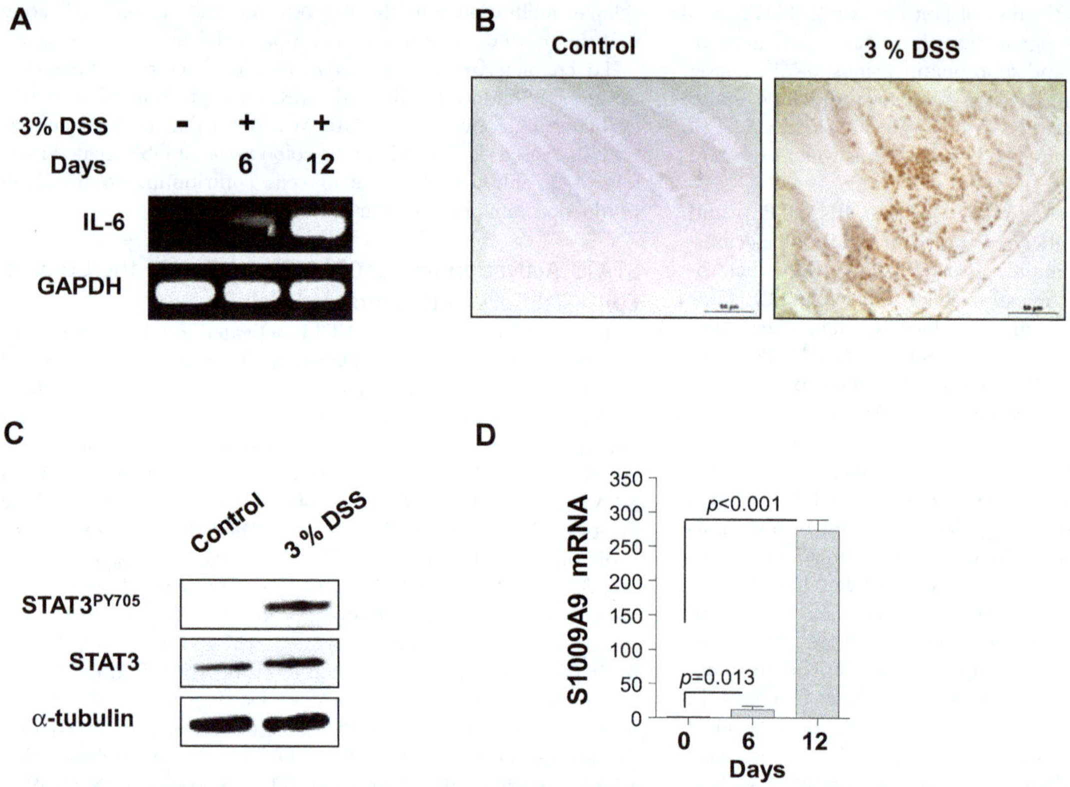

Figure 1. Increased IL-6 expression, activation of STAT3 in colon tissue, and S100A9 in isolated colonic epithelial cells (CECs), from a mouse model of dextran sulfate sodium (DSS)-induced colitis. (**A**) In control and DSS-treated mice at 6 or 12 days after DSS administration, colon tissues were homogenized using a tissue homogenizer. *IL-6* and *GAPDH* mRNA levels in each group of colonic tissue samples was analyzed by conventional reverse-transcription polymerase chain reaction assays. Data are representative of three independent experiments. (**B**) Activation of STAT3 ($STAT3^{PY705}$) in colon sections on day 6 from mice treated with 0% or 3% DSS was determined by immunohistochemistry. Scale bars = 100 μm. Data are representative of four independent experiments. (**C**) CECs from mice treated with 0% or 3% DSS were purified on day 6. Expressions of $STAT3^{PY705}$, total STAT3, and alpha-tubulin were analyzed by immunoblotting. Data are representative of four independent experiments. (**D**) CECs from mice treated with 3% DSS for 0, 6, or 12 days were prepared, and *S100A9* mRNA expression was analyzed by quantitative reverse-transcription polymerase chain reaction (qRT-PCR). The qRT-PCR data were analyzed by comparative C_t quantification. Data are presented as means ± standard deviations of values from six mice per group. *P* values were obtained using the two-tailed Student's *t*-test.

treated with si-STAT3/CH-NPs, resulting that STAT3 regulated the expression level of S100A9 in the CECs in DSS-induced colitis (Fig. 3C).

IL-6/STAT3 Signaling Cascades Induce S100A9 Expression in Caco-2 Cells *In Vitro*

To further confirm whether IL-6 directly triggers S100A9 expression through STAT3 activation, *in vitro* experiments were performed using a human IEC line (Caco-2). Sustained STAT3 activation was observed until 60 min (Fig. 4A) and S100A9 expression was significantly increased at mRNA levels after IL-6 stimulation for 3 or 6 h (Fig. 4B). S100A9 was released in the cell culture supernatant up to 24 h after stimulation of these cells with IL-6 (Fig. 4B). Thus, IL-6 can be postulated to mediate phosphorylated STAT3 and up-regulate S100A9 expression in Caco-2 cells.

IL-6-mediated S100A9 expression was further investigated to determine whether it is dependent on STAT3 activation using various agents that inhibit STAT3 signaling cascades. S3I and the STAT3 inhibitor, which inhibit phosphorylation by targeting a tyrosine residue or by dimerizing STAT3, respectively were incubated for 3 h prior to IL-6 stimulation. After 6 h, the expression of S100A9 at both mRNA and protein levels was measured. The expression of S100A9, which increased in response to IL-6 stimulation, was returned to resting levels by the two types of STAT3 inhibitors (Fig. 4C). These findings indicate that S100A9 expression by IL-6 in Caco-2 cells was directly mediated via the STAT3 signaling pathway.

To investigate whether STAT3 regulates the transcription of S100A9 upon IL-6 stimulation through direct binding to its promoter region, we performed a ChIP assay. Increased binding of $STAT3^{PY705}$ to the *S100A9* promoter in response to IL-6 was observed (Fig. 4D). Taken together, these data suggest that STAT3 activated in the presence of IL-6 interacts directly with the *S100A9* promoter, resulting in the production of S100A9.

Leukocytes Infiltration, Presumably Mediated by S100A9, in the Colonic Epithelium in DSS-Induced Colitis

Lastly, we explored the effects of S100A9 protein in CECs on DSS-induced colitis. Because the up-regulation of S100A9 is associated exclusively with the recruitment of leukocytes [21,22,38], we investigated whether IL-6-mediated S100A9 expression in CECs is associated with the recruitment of immune cell in the colonic epithelial area in DSS-treated mice using immunofluorescence staining for Gr-1 and CD11c. In fact, human recombinant S100A9 were evaluated *in vitro* in chemotaxis assy for human promyelocytic leukemia (HL-60) cell line at concentrations varying from 32 to 1,024 ng/ml. Cell migration was induced

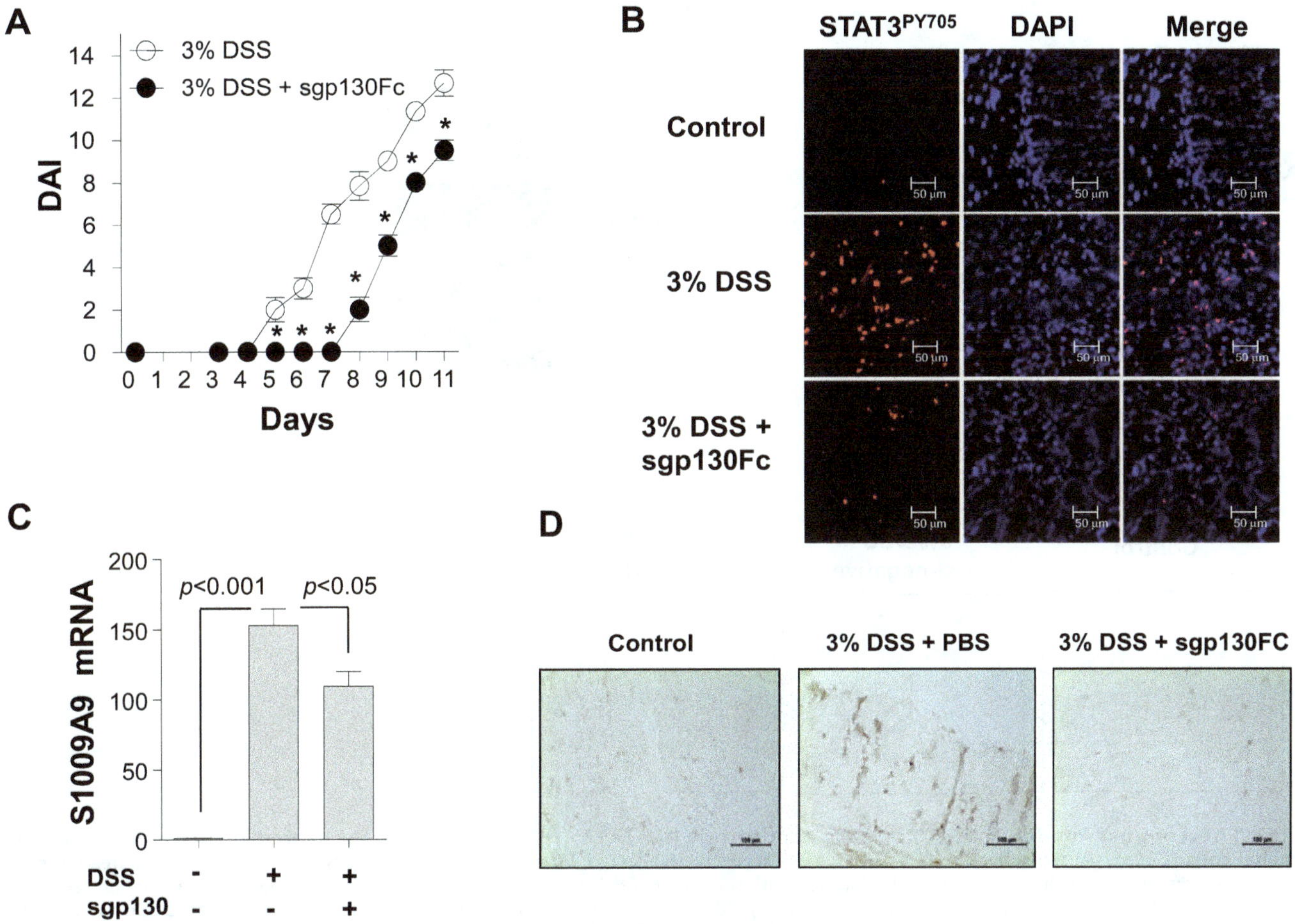

Figure 2. Effect of soluble gp130-Fc (sgp130Fc) injection on the expression of S100A9 in colonic epithelial cells (CECs) from mice with dextran sulfate sodium (DSS)-induced colitis. (**A**) Changes in the disease activity indices (DAI) of mice treated with DSS + phosphate-buffered saline (PBS) or DSS + sgp130Fc were assessed daily. Data are presented as means ± standard deviations of values from six mice per group. *$p<0.01$ vs. control mice (two-tailed Student's *t*-test). (**B**) Colon sections from mice in each group were examined for STAT3PY705 (red) levels by immunofluorescence on day 6 of DSS treatment. Data are representative of three independent experiments. DAPI, 4′,6-diamidino-2-phenylindole. Scale bars = 50 µm. (**C**) CECs from mice treated with or without 3% DSS for 8 days and a subsequent sgp130Fc or PBS injection were prepared, and *S100A9* mRNA expression was analyzed by quantitative reverse-transcription polymerase chain reaction (qRT-PCR). Data are presented as means ± standard deviations of values from six mice per group. *P* values were obtained using the two-tailed Student's *t*-test. (**D**) Expression of S100A9 in colon sections from mice treated with 0% or 3% DSS for 10 days was determined by immunohistochemistry. Scale bars = 100 µm. Data are representative of four independent experiments.

directional migration, depending on concentration of S100A9 (Fig. S4). We noticed a significant infiltration of Gr-1$^+$ cells in the epithelial lining, but found no expansion of CD11c$^+$ cells in DSS-induced colitis (Fig. 5A, E). Importantly, the infiltration of leukocytes in the colonic epithelium (Fig. 5A) was markedly suppressed when IL-6 was blocked by sgp130Fc injection (Fig. 5C). In order to confirm the possibility whether inflammatory chemokine is involved in recruitment of immune cells at inflammatory site, we measured CXCL10 (IP-10) expression. The expression of CXCL10 mRNA was mildly decreased but not significant statistically (Fig S3), suggesting that leukocytes infiltration is secondary to S100A9 expression not chemokine. Moreover, tissue damage in sgp130Fc injected colitis mice was restored to the level of normal mice with alleviated mucosal ulceration and degeneration, a decreased number of goblet cells, inflammatory cellular infiltration, and submucosal edema (Fig. 5B).

To further confirm whether these findings result from S100A9 expression in CECs from mice with DSS-induced colitis, we suppressed S100A9 expression by si-S100A9/CH-NP injection. The expression of S100A9 was markedly reduced by treatment with si-S100A9/CH-NPs (Fig. 5D). In particular, disease activities were significantly decreased on day 8 of DSS exposure in the S100A9 suppression group compared to the negative si-RNA-treated mice (Fig. 5G). The infiltration of GR-1$^+$ cells and histopathology of colon tissue were consistently and notably reduced when S100A9 expression was down-regulated (Fig. 5E–F), suggesting that the recruitment of immune cells in the colonic epithelium results from IL-6-induced S100A9 expression in CECs in DSS-induced colitis.

Discussion

We demonstrated a novel mechanism in which IL-6 increases S100A9 levels via STAT3 activation in CECs in an experimental murine model of DSS-induced colitis. S100A9 expressed in the CECs may contribute to the disease progression of active colitis by recruiting leukocytes within the colonic epithelia, presumably resulting in the breakdown of the epithelial lining and intestinal

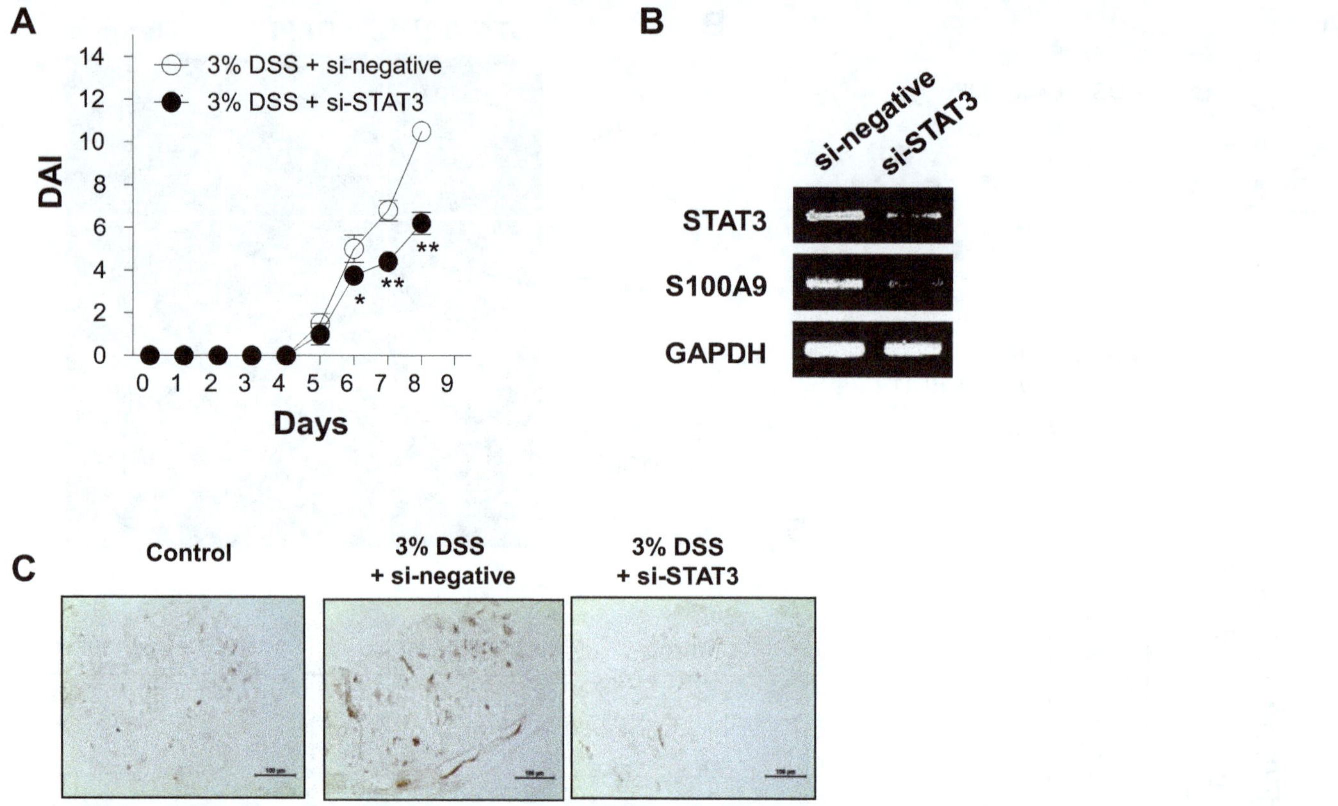

Figure 3. Effect of small interfering STAT3 chitosan nanoparticle (si-STAT3/CH-NP) injection on the expression of S100A9 in colonic epithelial cells (CECs). (**A**) si-negative/CH-NPs or si-STAT3/CH-NPs were injected intravenously twice on days 2 and 3 into 3% DSS-treated mice. Changes in the disease activity indices (DAI) of mice injected with si-negative/CH-NPs or si-STAT3/CH-NPs were assessed daily. Data are presented as means ± standard deviations of values from six mice per group. *$p<0.01$, **$p<0.001$ vs. control mice (two-tailed Student's *t*-test). (**B**) On day 8 of DSS exposure, CECs from each group of mice were purified and mRNA levels of *STAT3*, *S100A9*, and *GAPDH* were analyzed by conventional RT-PCR. Data are representative of three independent experiments. (**C**) Expression of S100A9 in colon sections from mice treated with si-negative/CH-NPs or si-STAT3/CH-NPs at 8 days was determined by immunohistochemistry. Scale bars = 100 μm. Data are representative of four independent experiments.

homeostasis. Our finding that non-immune cells, including mucosal epithelial cells, trigger immune responses through the release of damage-associated signals, such as S100A9, expands our understanding of the pathogenesis of UC in humans.

Although S100A9 is highly up-regulated in patients with UC, and is considered a fecal marker of gastrointestinal inflammation, previous studies have not determined whether CECs express S100A9 in colonic inflammation [22,45]. A growing body of evidence indicates that ECs help to maintain homeostasis in the gut by acting as physiological barriers against pathogenic bacteria or by generating anti-inflammatory signals. In contrast, our results suggest that ECs can also trigger inflammatory responses by secreting S100A9 in mice with colitis (Fig. 5E–G). Once the epithelial barrier is disrupted, ECs actively secrete damage-associated signals (i.e., S100A9) to prevent potentially pathogenic microorganisms from entering the systemic circulation, which can lead to severe infections, such as peritonitis or sepsis. S100A9, which has been identified as a danger-associated molecular pattern, is recognized by TLR4 in both dendritic cells (DCs) and ECs [21,22,46]. The S100A8/S100A9 heterodimer is also an active component that induces a complex signaling cascade comprising the translocation of myeloid differentiation primary response protein 88 and the activation of IL-1 receptor-associated kinase-1, mitogen-activated protein kinases, and the inhibitor of κB kinase by interacting with TLR4-myeloid differentiation factor 2, promoting lethality during septic shock by elevating tumor necrosis factor-α [35]. In addition, S100A9 triggers the infiltration of leukocytes, including granulocytes, which rapidly engulf invaders, damaged cells, or cellular debris [21,22,38,47]. Neutrophil granules also serve as reservoirs for digestive enzymes before delivery into the phagosome. Among them, azurophilic granule contents possess microbicidal activity and play an important role in tissue destruction during inflammation [47–49]. Consequently, the infiltration of granulocytes can facilitate the disintegration of the colonic epithelia and exacerbate colitis-associated symptoms in active UC. Moreover, our results suggest that S100A9 blockades, in combination with appropriate antibiotics, may be considered a treatment strategy for patients with UC.

In the present study, we found increased IL-6 expression in CECs from mice with DSS-induced colitis (Fig. 1A) and demonstrated directly that IL-6 induced S100A9 expression in both CECs from mice with colitis and in a human IEC cell line (Fig. 1D, 4B). The activation of TLR4 leads to the induction of IL-6 through the NF-κB signaling pathway [50]. Although CECs express low levels of TLR4 under normal conditions, the expression of TLR4 and IL-6 is increased in CECs from patients with UC, as well as in leukocytes and ECs [12,51], suggesting that intestinal ECs may produce IL-6 through TLR4 expression during inflammation [52].

Our results provide supporting evidence for the crucial role of IL-6 in the generation of colonic inflammation, as IL-6 blockade delayed disease onset and attenuated colitis-associated symptoms

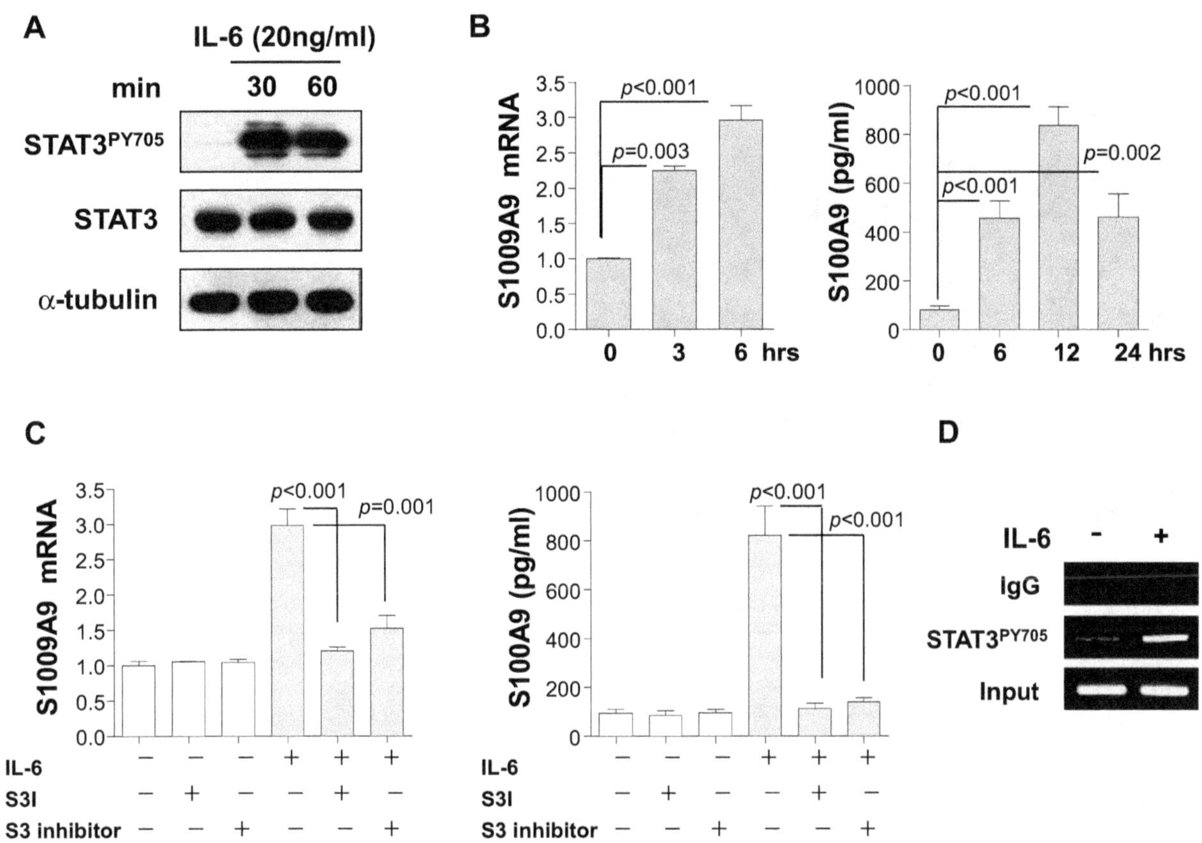

Figure 4. The role of the interleukin-6 (IL-6)/STAT3 axis in the expression of S100A9 in the Caco-2 cell line. (**A**) Caco-2 cells were stimulated with IL-6 (20 ng/ml) for 0, 30, or 60 min, and the cell lysates were analyzed by immunoblotting for $STAT3^{PY705}$ and total STAT3. Data are representative of three independent experiments. (**B**) The expression levels of *S100A9* in Caco-2 cells stimulated with IL-6 (20 ng/ml) for 0, 3, or 6 h were analyzed by quantitative reverse-transcription polymerase chain reaction (qRT-PCR, left panel). The qRT-PCR data were analyzed by comparative C_t quantification. S100A9 levels in the culture supernatants of Caco-2 stimulated with IL-6 for 0, 6, 12, or 24 h were determined by ELISA (right panel). Data are presented as means ± standard deviations of values from each group. (**C**) Up-regulation of IL-6-mediated S100A9 expression by STAT3 activation in Caco-2 cells. To measure the expression level of S100A9 in Caco-2 cells, the cells were pretreated with or without one of inhibitors for 3 h and then incubated in the presence or absence of IL-6 (20 ng/ml) for 6 h:S3I (20 μM); or STAT3 inhibitor peptide (5 μM). The transcriptional levels of S100A9 were analyzed by qRT-PCR (left panel) and secreted S100A9 were determined by ELISA (right panel). Data are presented as mean ± standard deviations of values from each group. *P* values were obtained using the two-tailed Student's *t*-test (**B, C**). (**D**) Caco-2 cells were stimulated with or without IL-6 (20 ng/ml) for 24 h. The cell lysates were prepared and sonicated (30 s on/1 min off for three cycles) to form a sheared, cross-linked chromatin. After incubation with anti-$STAT3^{PY705}$ or rabbit immunoglobulin G (IgG), the eluted DNA was amplified and analyzed by conventional polymerase chain reaction assay. Data are representative of four independent experiments.

in DSS-treated mice (Fig. 2A). This finding is consistent with Atreya et al. [13], who demonstrated that the blockade of IL-6 *trans*-signaling suppressed T-cell resistance to apoptosis in intestinal inflammation. Collectively, IL-6 elicits colonic inflammation in various ways, such as by stimulating innate immune organs (i.e., epithelial barrier), inducing the differentiation of adoptive immune cells (i.e., Th17 cells), and enhancing T-cell survival. This evidence provides insight into IL-6 function in multiple steps of UC generation and suggests a rationale for therapeutic approaches using IL-6 blockades, which could be effective treatment modalities for patients with UC.

However, IL-6 has a protective effect on enterocytes and IECs [14,17,53]. In the development of colitis-associated cancer (CAC), the IL-6/STAT3 axis acts as an oncogenic signal cascade in CECs by promoting BCL-$_{XL}$ and cyclin D [14]. In addition, it has been known that patients with active UC had significantly more IL6 and p-STAT3-positive epithelial cells than both patients with inactive UC and controls [53]. Notably, mice lacking IL-6 (IL-6 null) or STAT3 in IECs show reduced CAC tumorigenesis but develop more severe DSS-induced colitis, with pronounced colonic ulceration and body weight loss, than do wild-type counterparts [14]. Tebbutt et al. [54] also showed that IL-6 null mice or those harboring the reciprocal mutation ablating STAT1/3 signaling show impaired colonic mucosal wound healing after DSS administration.

There are several possible explanations for the difference between our findings and the results of previous studies of the blockade of IL-6 signaling or STAT3 activation. It could stem from the use of knockout mice, the administration of the soluble receptor blocker (sgp130Fc), or different methods of targeting the S100A9 molecule. In intestinal inflammation, S100A9 is an effector molecule that enhances TLR signaling [35] and recruits granulocytes [21,22,38,47]. Thus, the blockade of this molecule can ameliorate disease severity in DSS-induced colitis (Fig. 5A–C). Thus, our data and previous findings suggest that IL-6 can finely tune the balance between negative and positive signals during DSS-induced colitis by providing protective signals to IECs or by promoting inflammation via interaction with CECs and inflammatory cells.

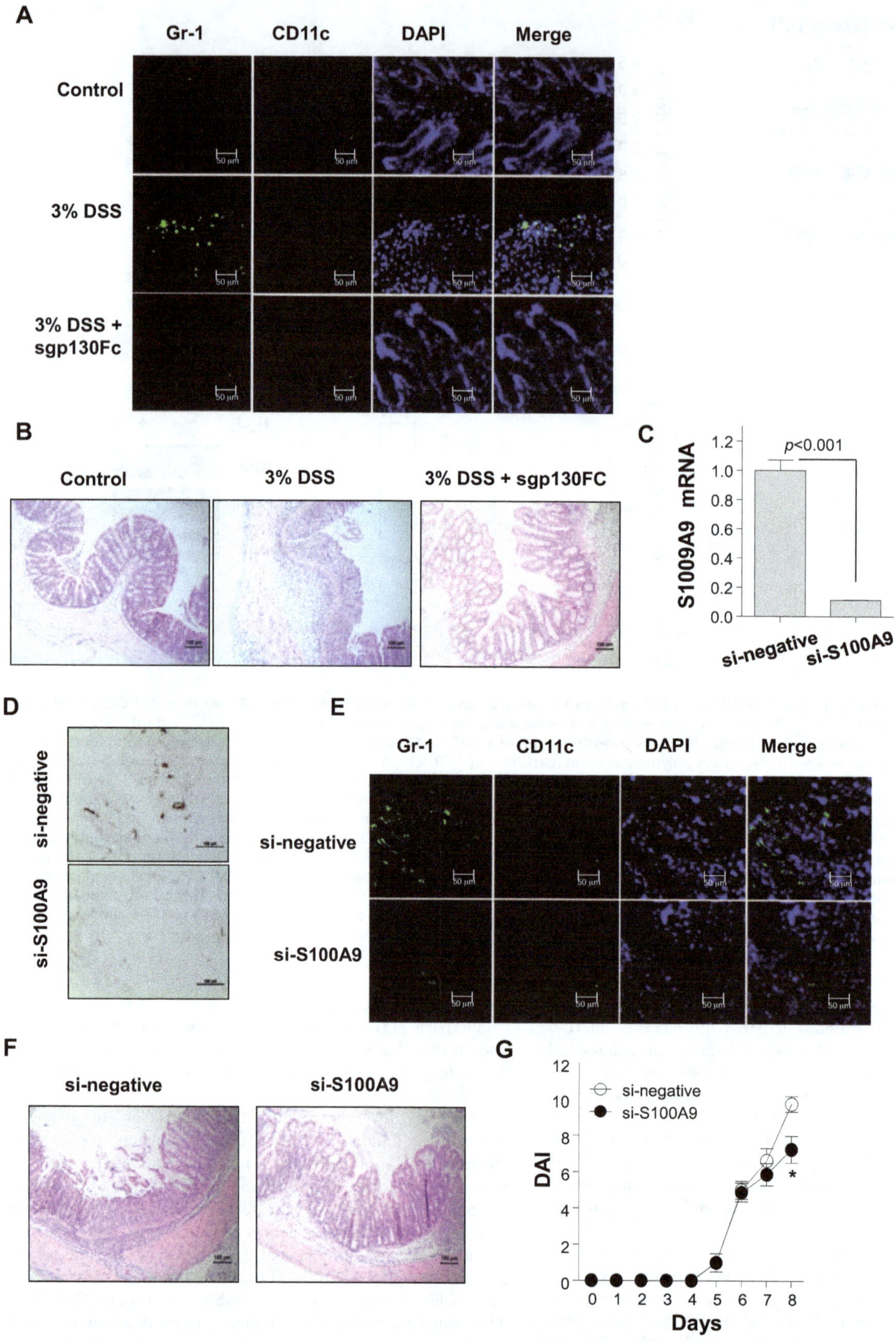

Figure 5. Gr-1⁺ cells infiltration in the colonic epithelial area of mice with dextran sulfate sodium (DSS)-induced colitis. (A) Colon sections from control mice and those treated with 3% DSS + phosphate-buffered saline (PBS) or 3% DSS + soluble gp130-Fc (sgp130Fc) were examined for Gr-1 (green), CD11c (red), and 4′,6-diamidino-2-phenylindole (DAPI; blue) expression by immunofluorescence on day 10 of DSS treatment. Data are representative of three independent experiments. Scale bars = 50 μm. (**B**) Colon histology was examined in control and DSS-

treated mice at 10 days after DSS or DSS + sgp130FC administration by hematoxylin and eosin staining of paraffin-embedded sections. Scale bars = 100 μm. Data are representative of three independent experiments. (**C–D**) Small interfering-negative chitosan nanoparticles (si-negative/CH-NPs) or si-S100A9/CH-NPs were injected intravenously twice on days 2 and 3 into 3% DSS-treated mice. On day 10 of DSS-exposure, expression of S100A9 in colon sections from mice was determined by qRT-PCR (C) and immunohistochemistry (D). qRT-PCR data are presented as mean ± standard deviations of values from each group. *P* values were obtained using the two-tailed Student's *t*-test Scale bars = 100 μm. Immunohistochemistry data are representative of four independent experiments. (**E**) The colon sections of DSS-exposed mice receiving si-negative/CH-NP or si-S100A9/CH-NP injections were examined for Gr-1 (green), CD11c (red), and DAPI (blue) expression by immunofluorescence on day 10 of DSS treatment. Data are representative of three independent experiments. Scale bars = 50 μm. (**F**) Colon histology was examined in control and DSS-treated mice at 10 days after si-negative/CH-NP or si-S100A9/CH-NP injections by hematoxylin and eosin staining of paraffin-embedded sections. Scale bars = 100 μm. Data are representative of three independent experiments. (**G**) Changes in the disease activity indices (DAI) of DSS-exposed mice receiving si-negative/CH-NP or si-S100A9/CH-NP injections were assessed daily. Data are presented as mean ± standard deviations of values from six mice per group. $^*p<0.01$ vs. control (two-tailed Student's *t*-test).

In conclusion, our results suggest the existence of an immune-triggering mechanism mediated by S100A9 released by CECs that helps to scavenge invading microorganisms when epithelial barriers are impaired. This mechanism may also induce further undesirable destruction in epithelial linings, leading to the exacerbation of colitis symptoms. Further studies should investigate how this mechanism can be controlled without interfering with immune surveillance in CECs. Our findings suggest that drugs inhibiting STAT3 signals may be good candidates for controlling disease activities in patients with UC while avoiding CAC development.

Materials and Methods

Cell Culture

A Caco-2 human IEC line was obtained from the Korean Cell Line Bank (Seoul, Republic of Korea). Human embryonic kidney cell line 293T and human colon cancer cell line HCT116 were purchased from the American Type Culture Collection (Manassas, VA, USA). The cells were cultured in appropriate media with 10% heat-inactivated fetal bovine serum (Lonza, Walkersville, MD, USA).

Reagents and Inhibitors

DSS (molecular weight, 35,000–50,000 Da; United States Biochemical, Cleveland, OH, USA) was used to induce experimental colitis in mice. IL-6 (PeproTech, Rocky Hill, NJ, USA) was used to stimulate Caco-2 cells. The following inhibitors were used to treat Caco-2 cells throughout IL-6 stimulation: S3I and STAT3 inhibitor peptide (Merck) to block phosphorylation by targeting a tyrosine residue and to dimerize STAT3, respectively [55,56].

To prepare small interfering (si) RNA-incorporated chitosan nanoparticles (CH-NPs), siRNAs for STAT3 and S100A9 were purchased from Bioneer Corporation (Daejeon, Republic of Korea). siRNA-incorporated CH-NPs were prepared according to a previously described method [44] by ionic gelation of anionic tripolyphosphate (TPP; Sigma Chemical, St. Louis, MO, USA) and siRNA with cationic chitosan (Sigma Chemical). The weight ratio of chitosan to TPP was set to 3:1 to generate particles about 200:nm in size. The prepared siRNA/CH-NPs (si-STAT3/CH-NPs and si-S100A9/CH-NPs) were injected intravenously twice into mice with DSS-induced colitis.

Establishment of an Experimental DSS-Induced Colitis Mouse Model

Six-week-old male C57BL/6 mice were purchased from Joongang Laboratory Animal Co. (Seoul, Republic of Korea) and maintained under specific pathogen-free conditions. As described previously [57], colitis was induced with water containing 3% DSS. The disease activity index (DAI) represents the combined scores of weight loss, stool consistency, and bleeding, according to scoring criteria described previously [58,59]. Body weight loss (scores: 0, none; 1, 1–10%; 2, 11–20%), stool consistency (scores: 0, normal; 1, soft; 2, liquid), hemoccult positivity, and the presence of blood (scores: 0, negative fecal occult blood; 1, positive fecal occult blood; 2, visible rectal bleeding) were assessed daily in each group of mice. In some experiments, mice were injected intraperitoneally with soluble gp130-FC fusion protein (sgp130Fc, 0.5 mg/kg; R&D Systems, Minneapolis, MN, USA) or phosphate-buffered saline (PBS). All surgical and experimental procedures were reviewed and approved by the Institutional Animal Care and Use Committee (IACUC) in College of Medicine, Seoul National University.

Isolation of Colonic Epithelial Cells

CECs were isolated using a modified version of previously described methods [60,61]. In brief, colon pieces were incubated in Ca^{2+}- and Mg^{2+}-free Hanks Balanced Salt Solution (HBSS; Sigma Chemical) containing 2% calf serum at 37°C for 30 min while stirring. After collecting the supernatant, remaining tissue was resuspended in HBSS with 3 mM ethylenediaminetetraacetic acid (EDTA). The tissues were incubated while stirring at 37°C for 30 min. The supernatant was then collected and centrifuged at 300×g for 10 min.

Histopathology and Immunohistochemistry of Colon Tissue

Large intestine specimens were fixed in 10% neutralized formalin for 24 h, embedded in paraffin, and sectioned at 4 μm. Colon sections were stained with hematoxylin and eosin (H&E) for histopathological analysis, and stained immunohistochemically as described previously to investigate the expression of phospho-STAT3 ($STAT3^{PY705}$) [62]. Briefly, paraffin-embedded slides were hydrated with ethanol and distilled water, followed by antigen retrieval in 10 mM sodium citrate buffer. Sections were incubated with anti-S100A9 (Abcam, Cambridge, MA, USA) and anti-$STAT3^{PY705}$ immunoglobulin G (IgG; Cell Signaling Technology, Danvers, MA, USA) and stained with 3,3-diaminobenzidine substrate. Image acquisition and processing were performed using a Leica microscope and the Leica Application Suite (Leica Microsystems, Buffalo Grove, IL, USA).

Immunofluorescence of Colon Tissue

To perform immunofluorescence analyses, mouse large intestine specimens were embedded in optimal cutting temperature compound (Sakura Finetek Japan, Tokyo, Japan) and sectioned at 10 μm by cryostats (Leica Microsystems). The sections were incubated with a combination of anti-Gr-1-biotin and purified anti-CD11c antibodies (BD Biosciences) or with rabbit anti-$STAT3^{PY705}$ IgG at 4°C overnight, followed by incubation with appropriate secondary antibodies. Stained sections were mounted in VectaShield 4′, 6-diamidino-2-phenylindole (DAPI) mounting medium (Vector Laboratories, Burlingame, CA, USA) and analyzed under a confocal laser scanning microscope (LSM 510; Carl Zeiss, Gottingen, Germany). Images were taken under a confocal microscope using a 40× objective.

Immunoblotting

Cells were harvested in a lysis solution (Santa Cruz Biotechnology, Santa Cruz, CA, USA) in the presence of a protease inhibitor cocktail (Roche, Basel, Switzerland) and phosphatase inhibitor (Santa Cruz Biotechnology). After incubation for 30 min on ice, insoluble debris was removed by centrifugation for 15 min at 4°C. Total protein was resolved by sodium dodecyl sulfate polyacrylamide gel electrophoresis and transferred to nitrocellulose membranes (GE Healthcare, Pittsburgh, PA, USA). The membranes were then probed with antibodies against α-tubulin (Thermo Fisher Scientific, Fremont, CA, USA), STAT3 (Cell Signaling Technology), or $STAT3^{PY705}$ and visualized using SuperSignal West Femto Chemiluminescent Substrate (Thermo Fisher Scientific).

Quantitative and Conventional Reverse-Transcription Polymerase Chain Reaction Assays

Total RNA was isolated from colon tissues and cDNA was synthesized using a QuantiTech Reverse Transcription Kit (QIAGEN, Valencia, CA, USA), then mixed with QuantiFast SYBR Green polymerase chain reaction (PCR) master mix (QIAGEN) and specific primers. Quantitative reverse-transcription PCR (qRT-PCR) was performed with an Applied Biosystems 7300 Real-Time PCR System (Life Technologies, Carlsbad, CA, USA) and analyzed by comparative C_t quantification [63]. The conventional PCR products were generated by *AccuPower* PCR Premix (Bioneer). The specific primers for genes used in this study were obtained from QIAGEN.

Enzyme-linked Immunosorbent Assay (ELISA)

Cell culture supernatants were analyzed for S100A9 levels using an S100A9 ELISA kit (Cyclex Co., Ltd, Nagano, Japan) according to the manufacturer's instructions.

Chromatin Immunoprecipitation

Chromatin immunoprecipitation (ChIP) assays were performed using a Chromatin Immunoprecipitation Assay Kit (Millipore, Billerica, MA, USA) according to the manufacturer's instructions. Briefly, Caco-2 cells were fixed with formaldehyde for 10 min at room temperature. After sonication (30 s on/1 min off for three cycles), the fragmented soluble chromatin was immunoprecipitated with anti-$STAT3^{PY705}$ IgG or rabbit IgG. Cross-links were reversed by incubating at 65°C. Precipitated DNA was amplified by conventional PCR using specific primers covering the canonical STAT3 binding motif within the *S100A9* promoter: forward, 5′-ACACATCTTGCCCACCAGGAGGCTA-3′; reverse, 5′-AAATCCTGCTCCCAGCAAGGGTTCC-3′.

Statistical Analysis

Data are presented as means ± standard deviations (SDs). *P* values <0.05 were considered statistically significant. Two-tailed Student's *t*-tests were conducted using the GraphPad Prism software (ver. 5.01; GraphPad Software, La Jolla, CA, USA).

Supporting Information

Figure S1 Changes in interleukin-6 (IL-6) expression in the colons of an experimental ulcerative colitis mouse model established by dextran sulfate sodium (DSS) treatment. (**A**) The difference (%) between baseline and subsequent body weight was measured daily for 11 days (left). Changes in clinical symptoms are represented by the disease activity index (DAI; right). Data are presented as means ± standard deviations of values from six mice per group. *$p<0.01$, **$p<0.001$ vs. control mice (two-tailed Student's *t*-test). PBS, phosphate-buffered saline. (**B**) Colon histology was examined in control and DSS-treated mice at 6 or 12 days after DSS administration by hematoxylin and eosin (H&E) staining of paraffin-embedded sections. Scale bars = 100 μm. Data are representative of three independent experiments. (**C**) In each of three groups, colon tissues were homogenized using a tissue homogenizer. *IL-6* and *GAPDH* mRNA levels in each group of colonic tissue samples was analyzed by conventional reverse-transcription polymerase chain reaction assays. Data are representative of three independent experiments.

Figure S2 The purity of the isolated colonic epithelial cells (CECs) from a mouse model of dextran sulfate sodium (DSS)-induced colitis. (**A**) Epithelial cells were isolated from colon tissue specimens from DSS-treated or control mice, and the purity of the isolated CECs was confirmed by staining with fluorescein isothiocyanate-labeled antibodies against E-cadherin (BD Biosciences, San Diego, CA, USA) by flow cytometry. Numbers indicate the percentage of positive cells in the histogram. Data are representative of three independent experiments. (**B**) *CD45* and *villin* mRNA expression was analyzed by conventional reverse-transcription polymerase chain reaction (RT-PCR) for isolated CECs and intraepithelial lymphocyte (IEL), which is control cell expressing CD45.

Figure S3 Effect of soluble gp130-Fc (sgp130Fc) injection on the expression of CXCL10 in colonic epithelial cells (CECs) from mice with dextran sulfate sodium (DSS)-induced colitis. CECs from mice treated with or without 3% DSS for 8 days and a subsequent sgp130Fc or PBS injection were prepared, and *CXCL10* mRNA expression was analyzed by quantitative reverse-transcription polymerase chain reaction (qRT-PCR). Data are presented as means ± standard deviations of values from six mice per group. *P* values were obtained using the two-tailed Student's *t*-test.

Figure S4 S100A9 is potent chemotactic factors for human promyelocytic leukemia (HL-60) *in vitro*. Chemotaxis assays were performed using CytoSelect Cell migratory Assay Kit (Cell Biolabs, San Diego, CA, USA). Media (control) or increasing concentration of S100A9 (Cyclex Co. Nagano, Japan) were added to the lower chamber. HL-60 cells were added to the upper chamber (5×10^3 cells) and allowed to migrate through the membrane (5 μm pore size) for 6 h. Migrated cells were stained with trypan blue and counted with hemocytometer. Results are the mean % of migrated cells. Data are presented as means ± standard deviations of values from triplicate experiments. *P* values were obtained using the two-tailed Student's *t*-test.

Acknowledgments

We thank Dr. Tae Woo Kim for preparation of siRNA-incorporated chitosan nanoparticles (CH-NPs). We also thank the Institute for Experimental Animals of Seoul National University, College of Medicine.

The English in this document has been checked by at least two professional editors, both native speakers of English. For a certificate, please see:

http://www.textcheck.com/certificate/ZzjI38.

Author Contributions

Conceived and designed the experiments: MJL JKL JWC CL JHS CC KL MC HK SKY. Performed the experiments: MJL JKL IHC. Analyzed the data: MJL JKL JWC CL JHS CC KL MC HK SKY IHC. Contributed reagents/materials/analysis tools: MJL JKL JWC CL JHS CC KL MC HK SKY IHC. Wrote the paper: MJL JKL HK SKY.

References

1. Podolsky DK (1991) Inflammatory bowel disease (1). N Engl J Med 325: 928–937.
2. Maloy KJ, Powrie F (2011) Intestinal homeostasis and its breakdown in inflammatory bowel disease. Nature 474: 298–306.
3. Kaser A, Zeissig S, Blumberg RS (2010) Inflammatory bowel disease. Annu Rev Immunol 28: 573–621.
4. Garud S, Peppercorn MA (2009) Ulcerative colitis: current treatment strategies and future prospects. Therap Adv Gastroenterol 2: 99–108.
5. Baumgart DC, Carding SR (2007) Inflammatory bowel disease: cause and immunobiology. Lancet 369: 1627–1640.
6. Eaden JA, Abrams KR, Mayberry JF (2001) The risk of colorectal cancer in ulcerative colitis: a meta-analysis. Gut 48: 526–535.
7. Suzuki Y, Saito H, Kasanuki J, Kishimoto T, Tamura Y, et al. (1990) Significant increase of interleukin 6 production in blood mononuclear leukocytes obtained from patients with active inflammatory bowel disease. Life Sci 47: 2193–2197.
8. Mudter J, Neurath MF (2007) Il-6 signaling in inflammatory bowel disease: pathophysiological role and clinical relevance. Inflamm Bowel Dis 13: 1016–1023.
9. Reinecker HC, Steffen M, Witthoeft T, Pflueger I, Schreiber S, et al. (1993) Enhanced secretion of tumour necrosis factor-alpha, IL-6, and IL-1 beta by isolated lamina propria mononuclear cells from patients with ulcerative colitis and Crohn's disease. Clin Exp Immunol 94: 174–181.
10. Umehara Y, Kudo M, Nakaoka R, Kawasaki T, Shiomi M (2006) Serum proinflammatory cytokines and adhesion molecules in ulcerative colitis. Hepatogastroenterology 53: 879–882.
11. Matsumoto S, Hara T, Mitsuyama K, Yamamoto M, Tsuruta O, et al. (2010) Essential roles of IL-6 trans-signaling in colonic epithelial cells, induced by the IL-6/soluble-IL-6 receptor derived from lamina propria macrophages, on the development of colitis-associated premalignant cancer in a murine model. J Immunol 184: 1543–1551.
12. Cammarota R, Bertolini V, Pennesi G, Bucci EO, Gottardi O, et al. (2010) The tumor microenvironment of colorectal cancer: stromal TLR-4 expression as a potential prognostic marker. J Transl Med 8: 112.
13. Atreya R, Mudter J, Finotto S, Mullberg J, Jostock T, et al. (2000) Blockade of interleukin 6 trans signaling suppresses T-cell resistance against apoptosis in chronic intestinal inflammation: evidence in crohn disease and experimental colitis in vivo. Nat Med 6: 583–588.
14. Grivennikov S, Karin E, Terzic J, Mucida D, Yu GY, et al. (2009) IL-6 and Stat3 are required for survival of intestinal epithelial cells and development of colitis-associated cancer. Cancer Cell 15: 103–113.
15. Neurath MF, Finotto S, Fuss I, Boirivant M, Galle PR, et al. (2001) Regulation of T-cell apoptosis in inflammatory bowel disease: to die or not to die, that is the mucosal question. Trends Immunol 22: 21–26.
16. Bettelli E, Carrier Y, Gao W, Korn T, Strom TB, et al. (2006) Reciprocal developmental pathways for the generation of pathogenic effector TH17 and regulatory T cells. Nature 441: 235–238.
17. Jin X, Zimmers TA, Zhang Z, Pierce RH, Koniaris LG (2010) Interleukin-6 is an important in vivo inhibitor of intestinal epithelial cell death in mice. Gut 59: 186–196.
18. Kishimoto T (2005) Interleukin-6: from basic science to medicine–40 years in immunology. Annu Rev Immunol 23: 1–21.
19. Cenit MC, Alcina A, Marquez A, Mendoza JL, Diaz-Rubio M, et al. (2010) STAT3 locus in inflammatory bowel disease and multiple sclerosis susceptibility. Genes Immun 11: 264–268.
20. Odink K, Cerletti N, Bruggen J, Clerc RG, Tarcsay L, et al. (1987) Two calcium-binding proteins in infiltrate macrophages of rheumatoid arthritis. Nature 330: 80–82.
21. Foell D, Wittkowski H, Vogl T, Roth J (2007) S100 proteins expressed in phagocytes: a novel group of damage-associated molecular pattern molecules. J Leukoc Biol 81: 28–37.
22. Foell D, Wittkowski H, Roth J (2009) Monitoring disease activity by stool analyses: from occult blood to molecular markers of intestinal inflammation and damage. Gut 58: 859–868.
23. Thorey IS, Roth J, Regenbogen J, Halle JP, Bittner M, et al. (2001) The Ca2+-binding proteins S100A8 and S100A9 are encoded by novel injury-regulated genes. J Biol Chem 276: 35818–35825.
24. Rammes A, Roth J, Goebeler M, Klempt M, Hartmann M, et al. (1997) Myeloid-related protein (MRP) 8 and MRP14, calcium-binding proteins of the S100 family, are secreted by activated monocytes via a novel, tubulin-dependent pathway. J Biol Chem 272: 9496–9502.
25. Katz AB, Taichman LB (1999) A partial catalog of proteins secreted by epidermal keratinocytes in culture. J Invest Dermatol 112: 818–821.
26. Wilkinson MM, Busuttil A, Hayward C, Brock DJ, Dorin JR, et al. (1988) Expression pattern of two related cystic fibrosis-associated calcium-binding proteins in normal and abnormal tissues. J Cell Sci 91 (Pt 2): 221–230.
27. Roth J, Burwinkel F, van den Bos C, Goebeler M, Vollmer E, et al. (1993) MRP8 and MRP14, S-100-like proteins associated with myeloid differentiation, are translocated to plasma membrane and intermediate filaments in a calcium-dependent manner. Blood 82: 1875–1883.
28. Frosch M, Metze D, Foell D, Vogl T, Sorg C, et al. (2005) Early activation of cutaneous vessels and epithelial cells is characteristic of acute systemic onset juvenile idiopathic arthritis. Exp Dermatol 14: 259–265.
29. Lugering N, Stoll R, Kucharzik T, Schmid KW, Rohlmann G, et al. (1995) Immunohistochemical distribution and serum levels of the Ca(2+)-binding proteins MRP8, MRP14 and their heterodimeric form MRP8/14 in Crohn's disease. Digestion 56: 406–414.
30. Li C, Zhang F, Lin M, Liu J (2004) Induction of S100A9 gene expression by cytokine oncostatin M in breast cancer cells through the STAT3 signaling cascade. Breast Cancer Res Treat 87: 123–134.
31. Cheng P, Corzo CA, Luetteke N, Yu B, Nagaraj S, et al. (2008) Inhibition of dendritic cell differentiation and accumulation of myeloid-derived suppressor cells in cancer is regulated by S100A9 protein. J Exp Med 205: 2235–2249.
32. Guignard F, Mauel J, Markert M (1995) Identification and characterization of a novel human neutrophil protein related to the S100 family. Biochem J 309 (Pt 2): 395–401.
33. Newton RA, Hogg N (1998) The human S100 protein MRP-14 is a novel activator of the beta 2 integrin Mac-1 on neutrophils. J Immunol 160: 1427–1435.
34. Viemann D, Barczyk K, Vogl T, Fischer U, Sunderkotter C, et al. (2007) MRP8/MRP14 impairs endothelial integrity and induces a caspase-dependent and -independent cell death program. Blood 109: 2453–2460.
35. Vogl T, Tenbrock K, Ludwig S, Leukert N, Ehrhardt C, et al. (2007) Mrp8 and Mrp14 are endogenous activators of Toll-like receptor 4, promoting lethal, endotoxin-induced shock. Nat Med 13: 1042–1049.
36. Viemann D, Strey A, Janning A, Jurk K, Klimmek K, et al. (2005) Myeloid-related proteins 8 and 14 induce a specific inflammatory response in human microvascular endothelial cells. Blood 105: 2955–2962.
37. Croce K, Gao H, Wang Y, Mooroka T, Sakuma M, et al. (2009) Myeloid-related protein-8/14 is critical for the biological response to vascular injury. Circulation 120: 427–436.
38. Ryckman C, Vandal K, Rouleau P, Talbot M, Tessier PA (2003) Proinflammatory activities of S100: proteins S100A8, S100A9, and S100A8/A9 induce neutrophil chemotaxis and adhesion. J Immunol 170: 3233–3242.
39. Bogumil T, Rieckmann P, Kubuschok B, Felgenhauer K, Bruck W (1998) Serum levels of macrophage-derived protein MRP-8/14 are elevated in active multiple sclerosis. Neurosci Lett 247: 195–197.
40. Kuruto R, Nozawa R, Takeishi K, Arai K, Yokota T, et al. (1990) Myeloid calcium binding proteins: expression in the differentiated HL-60 cells and detection in sera of patients with connective tissue diseases. J Biochem 108: 650–653.
41. Wang L, Walia B, Evans J, Gewirtz AT, Merlin D, et al. (2003) IL-6 induces NF-kappa B activation in the intestinal epithelia. J Immunol 171: 3194–3201.
42. Becker C, Fantini MC, Schramm C, Lehr HA, Wirtz S, et al. (2004) TGF-beta suppresses tumor progression in colon cancer by inhibition of IL-6 trans-signaling. Immunity 21: 491–501.
43. Jostock T, Mullberg J, Ozbek S, Atreya R, Blinn G, et al. (2001) Soluble gp130 is the natural inhibitor of soluble interleukin-6 receptor transsignaling responses. Eur J Biochem 268: 160–167.
44. Lu C, Han HD, Mangala LS, Ali-Fehmi R, Newton CS, et al. (2010) Regulation of tumor angiogenesis by EZH2. Cancer Cell 18: 185–197.
45. Fagerhol MK (2000) Calprotectin, a faecal marker of organic gastrointestinal abnormality. Lancet 356: 1783–1784.
46. Ehrchen JM, Sunderkotter C, Foell D, Vogl T, Roth J (2009) The endogenous Toll-like receptor 4 agonist S100A8/S100A9 (calprotectin) as innate amplifier of infection, autoimmunity, and cancer. J Leukoc Biol 86: 557–566.
47. Dale DC, Boxer L, Liles WC (2008) The phagocytes: neutrophils and monocytes. Blood 112: 935–945.
48. Elsbach P, Weiss J (1998) Role of the bactericidal/permeability-increasing protein in host defence. Curr Opin Immunol 10: 45–49.
49. Ganz T, Selsted ME, Szklarek D, Harwig SS, Daher K, et al. (1985) Defensins. Natural peptide antibiotics of human neutrophils. J Clin Invest 76: 1427–1435.
50. Rose-John S, Mitsuyama K, Matsumoto S, Thaiss WM, Scheller J (2009) Interleukin-6 trans-signaling and colonic cancer associated with inflammatory bowel disease. Curr Pharm Des 15: 2095–2103.

51. Soliman A, Michelsen KS, Karahashi H, Lu J, Meng FJ, et al. (2010) Platelet-activating factor induces TLR4 expression in intestinal epithelial cells: implication for the pathogenesis of necrotizing enterocolitis. PLoS One 5: e15044.
52. Abreu MT, Thomas LS, Arnold ET, Lukasek K, Michelsen KS, et al. (2003) TLR signaling at the intestinal epithelial interface. J Endotoxin Res 9: 322–330.
53. Li Y, de Haar C, Chen M, Deuring J, Gerrits MM, et al. (2010) Disease-related expression of the IL6/STAT3/SOCS3 signalling pathway in ulcerative colitis and ulcerative colitis-related carcinogenesis. Gut 59: 227–235.
54. Tebbutt NC, Giraud AS, Inglese M, Jenkins B, Waring P, et al. (2002) Reciprocal regulation of gastrointestinal homeostasis by SHP2 and STAT-mediated trefoil gene activation in gp130 mutant mice. Nat Med 8: 1089–1097.
55. Miyamoto N, Sugita K, Goi K, Inukai T, Lijima K, et al. (2001) The JAK2 inhibitor AG490 predominantly abrogates the growth of human B-precursor leukemic cells with 11q23 translocation or Philadelphia chromosome. Leukemia 15: 1758–1768.
56. Turkson J, Ryan D, Kim JS, Zhang Y, Chen Z, et al. (2001) Phosphotyrosyl peptides block Stat3-mediated DNA binding activity, gene regulation, and cell transformation. J Biol Chem 276: 45443–45455.
57. Okayasu I, Hatakeyama S, Yamada M, Ohkusa T, Inagaki Y, et al. (1990) A novel method in the induction of reliable experimental acute and chronic ulcerative colitis in mice. Gastroenterology 98: 694–702.
58. Cooper HS, Murthy SN, Shah RS, Sedergran DJ (1993) Clinicopathologic study of dextran sulfate sodium experimental murine colitis. Lab Invest 69: 238–249.
59. Suzuki K, Sun X, Nagata M, Kawase T, Yamaguchi H, et al. (2011) Analysis of intestinal fibrosis in chronic colitis in mice induced by dextran sulfate sodium. Pathol Int 61: 228–238.
60. Montufar-Solis D, Klein JR (2006) An improved method for isolating intraepithelial lymphocytes (IELs) from the murine small intestine with consistently high purity. J Immunol Methods 308: 251–254.
61. Panja A, Blumberg RS, Balk SP, Mayer L (1993) CD1d is involved in T cell-intestinal epithelial cell interactions. J Exp Med 178: 1115–1119.
62. Oskouian B, Sooriyakumaran P, Borowsky AD, Crans A, Dillard-Telm L, et al. (2006) Sphingosine-1-phosphate lyase potentiates apoptosis via p53- and p38-dependent pathways and is down-regulated in colon cancer. Proc Natl Acad Sci U S A 103: 17384–17389.
63. Popivanova BK, Kitamura K, Wu Y, Kondo T, Kagaya T, et al. (2008) Blocking TNF-alpha in mice reduces colorectal carcinogenesis associated with chronic colitis. J Clin Invest 118: 560–570.

Up-Regulation of microRNA-126 may Contribute to Pathogenesis of Ulcerative Colitis via Regulating NF-kappaB Inhibitor IκBα

Xiao Feng[1]⁹, Hao Wang[1]⁹, Shicai Ye[1], Jiaxi Guan[1], Wenkai Tan[1], Si Cheng[1], Guoli Wei[1], Weiyun Wu[1], Feng Wu[2], Yu Zhou[1]*

1 Department of Gastroenterology, The Affiliated Hospital of Guangdong Medical College, Zhanjiang, Guangdong, People's Republic of China, **2** Department of Medicine, University of Chicago, Chicago, Illinois, United States of America

Abstract

Background: MicroRNAs (miRNAs) are important post-transcriptional regulators. Altered expression of miRNAs has recently demonstrated association with human ulcerative colitis (UC). In this study, we attempted to elucidate the roles of miR-126 in the pathogenesis of UC.

Methods: Expression of miR-126, miR-21, miR-375 and the potential targets NF-κB inhibitor alpha (IκBα, IKBA or NFKBIA), Polo-like kinase 2 (PLK2) and v-Crk sarcoma virus CT10 oncogene homolog (CRK) were assessed in 52 colonic biopsies from patients with active UC, inactive UC, irritable bowel syndrome (IBS) and from healthy subjects by quantitative RT-PCR and immunofluorescence analyses. Regulation of gene expression by miR-126 was assessed using luciferase reporter construct assays and specific miRNA mimic transfection.

Results: We found that the expression of miR-126 and miR-21 were significantly increased in active UC group compared to the inactive UC, IBS and healthy control groups ($P<0.05$). In contrast, the expression of IKBA mRNA and protein was remarkably decreased in the active UC group compared with the other three groups ($P<0.05$). The expression of miR-126 and IKBA mRNA were inversely correlated in active UC patients ($P<0.05$). However the expression of miR-375, PLK2 and CRK showed no difference between each group. Furthermore, we demonstrate that endogenous miR-126 and exogenous miR-126 mimic can inhibit IκBα expression. Finally, mutating the miR-126 binding site of the IKBA 3′-UTR reporter construct restored reporter gene expression.

Conclusion: miR-126 may play roles in UC inflammatory activity by down-regulating the expression of IKBA, an important inhibitor of NF-κB signaling pathway.

Editor: Alfred Lewin, University of Florida, United States of America

Funding: This study was supported by National Natural Science Foundation of China (grant number 30971350 to Yu Zhou) and the Planned Science and Technology Project of Guangdong Province, China (grant number 2009B030801332 to Yu Zhou). This research was also supported by the fund at The Affiliated Hospital of Guangdong Medical College. The funders had no role in study design, data collection and analysis, decision to publish, or preparation of the manuscript.

Competing Interests: The authors have declared that no competing interests exist.

* E-mail: ahdg2005@126.com

⁹ These authors contributed equally to this work.

Introduction

Ulcerative colitis (UC) is one of two major types of inflammatory bowel diseases (IBD) and is presented as a chronic, relapsing and remitting inflammatory disease limited to the mucosal layer of the rectum and colon. An increasing incidence of UC has recently been reported worldwide in the last 20 years, especially in China [1]. Pathogenesis of IBD is not yet fully understood. It is currently proposed that the pathogenesis of IBD involves genetic susceptibility variation, inappropriate immunoresponse to microbes in the gut and undetermined environmental factors. Furthermore, pathogenesis of UC may vary in different ethnic populations and demographic regions. Genome-wide association studies have identified multiple susceptibility loci with high risk of IBD development [2–5]. Gene expression studies found a significant set of genes differentially expressed in patients with UC compared to healthy individuals [6–9]. However, it is still unclear how such differential expression of genes is regulated.

microRNAs (miRNAs) have recently been recognized as important post transcriptional regulators. Mature miRNAs are a class of small, non-coding RNA molecules in length of 20–25 nucleotides(nt). miRNAs bind to sequences located in the 3′-untranslated region (3′-UTR) of target mRNAs in the RNA-induced silencing complex and regulate mRNA degradation or repress their translation. miRNAs have been proven to play critical roles in many biological processes such as cell differentiation, proliferation, apoptosis and tumorigenesis [10–11]. Mounting evidence has shown that miRNAs are critically involved in the regulation of inflammatory and immune responses. Inflammatory cytokines and microbial components (flagellin and lipopolysaccharide, LPS) induce expression of miRNAs such as miR-146a, miR-155 and miR-132, via the transcription factor nuclear factor-kappaB (NF-κB) pathway in myeloid cells [12,13]. It has been shown that miR-146a modulates Toll like receptors (TLR) and tumor necrosis factor-α (TNF-α) signaling pathways through a negative feedback loop, by reducing expression of Interleukin-1 receptor-associated kinase 1 (IRAK1), TNF receptor-associated factor 6 (TRAF6) and cyclooxygenase-2 [13–15]. miRNAs including miR-155 and miR-150 are shown to influence the fate of immune cells, and to regulate adaptive immune response such as antigen presentation and T-cell receptor signaling [12,16,17].

An interesting study first demonstrated the association of 11 miRNAs with active UC [18]. Since then, several research groups worldwide reported that various miRNAs are differentially expressed in colonic tissues of UC and Crohn's disease (CD), as well as in blood and stool samples from IBD patients [19–27].

The genome-wide microarray screening study identified a group of miRNAs differentially expressed in active UC in the American population, including 3 downregulated miRNAs (miR-192, miR-375 and miR-422b) and 8 unregulated miRNAs (miR-16, miR-21, miR-23a, miR-24, miR-29a, miR-126, miR-195 and Let-7f) in the colons of active UC patients [18]. However, the association of miR-126 with human IBD has not been further investigated.

In this study, we aimed to characterize the roles of miR-126 in the pathogenesis of human UC. We first found that miR-126 was significantly increased in the colons of active UC patients compared to other control groups. We also found that among three potential targets of miR-126, nuclear factor-kappaB inhibitor alpha (IκBα, also named as IKBA, NFKBIA) was decreased and inversely correlated with miR-126 expression in colons with active UC. Furthermore, we demonstrated that endogenous miR-126 and exogenous miR-126 mimic can inhibit IκBα expression. Our findings suggest that miR-126 may play an important role in the regulation of inflammation in chronic inflammatory disease, including UC.

Materials and Methods

Human Tissues

Colonoscopic pinch biopsies from the sigmoid colon of 52 patients with chronic active UC, chronic inactive UC, irritable bowel syndrome (IBS), and normal, healthy patients undergoing screening colonoscopies were obtained from The Affiliated Hospital of Guangdong Medical College, Zhanjiang, China. Biopsies from all patients were assessed between September 2008 and December 2009 and the clinical characteristics of the patients are indicated in Table 1. The diagnoses of active UC and inactive UC were confirmed by colonoscopy and pathological findings. Disease activities were determined using the Ulcerative Colitis Disease Activity Index (UCDAI) [28], which is a series of qualifiers about the symptoms of ulcerative colitis including stool frequency, rectal bleeding, appearance of the lining of the colon, and a physician rating of disease activity. Each of these items was given a number from 0 to 3, with 3 being the highest for rating of disease activity. Ratings of 0–2 were recorded as remission, 3–6 as mild, 7–10 as moderate,>10 as severe UC respectively. Patients with UCDAI >8 were included in the study.

Table 1. Clinical Characteristics of Patients.

	Control	Active UC	Inactive UC	IBS
No. of patients	15	12	10	15
No. of Male, (%)	7(46.7%)	5(41.7%)	4(40%)	9(60%)
Age(yrs)				
Mean±SE	47.1±14.1	48.8±21.3	37±12.4	40.2±9.9
Range	30~70	17~80	25~58	27~60
DAI score				
Mean±SE	-	8.91±0.9	0.9±0.88	-
Range	-	8–10	0–2	-
Diease duration(yrs)				
Mean±SE	-	1.8±1.0	4±1.2	3±1.6
Range		0.5–4	2–6	1–6

Isolation of Total RNA

Colonoscopic biopsies or cultured cells were rapidly transferred into 1.0 ml of TRIzol reagent (Invitrogen, Carlsbad, CA) and total RNA was extracted according to the manufacturer's instructions and stored at −80°C until used.

Real-time Quantitative Reverse Transcriptase-polymerase Chain Reaction (qRT-PCR)

The NCode™ VILO™ miRNA cDNA Synthesis Kit(Invitrogen, Carlsbad, CA)and ImProm-II™ Reverse Transcription System(Promege, Madison, USA)were used to reverse-transcribe the miRNA and mRNA, respectively. For qRT-PCR on biopsy tissues, 500 ng of total RNA was converted to cDNA. 2 µl of cDNA from each sample was amplified by real-time fluorescent qPCR, using SYBR Premix Ex Taq™ (Takara Bio, Inc., Tokyo, Japan). The expression of each target miRNA in tissues was calculated relative to U6B, a ubiquitously expressed small nuclear RNA used as internal control. Expression of beta-actin was used as normalization control in mRNA qPCR. For miRNA qPCR, the reverse primer was the NCode miRNA universal qPCR primer (Invitrogen, Carlsbad, CA). Forward miRNA primers and mRNA primers were compound by Sangon Biotech Co, Ltd (Shanghai, China) and are listed in Table 2. A comparative threshold cycle method was used to compare each condition with controls.

Immunofluorescence

Immunofluorescencet staining was performed according to standard protocol (Santa Cruz Biotechnology). Briefly, a 5-µm frozen section from each case was fixed in acetone at 4°C for 10 min and blocked with 10% goat serum albumin at room temperature (RT) for 30 min. the sections were incubated with rabbit anti-human IκBα primary antibody (1:400) (Santa Cruz Biotechnology) overnight at 4°C. After rinsing in phosphate-buffered saline (PBS) for three times, the sections were incubated with secondary polyclonal Cy3 labeled goat anti-rabbit-594 IgG (1:400) (Zhongshan Goldenbridge Biotechnology. Beijing, China) for one hour at RT in dark, and then washed with PBS. PBS replaced anti-IκBα antibody as a negative control. 4′,6-diamidino-2-phenylindole (DAPI) was used to counter-stain the nuclei for 5 min at RT. The staining was evaluated on a Leica converted fluorescence microscope and the fluorescence intensity was measured using Image-Pro Plus 6.0 software. We quantified the total Cy3-fluorescence intensity (as shown in red) of the mucosa and submucosal layers as representation of protein expression level of IκBα. Intensity of DAPI staining (blue) was used as an internal normalization control for adjusting fluorescence signals among different slides.

Table 2. Primers Used for Quantitative Real-time PCR in This Study.

Name	Direction	Primer (5′-3′)
For microRNA qPCR		
Universal qPCR primer	Reverse	NCode™ VILO™ miRNA cDNA Synthesis Kit (Invitrogen)
miR-126	Forward	TCGTACCGTGAGTAATAATGCG
miR-21	Forward	TAGCTTATCAGACTGATGTTGA
miR-375	Forward	CGGCTCGCGTGAAAAA
U6 snRNA	Forward	CTCGCTTCGGCAGCACA
For mRNA qPCR		
IKBA	Forward	CACTCCATCCTGAAGGCTACCAA
	Reverse	AAGGGCAGTCCGGCCATTA
PLK2	Forward	GAACACCCGCAGTAGAAAACA
	Reverse	GACCCACTGAAATGATGTGCT
CRK	Forward	AGGGTTATCCAGAAGCGAGTC
	Reverse	CTTCCCACTGACCACTCACAT
Beta-actin	Forward	GGCGGCAACACCATGTACCCT
	Reverse	AGGGGCCGGACTCGTCATACT

Identification of Potential Downstream Targets of miR-126

To predict potential targets of miR-126, three in silico analysis programs were used for microRNA targets prediction, including MicroCosm Targets (http://www.ebi.ac.uk/enright-srv/microcosm/htdocs/targets/v5/), Targetscan (http://www.targetscan.org/) and PicTar (http://pictar.mdc-berlin.de/).

IKBA 3′-UTR Wild Type and Mutant Constructs

The 3′-UTR of IKBA mRNA (RefSeq NM-020529) has a putative miRNA-126 binding site. In order to test the effects of miR-126 on the expression of IκBα, we created a dual-luciferase reporter construct containing two replicate miR-126 binding sequences corresponding to 1502–1538 nucleotides of IKBA mRNA sequence using an established method [29]. Briefly, the wild type sequence (5′-TGTATTGTTGGTAATTATTTTGG-TACTT TTATGATGTTGTATTGTTGGTAAT-TATTTTGGTACTTTTATGATGT-3′) was created by PCR with forward primer IKBA-XhoIF (5′-CCGCTCGAGTG-TATTGTTGGTAATTATTTTG GTACTTTTAT-GATGTTGTATTGTTGG-3′) and reverse primer IKBA-NotIR (5′-ATAAGAA TGCGGCCGCACATCATAAAAGTAC-CAAAATAA-TTACCAACAATACAACATCATAAAAG-3′). To generate a construct containing the miR-126 binding site mutants, we used a forward primer (Mut IKBA XhoIF: 5′-CCGCTCGAGTGTATTGTTGGTAATTATTTACCAT GTTTTATGATGTTGTATTGTTGG-3′) and a reverse primer (Mut IKBA NotIR: 5′-ATAAG AATGCGGCCGCACATCA-TAAAACATGGTAAATAATTACCAACAATACAACATCA-TAAAAC-3′) bearing six substituted nucleotides corresponding to the 5′-seeding region of the miR-126 binding site (shown as underlined in wild type sequence). The PCR parameters were as the followings: initial denature at 94°C for 5 min, 30 cycles of 30 sec at 94°C, 30 sec at 55°C and 20 sec at 72°C, and a final extension of 5 min at 72°C.

The wild type and mutant sequences were then cloned into the XhoI and NotI sites downstream of the Renilla luciferase gene of the dual-luciferase report vector psiCHECK-2 (Promega Corporation, Madison, USA) according to manufacturer's protocols. The wild type and the mutant constructs were named as psi-IKBA and psi-mutIKBA, respectively. The sequences of the constructs were verified by DNA sequencing. The constructs were transformed in E.coli JM109 and the plasmid DNA was purified using TIANpure MidiPrep kit (Tiangen Biotech, Beijing, China).

Construct Transfection and Luciferase Report Assay

Human colonic cancer cell line HT29 and HCT116 (Beijing Institute For Cancer Research, China) were maintained in DMEM containing 10% FBS at 37°C in a 5% CO_2 incubator. HT29 cells were seeded in 24-well plates overnight before transfections. Luciferase report constructs (100–250 ng/well) were transfected into cells using Lipofectamine 2000 (Invitrogen, Carlsbad, CA) according to the manufacturer's protocols. Cells were harvested at 24 hours after transfection. Renilla and Firefly luciferase activites were measured using the Dual Luciferase Reporter Assay System (Promega Corporation, Madison, USA) according to the manufacturer's instructions. Experiments were performed in quadruplicate wells and datas are represents of three independent experiments.

miRNA Mimic Transfection

HT29 cells were seeded into 24-well plates at 90% confluence and kept in a 37°C and 5% CO_2 incubator overnight. Varying amounts of miR-126 mimic or negative control mimic (RiBoBio, Guangzhou, China) were transfected into HT29 cells using Lipofectamine 2000. The transfected cells were incubated at 37°C in a 5% CO_2 incubator for 24 hours. Cellular total RNA and protein were harvested separately, and stored in −80°C until used.

To determine the specific effect of miR-126 on 3′-UTR of IKBA, the miR-126 mimic and the psi-IKBA luciferase construct were co-transfected into HT29 cells using Lipofectamine 2000. Renilla and Firefly luciferase levels were measured at 24 hours post-transfection using the Dual Luciferase Reporter Assay System. Experiments were performed in quadruplicate wells and datas are represents of three independent experiments.

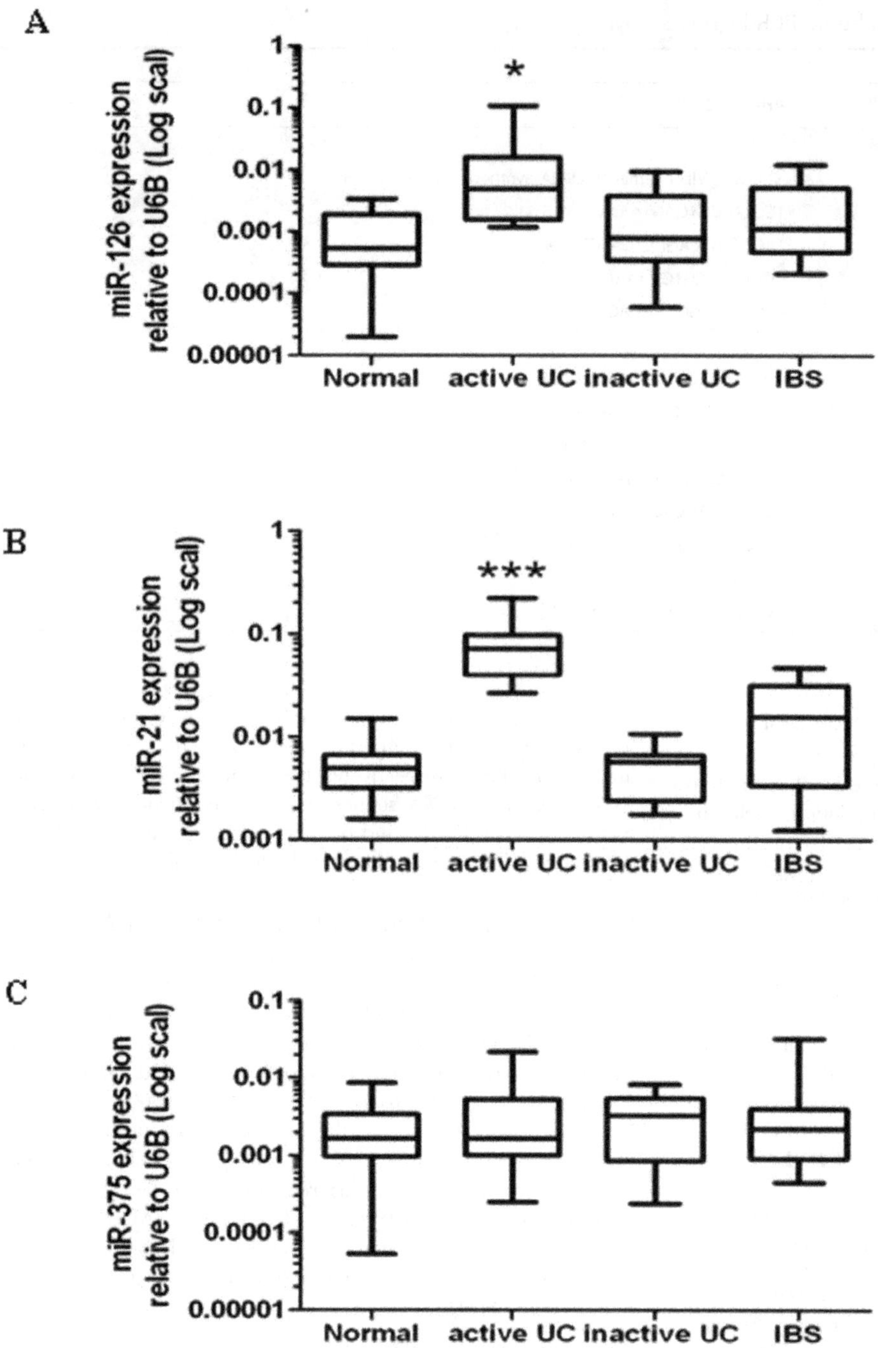

Figure 1. miRNAs expression in sigmoid colonic tissues. Expression of (A) miR-126, (B) miR-21 and (C) miR-375 were measured by quantitative RT-PCR in RNA samples of active UC tissues (n = 12), inactive UC samples (n = 10), IBS samples (n = 15) and healthy controls (n = 15), respectively. Data is presented as box-whisker plots (box - 25%–75%, whisker - 5%–95%; line - median). (*$P<0.05$, ***$P<0.001$, compared to that of normal healthy individuals).

Western Blot

Western blot was performed according to standard protocol. Briefly, 15 μg protein per samples were separated by sodium dodecyl sulfate-polyacrylamide gel electrophoresis (SDS-PAGE) and then transferred to polyvinylidene fluoride (PVDF) membrane. The membrane was probed with rabbit anti-human IκBα primary antibody (1:1000 dilution. SC-371. Santa Cruz Biotechnology, Santa Cruz, CA, USA) overnight at 4°C. The membrane was then incubated with HRP-labeled Goat Anti-Rabbit IgG (1:1000. Beyotime, Jiangsu, China) at RT for one hour. Mouse anti-human Tubulin antibody was used to detect tubulin as a loading control. The integral of optical density of bands was measured using Quantity One image analysis software (Bio-Red, Hercules, CA, USA).

Statistical Analysis

Experimental results are expressed as mean values ± standard error. Statistical analysis for qRT-PCR and Immunofluorescence

```
has-miR-126     gcgUAAUAAUGAGUGCCAUGcu -5'
                   :| ||||:|:  :|||||
IKBA 3'UTR      uugGUAAUUAUUU--UGGUACuu -3'

has-miR-126     gcguaauaaugAGUGCCAUGCU -5'
                           |  ::|||| |||
PLK2 3'UTR      agauggacaugUGGUGGUACGA -3'

has-miR-126     gcguaauaAUGAGUGCCAUGCU -5'
                        ||:|||  ||||||
CRK 3'UTR       |aauuaccaUAUUCAGGGUACGA -3'
```

Figure 2. Sequence alignments between miR-126 and target mRNAs. Base pairing complement suggested the putative miR-126 binding position at 445–465 of 3′-UTR of the IKBA mRNA sequence.

was performed with 1-way ANOVA for comparing all pairs of groups. The correlation between miR-126 and IKBA mRNA was calculated according to Pearson correlation analysis using SPSS software, v13.0 (International Business Machines Corporation). $P<0.05$ was considered significant.

Ethical Statement

The study was approved by Institutional Review Board of the Affiliated Hospital of Guangdong Medical College. All patients gave written informed consent for their participation.

Results

Differential Expression of miR-126, miR-21 and miR-375 in UC Tissues

A genome-wide microarray screening indicated that miR-126 and miR-21 are increased and miR-375 is decreased in sigmoid colons of active UC patients [18]. To determine whether miR-126, miR-21, and miR-375 are differentially expressed in UC patients from different ethnic groups, we analyzed the expression of these candidate miRNA in Chinese patients with active UC.

A total of 52 sigmoid colon pinch biopsies from patients with histologically confirmed active UC, inactive UC, IBS and normal healthy control subjects were obtained. Clinical characteristics of each patient group are listed in Table 1. We performed quantitative real-time PCR on total RNAs isolated from these biopsies. We found that expressions of miR-126 and miR-21 were significantly increased in active UC tissues compared to healthy control tissues (Figure 1 A and B). The expression of miR-126 was increased 18-fold ($P<0.05$), while the expression of miR-21 exhibited a 14.7-fold increase ($P<0.05$), in active UC tissues compared to healthy controls, respectively. However, expressions of miR-126 and miR-21 were not significant changed in either inactive UC or IBS tissues compared to healthy controls (both $P>0.05$ respectively) (Figure 1). The results are consistent with findings by previous microarray analysis [18]. However, there was no statistical significant difference in expression of miR-375 among the sample groups tested ($P>0.05$) (Figure 1C).

Selection of Potential Downstream Targets of miR-126

In order to identify downstream targets of miR-126, we used three miRNA targets prediction programs including MicroCosm Targets, Targetscan and PicTar. In silico analysis indicated approximately 900 mRNA targets of miR-126. Among these targets, Polo-like kinase 2 (PLK2, a tumor suppressor) and v-Crk sarcoma virus CT10 oncogene homolog (CRK) were shown as targets of miR-126 in previous studies [30–33]. However, there currently is no evidence that PLK2 and CRK are association with UC.

Interestingly, IκBα, an inhibitor of NF-κB pathway, is also one of the predicted targets of miR-126. A putative miR-126 binding site that encompasses 11 perfectly matched nucleotides was defined at the 3′-UTR (un-translated region) of IKBA (Figure 2).

In an effort to delineate potential downstream targets and further understand the mechanisms of miR-126 over-expression for pathogenesis of UC, we selected three putative targets (IKBA, PLK2, CRK) for further molecular and functional analyses.

Both IKBA mRNA and Protein Decreased in Active UC Tissues

To experimentally identify the targets of miR-126 in colon tissue, we performed qRT-PCR analysis on the expression of IKBA, PLK2, and CRK in total RNA from the same 52 sigmoid colon pinch biopsies. Among the three candidates, we found that only IKBA mRNA was markedly decreased in active UC tissues compared to healthy controls. A 32% decrease in IKBA mRNA expression was observed in active UC tissues relative to healthy controls ($P<0.05$) (Figure 3A). However, IκBα expression in either inactive UC or IBS tissues was not significantly changed as compared to healthy control tissues ($P>0.05$) (Figure 3A). No significant differences for the expression of PLK2 and CRK mRNAs were observed between active UC tissues and healthy controls (Figure 3B, C).

To determine whether the expression of IκBα protein was altered in colons with active UC, we further performed immunofluorescent staining on cryosections of sigmoid biopsies within each group. The staining results displayed that IκBα protein was clearly expressed in epithelial cells of normal colonic mucosa (Figure 4A and Figure S1). It was markedly decreased in active UC tissues, when compared to the other three groups ($P<0.05$) (Figure 4A, B and E). However, there was no differential expression of IκBα protein among inactive UC, IBS, and healthy control colon tissues ($P>0.05$) (Figure 4B, C, D and E).

Inverse Correlation of IKBA and miR-126 Expression

Our findings showed that miR-126 expression was significantly increased in active UC tissues as compared to healthy controls, inactive UC and IBS patients. In contrast, IκBα expression, mRNA and protein, were decreased markedly in active UC tissues. We found that the expression of miR-126 and IKBA mRNA were inversely correlated in active UC tissues and normal controls (Pearson correlation analysis $r=-0.466$, $P<0.01$) (Figure 5A). Such inverse correlation patterns were also present between miR-126 expression and IκBα protein level in active UC and normal control samples (Figure 5B). These results indicate that IκBα may be a target of miR-126 in the pathogenesis of active UC.

Inhibition of IKBA Expression by miR-126

To test whether miR-126 regulates endogenous IκBα expression, the miR-126 mimic was transiently transfected into HT29 cells and then IKBA mRNA expression was assessed. IKBA

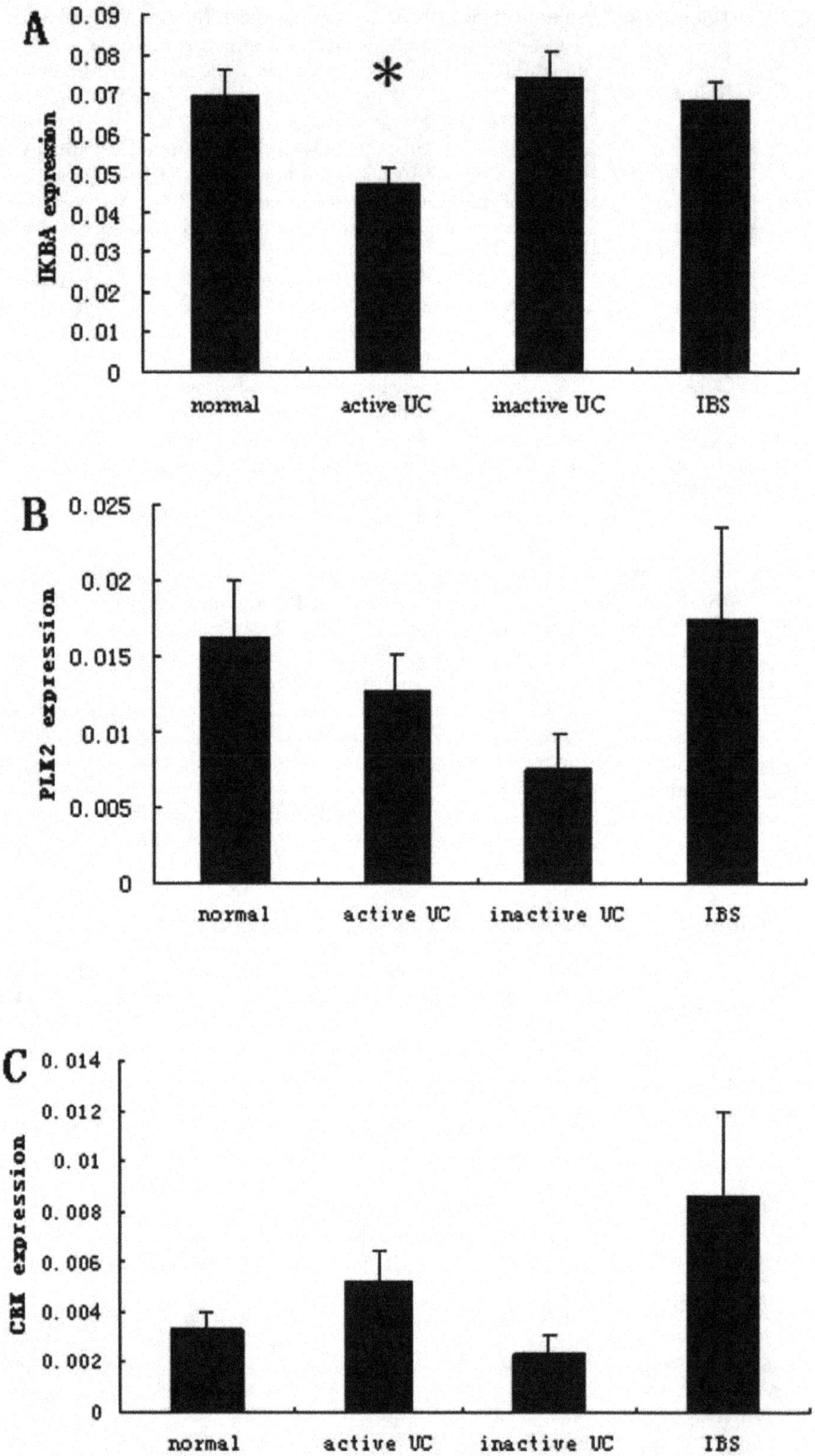

Figure 3. IKBA, PLK2 and CRK mRNA expression in sigmoid colonic tissues. Expression of (A) IKBA, (B) PLK2 and (C) CRK were measured by quantitative RT-PCR in RNA samples as indicated in Figure 1. Data is presented as mean ± SEM (*P<0.05 compared to that of normal healthy individuals).

mRNA expression was decreased by 20% and 40% in the cells transfected with 10 nM and 20 nM of miR-126 mimic, respectively (Figure 6A). However, the negative control mimic did not significantly reduce IKBA mRNA expression. In addition, we

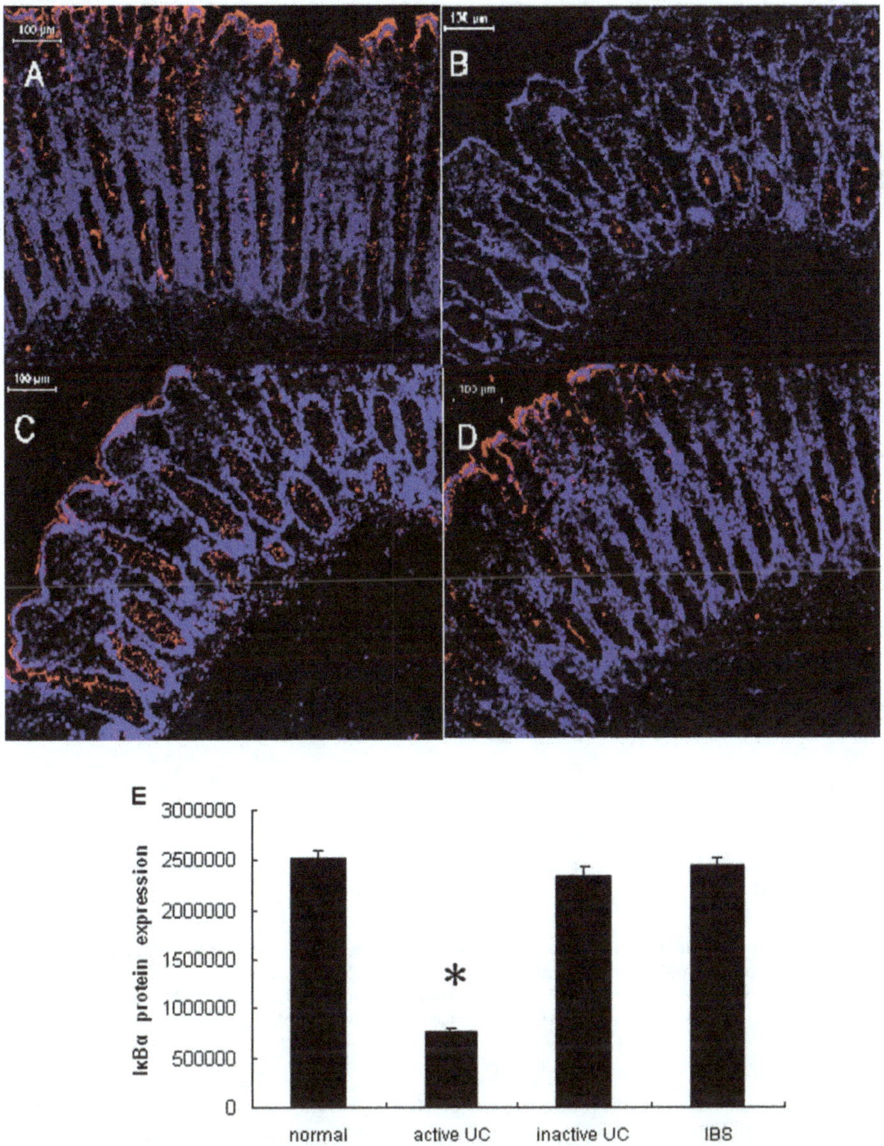

Figure 4. Localization of IκBα in human colon tissues. Representative frozen-sections were prepared from inflamed mucosa of an active UC patient (A), an inactive UC patient (B), a healthy control (C), and an IBS patient (D), and stained for IκBα by immunofluorescence. IκBα is significantly reduced in epithelial cells of active UC tissues, while it is detected in the epithelial cells of healthy controls, inactive UC and IBS tissues. Red, IκBα; blue, DAPI nuclear staining. Pictures were imaged at ×20 magnification on a Leica converted fluorescence microscope. (E) Fluorescence intensity of IκBα in each group was then calculated. Data is presented as mean ± SEM of 15 cases of healthy control, 12 cases of active UC, 10 cases of inactive UC and 15 cases of IBS (*$P<0.05$ compared to that of normal healthy individuals).

also checked the expression of CRK and PLK2 in these cells. The expression of CRK mRNA was not affected by the miR-126 mimic treatment, while PLK2 expression was reduced by about 35% in cells transfected with 20 nM of miR-126 mimic (Figure 6B, C). These results were consistent with previous reports [30–33].

Furthermore, we found that the IκBα protein expression in HT29 cells transfected with 20 nM miR-126 mimic, was significantly inhibited by 57% as detected by western blot analysis (Figure 6 D, E). Similar inhibitory effect of miR-126 mimic on IκBα protein expression was observed in the experiments using an additional colonic cell line HCT116 (Figure S2). These results suggest that miR-126 negatively regulates endogenous IκBα expression in colonic epithelia.

Regulation of IKBA 3′-UTR by miR-126

To determine whether miR-126 directly targets the 3′-UTR of IKBA mRNA, we transfected HT29 cells with an IKBA 3′-UTR luciferase reporter construct containing two wild type miR-126 putative binding sites (psi-IKBA) or a mutant construct bearing mutations on miR-126 binding sites (psi-mutIKBA). Compared to the parental luciferase reporter (psi-vector), the relative luciferase activity of the wild type psi-IKBA showed 35% reduction. Mutations of miR-126 binding sites in the IKBA 3′-UTR resulted in a restoration of luciferase activity to 92% of the parental reporter ($P<0.01$) (Figure 7A). These results indicate that endogenous miR-126 can regulate IκBα expression by directly targeting its 3′-UTR.

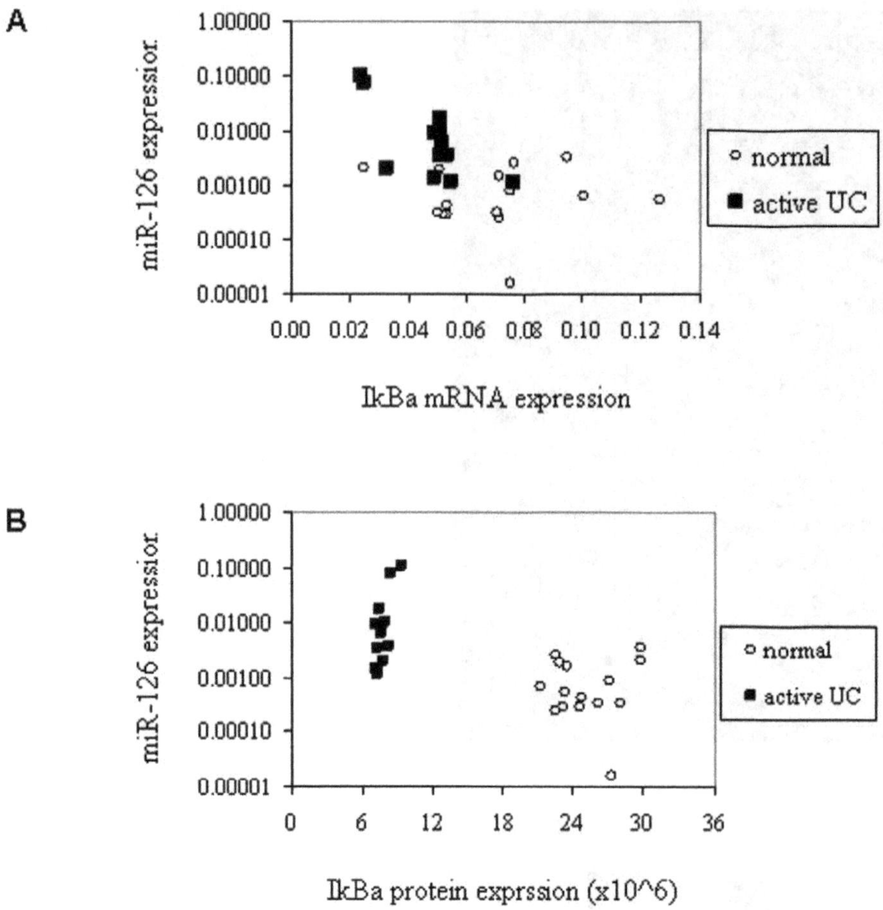

Figure 5. Correlation of IκBα expression and miR-126 expression in human colon tissues. (A) The expression of miR-126 and IKBA mRNA were detected by qRT-PCR in individual biopsy samples from normal healthy individuals (open circles, $n = 15$) and active UC (solid squares, $n = 12$), Pearson correlation analysis $r = -0.466$, $P < 0.01$. (B) The expression patterns of miR-126 and IκBα protein (detected by immunofluorescence analysis as shown in Figure 4E) in samples from normal healthy individuals (open circles, $n = 15$) and active UC patients (solid squares, $n = 12$).

To further confirm the findings, the miR-126 mimic was co-transfected with the above luciferase reporter constructs into HT29 cells. The miR-126 mimic dramatically reduced (>55%) the luciferase activity of the wild type IKBA 3′-UTR reporter construct psi-IKBA, while a negative control mimic had no effect on luciferase activity in any group (Figure 7B). The inhibitory effect of miR-126 mimic on the wild type psi-IKBA also showed a dose-dependent response, even though a relatively high amount of the wild type psi-IKBA construct was used (Figure 7C).

However, miR-126 mimic did not reduce the luciferase activity of mutant construct psi-mutIKBA (Figure 7B), indicating its specific recognition effect. These results further indicate that miR-126 can regulate IκBα expression by directly targeting its 3′-UTR.

Discussion

Numerous studies have demonstrated that different subtypes of IBD possess a distinct gene expression profile and identified a number of protein coding transcripts as molecular targets for pathogenesis of human IBD. Compared to protein coding genes, the roles of microRNAs, a subset of non-coding transcripts, in initiation and progression of IBD have not been extensively characterized. The involvement of microRNAs in pathological processes of IBD was first demonstrated in a recent study which revealed a strikingly unique signature of microRNA expression in different subtypes of IBD [18], later confirmed by several studies [19–27]. These findings suggest the critical roles of microRNA alterations in the development of chronic inflammatory processes of human IBD. From genome-wide microarray screening, miR-126 was previously identified as one of the up-regulated microRNAs detected in active UC patients in America [18]. In this study, we specifically analyzed alterations of miR-126 in a cohort of UC and IBS patients as well as healthy controls. Among three candidate microRNAs, we found that miR-126 and miR-21 were upregulated in colonic biopsies from patients with active UC, with 18- and 14.7-fold increases respectively. This finding was consistent with a previous study [18] and further suggests that miR-126 is a crucial molecular target for development of UC.

An inconsistent finding between previous genome-wide screening [18] and our current study was observed for miR-375 expression in UC patients, which may be attributed to patient populations with different ethnic and genetic backgrounds.

Our study provides the first evidence that upregulation of miR-126 is a novel mechanism in the development of UC. Although regulation of a number of molecular targets by miR-126 has been studied, involvement of pathways regulated by miR-126 in UC is completely unknown. In cancers, miR-126 has been found to possess paradoxical roles in different tumor types. miR-126 was found to target a tumor suppressor PLK2 and further inhibit

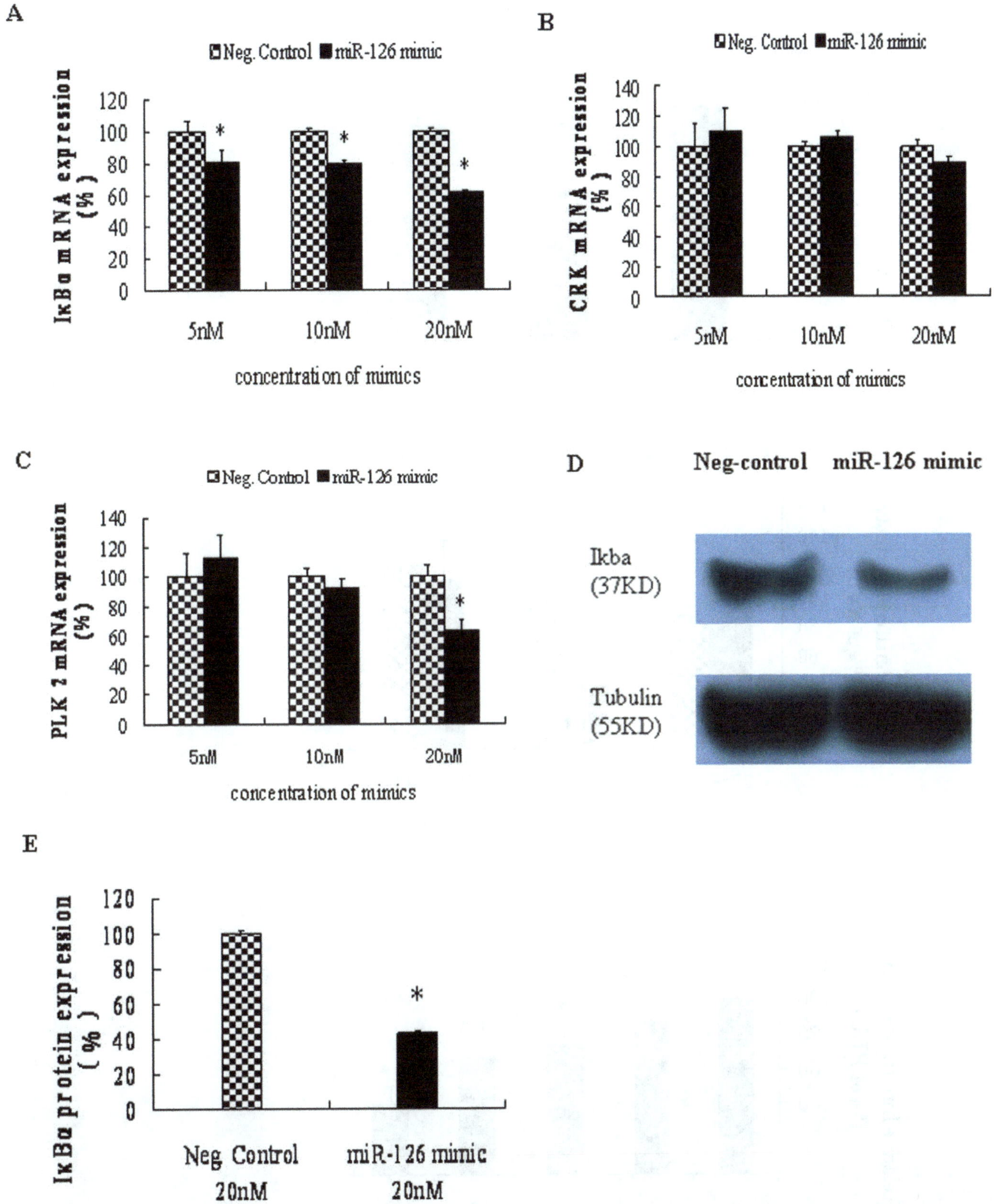

Figure 6. Effects of miR-126 mimic on expression of IKBA. HT29 cells were transfected with various amount miR-126 mimic or negative control mimic for 24 hours. Expression of (A) IKBA, (B) CRK and (C) PLK2 mRNA in total RNA of these cells were detected by qRT-PCR. (D) IκBα proteins of cells transfected with 20 nM of miR-126 mimic or the negative control were detected by Western Blot. Tubulin detection was served as loading reference. (E) The integral of optical density of (D) was measured using Quantity One program and normalized to corresponding density of Tubulin band. Data is presented as mean ± SEM of three independent experiments (*$P<0.05$, compared to that of negative control mimic treatment).

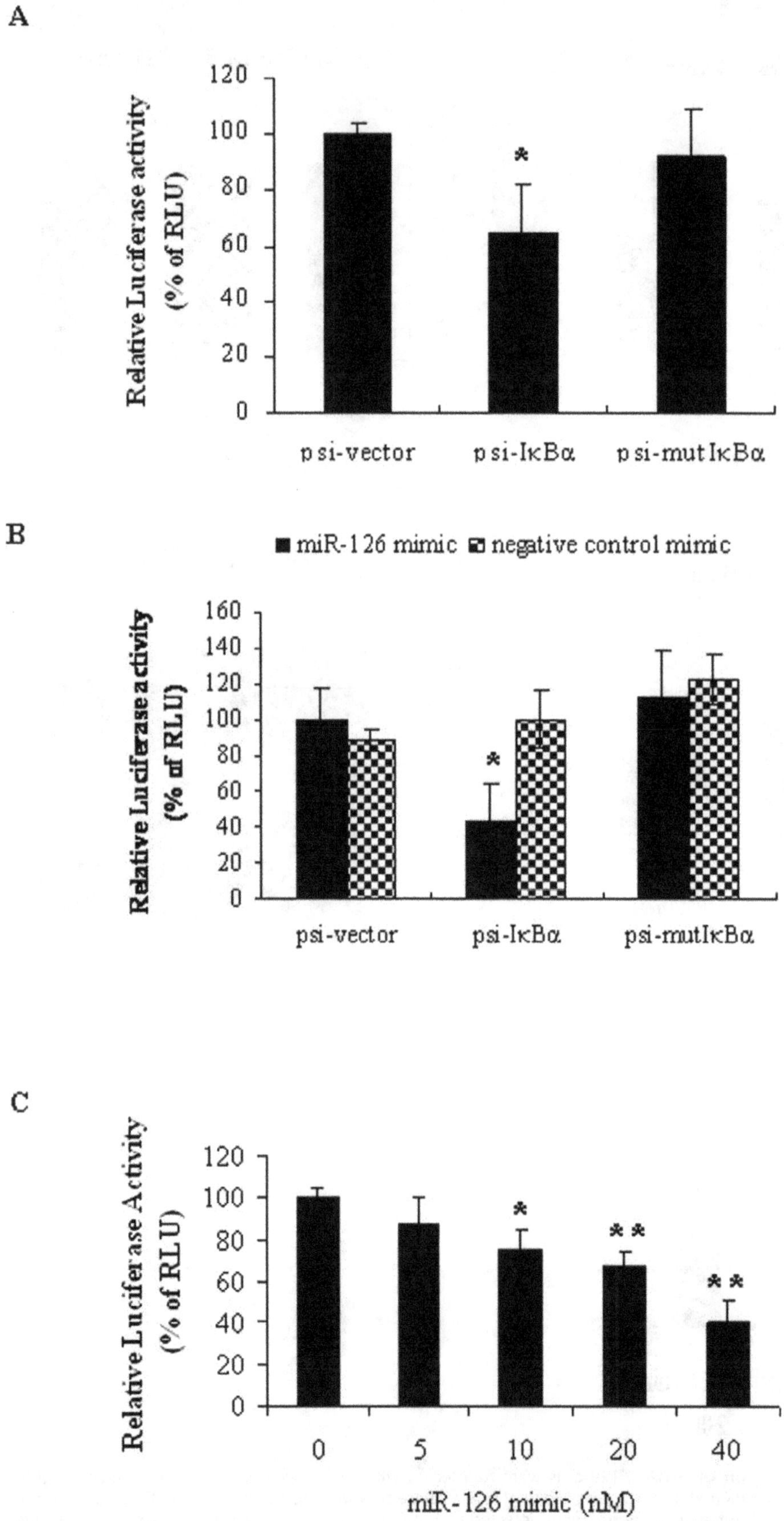

Figure 7. miR-126 targeting on 3′-UTR of IKBA. HT29 cells were transfected with either original dual luciferase reporter vector (psi-vector), or wild type miR-126 biding site of IKBA 3′-UTR construct (psi-IKBA) or mutated miR-126 biding site construct (psi-mutIKBA). Relative Renilla Luciferase

activity (normalized to Firefly luciferase activity) was measured 24 hours post-transfecting. (A) Relative Renilla luciferase activity was reduced in cells transfected with wild type IKBA 3′-UTR construct (psi-IKBA) compared to that with the psi-vector (100 ng/well of a 24-well-plate). Relative Renilla luciferase activity was restored in cells transfected with mutant construct (psi-mutIKBA). (*$P<0.05$, compared to that of psi-vector). (B) Co-transfecting 10 nM miR-126 mimic with various luciferase reporter constructs (100 ng/well) into HT29 cells reduced the relative Renilla luciferase activity. (*$P<0.05$, compared to that of psi-vector) (C) miR-126 mimic showed dose-dependent effects on relative Renilla luciferase activity in cells transfected with wild type psi-IKBA construct (250 ng/well) for 24 hours. (*$P<0.05$, **$P<0.01$, compared to that without miR-126 mimic treatment). Data is presented as mean ± SEM of three independent experiments.

apoptosis and increase the viability of acute myeloid leukemia cells [30]. On the other hand, miR-126 was shown to function as a tumor suppressor targeting on CRK in gastric cancer, mammary cancer and non-small cell lung carcinoma cell lines [31–33]. Recently, a few studies suggest that miR-126 is associated with human disorders other than cancers such as inflammation and fibrosis [34–36]. miR-126 was shown to down-regulate vascular cell adhesion molecule-1 (VCAM-1) expression and may provide additional control of vascular inflammation [34]. Selective blockade of miR-126 suppresses the asthmatic phenotype by diminishing TH2 responses [35]. These findings indicate that miR-126 regulates different molecular targets in different inflammatory processes.

To characterize the potential mechanism regulated by miR-126 in UC, we performed target scan analysis to identify the molecular targets of miR-126. We found that the 3′-UTR of IκBα mRNA possesses a miR-126 targeted sequence. IκBα is an important inhibitor for NF-κB. IκBα binds to the NF-κB complex and further inactivates NF-κB by retaining its cytoplasmic localization. The degradation of IκBα is in response to certain pro-inflammatory cytokine like TNF and results in dissociation of NF-κB from IκBα/p50/p65 complex. Consequentially NF-κB is translocated into the nucleus and activates NF-κB-mediated transcription of genes such as cytokines and chemokines. Constant activation of NF-κB activity has been a well-proven molecular event for human IBD including UC [37–39]. Several studies have established IκBα as a key inhibitor for NF-κB activity in IBD [37,40]. Viral IκBα expression vectors have been shown to produce a preventive effect on NF-κB activation in mucosal macrophages and T lymphocytes as a treatment option in IBD [41]. Moreover, Teaflavin-3,3′-digallate which stabilizes IκBα from degradation, can inhibit the activity of NF-κB in colon tissues [42].

Here we demonstrated that IκBα is abundantly expressed in normal colonic epithelia, but significantly reduced in active UC tissues. More interestingly, we found a significant inverse correlation between miR-126 over-expression and down-regulation of IκBα in active UC tissues. We then demonstrated that endogenous miR-126 and exogenous miR-126 mimic can inhibit IκBα expression. Finally, mutating the miR-126 binding site in the IKBA 3′-UTR in a reporter construct resulted in the restoration of reporter gene expression. Taken together, our results imply that over-expression of miR-126 leads to NF-κB activation via down-regulation of IκBα, which may contribute to the pathogenesis of human UC.

NF-κB mediated pathways are complex biological processes and signaling components including IκBα in this important pathway are regulated by a number of molecules playing essential roles in different cellular functions. It was shown that TNF-α and interleukin-1(IL-1)activated IkappaB kinase-beta (IKK-beta) and further phosphorylate IκBα [43]. In addition, phosphatidylinositol (PI) 3′-kinase (PI3′K) can also directly lead tyrosine phosphorylation of IκBα in breast cancer cell models [44]. IκBα phosphoration consequentially results in its ubiquitination and degradation, which ultimately leads to activation of NF-κB signaling. Therefore, multiple molecular mechanisms in addition to miR-126 overexpression may potentially contribute to the regulation of IκBα expression in inflammatory processes of UC.

Supporting Information

Figure S1 Localization of IκBα in human colon tissues. Representative frozen-section was prepared from a healthy control, and stained for IκBα by immunofluorescence. IκBα is detected in the epithelial cells of healthy colon tissues. Red, IκBα; blue, DAPI nuclear staining. Pictures were imaged at ×40 magnification on a Leica converted fluorescence microscope.

Figure S2 Effects of miR-126 mimic on expression of IKBA in HCT116. HCT116 cells were transfected with 20 uM of miR-126 mimic or negative control mimic for 24 hours. (A) Expression of IκBα proteins were detected by Western Blot. Tubulin detection was served as loading reference. (B) The integral of optical density of (A) was measured using Quantity One program and normalized to corresponding density of Tubulin band. Data is presented as mean ± SEM of three independent experiments (*$P<0.05$, compared to that of negative control mimic treatment).

Author Contributions

Conceived and designed the experiments: YZ FW. Performed the experiments: XF HW JxG. Analyzed the data: XF HW JxG YZ FW. Contributed reagents/materials/analysis tools: ScY WkT SC GlW WyW. Wrote the paper: XF YZ FW.

References

1. Jiang XL, Cui HF (2002) An analysis of 10218 ulcerative colitis cases in China. World J Gastroenterol 8: 158–161.
2. Hugot JP, Chamaillard M, Zouali H, Lesage S, Cézard JP, et al. (2001) Association of NOD2 leucine-rich repeat variants with susceptibility to Crohn's disease. Nature 411: 599–603.
3. Ogura Y, Bonen DK, Inohara N, Nicolae DL, Chen FF, et al. (2001) A frameshift mutation in NOD2 associated with susceptibility to Crohn's disease. Nature 411: 603–606.
4. Barrett JC, Hansoul S, Nicolae DL, Cho JH, Duerr RH, et al. (2008) Genome-wide association defines more than 30 distinct susceptibility loci for Crohn's disease. Nat Genet 40: 955–962.
5. McGovern DP, Gardet A, Törkvist L, Goyette P, Essers J, et al. (2010) Genome-wide association identifies multiple ulcerative colitis susceptibility loci. Nat Genet 42: 332–337.
6. Lawrance IC, Fiocchi C, Chakravarti S (2001) Ulcerative colitis and Crohn's disease: distinctive gene expression profiles and novel susceptibility candidate genes. Hum Mol Genet 10: 445–456.
7. Costello CM, Mah N, Häsler R, Rosenstiel P, Waetzig GH, et al. (2005) Dissection of the inflammatory bowel disease transcriptome using genome-wide cDNA microarrays. PLoS Med 2: e199.
8. Wu F, Dassopoulos T, Cope L, Maitra A, Brant SR, et al. (2007) Genome-wide gene expression differences in Crohn's disease and ulcerative colitis from endoscopic pinch biopsies: insights into distinctive pathogenesis. Inflamm Bowel Dis 13: 807–821.

9. Toedter G, Li K, Marano C, Ma K, Sague S, et al. (2011) Gene expression profiling and response signatures associated with differential responses to infliximab treatment in ulcerative colitis. Am J Gastroenterol 106: 1272–1280.
10. Carthew RW (2006) Gene regulation by microRNAs. Curr Opin Genet Dev 16: 203–208.
11. Bartel DP (2004) MicroRNAs: genomics, biogenesis, mechanism and function. Cell 116: 281–297.
12. Taganov KD, Boldin MP, Chang KJ, Baltimore D (2006) NF-kappaB-dependent induction of microRNA miR-146, an inhibitor targeted to signaling proteins of innate immune responses. Proc Natl Acad Sci U S A 103: 12481–12486.
13. Williams AE, Perry MM, Moschos SA, Larner-Svensson HM, Lindsay MA (2008) Role of miRNA-146a in the regulation of the innate immune response and cancer. Biochem Soc Trans 36: 1211–1215.
14. Lederhuber H, Baer K, Altiok I, Sadeghi K, Herkner KR, et al. (2010) MicroRNA-146: tiny player in neonatal Innate immunity? Neonatology 99: 51–56.
15. Sato T, Liu X, Nelson A, Nakanishi M, Kanaji N, et al. (2010) Reduced miR-146a increases prostaglandin E2 in chronic obstructive pulmonary disease fibroblasts. Am J Respir Crit Care Med 182: 1020–1029.
16. Sonkoly E, Stahle M, Pivarcsi A (2008) MicroRNAs and immunity: novel players in the regulation of normal immune function and inflammation. Semin Cancer Biol 18: 131–140.
17. Zhou B, Wang S, Mayr C, Bartel DP, Lodish HF (2007) MiR-150, a microRNA expressed in mature B and T cells, blocks early B cell development when expressed prematurely. Proc Natl Acad Sci U S A 104: 7080–7085.
18. Wu F, Zikusoka M, Trindade A, Dassopoulos T, Harris ML, et al. (2008) MicroRNAs are differentially expressed in ulcerative colitis and alter expression of macrophage inflammatory peptide-2 alpha. Gastroenterology 135: 1624–1635.
19. Takagi T, Naito Y, Mizushima K, Hirata I, Yagi N, et al. (2010) Increased expression of microRNA in the inflamed colonic mucosa of patients with active ulcerative colitis. J Gastroenterol Hepatol 25: S129–133.
20. Fasseu M, Tréton X, Guichard C, Pedruzzi E, Cazals-Hatem D, et al. (2010) Identification of restricted subsets of mature microRNA abnormally expressed in inactive colonic mucosa of patients with inflammatory bowel disease. PLoS One 5: e13160.
21. Wu F, Zhang S, Dassopoulos T, Harris ML, Bayless TM, et al. (2010) Identification of microRNAs associated with ileal and colonic Crohn's disease. Inflamm Bowel Dis 16: 1729–1738.
22. Olaru AV, Selaru FM, Mori Y, Vazquez C, David S, et al. (2011) Dynamic changes in the expression of MicroRNA-31 during inflammatory bowel disease-associated neoplastic transformation. Inflamm Bowel Dis 17: 221–231.
23. Bian Z, Li L, Cui J, Zhang H, Liu Y, et al. (2011) Role of miR-150-targeting c-Myb in colonic epithelial disruption during dextran sulphate sodium-induced murine experimental colitis and human ulcerative colitis. J Pathol 225: 544–553.
24. Wu F, Guo NJ, Tian H, Marohn M, Gearhart S, et al. (2011) Peripheral blood microRNAs distinguish active ulcerative colitis and Crohn's disease. Inflamm Bowel Dis 17: 241–250.
25. Ahmed FE, Jeffries CD, Vos PW, Flake G, Nuovo GJ, et al. (2009) Diagnostic microRNA markers for screening sporadic human colon cancer and active ulcerative colitis in stool and tissue. Cancer Genomics Proteomics 6: 281–295.
26. Wei B, Pei G (2010) MicroRNAs: critical regulators in Th17 cells and players in diseases. Cell Mol Immunol 7: 175–181.
27. Dalal SR, Kwon JH (2010) The Role of microRNA in inflammatory bowel disease. Gastroenterol Hepatol (N Y) 6: 714–722.
28. Sutherland LR, Martin F, Greer S, Robinson M, Greenberger N, et al. (1987) 5-Aminosalicylic acid enema in the treatment of distal ulcerative colitis, proctosigmoiditis, and proctitis. Gastroenterology 92: 1894–1898.
29. Shuo Gu, Lan Jin, Feijie Zhang, Sarnow P, Kay MA (2009) Biological basis for restriction of microRNA targets to the 3′untranslated region in mammalian mRNAs. Nat Struct Mol Biol 16: 144–150.
30. Li Z, Lu J, Sun M, Mi S, Zhang H, et al. (2008) Distinct microRNA expression profiles in acute myeloid leukemia with common translocations. Proc Natl Acad Sci U S A 105: 15535–15540.
31. Feng R, Chen X, Yu Y, Su L, Yu B, et al. (2010) miR-126 functions as a tumour suppressor in human gastric cancer. Cancer Lett 298: 50–63.
32. Li X, Shen Y, Ichikawa H, Antes T, Goldberg GS (2009) Regulation of miRNA expression by Src and contact normalization: effects on non-anchored cell growth and migration. Oncogene 28: 4272–4283.
33. Crawford M, Brawner E, Batte K, Yu L, Hunter MG, et al. (2008) MicroRNA-126 inhibits invasion in non-small cell lung carcinoma cell lines. Biochem Biophys Res Commun 373: 607–612.
34. Harris TA, Yamakuchi M, Ferlito M, Mendell JT, Lowenstein CJ (2008) MicroRNA-126 regulates endothelial expression of vascular cell adhesion molecule 1. Proc Natl Acad Sci U S A 105: 1516–1521.
35. Mattes J, Collison A, Plank M, Phipps S, Foster PS (2009) Antagonism of microRNA-126 suppresses the effector function of TH2 cells and the development of allergic airways disease. Proc Natl Acad Sci U S A 106: 18704–18709.
36. Murakami Y, Yasuda T, Saigo K, Urashima T, Toyoda H, et al. (2006) Comprehensive analysis of microRNA expression patterns in hepatocellular carcinoma and non-tumorous tissues. Oncogene 25: 2537–2545.
37. Visekruna A, Joeris T, Seidel D, Kroesen A, Loddenkemper C, et al. (2006) Proteasome-mediated degradation of IkappaBalpha and processing of p105 in Crohn's disease and ulcerative colitis. J Clin Invest 116: 3195–3203.
38. Tak PP, Firestein GS (2001) NF- kappa B: a key role in inflammatory diseases. J. Clin. Invest 107: 7–11.
39. Stevens C, Walz G, Singaram C, Lipman ML, Zanker B, et al. (1992) Tumor necrosis factor-alpha, interleukin-1 beta, and interleukin-6 expression in inflammatory bowel disease. Dig Dis Sci 37: 818–826.
40. Szamosi T, Lakatos PL, Hungarian IBD Study Group, Szilvasi A, Lakatos L, et al. (2009) The 3'UTR NFKBIA variant is associated with extensive colitis in Hungarian IBD patients. Dig Dis Sci 54: 351–359.
41. Dijkstra G, Moshage H, Jansen PL (2002) Blockade of NF-kappaB activation and donation of nitric oxide: new treatment options in inflammatory bowel disease? Scand J Gastroenterol Suppl 236: 37–41.
42. Ukil A, Maity S, Das PK (2006) Protection from experimental colitis by theaflavin-3,3′-digallate correlates with inhibition of IKK and NF-kappaB activation. Br J Pharmacol 149: 121–131.
43. Woronicz JD, Gao X, Cao Z, Rothe M, Goeddel DV (1997) IkappaB kinase-beta: NF-kappaB activation and complex formation with IkappaB kinase-alpha and NIK. Science 278: 866–869.
44. Mahabeleshwar GH, Kundu GC (2003) Syk, a protein-tyrosine kinase, suppresses the cell motility and nuclear factor kappa B-mediated secretion of urokinase type plasminogen activator by inhibiting the phosphatidylinositol 3′-kinase activity in breast cancer cells. J Biol Chem 278: 6209–6221.

10

Detection of *Campylobacter concisus* and Other *Campylobacter* Species in Colonic Biopsies from Adults with Ulcerative Colitis

Indrani Mukhopadhya, John M. Thomson, Richard Hansen, Susan H. Berry, Emad M. El-Omar, Georgina L. Hold*

Gastrointestinal Research Group, Division of Applied Medicine, University of Aberdeen, Foresterhill, Aberdeen, United Kingdom

Abstract

Introduction: The critical role of bacteria in the pathogenesis of ulcerative colitis (UC) is well recognized, but an individual causative microorganism has not been singled out so far. *Campylobacter concisus* and other non-*jejuni* species of *Campylobacter* have been implicated as putative aetiological agents in inflammatory bowel disease in children, but such studies have not been addressed in adults. This study investigated the prevalence of *Campylobacter* species in colonic biopsy samples from adults with UC and healthy controls.

Methods: Adult patients who were undergoing diagnostic colonoscopy were recruited for the study, which included 69 patients with histologically proven UC and 65 healthy controls. DNA was extracted from the biopsy samples and subjected to *Campylobacter* genus specific and *Campylobacter concisus* specific polymerase chain reaction and sequencing.

Results: Detection of all *Campylobacter* DNA utilising genus specific primers was significantly higher in cases of UC, with a prevalence of 73.9% (51/69) compared to 23.1% (15/65) in controls ($p = 0.0001$). Nested PCR for *C. concisus* DNA was positive in 33.3% (23/69) of biopsy samples from subjects with UC, which was significantly higher than the prevalence rate of 10.8% (7/65) from controls ($p = 0.0019$). Sequencing of the remaining *Campylobacter* positive samples revealed that *Campylobacter ureolyticus* was positive in 21.7% (15/69) of samples from UC subjects as opposed to 3.1% (2/65) in controls ($p = 0.0013$). Mixed *Campylobacter* species were more common in UC patients, 20.3% (14/69) as compared to controls 4.6% (3/65) ($p = 0.0084$).

Conclusion: The higher prevalence of *Campylobacter* genus and more specifically *C. concisus* and *C. ureolyticus* in biopsy samples from adults with UC suggests these genera of bacteria may be involved in the chronic inflammation that is characteristically seen in UC. To the best of our knowledge this is the first report of this association of *C. concisus* and *C. ureolyticus* with UC in adults.

Editor: Markus M. Heimesaat, Charité, Campus Benjamin Franklin, Germany

Funding: This work was funded by the Broad Medical Research Program (Grant number IBD-0178). JMT was supported by grants from the GI Research Unit, Aberdeen Royal Infirmary. The funders had no role in study design, data collection and analysis, decision to publish, or preparation of the manuscript.

Competing Interests: The authors have declared that no competing interests exist.

* E-mail: g.l.hold@abdn.ac.uk

Introduction

Ulcerative colitis (UC) and Crohn's disease (CD) are chronic diseases of the gastrointestinal tract that together are usually referred to as inflammatory bowel disease (IBD). During the last two decades there has been a significant increase in IBD associated hospitalization, outlining the enormous economic impact to health services [1]. It has been projected that at anytime up to 240,000 people are affected by IBD in the UK [2]. More specifically, the epidemiological pattern of UC has changed significantly with an increased incidence estimated at 10–20 per 100 000 per year. The incidence rate of juvenile onset UC has also risen in Scotland over the last twenty years, which translates into a longer period of monitored healthcare for affected individuals [3,4,5].

Ulcerative colitis has been traditionally observed in developed societies but with increasing westernization its prevalence has been on the rise in developing countries as well [6,7]. The current paradigm of the pathogenesis of UC revolves around an aberrant host immune response that is triggered by a poorly understood interaction between the microbiome and host genetic defects involved in the identification and clearance of microbes [8]. The genetic associations with UC are not as strong as CD suggesting a greater role of luminal factors influencing its pathogenesis. It is postulated that 'dysbiosis' or an imbalance between protective and harmful components of the luminal microbiota in favour of the latter plays a critical role in initiating and possibly perpetuating inflammation in UC [9].

Recent methodological advances in studying the gut microbiome have made clear distinctions between the mucosa-associated and faecal populations [10,11]. It is suggested that in healthy individuals the mucosal microbiome forms a synergistic and stable interaction with the host immune system, while the luminal or faecal microbiome varies based on diet or other environmental factors. This distinction is critical as it is therefore more likely that mucosa-associated bacteria will have the ability and proximity to invade the protective mucous layer and the intestinal epithelial barrier. *Helicobacter* and *Bacteroides* species are two groups of mucosa-associated bacteria that have been implicated in the pathogenesis of UC [12,13,14]. A recent epidemiological study demonstrated an increased risk of IBD in individuals with an episode of *Campylobacter* or *Salmonella* gastroenteritis, suggesting that infection with particular bacteria may trigger the process that ultimately leads to the chronic inflammation of IBD [15]. Other population-based studies have however refuted these findings and suggested that this association is perhaps a result of detection bias [16]. More recently, the role of non-*jejuni Campylobacter* species have evoked attention, predominantly in paediatric Crohn's disease [17,18].

The members of the *Campylobacter* genus comprise Gram negative, spiral, microaerophilic bacteria that reside in the small or large intestine of humans and animals. At least a dozen species of *Campylobacter* have been associated with human disease, with *Campylobacter jejuni* and *Campylobacter coli* the most commonly isolated strains. However, newer information suggests that non-*jejuni Campylobacter* species, most specifically *Campylobacter concisus*, may be responsible for infective gastroenteritis and septicaemia in children [19]. This species has also been isolated from stool samples of immunocompromised patients with diarrhoea suggesting that it may even be an opportunistic pathogen [20]. The recent reclassification of *Campylobacter ureolyticus* has added another species in the broader genus of *Campylobacter* having previously been within the *Bacteroides* [21]. The identification of this species in the faeces of subjects presenting with gastroenteritis suggests that it may also be an emerging enteric pathogen [22]. It appears that non-*jejuni Campylobacter* species are increasingly being identified as potential gastrointestinal pathogens. This study has for the first time aimed to delineate these mucosa-associated bacteria in biopsy samples from adults with ulcerative colitis.

Methods

Study Subjects

Patients were recruited from the department of gastroenterology at Aberdeen Royal Infirmary. These subjects were recruited for a previous study looking at the role of enterohepatic *Helicobacter* in UC [14]. Sixty-nine patients with a primary diagnosis of UC on the basis of a histological diagnosis from colonoscopic biopsies were recruited and assessed. The extent and severity of disease was scored according to the Montreal criteria [23]. A total of sixty-five healthy controls were recruited from the bowel cancer screening programme if they had documented absence of both macroscopic and microscopic inflammation. Subjects were excluded if they received antibiotics within six months prior to recruitment.

Colonic biopsies were obtained from colonoscopy procedures carried out at Aberdeen Royal Infirmary, Aberdeen, UK. Ethical approval for the study was granted by the North of Scotland Research Ethics Service, UK (reference number 04/S0802/8). Written informed consent was obtained from all subjects in the study.

Biopsy collection, Processing and Genomic DNA Extraction

Biopsy samples were collected from patients with UC and controls during colonoscopy using standard endoscopic forceps (Boston Scientific Nanterre Cedex France). The colonic mucosa was washed with sterile water via the colonoscope to remove residual faecal material. Biopsies were immediately snap-frozen in liquid nitrogen and then transferred to a -80°C freezer for storage pending DNA extraction and analysis.

Genomic DNA was extracted from the biopsies using the QIAamp DNA Mini Kit (Qiagen, Crawley, UK) according to an established modification of the manufacturer's instructions, optimised in-house for colonic biopsy tissue [14]. Biopsy samples were kept frozen until the addition of ATL buffer, thereafter they were allowed to equilibrate to room temperature. An additional 10 µl of Proteinase K was added for an initial lysis period of 18 hours to ensure complete lysis of the biopsy material prior to DNA extraction. DNA obtained from the biopsy samples was initially subjected to universal bacterial PCR to confirm the suitability of the DNA for further analysis [24].

PCR amplification

***Campylobacter* genus specific PCR.** The *Campylobacter* genus-specific primers, C412F and C1228 R, described by Linton *et al* in 1996 were used to amplify a ≈800 bp fragment within the 16S rRNA gene of *Campylobacter* species [25]. *Campylobacter* DNA was detected in the extracted biopsy samples by PCR using a 50 µl reaction mixture consisting of 10 pmol of each primer (C412F and C1228R [Sigma-Aldrich, UK]), 1× PCR buffer (Roche, UK), 250 nM of each deoxy-nucleotide-triphosphate (Bioline, UK), 2 mM MgCl2 (Roche, UK), 1 U of Taq polymerase (Roche,UK), and 40 ng of DNA. The PCR cycling conditions used were: 30 cycles of 94°C for 30 seconds, 55°C for 30 seconds, and 72°C for 2 minutes.

***Campylobacter concisus* specific PCR.** *C. concisus* specific primers, Concisus F and Concisus R, were used to amplify a 560 bp fragment within the 16S rRNA gene of *C. concisus* strains as per the protocol described by Ming Man *et al* in 2010 [18]. The sequences corresponding to the primer pair Concisus F/Concisus R were located within the region amplified by the *Campylobacter* genus specific primer C412F and C1228R and hence a nested PCR approach was used to identify the *C. concisus* strains - *Campylobacter* genus-specific PCR was therefore followed by *C. concisus* specific PCR. The composition of a 50 µl PCR reaction mixture was: 10 pmol of each primer (Concisus F and Concisus R [Sigma-Aldrich, UK]), 1× PCR buffer (Roche, UK), 250 nM of each deoxy-nucleotide-triphosphate (Bioline, UK), 2 mM MgCl2 (Roche, UK) and 1 U of Taq polymerase (Roche, UK). The optimum thermal cycling conditions for the *C. concisus*-specific nested PCR were: 94°C for 5 minutes, 40 cycles of 94°C for 30 seconds, 65°C for 30 seconds, and 72°C for 1 minute, followed by 72°C for 7 minutes.

Cloning and Sequencing

To enable the identification of other *Campylobacter* species, *Campylobacter* genus positive PCR products were first subjected to restriction fragment length polymorphism (RFLP) analysis by digestion with *Dde* I enzyme [26]. PCR products which did not show a mixed RFLP pattern were directly sequenced on an Applied Biosystems model 3730 automated capillary DNA sequencer using the *Campylobacter* genus specific primers C412F and C1228R. Samples with mixed RFLP profiles were analyzed by cloning the *Campylobacter* genus positive PCR products into JM109 competent cells with pGEM-T-easy vector and the sequence of the insert was established with M13 sequencing primers.

The sequences obtained were compared to those of the National Center for Biotechnology Information GenBank database using the basic local alignment search tool (BLAST) search program (http://www.ncbi.nlm.nih.gov).

Multiple alignments and phylogenetic analyses were performed using Bioedit (version 7.0.5.3) (http://www.mbio.ncsu.edu/BioEdit/bioedit.html) and a dendogram was constructed using MEGA version 4 software [27].

GenBank Sequence Submission

All 16S rRNA gene sequences derived from either direct sequencing or cloning of *Campylobacter* genus-specific PCR products were submitted to GenBank with the accession numbers from JF795865 to JF795912.

Statistical Analysis

Statistical analysis was performed using the Pearson Chi Squared, 2-tailed test or the Fisher's exact test wherever appropriate, utilising Graph Pad software (San Diego, CA).

Results

Patient characteristics

The prospective UC cohort (n = 69, male 46.4%) had a mean age of 45.3±17.9 years at the time of index colonoscopy. The control group (n = 65, male 59.3%) had a mean age of 61.4±8.5 years at the time of index colonoscopy. There was a statistically significant difference in age between the UC cohort and the control group (p<0.0001). A total of 115 biopsy sites were analysed from UC patients. Twenty four (34.8%) subjects had a single site analysed and 45 (65.2%) had more than one biopsy site assessed. Of the 115 biopsies analysed, 68 (59.1%) were from histologically inflamed sites, whereas 47 (40.9%) were from histologically normal sites A single biopsy site was analysed from each control subject. The clinical characteristics and Montreal classification of the patients with UC are summarised in Table 1.

Detection of *Campylobacter concisus* from mucosal biopsy samples of adults with UC and controls

Utilising the species-specific primers, *C. concisus* was detected in 23 of the 69 subjects with ulcerative colitis and 7 of the 65 controls. The prevalence of *C. concisus* in the UC population was 33.3% which was significantly higher than that in the controls, 10.8% (p = 0.0019) (Figure 1).

Table 1. Clinical characteristics of subjects with Ulcerative colitis.

	Ulcerative Colitis
Number of subjects	69
Age at diagnosis(Years) ± SD	45.6±27.8
Sex (Male %)	32 (46.4%)
Montreal classification (Extent)	
Proctitis E1 (%)	8 (11.6%)
Left sided UC E2 (%)	44 (63.8%)
Extensive UC E3 (%)	17 (24.6%)
Montreal classification (Severity)	
Clinical remission S0 (%)	7 (10.1%)
Mild UC S1 (%)	16 (23.2%)
Moderate UC S2 (%)	32 (46.4%)
Severe UC S3 (%)	14 (20.3%)

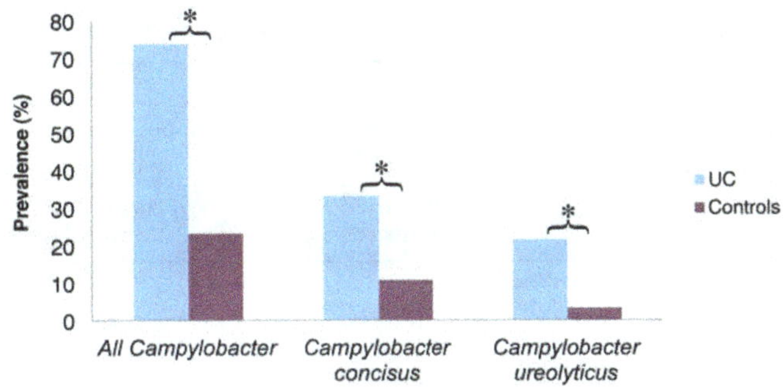

Figure 1. *Campylobacter species, Campylobacter concisus* and *Campylobacter ureolyticus* in subjects with ulcerative colitis and controls. The prevalence of all *Campylobacter species* was 73.9% (51/69) in subjects with UC as compared to 23.1% (15/65) in controls (p = 0.0001). *Campylobacter concisus* was detected in 33.3% (23/69) of subjects with UC, which was significantly higher than the prevalence rate of 10.8% (7/65) from controls (p = 0.0019). *Campylobacter ureolyticus* was positive in 21.7% (15/69) of samples from UC subjects as opposed to 3.1% (2/65) in controls (p = 0.0013).

Detection of all *Campylobacter* species from mucosal biopsy samples of adults with UC and controls

Utilising *Campylobacter* genus specific primers, *Campylobacter* DNA was detected in 51 of the 69 patients with UC, and 15 of the 65 controls. The prevalence of *Campylobacter* was significantly higher in cases of UC, with a prevalence of 73.9% compared to 23.1% in controls (p = 0.0001). Sequencing of the remaining *Campylobacter* positive samples revealed that *C. ureolyticus* was present in 21.7% (15/69) of samples from UC patients as opposed to 3.08% (2/65) from controls (p = 0.0013) (Figure 1). Detailed breakdown of all the species identified from both UC subjects and controls is summarised in Table 2. Other notable members of the *Campylobacter* genus that were identified include: *Campylobacter hominis*, *Campylobacter curvus*, *Campylobacter gracilis*, *Campylobacter showae* and *Campylobacter jejuni.*

Mixed *Campylobacter* species from mucosal biopsy samples of adults with UC and controls

Mixed *Campylobacter* species were more likely in UC patients, 20.3% (14/69) as compared to controls 4.6% (3/65) (p = 0.0084). The most commonly identified combination of *Campylobacter* species in adults with UC was *C.ureolyticus* and *C. hominis* seen in 8.7% of all cases. The most common mix in the controls was *C. concisus* and *C. hominis* accounting for 3.1% of cases. A variety of different *Campylobacter* combinations were noted in UC as opposed to controls wherein only two combinations involving *C. concisus/C. hominis* and *C. hominis/C. curvus* were found (Table 2).

Prevalence of *Campylobacter* species and *Campylobacter concisus* in relation to gender, site of disease and severity of symptoms

There were no significant differences noted between the prevalence of *Campylobacter* species or indeed *C. concisus* with respect to gender of subjects with UC or controls. The prevalence of all *Campylobacter* species and *C. concisus* with reference to extent and severity of disease is summarised in Table 3. There were no significant differences noted between the prevalence of *Campylo-*

Table 2. *Campylobacter* species identified by sequencing.

Campylobacter Species Identified	Number of Subjects Combination of Species identified in	
	Ulcerative Colitis (%)	Healthy Control (%)
Single species identified		
Campylobacter concisus	16 (23.2%)	5 (7.7%)
Campylobacter ureolyticus	7 (10.1%)	2 (3.1%)
Campylobacter hominis	7 (10.1%)	2 (3.1%)
Campylobacter curvus	1 (1.4%)	3 (4.6%)
Campylobacter gracilis	1 (1.4%)	0
Campylobacter showae	2 (2.9%)	0
Campylobacter jejuni	1 (1.4%)	0
Two or more species co-existing within Subject		
Campylobacter ureolyticus Campylobacter hominis	6 (8.7%)	0
Campylobacter showae Campylobacter concisus	2 (2.9%)	0
Campylobacter curvus Campylobacter concisus	2 (2.9%)	0
Campylobacter hominis Campylobacter concisus	1 (1.4%)	2 (3.1%)
Campylobacter rectus Campylobacter concisus	1 (1.4%)	0
Campylobacter ureolyticus Campylobacter concisus	1 (1.4%)	0
Campylobacter hominis Campylobacter curvus	0	1 (1.5%)
Campylobacter ureolyticus Campylobacter jejuni	1 (1.4%)	0

bacter species or specifically *C. concisus* with respect to extent of disease. The detection of *Campylobacter* species and *C. concisus* was also studied in relation to the severity of symptoms according to the Montreal classification, as summarised in Table 3. The only significant difference noted was with the prevalence of all *Campylobacter* species and disease severity between patients with moderate UC (87.5%) and those with severe UC (50%) ($p = 0.01$). No significant differences were noted between the prevalence of *Campylobacter concisus* with respect to severity of symptoms.

Prevalence of *Campylobacter* species and *Campylobacter concisus* in relation to inflamed and non-inflamed biopsy samples from subjects with UC

Of the 115 biopsy sites analysed from subjects with UC, 68 were from histologically inflamed sites whereas 47 were from sites that were histologically normal. The prevalence of all *Campylobacter* species was 66.2% (45/68) from inflamed biopsies and 46.8% from histologically normal biopsies (22/47) which was significant ($p = 0.038$). However, there was no significant difference noted between the prevalence of *Campylobacter concisus* in inflamed biopsies 25% (17/68) and that from normal biopsies 21.3%(10/47) ($p = 0.64$).

Comparison of *Campylobacter* and *Helicobacter* species from mucosal biopsies

As previously stated, *Helicobacteraceae* PCR positivity was significantly higher in UC than controls within this cohort: 32 of 69 (46.4%) versus 10 of 65 (15.4%) respectively ($p = 0.0002$) [14]. The majority of *Helicobacter* species were non-*pylori*, constituting 96.9% (31/32) of all PCR positive subjects with UC and 80% (8/10) of all PCR positive controls. We wanted to compare the previously published *Helicobacter* prevalence with *Campylobacter* positivity from the current study. The prevalence of *Campylobacter* in subjects with UC (51/69) was higher than the prevalence of all *Helicobacter* (32/69) but it did not reach statistical significance ($p = 0.252$). Similarly, the difference between the prevalence of *Campylobacter* (15/65) and *Helicobacter* (10/65) was not statistically significant in controls ($p = 0.374$). The prevalence of both these bacterial groups was significantly less in controls as opposed to patients with UC. Identification of mixed *Helicobacter* and *Campylobacter* species was noted in 34.8% of all patients with UC (24/69) and 47.1% (24/51) of the UC patients harbouring *Campylobacter*.

Phylogenetic Analysis

Sequence analysis ≈800 bp *Campylobacter* genus specific PCR amplicons, revealed a high nucleotide sequence similarity to various *Campylobacter* species with a maximum identity of 99–100%. *C. concisus* sequences analysed from the UC and HC group did not cluster into separate groups in the dendogram as shown in Figure 2.

Discussion

This study has investigated the prevalence of the *Campylobacter* genus of bacteria in UC and for the first time, a positive

Table 3. Distribution of *Campylobacter* species according to extent and severity of disease.

Subjects	Characteristic		Number	*Campylobacter* species	*Campylobacter concisus*
Ulcerative colitis	**Montreal extent**	**Proctitis**	8	5 (62.5%)	2 (25%)
		Left sided UC	44	35 (79.6%)	15 (34.1%)
		Pancolitis	17	11 (64.7%)	6 (35.3%)
	Montreal severity	**Remission**	7	4 (57.1%)	2 (28.6%)
		Mild	16	12 (75%)	6 (37.5%)
		Moderate	32	28 (87.5%)	13 (40.6%)
		Severe	14	7 (50%)	2 (14.3%)
Controls			65	15(23.1%)	7 (10.8%)

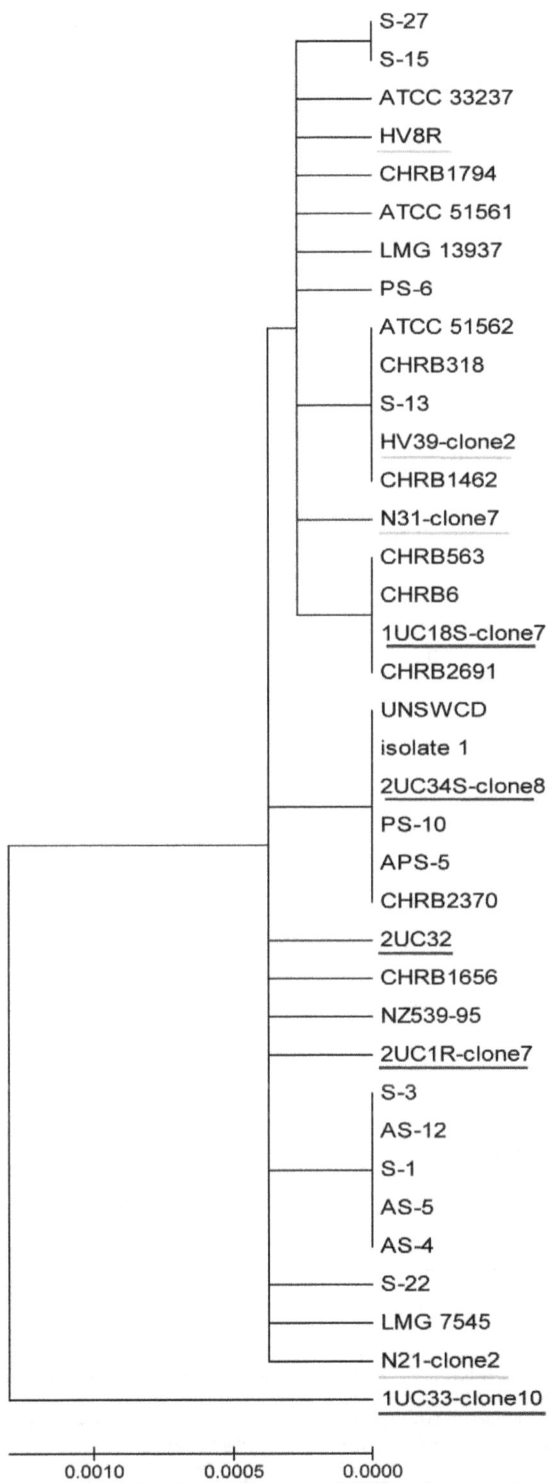

Figure 2. Phylogenetic tree constructed using sequences of the 16S rRNA gene of *C. concisus* strains from UC and controls and other strains available in GenBank. Strains from UC are underlined in red and those from HC are underlined in blue. The evolutionary history was inferred using the Neighbor-Joining method. The bootstrap consensus tree inferred from 500 replicates was taken to represent the evolutionary history of the taxa analysed. The evolutionary distances were computed using the Maximum Composite Likelihood method.

association has been noted between the presence of *Campylobacter* species and adult UC. *Campylobacter* was detected in a significantly larger proportion of UC patients as opposed to controls. Furthermore, two individual species, namely *C. concisus* and *C. ureolyticus* were found to have a significant association with UC. The control group comprised of a significantly older group of patients as they had been recruited from the bowel screening programme. A recent study found that the greatest incidence of *Campylobacter* infection was for those aged more than 60 years of age, making this difference even more clinically significant [28]. A study documenting prevalence of *C. concisus* in salivary samples from different age groups did not find any significant difference among various adult age groups but found the prevalence to be significantly lower in the children age 3–5 years [29].

In the last two years, *C. concisus* has been associated with paediatric CD, with two studies documenting this association from faecal and biopsy samples [17,18]. The reported prevalence of *C. concisus* from these two studies was 65% from faecal samples and 51% from biopsy samples. The prevalence of *C. concisus* in biopsy samples from adult UC in our study was lower than these studies at 31.9%. Our finding contrasts with these previous studies as it is based on adult subjects with UC as opposed to children with CD. Therefore, our findings have expanded the role of *C. concisus* to encompass both forms of IBD necessitating further studies to firstly validate our findings and secondly to delineate the exact mechanism of this association.

This study not only found an increased prevalence of *C. concisus* in mucosal biopsy samples from adults with UC but also identified DNA from this putative pathogen in one in ten controls. *C. concisus* is a common commensal in the oral mucosa and it has been associated with periodontitis [30]. A study by Zhang *et al* aimed to look at the relative rates of isolation and detection of *C. concisus* from salivary samples of healthy controls and patients with IBD but did not find any significant difference between the two groups (97% vs. 100%) [29]. Protein profiling of six of the oral strains were compared with an intestinal strain of *C. concisus* using SDS-PAGE. Interestingly only one of the six oral strains matched the intestinal strain, suggesting that different strains of the bacteria may exist in the oral cavity with some having the ability to colonise the intestine. The increased detection of this oral commensal in UC may be as a result of defective innate immunity, allowing easier access to an additional ecological niche where the organism may potentially cause disease. This hypothesis is supported by the detection of this pathogen during episodes of diarrhoea in immunocompromised adults [20]. Additionally, the finding of this bacterium in the extremes of age groups, who are characterized with poorer immunity, suggests that *C. concisus* may be an opportunistic pathogen [31].

There is an additional suggestion that *C. concisus* exists as a heterogeneous population with both pathogenic and non-pathogenic strains co-existing together, with disease being manifest following infection with a pathogenic genotype. This has been elegantly demonstrated by Aabenhus *et al* who utilized amplified fragment length polymorphism (AFLP) analysis from a variety of clinical isolates of *C. concisus* obtained from sixty-two immunocompetent and immunocompromised individuals over a period of five years [32]. Their analysis showed at least four distinct *C. concisus* genomospecies which exhibited differences in their spectra of virulence potential. In another similar study, analysis of SDS-PAGE protein profiles and PCR amplification of 23S rDNA assigned clinical *C. concisus* isolates into two distinct, but discordant groups [33]. Identification of two genetically distinct clusters have also been reported from a recent report utilizing analysis of amplified fragment length polymorphism profiles [34]. This study identified genomospecies A from healthy individuals and genomospecies B from patients with diarrhoea. More importantly they found that the pathogenic strains (genomospecies B) displayed greater epithelial invasion and translocation. This is possibly the first report of a genotype-phenotype correlation of pathogenicity of *C. concisus* isolates. During the current study, phylogenetic analysis was also undertaken to see if a similar clustering effect could be seen based on 16S rDNA sequence data. Our study cohort did not demonstrate a similar clustering effect, indicating that 16S rDNA sequence data is not as discriminatory as 23S rDNA for categorising *C. concisus* isolates. The debate on whether differing phenotypic characteristics of *C. concisus* can be identified by studying genetic composition still needs to be resolved.

In comparison to *C. concisus*, *C. ureolyticus* is a relatively unknown gastrointestinal pathogen. In its previous nomenclature as *Bacteroides ureolyticus* it was known to cause soft tissue infections and urethritis and it has only recently been implicated as a cause of diarrhoea [22,35,36]. Its significant association with UC in our study suggests that these patients may be susceptible to colonisation with *Campylobacter* and perhaps this is genus-specific rather than to any particular *Campylobacter* species. This is supported by the increased number of mixed *Campylobacter* (with relatively rare members of the *Campylobacter* genus, including *C. showae*, *C. curvus* and *C. gracilis*) in adults with ulcerative colitis as opposed to controls. This finding is similar to those in paediatric Crohn's disease reported by Man et al [18]. The increased diversity of *Campylobacter* species in UC may reflect a specific defect in the immunological handling of this genus in the intestinal mucosa of UC. The additional finding of mixed *Helicobacteraceae* and *Campylobacter* species in UC suggest that this defect may extend to the entire phylum of *Proteobacteria*.

A sub-group analysis of the patients with UC was performed which found no definite relationship between extent of disease and the prevalence of *Campylobacter* and specifically *C. concisus*. There was a significantly lower prevalence of all *Campylobacters* in subjects with severe colitis (50%) as opposed to moderate colitis (87.5%), but no such difference was noted with the prevalence of *C. concisus* infection. The obvious corollary to this finding is that our study did not have the power to detect differences between the various sub-groups of UC. This finding appears to be against the obvious premise that a greater exposure should generally lead to greater incidence of the effect. Contrary to this finding, a greater prevalence of *Campylobacter* species was noted in histologically inflamed biopsies as opposed to normal biopsy samples taken from UC patients. One can surmise that there can be regional changes in mucosal bacterial species, in this case *Campylobacter*, that may trigger an inflammatory cascade which then leads to ulceration and loss of the epithelial surface that harbours these organisms. This would paradoxically lead to reduced identification of the pathogen in the most severe phases of active disease. Future studies should also be conducted on non-IBD inflammatory colonic diseases to ensure that the presence of the bacteria is not merely a superinfection of inflamed tissue.

In the classic essay by Bradford Hill on the theory of causation he states that: "We must not be too ready to dismiss a cause and effect hypothesis merely on the grounds that the observed association appears to be slight" [37]. This doctrine is all the more relevant when considering the role of a solitary pathogen like *C. concisus* in the broader aetiopathogenesis of a multifactorial disease like UC. The pathogenic potential of *C. concisus* has been elegantly demonstrated in an *in-vitro* model wherein these strains were demonstrated to be invasive and also induced production of pro-inflammatory cytokines from epithelial cells, monocytes and macrophages [38]. A cytolethal distending toxin (CDT)-like effect on Vero cells has been shown by clinical isolates of *C. concisus* from subjects with diarrhoea [33]. The bacterium also produces cell-associated and secreted haemolysins that may have a role in pathogenicity [39]. It is obvious that this bacterium can cause tissue damage but whether it is the initiating trigger, the perpetuating factor or merely an epiphenomenon amidst the mucosal inflammatory cascade is a question that still needs to be answered.

Author Contributions

Conceived and designed the experiments: IM JMT RH EMEO GLH. Performed the experiments: IM JMT SHB. Analyzed the data: IM JMT RH GLH. Wrote the paper: IM EMEO GLH.

References

1. Sonnenberg A (2010) Temporal changes in the age distribution of inflammatory bowel disease hospitalization: data from England and Scotland. Eur J Gastroenterol Hepatol 22: 95–101.
2. Carter MJ, Lobo AJ, Travis SP (2004) Guidelines for the management of inflammatory bowel disease in adults. Gut 53 Suppl 5: V1–16.
3. Armitage E, Drummond HE, Wilson DC, Ghosh S (2001) Increasing incidence of both juvenile-onset Crohn's disease and ulcerative colitis in Scotland. Eur J Gastroenterol Hepatol 13: 1439–1447.
4. Benchimol EI, Fortinsky KJ, Gozdyra P, Van den Heuvel M, Van Limbergen J, et al. (2010) Epidemiology of pediatric inflammatory bowel disease: a systematic review of international trends. Inflamm Bowel Dis 17: 423–439.
5. Henderson P, Hansen R, Cameron FL, Gerasimidis K, Bisset WM, et al. (2011) The rising incidence of paediatric inflammatory bowel disease in Scotland. Inflamm Bowel Dis.
6. Loftus EV, Jr. (2004) Clinical epidemiology of inflammatory bowel disease: Incidence, prevalence, and environmental influences. Gastroenterology 126: 1504–1517.
7. Baumgart DC, Bernstein CN, Abbas Z, Colombel JF, Day AS, et al. (2011) IBD Around the world: comparing the epidemiology, diagnosis, and treatment: proceedings of the World Digestive Health Day 2010–Inflammatory Bowel Disease Task Force meeting. Inflamm Bowel Dis 17: 639–644.
8. Hansen R, Thomson JM, El-Omar EM, Hold GL (2010) The role of infection in the aetiology of inflammatory bowel disease. J Gastroenterol 45: 266–276.
9. Tannock GW (2010) The bowel microbiota and inflammatory bowel diseases. Int J Inflam 2010: 954051.
10. Eckburg PB, Bik EM, Bernstein CN, Purdom E, Dethlefsen L, et al. (2005) Diversity of the human intestinal microbial flora. Science 308: 1635–1638.
11. Momozawa Y, Deffontaine V, Louis E, Medrano JF (2011) Characterization of Bacteria in Biopsies of Colon and Stools by High Throughput Sequencing of the V2 Region of Bacterial 16S rRNA Gene in Human. PLoS One 6: e16952.
12. Bohr UR, Glasbrenner B, Primus A, Zagoura A, Wex T, et al. (2004) Identification of enterohepatic Helicobacter species in patients suffering from inflammatory bowel disease. J Clin Microbiol 42: 2766–2768.
13. Saitoh S, Noda S, Aiba Y, Takagi A, Sakamoto M, et al. (2002) Bacteroides ovatus as the predominant commensal intestinal microbe causing a systemic antibody response in inflammatory bowel disease. Clin Diagn Lab Immunol 9: 54–59.
14. Thomson JM, Hansen R, Berry SH, Hope ME, Murray GI, et al. (2011) Enterohepatic helicobacter in ulcerative colitis: potential pathogenic entities? PLoS One 6: e17184.
15. Gradel KO, Nielsen HL, Schonheyder HC, Ejlertsen T, Kristensen B, et al. (2009) Increased short- and long-term risk of inflammatory bowel disease after salmonella or campylobacter gastroenteritis. Gastroenterology 137: 495–501.
16. Jess T, Simonsen J, Nielsen NM, Jorgensen KT, Bager P, et al. (2010) Enteric Salmonella or Campylobacter infections and the risk of inflammatory bowel disease. Gut 60: 318–324.
17. Zhang L, Man SM, Day AS, Leach ST, Lemberg DA, et al. (2009) Detection and isolation of Campylobacter species other than C. jejuni from children with Crohn's disease. J Clin Microbiol 47: 453–455.
18. Man SM, Zhang L, Day AS, Leach ST, Lemberg DA, et al. (2010) Campylobacter concisus and other Campylobacter species in children with newly diagnosed Crohn's disease. Inflamm Bowel Dis 16: 1008–1016.
19. Lastovica AJ (2009) Clinical relevance of Campylobacter concisus isolated from pediatric patients. J Clin Microbiol 47: 2360.

20. Aabenhus R, Permin H, On SL, Andersen LP (2002) Prevalence of Campylobacter concisus in diarrhoea of immunocompromised patients. Scand J Infect Dis 34: 248–252.
21. Vandamme P, Debruyne L, De Brandt E, Falsen E (2010) Reclassification of Bacteroides ureolyticus as Campylobacter ureolyticus comb. nov., and emended description of the genus Campylobacter. Int J Syst Evol Microbiol 60: 2016–2022.
22. Bullman S, Corcoran D, O'Leary J, Lucey B, Byrne D, et al. (2011) Campylobacter ureolyticus: an emerging gastrointestinal pathogen? FEMS Immunol Med Microbiol 61: 228–230.
23. Silverberg MS, Satsangi J, Ahmad T, Arnott ID, Bernstein CN, et al. (2005) Toward an integrated clinical, molecular and serological classification of inflammatory bowel disease: Report of a Working Party of the 2005 Montreal World Congress of Gastroenterology. Can J Gastroenterol 19 Suppl A: 5–36.
24. Hold GL, Pryde SE, Russell VJ, Furrie E, Flint HJ (2002) Assessment of microbial diversity in human colonic samples by 16S rDNA sequence analysis. FEMS Microbiol Ecol 39: 33–39.
25. Linton D, Owen RJ, Stanley J (1996) Rapid identification by PCR of the genus Campylobacter and of five Campylobacter species enteropathogenic for man and animals. Res Microbiol 147: 707–718.
26. Marshall SM, Melito PL, Woodward DL, Johnson WM, Rodgers FG, et al. (1999) Rapid identification of Campylobacter, Arcobacter, and Helicobacter isolates by PCR-restriction fragment length polymorphism analysis of the 16S rRNA gene. J Clin Microbiol 37: 4158–4160.
27. Tamura K, Dudley J, Nei M, Kumar S (2007) MEGA4: Molecular Evolutionary Genetics Analysis (MEGA) software version 4.0. Mol Biol Evol 24: 1596–1599.
28. Gillespie IA, O'Brien SJ, Bolton FJ (2009) Age patterns of persons with campylobacteriosis, England and Wales, 1990–2007. Emerg Infect Dis 15: 2046–2048.
29. Zhang L, Budiman V, Day AS, Mitchell H, Lemberg DA, et al. (2010) Isolation and detection of Campylobacter concisus from saliva of healthy individuals and patients with inflammatory bowel disease. J Clin Microbiol 48: 2965–2967.
30. Macuch PJ, Tanner AC (2000) Campylobacter species in health, gingivitis, and periodontitis. J Dent Res 79: 785–792.
31. Engberg J, On SL, Harrington CS, Gerner-Smidt P (2000) Prevalence of Campylobacter, Arcobacter, Helicobacter, and Sutterella spp. in human fecal samples as estimated by a reevaluation of isolation methods for Campylobacters. J Clin Microbiol 38: 286–291.
32. Aabenhus R, On SL, Siemer BL, Permin H, Andersen LP (2005) Delineation of Campylobacter concisus genomospecies by amplified fragment length polymorphism analysis and correlation of results with clinical data. J Clin Microbiol 43: 5091–5096.
33. Engberg J, Bang DD, Aabenhus R, Aarestrup FM, Fussing V, et al. (2005) Campylobacter concisus: an evaluation of certain phenotypic and genotypic characteristics. Clin Microbiol Infect 11: 288–295.
34. Kalischuk LD, Inglis GD (2011) Comparative genotypic and pathogenic examination of Campylobacter concisus isolates from diarrheic and non-diarrheic humans. BMC Microbiol 11: 53.
35. Woolley PD (2000) Anaerobic bacteria and non-gonococcal urethritis. Int J STD AIDS 11: 347–348.
36. Duerden BI, Eley A, Goodwin L, Magee JT, Hindmarch JM, et al. (1989) A comparison of Bacteroides ureolyticus isolates from different clinical sources. J Med Microbiol 29: 63–73.
37. Hill AB (1965) The Environment and Disease: Association or Causation? Proc R Soc Med 58: 295–300.
38. Man SM, Kaakoush NO, Leach ST, Nahidi L, Lu HK, et al. (2010) Host attachment, invasion, and stimulation of proinflammatory cytokines by Campylobacter concisus and other non-Campylobacter jejuni Campylobacter species. J Infect Dis 202: 1855–1865.
39. Istivan TS, Smith SC, Fry BN, Coloe PJ (2008) Characterization of Campylobacter concisus hemolysins. FEMS Immunol Med Microbiol 54: 224–235.

Delayed Resolution of Acute Inflammation in Ulcerative Colitis is Associated with Elevated Cytokine Release Downstream of TLR4

Farooq Z. Rahman[1§], Andrew M. Smith[1*§], Bu'Hussain Hayee[1], Daniel J. B. Marks[1], Stuart L. Bloom[2], Anthony W. Segal[1]

1 Departments of Medicine, University College London, London, United Kingdom, **2** Department of Gastroenterology, University College London Hospital, London, United Kingdom

Abstract

Background: Ulcerative colitis (UC) is widely viewed as a leukocyte-mediated disorder. Although strong evidence implicates an exuberant response to microbial components in its pathogenesis, no intrinsic immune defect has been identified and the underlying pathogenic mechanisms remain obscure.

Methodology/Principal Findings: The acute immune response to bacterial injection was determined in UC patients with quiescent disease and directly compared to healthy control subjects. Monocyte-derived macrophages were used to investigate bacterial recognition mechanisms *in vitro*. An exuberant and protracted acute inflammatory response to bacteria was evident in patients with UC, which coincides with increased systemic levels of CXCL10. Macrophages stimulated with bacteria and Toll-like receptor (TLR) ligands revealed a specific defect in the TLR4 response in UC. The defect resulted in the over-expression of a number of pro-inflammatory molecules under transcriptional control of the adaptor TIR-domain containing adaptor inducing interferon-β (TRIF).

Conclusion: These findings highlight a dysregulated innate immune response with over-expression of molecules associated with leukocyte recruitment and activation that may eventuate in the hallmark chronic immune-mediated inflammation of UC.

Editor: Stefan Bereswill, Charité-Universitätsmedizin Berlin, Germany

Funding: This work was supported by The Wellcome Trust (GHACB) (www.wellcome.ac.uk) and The Broad Medical Research Program (GHADY) (www.broadmedical.org). The funders had no role in study design, data collection and analysis, decision to publish, or preparation of the manuscript.

Competing Interests: The authors have declared that no competing interests exist.

* E-mail: andrew.m.smith@ucl.ac.uk

§ These authors contributed equally to this work.

Introduction

Ulcerative colitis (UC) is a chronic inflammatory bowel disease (IBD) characterised by intermittent florid, continuous superficial colonic inflammation. It has an incidence of 1 in 1,000 and is associated with considerable morbidity including an increased long-term risk of colorectal cancer. UC is most commonly confined to the rectum or left colon, but involves the whole colon in 20% of cases. A small proportion of patients (5%) have rectal sparing and/or backwash ileitis. Aminosalicylates (5-ASA), corticosteroids and immunomodulators thought to intervene at various points along the immune and inflammatory cascade are the mainstay of medical therapy. Colectomy for severe or recalcitrant disease is required in 20% of patients[1].

It is currently believed that an aberrant innate immune response to commensal colonic microbiota in genetically susceptible individuals is a prerequisite for excessive activation of adaptive immunity within the lamina propria[2]. Although this concept is supported by extensive evidence from human and animal studies, neither an intrinsic immune defect nor the underlying mechanism(s) have been identified to date. The pathogenesis of UC is clearly complex and likely to involve multiple genetic, environmental and immunological factors[3]. Furthermore, recent genome wide association (GWA) studies in UC[4,5,6] have provided few direct clues as to the aetiology. Macrophages are crucially important in orchestrating innate and adaptive immune responses to microbes via pattern recognition receptors (TLRs and NOD-like receptors). These sentinels of the cellular innate immune system recognise pathogen associated microbial patterns and mediate diverse immune responses through interconnected, but subtly distinct, signalling pathways[7]. Colonic microbiota provide the innate immune system, and specifically TLRs, with the complex challenge of balancing tolerance and immunological responsiveness to infection. A dysregulated TLR-mediated innate immune response may be central to the pathogenesis of UC and produce the immune cell-mediated inflammation characteristic of this disease.

In this study, we examined the acute inflammatory response to bacterial challenge in UC. Using an *in vivo* model of acute inflammation, we demonstrate dysregulated innate immunity in

UC with an exuberant, protracted acute inflammatory response to subcutaneously injected heat killed *E.coli* (HkEc), with a concurrent elevation in CXCL10 in the circulation. To elucidate the underlying cellular mechanism we then examined cytokine secretion and gene expression in primary monocyte-derived macrophages stimulated with HkEc and individual TLR ligands. These *in vitro* studies identify a specific defect relating to TLR4, which results in over-expression of a number of pro-inflammatory molecules associated with leukocyte recruitment and activation.

Materials And Methods

Ethics Statement

These studies were approved by the Joint UCL/UCLH Committee for the Ethics of Human Research (project number 04/0324 and 05/Q0505/115). Written informed consent was obtained from all volunteers.

Subjects

Adult patients with definitive diagnoses of UC confirmed using standard diagnostic criteria, who met inclusion criteria, were recruited from the Gastroenterology outpatient clinic at University College London Hospitals NHS Foundation Trust (UCLH). All patients had quiescent disease (Mayo score <3 and serum inflammatory markers within normal limits) and were on either no medication or mesalazine alone (≤ 2.4 g/day) at a stable dose for at least 3 months prior to recruitment. No patient had received corticosteroid or biological therapy within three months of inclusion. Healthy controls were approximately matched for age, sex and smoking history. No subject was studied more than once in any of the different sets of experiments.

Subcutaneous injection of heat killed E. coli

For bacterial injection experiments, a fully antibiotic-sensitive clinical isolate of *E. coli* was grown overnight in minimal citrate medium supplemented with 1.25 g/L yeast extract (Oxoid), then killed by heating to 80°C for 30 minutes. Bacteria were washed twice in sterile PBS, aliquoted, centrifuged and the pellets were snap-frozen and stored at −70°C. Sterility was confirmed by culture. Bacteria were resuspended in injection grade normal saline. Initial dose response was carried out using 2.5×10^8, 6×10^7, 3×10^7, 1.5×10^7 and 7.5×10^6 *E. coli* per 100 µl. Four HC subjects were injected subcutaneously into the volar aspect of each forearm with four of the doses. From the dose response results all subsequent studies used 3×10^7 per 100 µl. Blood was collected before and 24, 48 and 72 h after injection, for full blood counts and measurements of C-reactive protein (CRP) and serum cytokines (see below). Blood flow was measured at the injection sites by laser Doppler imaging, and the mean reading of the two forearms taken (MoorLDI2; Moor Instruments, Axminster, UK).

Serum cytokine measurements

The expression profile of a panel of cytokines in serum samples collected at 24, 48 and 72 h post inoculation were measured using the Beadlyte Bio-Plex^{TM} human cytokine assay (Bio-Rad), according to the manufacturer's instructions.

Macrophage isolation and culture and stimulation

Peripheral venous blood was collected from subjects into syringes containing 5 U/ml heparin. Mononuclear cells were isolated by differential centrifugation (900 g, 30 minutes, 20°C) over Lymphoprep and washed twice with sterile phosphate-buffered saline (PBS; GIBCO, Paisley, UK) at 300 g (5 minutes, 20°C). Cells were resuspended in 10 ml RPMI-1640 medium (Invitrogen) supplemented with 100 U/ml of penicillin (GIBCO), 100 µg/ml streptomycin (GIBCO) and 20 mM HEPES pH 7.4 (Sigma-Aldrich), and plated at a density of approximately 5×10^6 cells/ml in 8 cm^2 NunclonTM Surface tissue culture dishes (Nunc, Roskilde, Denmark) at 37°C, 5% CO_2. After 2 h, non-adherent cells were discarded and 10 ml of fresh RPMI supplemented with 10% foetal bovine serum (FBS; Sigma) added to each tissue culture dish. Cells were then cultured for 5 days at 37°C, 5% CO_2, with the addition of a further 10 mls of fresh 10% FBS/RPMI after 24 h.

Adherent cells were scraped on day 5 and re-plated in 96-well culture plates at equal densities (10^5/well) in X-Vivo-15 medium (Cambrex, Walkersville, MD, USA). These primary monocyte-derived macrophages were incubated overnight at 37°C, 5% CO_2 to adhere, and then stimulated for up to 24 h with either 2.5×10^5 HkEc, (preparation method same as above), Pam_2CSK_4 (2 µg/ml), Pam_3CSK_4 (2 µg/ml), smooth LPS (sLPS, 200 ng/ml), rough LPS (rLPS, 200 ng/ml) Poly I:C (125 µg/ml) or flagellin (500 ng/ml) (Alexis Biochemicals, San Diego, US).

Cytokine secretion assays

Macrophage supernatants were collected after 24 h stimulation of primary monocyte-derived macrophages with HkEc, Pam_2-CSK_4, Pam_3-CSK_4, sLPS, rLPS, poly I:C or flagellin as described previously. The expression profile of a panel of cytokines in macrophage supernatants was measured using the Beadlyte Bio-Plex^{TM} human cytokine assay (IL-1Ra, IL-4, IL-5, IL-6, IL-10, IL-12, IL-13, IL-15, IL-17, G-CSF, GM-CSF, IFN-γ, CXCL10 and MCP-1) (Bio-Rad), according to the manufacturer's instructions. IL-8 secretion was measured using commercially available sandwich ELISA Development kits (R&D Systems, Abingdon, UK).

TNF-α release was measured using a cytotoxicity bioassay (obtained from Prof. B. Beutler, The Scripps Institute, CA, USA). Murine L929 fibroblast cells were grown in DMEM (GIBCO), supplemented with 10% FBS (Sigma), 100 U/ml of penicillin (GIBCO) and 100 µg/ml streptomycin (GIBCO), at 37°C, 5% CO_2. A confluent monolayer of murine L929 fibroblasts was trypsinised and resuspended to 4×10^5 cells/ml in DMEM. L929 cells were seeded into 96-well flat bottomed tissue culture plates (4×10^4 cells/well), and incubated overnight at 37°C, 5% CO_2. After overnight culture, the medium was discarded, replaced by 50 µl DMEM containing cyclohexamide (0.04 mg/ml) and incubated for 20 minutes at 37°C, 5% CO_2. 50 µl of cell-free supernatant (diluted 1:50 in DMEM), collected from primary macrophages as already described, were added to individual wells. Serially diluted recombinant human TNF-α (100-0 pg/ml) was used to determine the standard curve for the assay.

IFN-β release was determined using an L-929 cell line (4×10^5 cells/well) transfected with an IFN-sensitive luciferase construct (obtained from Prof B. Beutler)[8]. Results expressed as relative luminescence per ml (rl/ml).

Cytokine release into culture supernatants was normalized for the numbers of viable cells in each well, ascertained with the MTT (3-[4,5-dimethylthiazol-2-yl]-2,5-diphenyl tetrozolium bromide, tetrazolium salt) assay (Boehringer Ingelheim, Berkshire, UK). 20 µl of 2.5 ng/ml MTT was added to each well and incubated for 4 h at 37°C, 5% CO_2. Supernatants were carefully discarded and 100 µl/well of lysis solution (90% isopropanol, 0.5% sodium dodecyl sulphate, 0.04 N HCl, 10% H_20) added to each well for 1 h at room temperature. The absorbance was read at 570 nm using a microplate reader (FLUOstar-omega, BMG labtech, UK).

RNA purification

Total RNA was prepared from monocyte-derived macrophages after 4 h stimulation with HkEc, using the RNeasy Mini Kit with RNase–free DNase treatment (Qiagen GmbH, Hilden, Germany). Optical density readings were determined for OD_{260}/OD_{280} and OD_{260}/OD_{230} using a NanoDrop ND-1000 spectrophotometer (Fisher Scientific, Loughborough, UK) to assess protein and solvent contamination respectively.

Toll-like receptor pathway OligoGEarray chips

Macrophage total RNA was prepared as previously described, both unstimulated and following incubation with HkEc. Total RNA (1 µg) was processed to produce biotinylated cRNA targets, using the TrueLabeling-AMP™ 2.0 Kit (Superarray Bioscience, MD, USA), according to the manufacturer's instructions. Double-stranded cDNA was synthesized by reverse transcription of twice-purified mRNA using Truelabeling primers and cDNA Synthesis Master Mix (Superarray Bioscience, MD, USA). The cDNA was used as a template to generate biotin-labelled *in vitro* transcription products using an Amplification Master Mix (Superarray Bioscience, MD, USA), and biotin-11-UTP (PerkinElmer, MD, USA). Biotinylated cRNA products were purified using a Superarray ArrayGrade cRNA Cleanup Kit and quantified using a Nano-drop® spectrophotometer as previously described. Biotinylated cRNA (2 µg) was hybridzed to Oligo GEArrays® following standard Superarray protocol. Microarrays were analyzed using the manufacturer's web-based integrated data analysis software (GEArray Expression Analysis Suite).

Statistical analysis

All data are presented as mean ± SEM. Statistical significance between groups was evaluated using an unpaired two-tailed Student's t-test. Mean differences were considered significant when $p<0.05$.

Results

E. coli challenge in vivo

Previously, one UC patient we studied developed a severe reaction to injected bacteria with persistent local inflammation leading to ulceration at both inoculation sites[9]. This reaction occurred after an injection of 10^9 HkEc, so further studies were only permissible at the lowest dose capable of eliciting a detectable response in healthy controls (HC), this corresponded to 3×10^7 organisms per inoculation (Figure S1). The subsequent local and systemic acute inflammatory responses in 21 UC patients and 15 HC subjects (Table S1) were determined.

Local blood flow

The magnitude of the acute inflammatory response was quantified by measuring elevation in local blood flow following bacterial challenge. This was maximal in both groups at 24 h, returning to baseline by 72 h in HC, with no difference in peak response between patients and controls (Figure 1). UC patients demonstrated a prolonged response with significantly elevated blood flow at 48 ($p=0.04$) and 72 ($p=0.002$) h. Results were not significantly different in UC patients with intact colons ($n=16$) compared to those that had undergone colectomy ($n=5$) (Figure S2). These findings provide strong evidence for an abnormal systemic inflammatory response to bacteria in UC patients, mediated by circulating marrow factors rather than colonic tissue.

Systemic acute phase inflammatory response to E. coli challenge

The systemic acute phase response was similar in the two groups: CRP levels were elevated in both and maximal at 48 h (Figure 2A). White cell and neutrophil counts peaked at 24 h before returning to baseline after 72 h (Figure 2B, C) in both groups.

Serum cytokine/chemokine changes after E. coli challenge

We next measured systemic cytokine/chemokine levels in the serum (Figure 2 D–F). Circulating CXCL10 levels were significantly greater at 48 ($p=0.02$) and 72 h ($p=0.03$) after HkEc inoculation in UC, which coincided with elevated blood flow. IL-6 and MCP-1 levels were not significantly different between the two groups over the 72 h period. TNF, IFN-γ, IL-8, IL-10, IL-13, IL-17 and MIP-1α were undetectable in serum samples at all time-points.

Macrophage cytokine release after E. coli stimulation

Our results show a prolonged local inflammatory response with elevated systemic CXCL10 levels in UC patients following bacterial stimulation. To investigate these phenomena in more detail we studied monocyte-derived macrophages from UC ($n=17$) and HC ($n=11$) subjects. Cells were exposed to HkEc for 24 h and the cytokine/chemokine profile determined (Figure 3). Release of CXCL10, RANTES, IL-12_{p70}, IL-13 and IL-6 was significantly elevated in UC. In contrast, no significant differences were observed in the secretion levels of TNF, GM-CSF, G-CSF, IFN-γ, IL-8, MCP-1, IL-4, IL-5, IL-15, IL-17, IL-10 and IL-1ra between the two groups. These results provide evidence that macrophages from UC patients release significantly higher amounts of a selective group of chemokines/cytokines following bacterial stimulation.

Macrophage cytokine/chemokine secretion following TLR stimulation

Whole bacteria are capable of activating a number of macrophage receptors including TLR and NOD-like receptors. It is possible that the defective cytokine release is due to an abnormality in the signalling pathways associated with one or more of these receptors. Highly purified bacterial-derived TLR ligands were used to investigate the nature of the defective immune response to bacteria, these included; rough-LPS (rLPS) (TLR4), smooth-LPS (sLPS) (TLR4/CD14), Pam_3-CSK_4 (TLR2/1) Pam_2-CSK_4 (TLR2/6) and flagellin (TLR5). Macrophages from UC patients released significantly elevated levels of CXCL10 following sLPS and rLPS (Figure 4A). Exposure to Pam_3-CSK_4, Pam_2-CSK_4 and flagellin resulted in low CXCL10 secretion with equivalent levels in both UC and HC (Figure 4A). The fact that both sLPS and rLPS resulted in elevated CXCL10 suggests that the defective TLR4 response is not CD14-dependent. In contrast to CXCL10, release of IL-8 and TNF-α were not significantly different in the two groups following stimulation with any of the TLR ligands (Figure 4B and C). This result suggests that defective macrophage cytokine secretion in UC results from an abnormality of TLR4, and not TLR 1, 2, 5 or 6, signalling.

Elevated Type I interferon release downstream of TLR4

TLR4, unlike other TLRs, is unique in its ability to activate MyD88-dependent and TRIF-dependent signalling pathways[10]. TRIF activates the transcription factor IRF3, which induces genes that contain interferon-sensitive response elements (ISRE). Genes

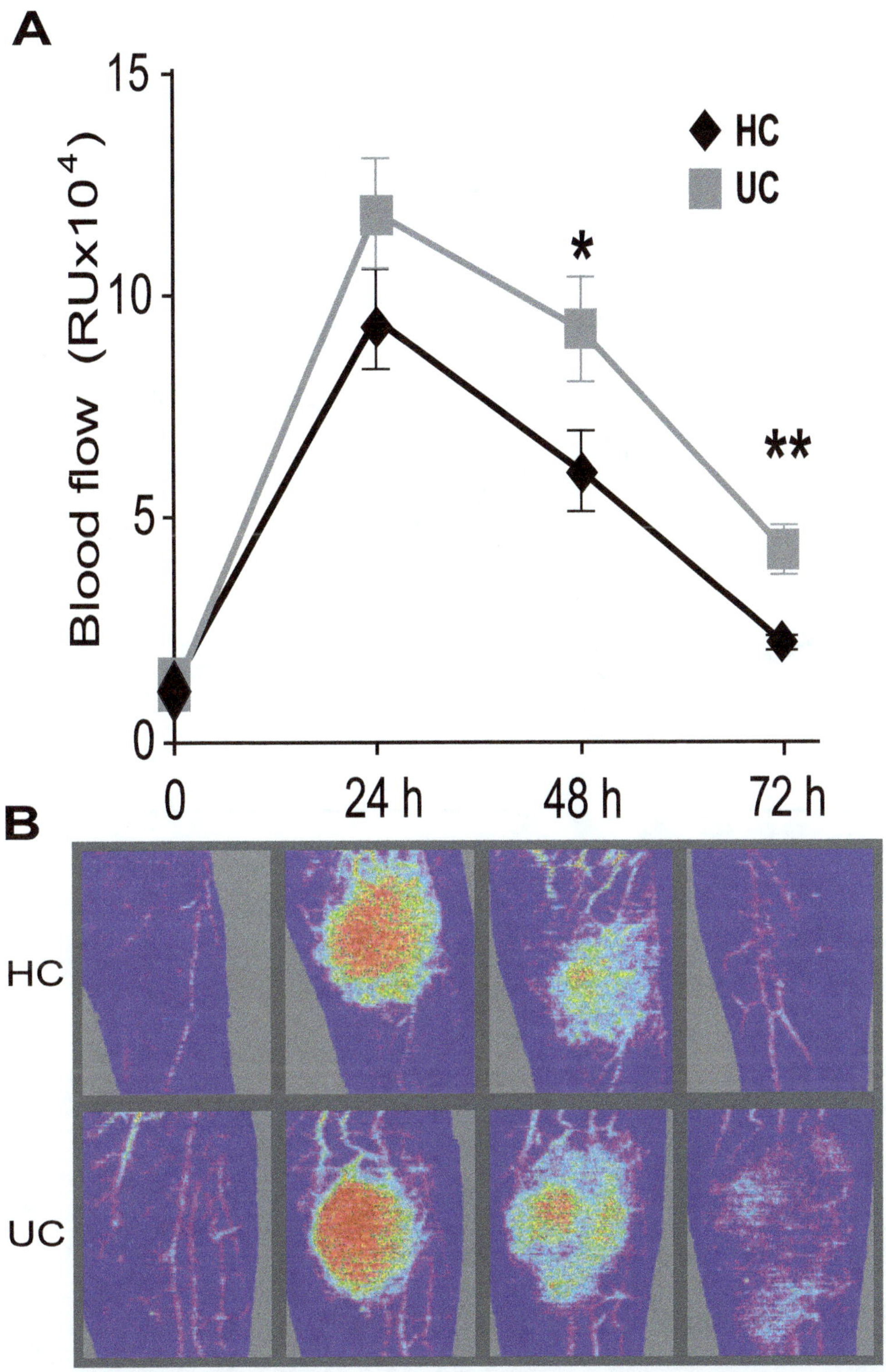

Figure 1. Local inflammation was protracted in UC patients after subcutaneous injection of HkEc. (**A**) Blood flow at the injection site was elevated and prolonged in patients with UC (n = 21) at 48 (p = 0.04) and 72 h (p = 0.002) compared to HC (n = 15). (**B**) Laser Doppler images showing elevated and prolonged local blood flow in a UC patient after HkEc inoculation (Red represents high and purple low blood flow).

which are dependent on IRF3 include the type I interferons (IFN-α and -β) which are release within hours after TLR stimulation[11]. In order to determine whether the abnormal TLR4 response in UC relates to a defective TRIF pathway, macrophages were stimulated for 6 h with LPS and Pam_3-CSK_4 and the level of IFN-β determined using an ISRE-luciferase reporter assay (Figure 5). Induction of the MyD88-dependent pathway via TLR2/1 resulted in minimal IFN-β release in both UC and HC

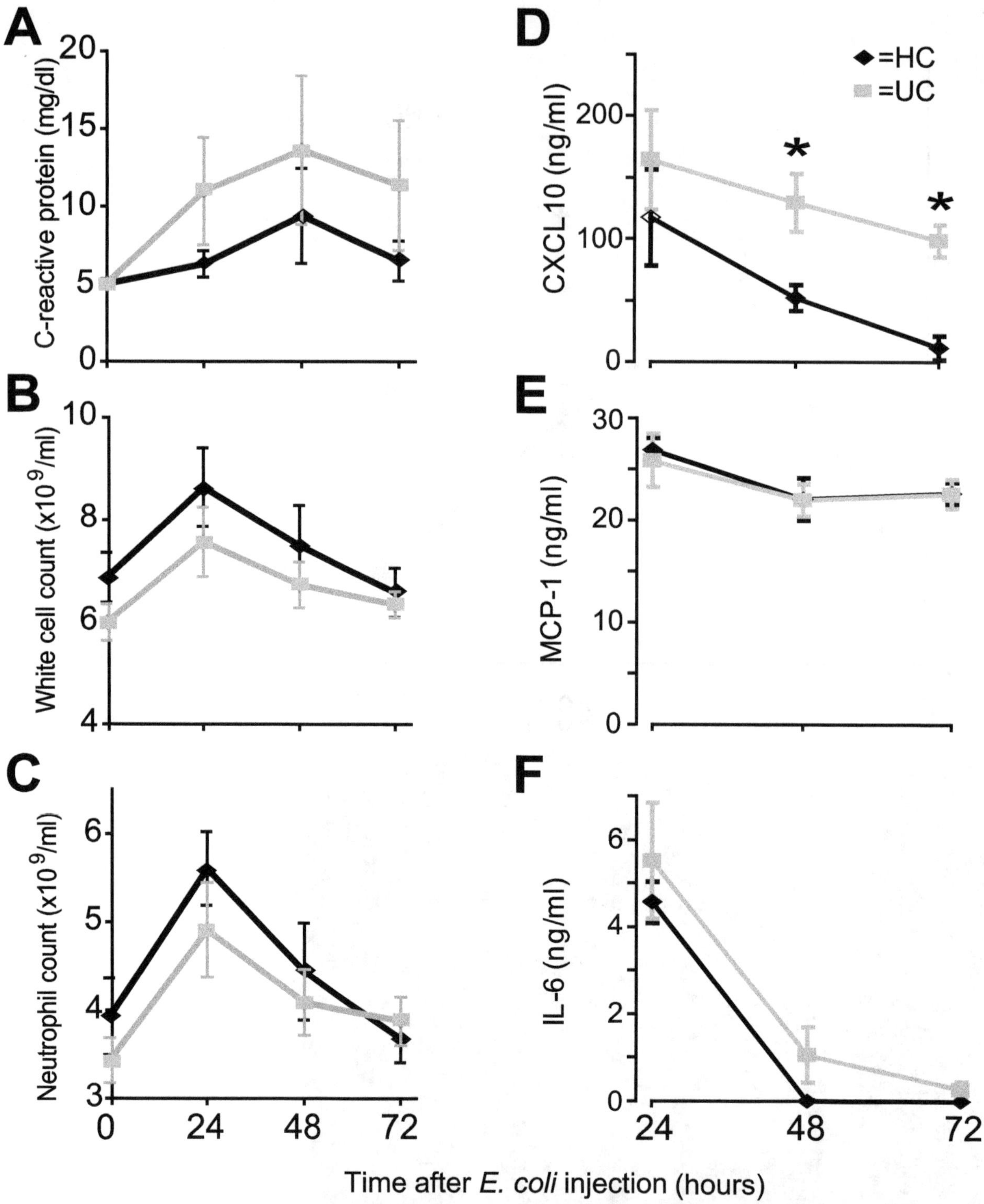

Figure 2. Systemic CXCL10 levels were elevated in UC patients. Effects of subcutaneous injection of HkEc on, (**A**) C-reactive protein (all subjects had baseline CRP levels of <5 mg/dl), (**B**) white cell count, (**C**) circulating neutrophil numbers, (**D**) CXCL10, (**E**) MCP and (**F**) -1 IL-6. TNF-α, IFN-γ, IL-8, IL-10, IL-13, IL-17 and MIP-1α were undetectable in serum samples at all time-points. Results are expressed as a mean ± SEM (*$p<0.05$).

subjects. In contrast, simultaneous activation of both TRIF- and MyD88-dependent pathways through TLR4 resulted in the induction of IFN-β in both HC and UC. Macrophages from UC subjects released significantly more IFN-β than HC ($p = 0.00006$). To ascertain whether TRIF-dependent signalling is generally abnormal in macrophages from UC subjects, we stimulated cells with poly I:C, a TLR3 ligand (Figure 5). Activation of TLR3, which results in selective activation of the TRIF-dependent pathway resulted in release of equivalent levels of IFN-β in HC and UC, suggesting a TLR4-specific macrophage defect in UC.

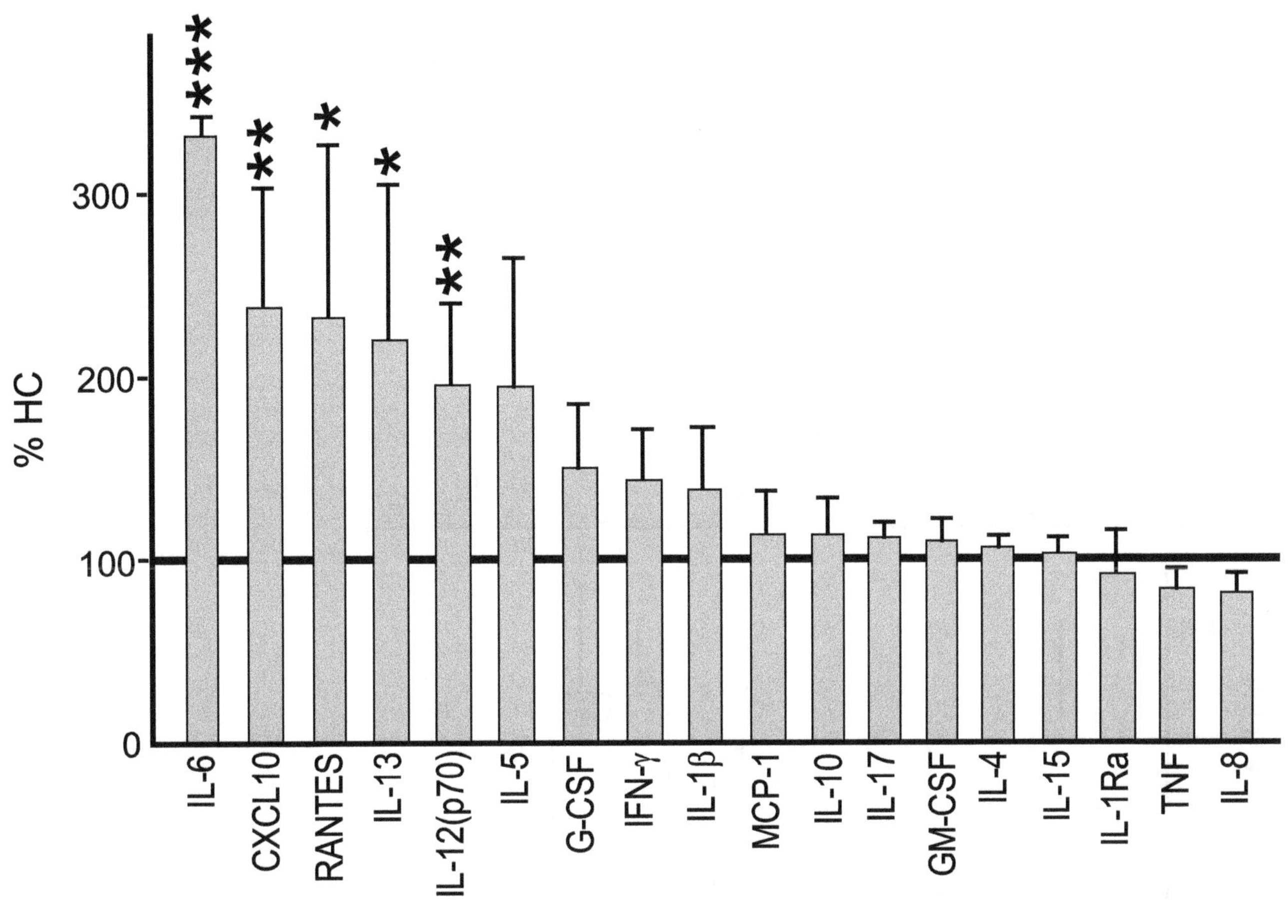

Figure 3. Pro-inflammatory cytokine secretion by UC macrophages (n = 11) in response to HkEc. Results are expressed as a percentage (mean ± SEM) of that secreted by HC cells (absolute values for HC shown in Table S1). (*$p<0.05$, **$p<0.01$ and ***$p<0.001$).

Macrophage gene expression after heat killed E.coli stimulation.

In order to discover if the hyperactive TLR4-TRIF dependent pathway was still evident when macrophages were exposed to whole bacteria transcription profiles following HkEc stimulation for 4 h were studies (Figure 6). We identified significant ($p<0.05$) over-expression (fold change >2) of a relatively small group of TLR-related genes (9 out of 123) in UC (n = 8) following stimulation with HkEc compared to HC (n = 8) (Figure 6). The abnormal gene list included the cytokines IFN-α, IFN-β, IL-12(p35), IL-10, MCP-1, heat shock protein HSPA6, cyclooxygenase 2 (COX2/PTGS2), as well as the T cell co-stimulatory molecules CD80 and CD86. The elevation in type I IFN expression provides evidence that exposure to whole bacterial results in over-activation of the TLR4-TRIF-dependent pathway. Interestingly, all of the over-expressed genes have previously been shown to be induced by TLR4-TRIF-dependent signaling[12,13,11,14,15].

Discussion

In this study we have identified a dysfunctional systemic innate immune response to bacterial challenge in patients with UC. The abnormal acute inflammatory response in these patients manifests as an exuberant and protracted inflammatory response following bacterial challenge. Detailed *in vitro* studies identified TLR4 as the defective bacterial receptor on macrophages, more specifically, related to regulation of the TRIF-dependent signaling pathway. Defective signaling resulted in the elevation in type I IFNs as well as antigen presentation and co-stimulatory genes which have been associated with leukocyte recruitment and activation. This abnormal immune response to bacteria may play a role in the induction of the chronic inflammatory state characteristic of UC.

Although leukocyte-mediated chronic inflammation is a hallmark of UC, no intrinsic defect has been identified in leukocytes from these patients. GWA studies have recently uncovered susceptibility loci which may play a role in the pathogenesis of UC[4,5,6]. A high proportion of these contain genes involved in T cell-mediated immunity[16]. Although this further strengthens the concept of an aberrant immune response in UC, the pathogenic mechanism remains unclear. It is becoming increasingly apparent that UC and Crohn's disease (the other major inflammatory bowel disorder) arise from distinctly different immune defects. We have previously demonstrated an attenuated innate immune response in Crohn's which results from diminished cytokine secretion and the retention of bacteria in the tissue[17,18]. This contrasts entirely with UC, where acute inflammation is prolonged after bacterial stimulation. For this reason, the exuberant response in UC patients is unlikely to be secondary to prior bacterial exposure or chronic bowel inflammation as the same argument should apply in Crohn's disease, in which bowel ulceration and exposure to coliform bacteria is similar[17].

Raised levels of numerous cytokines and chemokines have previously been reported in the serum and biopsies of patients with

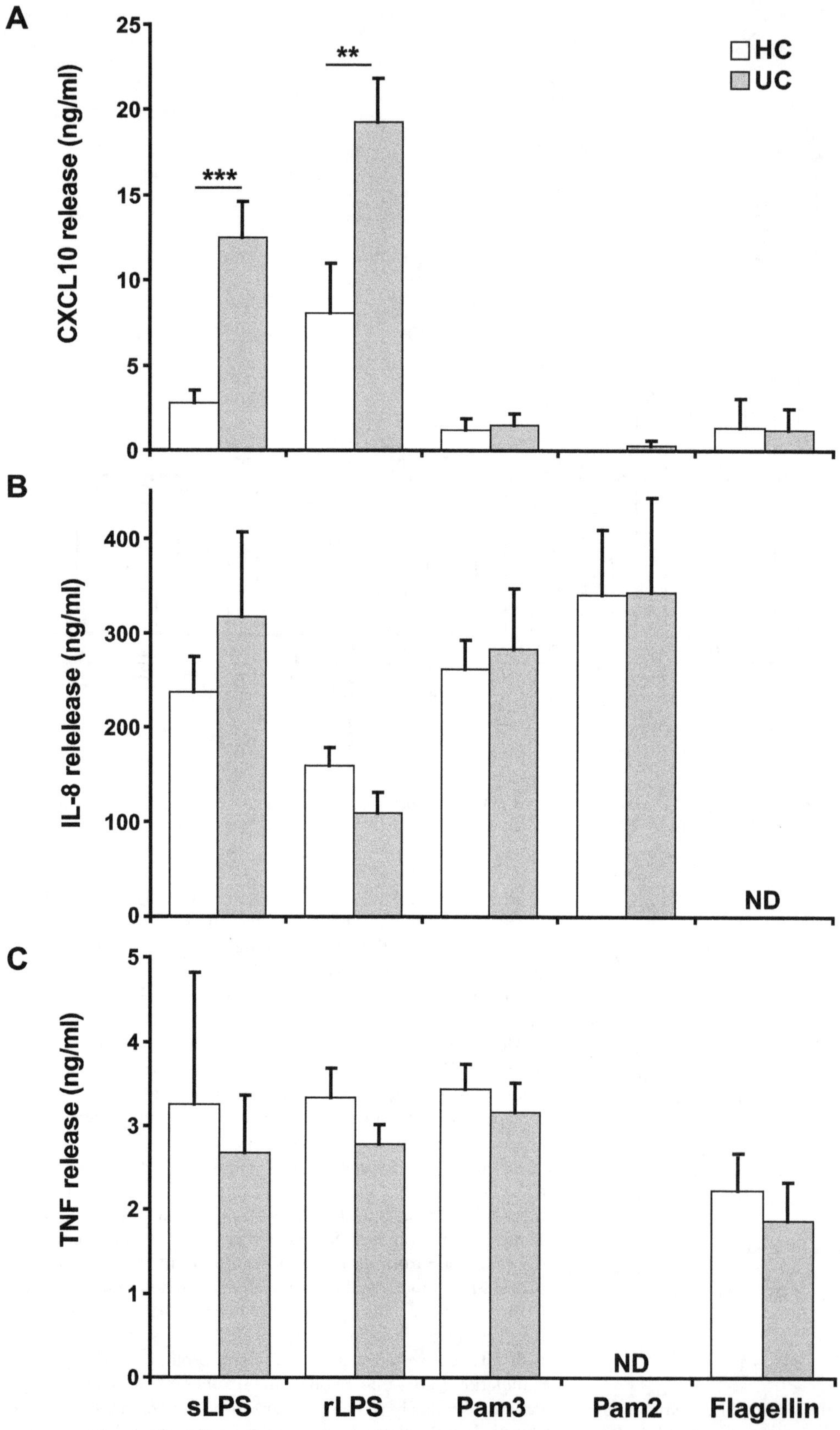

Figure 4. Macrophages from UC patients demonstrate defective cytokine release downstream of TLR4. Macrophages from UC (n = 12) and HC (n = 8) were stimulated for 24 h with sLPS (TLR4/CD14), rLPS (TLR4), Pam_3CSK_4 (TLR2/1), Pam_2CSK_4 (TLR2/6) and flagellin (TLR5). Secreted levels of (**A**) CXCL10, (**B**) IL-8 and (**C**) TNF-α were measured. Results are expressed as a mean ± SEM (**$p<0.01$, ***$p<0.001$) (ND = not determined).

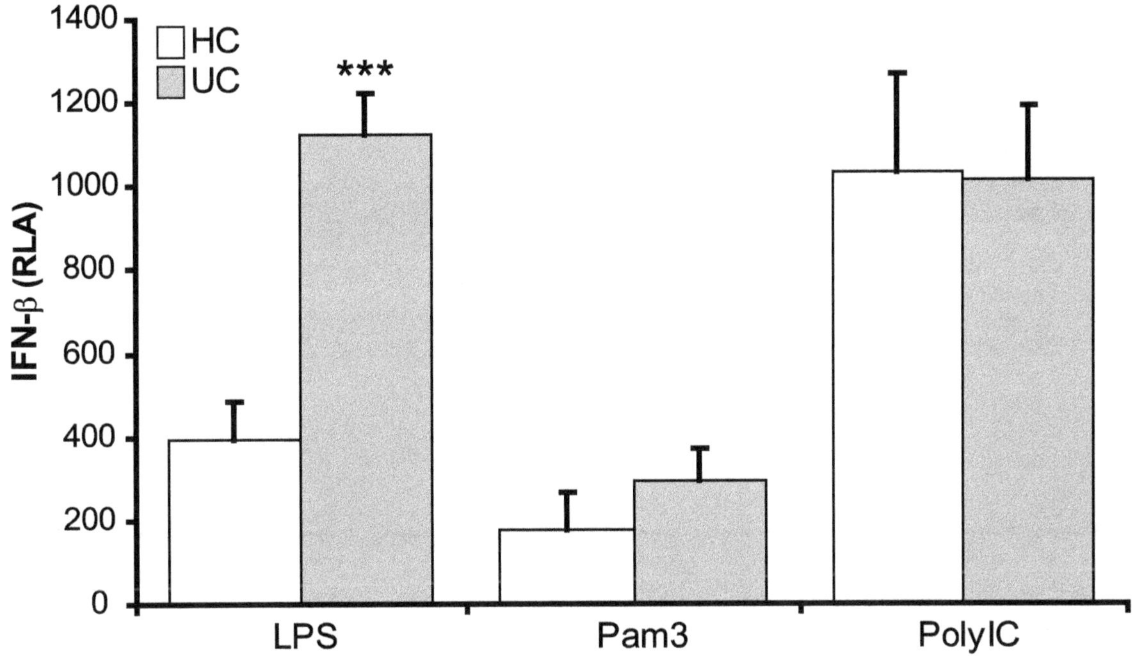

Figure 5. TLR4 activation results in an elevation in TRIF signaling and subsequent IFN-β release by macrophage from UC patients. Macrophages from UC (n = 11) and HC (n = 7) were stimulated for 6 h with rLPS (TLR4), Pam_3CSK_4 (TLR2/1) or Poly I:C (TLR3) and the levels of IFN-β release in determined. Results are expressed as relative luciferase activity (RLA) (mean ± SEM, ***$p<0.001$).

active UC[19,20,21,22]. Of the serum cytokines measured following HkEc injection, only CXCL10 was shown to be upregulated systemically in UC subjects (the majority of cytokines were below detectable limits). Local blood flow and CXCL10 were both significantly elevated at 48 and 72 h post HkEc injection. CXCL10 is a potent chemoattractant secreted mainly by monocytes and macrophages within inflamed bowel[22]. CXCR3, the only known receptor for CXCL10, is present on lymphoid, epithelial and endothelial cells. $CXCR3^+$ T cells are activated and recruited into inflammatory sites by CXCL10 and have been previously associated with colitis in mice[23,24,25]. Raised CXCL10 levels have been described both locally in colonic mucosal biopsies[22], and systemically in serum of patients with UC[26]. Interestingly, *ex vivo* studies on colonic biopsies identified macrophages rather than epithelial cells as the major source of CXCL10[22]. Our results support the notion that macrophages exposed to gram-negative bacteria alone have the potential to cause an exuberant and protracted inflammatory response and raised CXCL10 levels in UC patients.

Mouse models of colitis provide further support for a pathogenic role of CXCL10 in UC. CXCL10 and its receptor CXCR3 have been shown to be upregulated in IL-10 knockout ($IL\text{-}10^{-/-}$) mice and those with dextran sulphate sodium (DSS)-induced colitis. Blockade of the CXCL10-CXCR3 axis with monoclonal anti-CXCL10 antibodies ameliorates colitis in $IL\text{-}10^{-/-}$ mice by decreasing infiltrating T cells[25], and confers protection from DSS-induced colitis[23]. These findings have resulted in the development of novel therapeutics which target either CXCL10 or its receptor CXCR3[24]. A fully humanised anti-CXCL10 monoclonal antibody is currently undergoing phase 2 clinical trials in active UC.

Our results clearly show that the aberrant macrophage response to microbial challenge in UC relates specifically to TLR4 pathway dysregulation. In addition to CXCL10, UC macrophages also secrete elevated levels of a number of chemokines/cytokines following both HkEc and LPS stimulation. This contrasts with normal cytokine secretion following stimulation with other TLR ligands supporting a TLR4 specific defect in UC. TLR4 is unique as the only TLR capable of activating both MyD88- and TRIF-dependent signaling pathways[14]. The signalling defect in UC seems to lie specifically downstream of TLR4 TRIF-dependent pathway, with normal MyD88-dependent pathway gene expression. Stimulation of the TRIF-dependent pathway downstream of TLR3 results in normal cytokine production confirms a TLR4 TRIF-pathway defect in UC. Increased secretion of type I IFN could explain the elevation in CXCL10, RANTES, CD80 and CD86 expression due to IFN receptor (IFNR)-mediated auto-/paracrine feedback mechanisms[27,28,11,14]. IL-6 and IL-12 expression has been shown to be controlled by a TLR4-TRIF-dependent/IFNR-independent signal[14]. Collectively these results suggest UC macrophages possess a defect in the TLR4-TRIF-dependent pathway that may be amplified by IFNR signalling.

TRIF-dependent genes over-expressed in UC macrophages following HkEc stimulation, include the Type I IFNs (IFNα1 and IFNβ1) and the T cell co-stimulatory molecules CD80 and CD86[8]. These molecules have been previously linked to bowel inflammation. Interestingly, *de novo* cases of bowel inflammation resembling UC have been described following recombinant Type I IFN treatment of chronic hepatitis and multiple sclerosis[29,30,31]. Type I IFN therapy have previously been trialed in UC yielding equivocal results[32,33]. In addition, a direct pathological role for CD80 and CD86 in UC has been postulated[34], and blockade of CD80 suppresses colonic inflammation in a murine colitis model[35]. It is possible that dysregulated TLR4-TRIF signaling in UC distorts the immune response to bacteria with pathological consequences. Although the precise underlying mechanisms controlling the TRIF-dependent pathway downstream of TLR4 are still unclear, microbial and

A

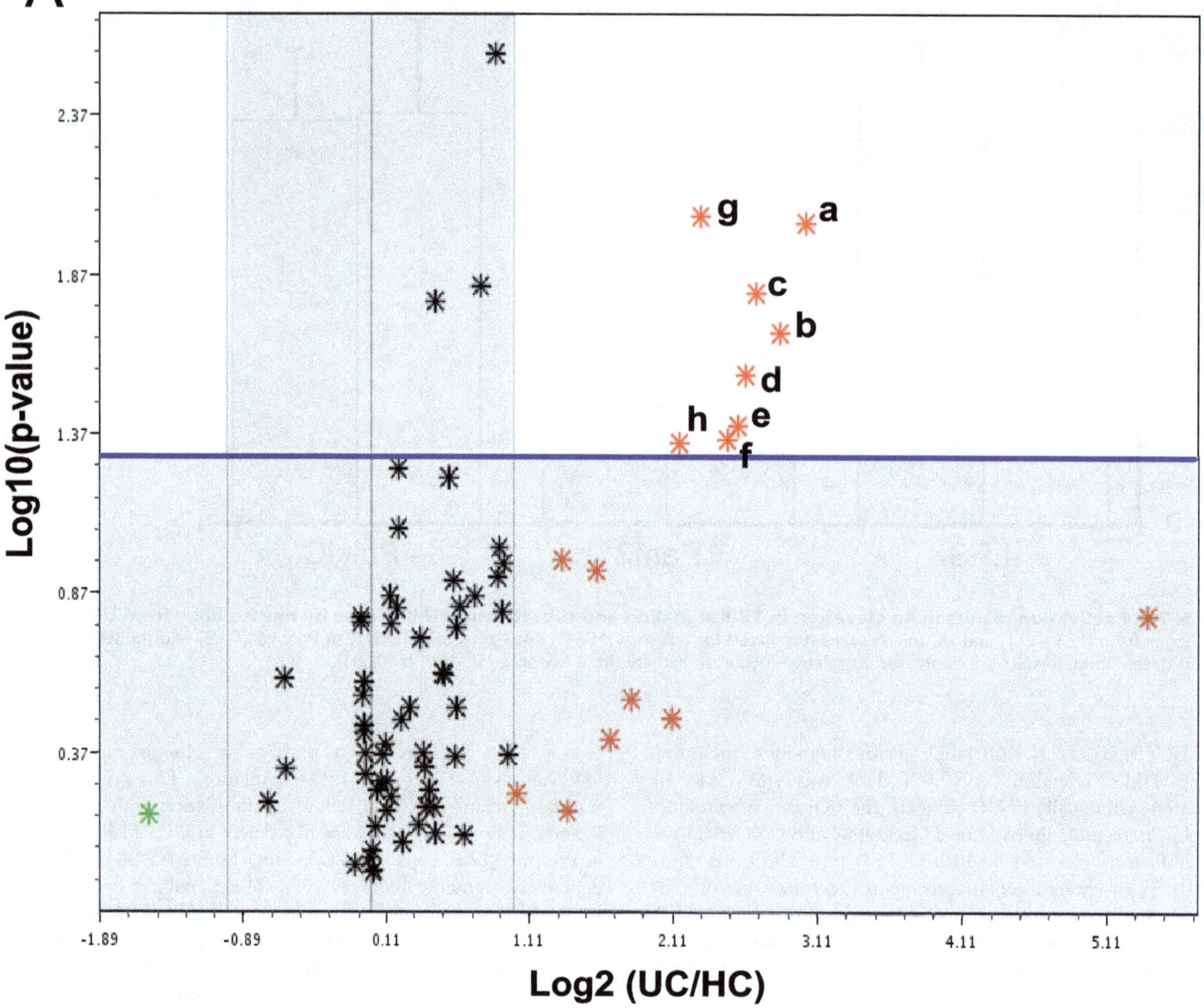

B

	Symbol	Fold change	p value
a	CD80	8.16	0.009
b	IL12A	7.21	0.020
c	IFNβ1	6.41	0.015
d	IFNα1	6.09	0.028
e	PTGS2	5.88	0.040
f	IL10	5.61	0.044
g	HSPA6	4.94	0.009
h	CD86	4.46	0.045

Figure 6. TLR-specific gene transcription profiles reveal increased expression of TRIF-responsive genes in macrophages from UC patients after stimulation with HkEc. Macrophages from UC (n = 8) and HC (n = 8) were stimulated for 4 h with HkEc followed by gene array analysis. (**A**) Volcano plot showing the alteration in expression levels between UC and HC after HkEc stimulation. Only eight genes ($p<0.05$ (blue line) and fold change >2) demonstrated significantly different expression levels after stimulation (labeled a–h). (**B**) Identification of the abnormally expressed genes with the corresponding fold change and p-value.

environmental stress have been shown to play a major role[36,37]. It is therefore probable that directly targeting molecules associated with the TRIF-pathway may prove advantageous in the treatment of UC.

In conclusion, prolonged inflammation and elevated cytokine release are associated with an abnormal response to bacterial exposure downstream of TLR4 signalling. Macrophages from patients with UC have an aberrant TLR4-mediated LPS response that relates to dysregulated TRIF-dependent gene activation, resulting in the over-expression of molecules associated with leukocyte recruitment and activation. The abnormalities identified might eventuate in the chronic T cell-mediated inflammation that is a hallmark of UC. Future challenges include further characterization of the abnormal TLR4 TRIF-dependent signaling pathway in UC and identification of the precise molecular defects in UC, paving the way for novel therapeutics for this debilitating condition.

Supporting Information

Figure S1 Dose response of local blood flow in HC subjects to a subcutaneous injection of E. coli.(A) Laser Doppler images of blood flow levels 24 h post injection. The dose, indicated above each panel, represents the total amount of bacteria injected. (B) Change in blood flow at the inoculation site over a 72 h period.

Figure S2 Comparing the effects of subcutaneous injection of E. coli on local inflammation in UC patients who have undergone colectomy surgery (n = 5) or have an intact colon (n = 16).

Table S1 HkEc injection study subject demographics;(A) Cumulative data, (B) HC, (C) UC. (*panproctocolectomy + ileoanal pouch).

Acknowledgments

We thank Sara McCartney and Louise Langmead for allowing us to study patients under their care; Gavin Sewell and Christine Palmer for help with tissue culture, critical discussion and comments on the manuscript; Jane Tempero and Penny Harrison for technical assistance; and all volunteers for participating in these studies.

Author Contributions

Conceived and designed the experiments: FZR AMS AWS. Performed the experiments: FZR AMS BH. Analyzed the data: FZR AMS BH DJM AWS. Contributed reagents/materials/analysis tools: SLB. Wrote the paper: FZR AMS BH.

References

1. Brain O, Travis SP (2008) Therapy of ulcerative colitis: state of the art. Curr Opin Gastroenterol 24: 469–474.
2. Xavier RJ, Podolsky DK (2007) Unravelling the pathogenesis of inflammatory bowel disease. Nature 448: 427–434.
3. Farrell RJ, Peppercorn MA (2002) Ulcerative colitis. Lancet 359: 331–340.
4. Fisher SA, Tremelling M, Anderson CA, Gwilliam R, Bumpstead S, et al. (2008) Genetic determinants of ulcerative colitis include the ECM1 locus and five loci implicated in Crohn's disease. Nat Genet 40: 710–712.
5. Franke A, Balschun T, Karlsen TH, Hedderich J, May S, et al. (2008) Replication of signals from recent studies of Crohn's disease identifies previously unknown disease loci for ulcerative colitis. Nat Genet 40: 713–715.
6. Silverberg MS, Cho JH, Rioux JD, McGovern DP, Wu J, et al. (2009) Ulcerative colitis-risk loci on chromosomes 1p36 and 12q15 found by genome-wide association study. Nat Genet 41: 216–220.
7. O'Neill LA (2008) The interleukin-1 receptor/Toll-like receptor superfamily: 10 years of progress. Immunol Rev 226: 10–8.:10–18.
8. Jiang Z, Georgel P, Du X, Shamel L, Sovath S, et al. (2005) CD14 is required for MyD88-independent LPS signaling. Nat Immunol 6: 565–570.
9. Marks DJ, Rahman FZ, Novelli M, Yu RC, McCartney S, et al. (2006) An exuberant inflammatory response to E coli: implications for the pathogenesis of ulcerative colitis and pyoderma gangrenosum. Gut 55: 1662–1663.
10. O'Neill LA, Bowie AG (2007) The family of five: TIR-domain-containing adaptors in Toll-like receptor signalling. Nat Rev Immunol 7: 353–364.
11. Hoebe K, Janssen EM, Kim SO, Alexopoulou L, Flavell RA, et al. (2003) Upregulation of costimulatory molecules induced by lipopolysaccharide and double-stranded RNA occurs by Trif-dependent and Trif-independent pathways. Nat Immunol 4: 1223–1229.
12. Cekic C, Casella CR, Eaves CA, Matsuzawa A, Ichijo H, et al. (2009) Selective activation of the p38 MAPK pathway by synthetic monophosphoryl lipid A. J Biol Chem.
13. Hacker H, Redecke V, Blagoev B, Kratchmarova I, Hsu LC, et al. (2006) Specificity in Toll-like receptor signalling through distinct effector functions of TRAF3 and TRAF6. Nature 439: 204–207.
14. Weighardt H, Jusek G, Mages J, Lang R, Hoebe K, et al. (2004) Identification of a TLR4- and TRIF-dependent activation program of dendritic cells. Eur J Immunol 34: 558–564.
15. Youn HS, Lee JY, Fitzgerald KA, Young HA, Akira S, et al. (2005) Specific inhibition of MyD88-independent signaling pathways of TLR3 and TLR4 by resveratrol: molecular targets are TBK1 and RIP1 in TRIF complex. J Immunol 175: 3339–3346.
16. Cho JH (2008) The genetics and immunopathogenesis of inflammatory bowel disease. Nat Rev Immunol 8: 458–466.
17. Marks DJ, Harbord MW, MacAllister R, Rahman FZ, Young J, et al. (2006) Defective acute inflammation in Crohn's disease: a clinical investigation. Lancet 367: 668–678.
18. Smith AM, Rahman FZ, Hayee B, Graham SJ, Marks DJ, et al. (2009) Disordered macrophage cytokine secretion underlies impaired acute inflammation and bacterial clearance in Crohn's disease. J Exp Med 206: 1883–1897.
19. Ansari N, Abdulla J, Zayyani N, Brahmi U, Taha S, et al. (2006) Comparison of RANTES expression in Crohn's disease and ulcerative colitis: an aid in the differential diagnosis? J Clin Pathol 59: 1066–1072.
20. Heller F, Florian P, Bojarski C, Richter J, Christ M, et al. (2005) Interleukin-13 is the key effector Th2 cytokine in ulcerative colitis that affects epithelial tight junctions, apoptosis, and cell restitution. Gastroenterology 129: 550–564.
21. Mudter J, Neurath MF (2007) Il-6 signaling in inflammatory bowel disease: pathophysiological role and clinical relevance. Inflamm Bowel Dis 13: 1016–1023.
22. Uguccioni M, Gionchetti P, Robbiani DF, Rizzello F, Peruzzo S, et al. (1999) Increased expression of IP-10, IL-8, MCP-1, and MCP-3 in ulcerative colitis. Am J Pathol 155: 331–336.
23. Sasaki S, Yoneyama H, Suzuki K, Suriki H, Aiba T, et al. (2002) Blockade of CXCL10 protects mice from acute colitis and enhances crypt cell survival. Eur J Immunol 32: 3197–3205.
24. Singh UP, Venkataraman C, Singh R, Lillard JW, Jr. (2007) CXCR3 axis: role in inflammatory bowel disease and its therapeutic implication. Endocr Metab Immune Disord Drug Targets 7: 111–123.
25. Singh UP, Singh S, Singh R, Cong Y, Taub DD, et al. (2008) CXCL10-producing mucosal CD4+ T cells, NK cells, and NKT cells are associated with chronic colitis in IL-10(-/-) mice, which can be abrogated by anti-CXCL10 antibody inhibition. J Interferon Cytokine Res 28: 31–43.
26. Noguchi A, Watanabe K, Narumi S, Yamagami H, Fujiwara Y, et al. (2007) The production of interferon-gamma-inducible protein 10 by granulocytes and monocytes is associated with ulcerative colitis disease activity. J Gastroenterol 42: 947–956.
27. Davidson NJ, Leach MW, Fort MM, Thompson-Snipes L, Kuhn R, et al. (1996) T helper cell 1-type CD4+ T cells, but not B cells, mediate colitis in interleukin 10-deficient mice. J Exp Med 184: 241–251.
28. Fitzgerald KA, Rowe DC, Barnes BJ, Caffrey DR, Visintin A, et al. (2003) LPS-TLR4 signaling to IRF-3/7 and NF-kappaB involves the toll adapters TRAM and TRIF. J Exp Med 198: 1043–1055.
29. Mavrogiannis C, Papanikolaou IS, Elefsiniotis IS, Psilopoulos DI, Karameris A, et al. (2001) Ulcerative colitis associated with interferon treatment for chronic hepatitis C. J Hepatol 34: 964–965.
30. Schott E, Paul F, Wuerfel JT, Zipp F, Rudolph B, et al. (2007) Development of ulcerative colitis in a patient with multiple sclerosis following treatment with interferon beta 1a. World J Gastroenterol 13: 3638–3640.
31. Tursi A (2007) Rapid onset of ulcerative colitis after treatment with PEG-interferon plus ribavirin for chronic hepatitis C. Inflamm Bowel Dis 13: 1189–1190.
32. Pena-Rossi C, Schreiber S, Golubovic G, Mertz-Nielsen A, Panes J, et al. (2008) Clinical trial: a multicentre, randomized, double-blind, placebo-controlled, dose-finding, phase II study of subcutaneous interferon-beta-la in moderately active ulcerative colitis. Aliment Pharmacol Ther 28: 758–767.
33. Seow CH, Benchimol EI, Griffiths AM, Steinhart AH (2008) Type I interferons for induction of remission in ulcerative colitis. Cochrane Database Syst Rev CD006790.

34. Scarpa M, Behboo R, Angriman I, Termini B, Barollo M, et al. (2004) The role of costimulatory molecules CD80 and CD86 and IFNgamma in the pathogenesis of ulcerative colitis. Dig Dis Sci 49: 1738–1744.

35. Eri R, Kodumudi KN, Summerlin DJ, Srinivasan M (2008) Suppression of colon inflammation by CD80 blockade: Evaluation in two murine models of inflammatory bowel disease. Inflamm Bowel Dis 14: 458–470.

36. Hardarson HS, Baker JS, Yang Z, Purevjav E, Huang CH, et al. (2007) Toll-like receptor 3 is an essential component of the innate stress response in virus-induced cardiac injury. Am J Physiol Heart Circ Physiol 292: H251–H258.

37. Smith JA, Turner MJ, DeLay ML, Klenk EI, Sowders DP, et al. (2008) Endoplasmic reticulum stress and the unfolded protein response are linked to synergistic IFN-beta induction via X-box binding protein 1. Eur J Immunol 38: 1194–1203.

12

Identification of Unique Gene Expression Profile in Children with Regressive Autism Spectrum Disorder (ASD) and Ileocolitis

Stephen J. Walker[1]*, John Fortunato[2], Lenny G. Gonzalez[3], Arthur Krigsman[4]

1 Wake Forest Institute for Regenerative Medicine, Wake Forest University Health Sciences, Winston Salem, North Carolina, United States of America, **2** Department of Pediatrics Section on Gastroenterology, Wake Forest University Health Sciences, Winston Salem, North Carolina, United States of America, **3** Pediatric Gastroenterology Department, Dr. Miguel Perez Carreño Hospital, Caracas, Venezuela, **4** Pediatric Gastroenterology Resources of New York & Texas, Far Rockaway, New York, United States of America

Abstract

Gastrointestinal symptoms are common in children with autism spectrum disorder (ASD) and are often associated with mucosal inflammatory infiltrates of the small and large intestine. Although distinct histologic and immunohistochemical properties of this inflammatory infiltrate have been previously described in this ASD^{GI} group, molecular characterization of these lesions has not been reported. In this study we utilize transcriptome profiling of gastrointestinal mucosal biopsy tissue from ASD^{GI} children and three non-ASD control groups (Crohn's disease, ulcerative colitis, and histologically normal) in an effort to determine if there is a gene expression profile unique to the ASD^{GI} group. Comparison of differentially expressed transcripts between the groups demonstrated that non-pathologic (normal) tissue segregated almost completely from inflamed tissue in all cases. Gene expression profiles in intestinal biopsy tissue from patients with Crohn's disease, ulcerative colitis, and ASD^{GI}, while having significant overlap with each other, also showed distinctive features for each group. Taken together, these results demonstrate that ASD^{GI} children have a gastrointestinal mucosal molecular profile that overlaps significantly with known inflammatory bowel disease (IBD), yet has distinctive features that further supports the presence of an ASD-associated IBD variant, or, alternatively, a prodromal phase of typical inflammatory bowel disease. Although we report qPCR confirmation of representative differentially expressed transcripts determined initially by microarray, these findings may be considered preliminary to the extent that they require further confirmation in a validation cohort.

Editor: Wenhui Hu, Temple University School of Medicine, United States of America

Funding: The authors are grateful to the Jane Botsford Johnson Foundation for financial support. The funders had no role in study design, data collection and analysis, decision to publish, or preparation of the manuscript.

Competing Interests: AK served as an expert witness in the role of treating pediatric gastroenterologist in the Autism Omnibus Hearings of 2007. AK has also served as expert witness on behalf of children with ASD associated bowel disease in Child Protective Services legal actions.

* E-mail: swalker@wakehealth.edu

Introduction

Gastrointestinal (GI) symptoms are common in children with autism spectrum disorders (ASD). Recent studies report an increased frequency of GI symptoms in ASD children compared with typically developing children and those with other developmental delays [1–4]. Prospective, controlled studies suggest that as many as 70% of autistic children exhibit chronic GI-related symptoms [1,5,6] including diarrhea, laxative-dependent constipation, abdominal distension, failure to thrive, weight loss, feeding problems, and abdominal pain related to extreme irritability, aggression, and self-injury. These symptoms can be minimized or disappear following treatment of the underlying GI disorder [7]. Retrospective chart review studies have shown no increase in GI symptoms in ASD children compared to neurotypical children [8].

In ASD children with GI symptoms who undergo endoscopic and histologic examinations, inflammatory pathology is reported with high frequency [9–12]. Features of the GI disease reported originally – ileocolonic lymphoid nodular hyperplasia (LNH) and ileocolitis – have since been expanded to include esophagitis [9], atypical focal gastritis [13], and enteritis [12,14,15]. Further analyses of the inflammatory infiltrate in the mucosa and the associated mucosal cytokine profiles have not only confirmed the presence of disease, but suggest characteristic features that distinguish the lesions in ASD children from the more well-described inflammatory bowel diseases (IBDs), i.e. Crohn's disease and ulcerative colitis [10,13,14,16]. In parallel, disturbances in mucosal function [17,18] and intestinal microflora [19,20] have been reported and may contribute to the GI pathology in ASD. A recent consensus report regarding GI disorders in individuals with ASDs concluded that ASD children with classic gastrointestinal symptoms often have a chronic inflammatory process "characterized by nodular lymphoid hyperplasia (NLH), enterocolitis, and mucosal infiltration by immune cells along the length of the gastrointestinal tract" [3]. While the clinical significance of these findings is still under investigation, it appears that the immunologic and inflammatory activity in the bowel may be part of a larger, systemic multi-organ immunopathology [21–23].

Currently, it is not clear whether the mucosal inflammatory changes seen in ASD^{GI} children represent a milder variant of inflammatory bowel disease or whether a novel pathogenic process is underway. It is possible that a thorough molecular character-

Table 1. Characteristics of Study Population.

Case Status	measure	Age (years)	Gender M(%) F (%)
ASD with GI symptoms (n = 25)	Mean (SD)	5.08 (2.06)	23 (92) 2 (8)
	Range	1.8–10.9	
non-ASD with Crohn's disease (n = 8)	Mean (SD)	12.97 (3.07)	3 (37) 5 (67)
	Range	4–17	
non-ASD with ulcerative colitis (n = 5)	Mean (SD)	12.0 (3.98)	0 (0) 5 (100)
	Range	5–15	
non-ASD – no IBD diagnosis (n = 15)	Mean (SD)	12.2 (3.07)	6 (40) 9 (60)
	Range	6–16	

ization of inflamed gastrointestinal tissue from ASD children and children with established IBD will help to answer this question. Several studies have described the use of gene expression profiling of biopsy-derived gastrointestinal tissue to provide molecular signatures for, and to distinguish between, Crohn's disease and ulcerative colitis [24–27]. Using this approach, one group identified a biomarker panel that could be used to distinguish IBD (Crohn's disease (CD) and ulcerative colitis (UC)) from "non-IBD" (in this case irritable bowel syndrome; IBS). The study further identified a subset of transcripts, consisting of seven genes, whose differential expression was useful in distinguishing the IBD subtypes, Crohn's disease and ulcerative colitis, with a high degree of sensitivity and specificity [28]. Gene expression analysis has been recently utilized in the investigation of gastrointestinal dysfunction in ASD children. Building upon prior findings of mucosal brush border enzyme deficiencies in GI symptomatic ASD children, transcript levels of ileal disaccharidases were measured and found to be deficient in those patients [20]. Using pyrosequencing analysis of mucoepithelial bacteria, a significant multi-component dysbiosis in the same ASD cohort was also reported.

Despite the published evidence [9–14,16], the debate still continues [3,29,30] as to whether children with ASD and GI symptoms and non-specific mucosal infiltrates have conventionally recognized forms of IBD, a novel IBD phenotype, or no disease at all.

Detailed molecular information, generated from clinical specimens derived from ASD^{GI} children, has the potential to provide valuable clarification of some of these issues. At a minimum, the analysis of differential gene expression in relevant tissue from this group of affected children will lead to a better understanding of the molecular processes involved in their inflammatory disease, including pathways that have been significantly impacted. This in turn may provide a more detailed understanding of the biology that underlies this condition. We report preliminary findings from a large on-going study designed to explore this hypothesis.

The purpose of this study was to compare gene expression profiles (differentially expressed transcripts – DETs) in both ileal and colonic tissues in GI symptomatic ASD children (ASD^{GI}) and three non-ASD control groups (Crohn's disease, ulcerative colitis, and normal). The hypotheses being tested were that: (a) DETs in ASD^{GI} distinguish this group from non-inflamed controls, as further evidence of an inflammatory bowel disease (IBD) in the former group; (b) DETs in the Crohn's disease and ulcerative colitis groups also distinguish them from non-inflamed controls; and (c) DETs in ASD^{GI} cases are distinct from those in groups with established IBD.

Results

Demographics of Cases and Controls

ASD^{GI} samples. A total of twenty five consecutive ASD^{GI} cases (6 *autism*; 19 *autism spectrum disorder*) with histopathologic findings of ileitis, colitis, or both were selected for inclusion in this study (Table 1; Table **S1**). All cases underwent routine diagnostic ileocolonoscopy for chronic gastrointestinal symptoms (Table 2) and demonstrated the histologic presence of ileal infiltrates (ileitis), colonic infiltrates (colitis) or both (ileocolitis). For twenty one of the individuals, both a terminal ileum and a colonic biopsy specimen provided usable RNA. For the remaining four individuals, only a terminal ileum specimen was processed and assayed because the RNA from the corresponding colonic specimens was of insufficient quantity and/or quality.

Non-ASD samples

Crohn's disease. Eight children with a diagnosis of Crohn's disease were included in this study; seven with active disease (Table 1: Table **S2**). For each individual, a terminal ileum and a colonic biopsy was processed. Pathologic cellular infiltrates were present in either the ileum, colon, or at both locations.

Ulcerative colitis. Five children with a diagnosis of ulcerative colitis were included in this study; four with active disease (Table 1; Table **S2**). For each individual, a terminal ileum and a colonic biopsy was processed. Pathologic cellular infiltrates were present in the colon or, in some cases, both ileum and colon.

Controls. Fifteen children without identifiable gastrointestinal pathology were included in this study (Table 1; Table **S2**). For each control individual, a terminal ileum and a colonic biopsy specimen was processed. No pathologic infiltrates were seen in either the ileum or colon.

Principal Component Analysis (PCA)

PCA and unsupervised hierarchical clustering of the sample level data were performed to determine similarity among biological replicates. No filtering was applied to the profile level data prior to PCA. This analysis supports *disease state* as the largest source of variation in these samples (Figures 1 and 2). In an additional analysis of the entire dataset, applying Kruskal-Wallis (@ fold change $\geq$2; adjusted p$\leq$0.001) with Benjamini and Hochberg FDR, hierarchial clustering demonstrated that: (1) groups of samples cluster by tissue type and, (2) known IBD

Table 2. Gastrointestinal Symptoms in ASD Study Population.

GI Symptom	ASD^{GI} N = 25 n (%)
Chronic diarrhea	18 (72)
Abdominal pain	14 (56)
Abdominal distention/gas	3 (12)
Constipation	3 (12)
Diarrhea alternating with constipation	2 (8)
Vomiting	2 (8)

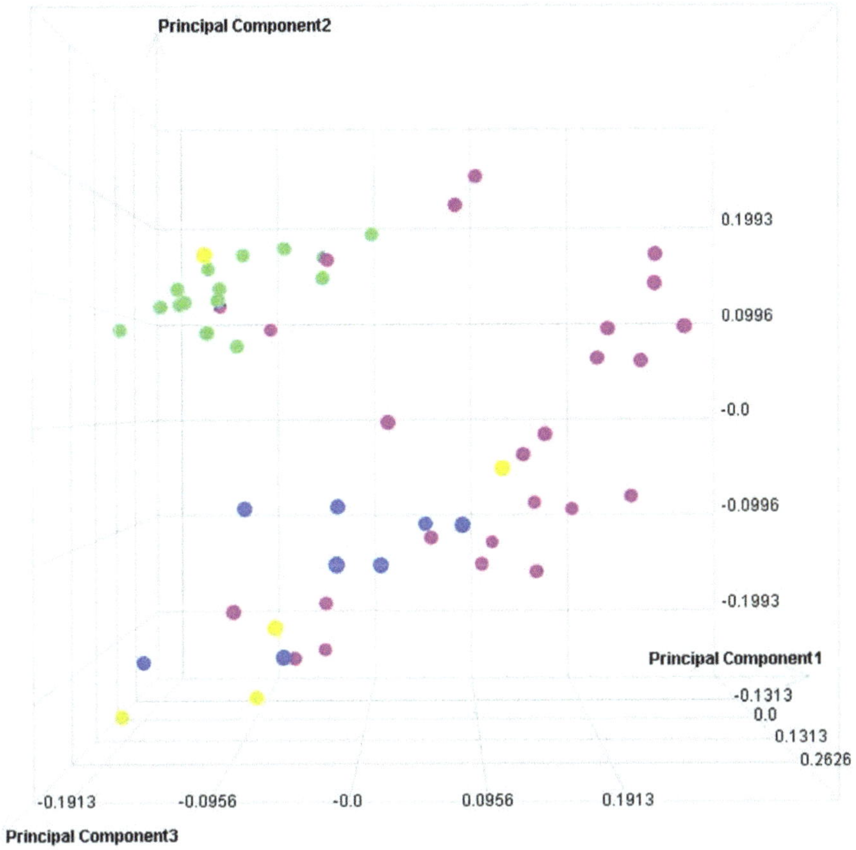

Figure 1. Principal Component Analysis (PCA) scatterplot representing 53 individual microarray datasets from terminal ileum tissues. Each circle represents the cumulative gene expression profile for an individual sample. Samples with similar profiles cluster together in the three-dimensional space.

samples (CD and UC) are more similar to each other than to ASD^{GI} samples (Figure 3).

Ileal mucosa gene expression profiles. In the PCA that illustrates findings in ileal mucosa, the 15 control children without identifiable GI disease cluster tightly together while gene expression profiles from inflamed mucosa representing the other groups show broader distribution (variability). Gene expression profiles for the ASD^{GI} samples show the broadest variability in the PCA, suggestive of some potential subgroup(s) (Figure 1). Significant overlap between ASD^{GI} and both Crohn's disease and ulcerative colitis is evident. Gene expression profiles for the Crohn's disease mucosa showed relatively tight clustering that was completely non-overlapping with the histologically normal control group (Figure 1). Interestingly, the majority (80%) of ileal mucosa profiles from children with ulcerative colitis segregated with the profiles for Crohn's disease ileal mucosa.

Colonic mucosa gene expression profiles. In the PCA displaying gene expression profiles in colonic mucosa (Figure 2), the 15 control children without identifiable GI disease once again cluster relatively tightly together, and apart from *all* other samples, while inflamed mucosa representing the other groups show broader distribution (variation). Gene expression profiles for the ASD^{GI} samples show the broadest distribution in the PCA (Figure 2). There is some degree of overlap with Crohn's disease and ulcerative colitis but no such overlap with non-inflamed controls. Once again, gene expression profiles for the Crohn's disease mucosa were quite distinct from those in the histologically normal control group. Likewise, for ulcerative colitis mucosa there was considerable overlap with the Crohn's disease profiles but no overlap with histologically normal controls.

Pairwise Comparisons

Following a determination of the overlap between DETs for three comparisons in each of the two tissues (six comparisons total), each list of DETs unique to a particular comparison (e.g. ASD^{GI} versus *control* in the terminal ileum) was imported into Ingenuity Pathway Analysis software (IPA: Ingenuity Systems, Inc.; Redwood City, CA) for gene ontology and pathway analysis. The IPA analysis returns significant ($p \leq 0.05$) 'hits' for each of several categories related to gene networks, biological functions, canonical pathways, and transcription factors. The results that follow focus on findings in the *Diseases and Disorders* (Table 3) and *Physiological System Development and Function* (Table 4) categories, and the *Top Canonical Pathway* (Table 5) involvement category.

Differentially-Expressed Transcripts in Ileal Mucosa

Gene expression profiles in ileal mucosa from ASD^{GI} children compared with histologically normal ileal mucosa from typically developing controls. Pair-wise analyses between ileal mucosa from ASD^{GI} and non-inflamed control samples resulted in 2570 DETs. Seventy-three percent (1862) of DET's were down-regulated in the ASD group compared with the control group while the remainder were up-regulated (@ fold change ≥ 2; adjusted $p \leq 0.05$). Of these, there were 1409 DETs unique to ASD-GI samples (Figure 4A).

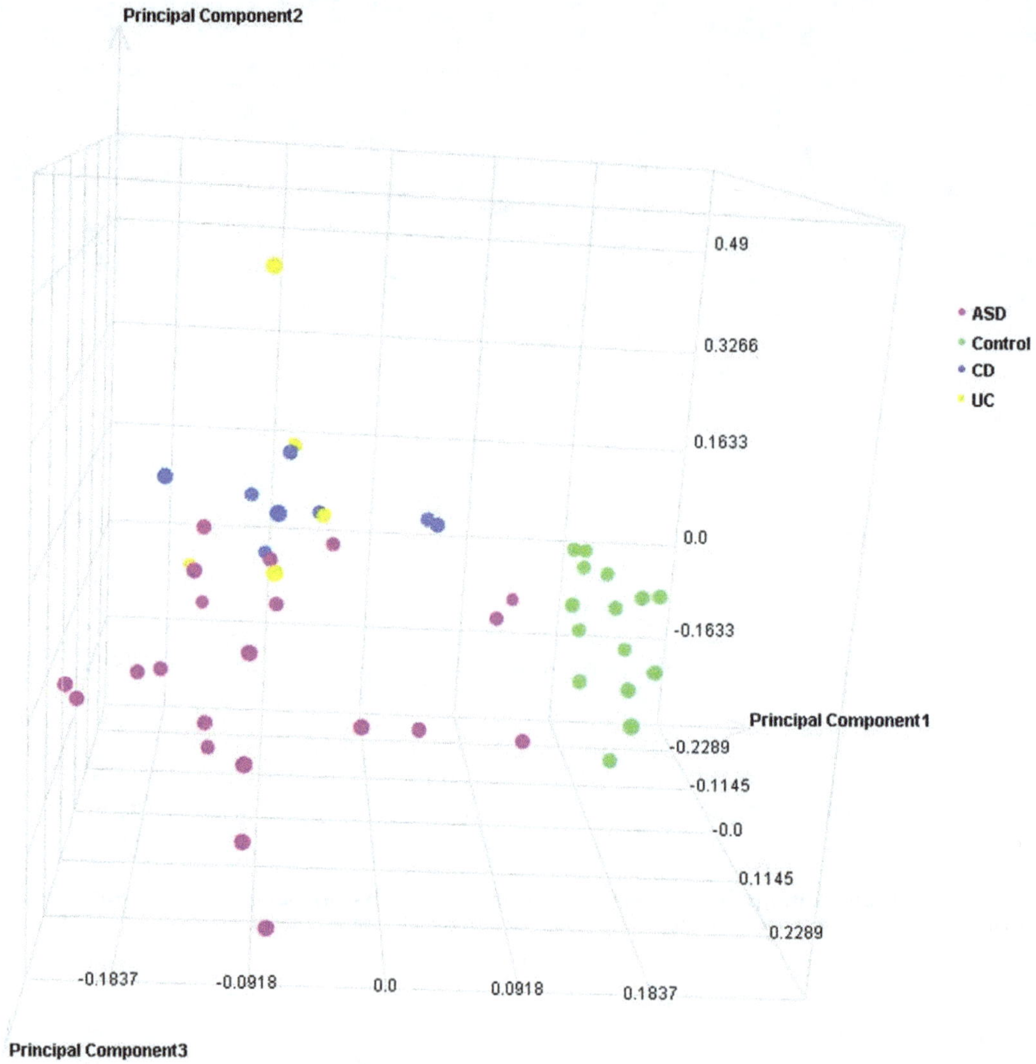

Figure 2. Principal Component Analysis (PCA) scatterplot representing 49 individual microarray datasets from colonic tissues. Each circle represents the cumulative gene expression profile for an individual sample. Samples with similar profiles cluster together in the three-dimensional space.

For this list of 1409 DETs unique to the ASD^{GI} ileal biopsies, the *Diseases and Disorders* category returned highly significant associations with: (1) *gastrointestinal disease* [217 genes; $p = 1.4 \times 10^{-08}$] including *inflammatory bowel disease* [42 genes; $p = 3.2 \times 10^{-05}$] and *colitis* [25 genes; $p = 8{,}8 \times 10^{-04}$] and (2) *inflammatory response* [198 genes; $p = 3.8 \times 10^{-07}$] including *inflammation of organ* [88 genes; $p = 3.8 \times 10^{-7}$], *antibody response* [27 genes; $p = 2.1 \times 10^{-6}$] and *activation of leukocytes* [74 genes; $p = 4.9 \times 10^{-6}$].

The *Physiological System Development and Function* category returned highly significant associations with: (1) *humoral immune response* [91 genes; $p = 2.2 \times 10^{-10}$] including *production of antibody* [52 genes; $p = 9.9 \times 10^{-10}$] and *function of B lymphocytes* [23 genes; $p = 4.4 \times 10^{-09}$]; (2) *tissue morphology* [208 genes; $p = 1.8 \times 10^{-09}$] including *quantity of leukocytes* [109 genes; $p = 1.7 \times 10^{-8}$], *quantity of blood cells* [113 genes; $p = 1.4 \times 10^{-6}$], *quantity of lymph node cells* [8 genes; $p = 3.6 \times 10^{-4}$] and *morphology of epithelial cells* [22 genes; $p = 4.5 \times 10^{-4}$]; and (3) *digestive system development and function* [87 genes; $p = 3.1 \times 10^{-09}$] including *morphology of digestive system* [78 genes; $p = 3.1 \times 10^{-9}$] and *development of gastrointestinal tract* [15 genes; $p = 1.8 \times 10^{-3}$].

Significant numbers of DETs were found in a number of canonical pathways including: *O-Glycan Biosynthesis* [9 genes; $p = 1.3 \times 10^{-4}$], *Propanoate Metabolism* [11 genes; $p = 4.6 \times 10^{-4}$], *Arginine and Proline Metabolism* [13 genes; $p = 4.8 \times 10^{-4}$], and *Alanine and Aspartate Metabolism* [9 genes; $p = 5.0 \times 10^{-4}$].

Gene expression profiles in ileal mucosa from typically developing children with Crohn's disease compared with histologically normal ileal mucosa from typically developing controls. Pair-wise analyses between inflamed ileal mucosa from Crohn's Disease samples and non-inflamed control mucosa resulted in 2104 DETs, 71% (1494) which were down-regulated in Crohn's disease mucosa compared to 29% of the DETs that were up-regulated (@ fold change ≥ 2; adjusted $p \leq 0.05$). Of these, there were 723 DETs unique to CD samples (Figure 4A).

The Ingenuity profile for Crohn's disease mucosa versus control mucosa for these unique DETs returned functional category results almost entirely related to inflammation and immune response. The *Diseases and Disorders* category returned a highly a significant association with: (1) *dematologic diseases and conditions* [58

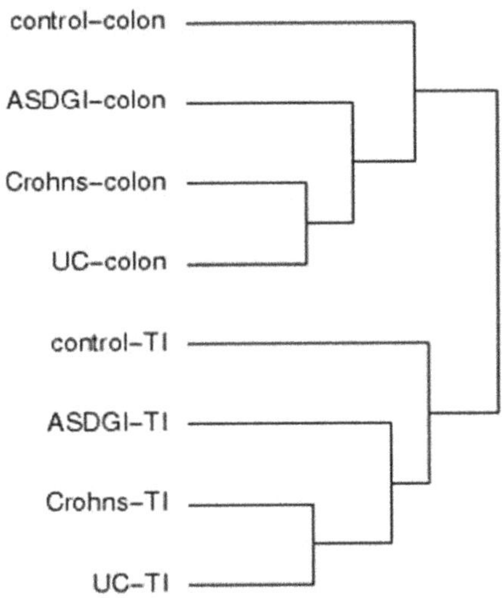

Figure 3. Hierarchial clustering analysis of all samples in all groups. A Kruskal-Wallis test with Benjamini and Hochberg FDR resulted in 5008 DETs (@ fold change ≥2; adjusted p≤0.001) between the 8 groups. In this dendogram, related groups are indicated by the length of the horizontal line (shorter = more related), joined by the vertical lines (e.g. in the colon: UC and Crohn's samples are most similar to each other, followed by ASDGI, and then the control group. This pattern is identical in the terminal ileum sample groups).

genes; $p=1.8\times10^{-7}$] including *exanthem* [15 genes; $p=1.8\times10^{-07}$] and *psoriasis* [38 genes; $p=3.0\times10^{-06}$]; (2) *inflammatory disease* [82 genes; $p=2.6\times10^{-7}$] including *rheumatic disease* [62 genes; $p=2.6\times10^{-07}$] and *dermatitis* [24 genes; $p=9.7\times10^{-05}$]; and (3) *inflammatory response* [69 genes; $p=4.8\times10^{-7}$] including *cell movement of phagocytes* [34 genes; $p=1.5\times10^{-06}$] and *migration of neutrophils* [12 genes; $p=8.5\times10^{-06}$].

The *Physiological System Development and Function* category returned highly significant associations with: (1) *immune cell trafficking* [57 genes; $p=4.8\times10^{-7}$] including *cell movement of myeloid cells* [33 genes; $p=2.7\times10^{-06}$] and *homing of leukocytes* [24 genes; $p=3.8\times10^{-5}$] and (2) *cell-mediated immune response* [18 genes; $p=7.7\times10^{-05}$] including *T cell migration* [15 genes; $p=4.3\times10^{-4}$] and *development of Th17 cells* [4 genes; $p=6.9\times10^{-4}$].

Significant numbers of DETs were found in several canonical pathways: Differential Regulation of Cytokine Production in Intestinal Epithelial Cells by IL-17A and IL17F [7 genes; $p=9.7\times10^{-7}$], Differential Regulation of Cytokine Production in Macrophages and T Helper Cells by IL-17A and IL-17F [5 genes; $p=6.1\times10^{-5}$], and LXR/RXR Activation [11 genes; $p=2.2\times10^{-4}$].

Gene expression profiles in ileal mucosa from typically developing children with ulcerative colitis compared with histologically normal ileal mucosa from typically developing controls. Pair-wise analyses between inflamed ileal mucosa from ulcerative colitis samples and non-inflamed control mucosa resulted in 1475 DETs, 59% (870) which were down-regulated in ulcerative colitis mucosa compared controls while the remainder were up-regulated (@ fold change ≥2; adjusted p≤0.05). Of these, there were 404 DETs unique to UC samples (Figure 4A).

For this analysis, in spite of the comparatively small number of DETs, the *Diseases and Disorders* category returned a highly significant associations with: (1) *cardiovascular disease* [25 genes; $p=7.2\times10^{-5}$] including *vascular disease* [21 genes; $p=5.4\times10^{-4}$] and (2) *connective tissue disorders* [32 genes; $p=6.5\times10^{-4}$] including *rheumatic disease* [29 genes; $p=1.9\times10^{-03}$].

Table 3. Summary for IPA Diseases and Disorders Category.

Diseases and Disorders	Ileum			colon		
	ASD^{GI}	CD	UC	ASD^{GI}	CD	UC
gastrointestinal disease	*			*	*	
inflammatory bowel disease	*				*	
Colitis	*					
inflammatory response	*	*				
inflammation of organ	*					
antibody response	*					
activation of leukocytes	*					
dermatologic diseases and conditions		*				
Exanthema		*				
Psoriasis		*				
inflammatory disease		*			*	
rheumatic disease		*	*		*	
Dermatitis		*				
cell movement of phagocytes		*				
migration of neutrophils		*				
cardiovascular disease			*			
vascular disease			*			
connective tissue disorder			*			
digestive organ tumor				*		
gastrointestinal tract cancer				*		
colon tumor				*		
neurological disease				*		
Schizophrenia				*		
hyperactive disorder				*		
necrotizing enterocolitis					*	
immunological disease					*	
autoimmune disease					*	
hypersensitive reaction					*	
Sjogren's syndrome					*	
organismal injury and abnormalities						*
Pain						*
Bleeding						*
nutritional disease						*
eating disorder						*
iron deficiency						*
failure to thrive						*

The *Physiological System Development and Function* category returned highly significant associations with: (1) *nervous system development and function* [32 genes; $p=6.4\times10^{-4}$] including *long-term potentiation* [10 genes; $p=6.4\times10^{-04}$] and *morphology of nervous tissue* [16 genes; $p=7.5\times10^{-3}$] and (2) *cardiovascular system development and function* [21 genes; $p=7.4\times10^{-04}$] including *migration of endothelial cell line* [5 genes; $p=7.4\times10^{-4}$] and *angiogenesis* [16 genes; $p=1.8\times10^{-2}$].

Significant numbers of DETs were found in a number of canonical pathways including: *Antigen Presentation Pathway* [5 genes;

Table 4. Summary for IPA Physiologic System Development and Function Category.

Physiologic System Development and Function	ileum			colon		
	ASD^{GI}	CD	UC	ASD^{GI}	CD	UC
humoral immune response	*					
production of antibody	*					
function of B lymphocytes	*					
tissue morphology	*					
quantity of leukocytes	*					
quantity of blood cells	*					
quantity of lymph node cells	*					
morphology of epithelial cells	*					
digestive system development and function	*					
morphology of digestive system	*					
development of gastrointestinal tract	*					
immune cell trafficking		*				
cell movement of myeloid cells		*				
homing of leukocytes		*				
cell-mediated immune response		*			*	
T cell migration		*				
development of Th17 cells		*				
nervous system development and function			*			
long-term potentiation			*			
morphology of nervous tissue			*			
cardiovascular system development and function			*			
migration of endothelial cell line			*			
Angiogenesis			*			
Behavior				*		
social behavior				*		
Learning				*		
Cognition				*		
organ development				*		
growth of intestinal villus				*		
development of brain				*		
lymphoid tissue structure and development					*	
tissue development						*
development of epidermis						*

$p = 1 \times 10^{-4}$], *Cysteine Metabolism* [4 genes; $p = 4.7 \times 10^{-3}$] and *B Cell Development* [3 genes; $p = 7.8 \times 10^{-3}$].

Differentially-Expressed Transcripts in Colonic Mucosa

Gene expression profiles in inflamed colonic mucosa from ASD^{GI} children compared with non-inflamed colonic mucosa from typically developing controls. Pair-wise analyses between inflamed colonic mucosa from ASD^{GI} children and non-inflamed control mucosa resulted in 2393 DETs, 69% (1657) that were down-regulated in ASD^{GI} mucosa compared with those in the control group, while the remainder were up-regulated (@ fold change ≥ 2; adjusted $p \leq 0.05$). Of these, there were 1189 DETs unique to ASD-GI samples (Figure 4B).

For this comparison, the *Diseases and Disorders* category returned highly significant associations with: (1) *gastrointestinal disease* [152 genes; $p = 2.4 \times 10^{-10}$] including *digestive organ tumor* [147 genes; $p = 2.4 \times 10^{-10}$], *gastrointestinal tract cancer* [106 genes; $p = 6.5 \times 10^{-10}$] and *colon tumor* [56 genes; $p = 5.6 \times 10^{-9}$] and (2) *neurological disease* [152 genes; $p = 9.3 \times 10^{-5}$] including *schizophrenia* [50 genes; $p = 9.3 \times 10^{-5}$] and *hyperactive disorder* [16 genes; $p = 8.8 \times 10^{-4}$].

The *Physiological System Development and Function* category returned highly significant associations with: (1) *behavior* [98 genes; $p = 4.3 \times 10^{-7}$] including *social behavior* [8 genes; $p = 5.3 \times 10^{-3}$], *learning* [23 genes; $p = 1.4 \times 10^{-2}$] and *cognition* [25 genes; $p = 1.5 \times 10^{-02}$] and (2) *organ development* [98 genes; $p = 6.1 \times 10^{-06}$] including *growth of intestinal villus* [2 genes; $p = 2.5 \times 10^{-3}$] and *development of brain* [37 genes; $p = 1.4 \times 10^{-2}$].

Significant numbers of DETs were found in a number of canonical pathways including: *Atherosclerosis Signaling* [14 genes;

Table 5. Summary for IPA Canonical Pathways Category.

Canonical Pathways	ileum			Colon		
	ASD[GI]	CD	UC	ASD[GI]	CD	UC
O-Glycan Biosynthesis	*					
Propanoate Metabolism	*					
Arginine and Proline Metabolism	*					
Alanine and Aspartate Metabolism	*					
Differential Regulation of Cytokine Production in Intestinal Epithelial Cells by IL-17A and IL17F		*				
Differential Regulation of Cytokine Production in Macrophages and T Helper Cells by IL-17A and IL-17F		*				
LXR/RXR Activation		*				
Antigen Presentation Pathway			*		*	
Cysteine Metabolism			*			
B Cell Development			*			
Atherosclerosis Signaling				*	*	*
Factors Promoting Cardiogenesis in Vertebrates				*		
Mitotic Roles of Polo-Like Kinase				*		
T Helper Cell Differentiation					*	
Interferon Signaling					*	
Il-12 Signaling and Production in Macrophages					*	
cAMP-mediated signaling						*
G-Protein Coupled Receptor Signaling						*

$p=2.4\times10^{-3}$], *Factors Promoting Cardiogenesis in Vertebrates* [11 genes; $p=4.1\times10^{-3}$] and *Mitotic Roles of Polo-Like Kinase* [9 genes; $p=5.5\times10^{-3}$].

Gene expression profiles in inflamed colonic mucosa from typically developing children with Crohn's disease compared with non-inflamed colonic mucosa from typically developing controls. Pair-wise analyses between inflamed colonic mucosa from Crohn's disease samples and non-inflamed colonic mucosa from typically developing children resulted in 1871 DETs, 35% (657) which were down-regulated in Crohn's disease mucosa compared with those in the control group while the rest were up-regulated (@ fold change ≥2; adjusted $p\leq0.05$). Of these, there were 371 DETs unique to CD samples (Figure 4B).

The Ingenuity profile for Crohn's disease mucosa versus control colonic mucosa resulted in three highly relevant *Diseases and Disorders* categories that returned several significant associations: (1) *inflammatory disease* [58 genes; $p=1.6\times10^{-10}$] including *rheumatic disease* [47 genes; $p=1.6\times10^{-10}$] and *necrotizing enterocolitis* [2 genes; $p=2.6\times10^{-3}$]; (2) *immunological disease* [53 genes; $p=3.5\times10^{-9}$] including *autoimmune disease* [47 genes; $p=3.5\times10^{-9}$] and *hypersensitive reaction* [15 genes; $p=2.8\times10^{-3}$] and (3) *gastrointestinal disease* [40 genes; $p=1.7\times10^{-7}$] including *Sjogren's syndrome* [11 genes; $p=1.7\times10^{-7}$] and *inflammatory bowel disease* [11 genes; $p=8.4\times10^{-3}$].

The *Physiological System Development and Function* category returned highly significant associations with: (1) *cell-mediated immune response* [21 genes; $p=9.3\times10^{-6}$] and (2) *lymphoid tissue structure and development* [28 genes; $p=9.3\times10^{-06}$].

Significant numbers of DETs are highlighted from five canonical pathways: *Antigen Presentation Pathway* [5 genes; $p=1.3\times10^{-4}$], *T Helper Cell Differentiation* [6 genes; $p=3.3\times10^{-4}$], *Interferon Signaling* [4 genes; $p=1.1\times10^{-3}$], *Atherosclerosis Signaling* [7 genes; $p=1.1\times10^{-3}$] and *Il-12 Signaling and Production in Macrophages* [7 genes; $p=2.2\times10^{-3}$].

Gene expression profiles in inflamed colonic mucosa from typically developing children with ulcerative colitis compared with non-inflamed colonic mucosa from typically developing controls. Pair-wise analyses between inflamed colonic mucosa from the ulcerative colitis group and non-inflamed mucosa from the control group resulted in 2491 DETs of which 32% (795) were down-regulated transcripts in the ulcerative colitis group compared with controls (@ fold change ≥2; adjusted $p\leq0.05$) and the majority 68% (1696) were up-regulated. Of these DETs, there were 957 unique to ulcerative colitis samples (Figure 4B).

For this comparison, the *Diseases and Disorders* category returned a highly a significant association with: (1) *organismal injury and abnormalities* [52 genes; $p=5\times10^{-7}$] including *pain* [23 genes; $p=5\times10^{-7}$] and *bleeding* [25 genes; $p=8.8\times10^{-4}$] and (2) *nutritional disease* [53 genes; $p=5\times10^{-6}$] including *eating disorder* [10 genes; $p=3.1\times10^{-4}$], *iron deficiency* [2 genes; $p=4.9\times10^{-3}$] and *failure to thrive* [2 genes; $p=1.2\times10^{-2}$].

The *Physiological System Development and Function* category returned a highly significant association with *tissue development* [94 genes; $p=4.1\times10^{-7}$] including *development of epidermis* [14 genes; $p=6.2\times10^{-04}$].

Significant numbers of DETs were found in a number of canonical pathways including: *cAMP-mediated signaling* [17 genes; $p=1.7\times10^{-4}$], *G-Protein Coupled Receptor Signaling* [27 genes; $p=2.1\times10^{-3}$], and *Atherosclerosis Signaling* [10 genes; $p=2.4\times10^{-3}$].

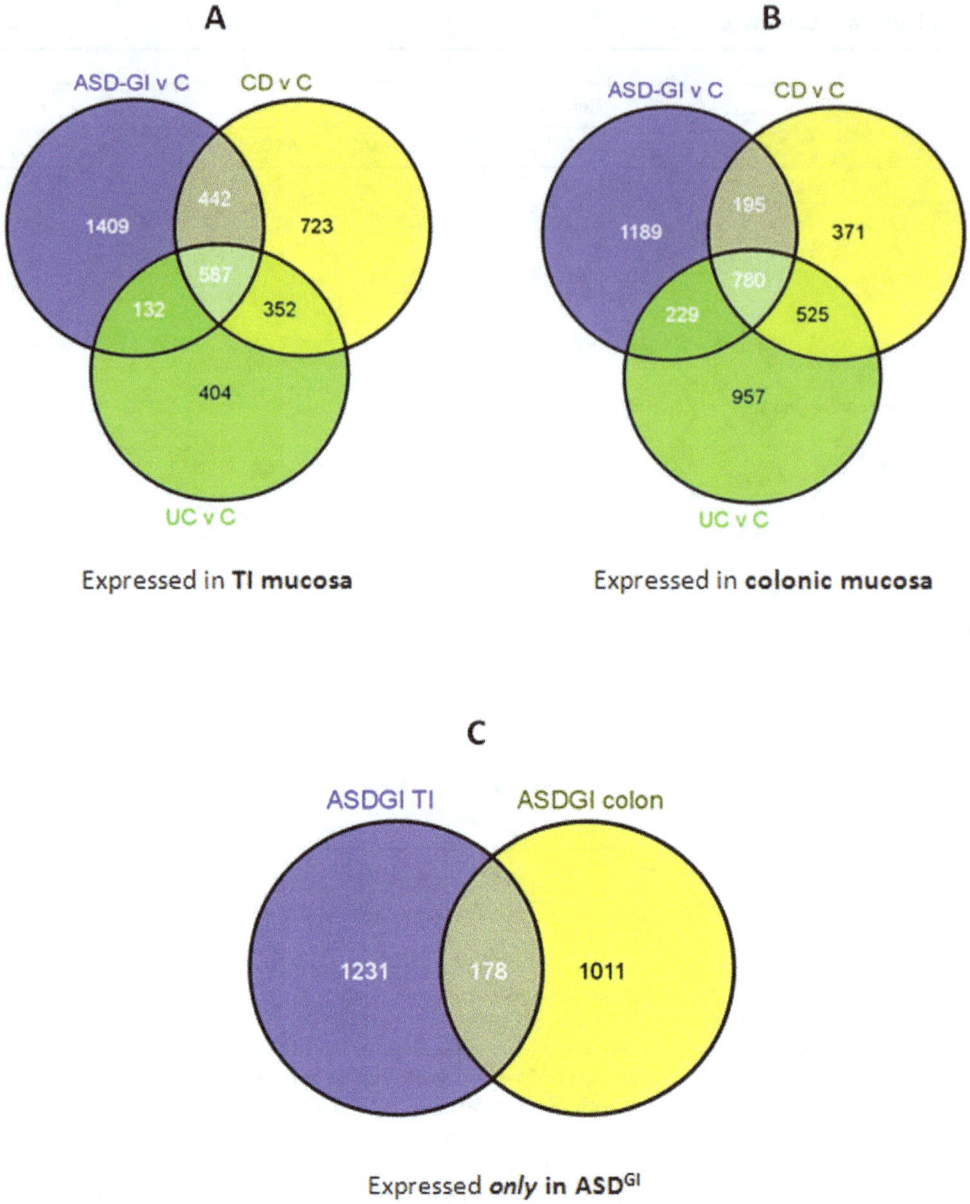

Figure 4. Overlapping unique ASD^{GI} gene expression from TI and colon. Pair-wise comparisons were performed between each of the disease groups (ASD^{GI}, CD and UC) and the control (non-histopathologic tissue) samples. **A.** There were 1409 unique DETs (differentially-expressed transcripts) in the ASD^{GI} versus control comparison in TI mucosa. **B.** There were 1189 unique DETs in the ASD^{GI} versus control comparison in colonic mucosa. **C.** The overlap between those two lists is displayed in this Venn diagram. There are a total of 178 DETs shared in ASD^{GI} tissues (Table **S4**). This list of 178 DETs was imported into Ingenuity Pathway Analysis software for further analysis.

Comparison of DETs in ASD^{GI} Sub-groups

Differential gene expression unique to tissues from ASD^{GI} children. In order to identify DETs that uniquely occur in the ASD^{GI} tissues, pair-wise comparisons were made between control samples and ASD^{GI} samples in each of the two tissues (terminal ileum and colon; Figure 4A&B). In these two groups of pair-wise comparisons there were 1409 DETs unique to the ASD^{GI} cases in terminal ileum and 1189 DETs unique to the colon in ASD^{GI} cases. The overlap between these two sets of DETs yielded 178 transcripts that are exclusively differentially-expressed in *both* TI and colonic tissues derived from the ASD^{GI} population, but not the others (Figure 4C). When these 178 DETs (Table **S3**) were analyzed using the Ingenuity Pathway Software, three of the top associated biological functions were *inflammatory disease* (7 genes; $p = 3.1 \times 10^{-3}$), *endocrine system development and function* (17 genes; $p = 6.6 \times 10^{-5}$), *and digestive system development and function* (13 genes; $p = 2 \times 10^{-4}$). Significant numbers of DETs were found in a number of metabolic and signaling pathways including: *Granzyme A Signaling* [2 genes; $p = 1 \times 10^{-2}$], *Athersclerosis Signaling* [4 genes; $p = 1.6 \times 10^{-2}$], *Valine, Leucine and Isoleucine Degradation* [3 genes; $p = 1.6 \times 10^{-2}$] and *Clathrin-mediated Endocytosis Signaling* [5 genes; $p = 1.7 \times 10^{-2}$].

A subset of transcripts determined by microarray analysis to be differentially expressed in both TI and colonic tissues in ASG^{GI} cases was verified by quantitative real-time PCR. Twelve transcripts were chosen from the 178 DETs listed in Table **S3** for analysis by PCR. Of these twelve, six transcripts were up-regulated in both the TI and colon, five transcripts were down-regulated in both tissues, and one transcript was up-regulated in colonic tissue but down-regulated in the terminal ileum. Analysis by quantitative PCR confirmed the microarray findings for 11 of 12 transcripts in each of the two tissues (Table 6).

Gene expression profiles in ileal mucosa from ASD children with LNH only (17) compared with ileal mucosa from ASD children with LNH & ileitis (8). Of the children in the ASD^{GI} group, all 25 had LNH while 8 of the 25 also had histologically confirmed ileitis. A comparison was performed in order to examine the additional effect of ileal inflammation on gene expression within the ASD^{GI} group. Comparison of results from pair-wise analyses between ASD^{GI} cases with LNH only versus ASD^{GI} cases with LNH *and* ileitis resulted in 41 DETs that were unique to the LNH + ileitis group (Table **S4**). When this list of DETs was analyzed in IPA, the *Diseases and Disorders* category returned a highly a significant association with *inflammatory response* [16 genes; $p = 5.8 \times 10^{-13}$], *immunologic disease* [17 genes; $p = 1.9 \times 10^{-11}$] and *dermatological diseases and conditions* [16 genes; $p = 2.9 \times 10^{-11}$]. The *Physiological System Development and Function* category returned a highly significant association with *immune cell trafficking* [13 genes; $p = 3.4 \times 10^{-14}$]. Significant numbers of DETs were highlighted in three key pathways: *IL-17 Signaling* [3 genes; $p = 3.1 \times 10^{-4}$], *Il-17A Signaling in Gastric Cells* [2 genes; $p = 9.6 \times 10^{-4}$] and *Role of IL-17A in Arthritis* [2 genes; $p = 4.4 \times 10^{-3}$].

Discussion

In these analyses of the gene expression profiles of ASD^{GI} tissue and their comparison to three non-ASD control groups, we have, for the first time, provided molecular characterization of inflamed GI biopsy tissue previously described only in terms of its histologic and immunohistochemical staining properties. Employing differential expression and principle component analysis methodologies we have addressed the three stated hypotheses and found that: (a) DETs in ASD^{GI} distinguish this group from non-inflamed controls (i.e. non-specific ileocolonic cellular infiltrate in GI symptomatic ASD children is not "normal"), (b) previously published data that demonstrate characteristic DETs in Crohn's disease and ulcerative colitis, as compared to non-inflamed controls, was reaffirmed and, (c) DETs in ASD^{GI} cases are distinct from both IBD and non-inflamed typically developing controls, though overlap exists between ASD^{GI} and IBD gene expression profiles.

An analysis of the three groups consisting of inflamed GI tissue demonstrated extensive intergroup DET overlap in both ileum and colon when compared to non-inflamed controls. The finding of overlap between the Crohn's disease and ulcerative colitis samples was expected based on previous comparisons of gene expression in mucosal tissue in IBD patients, however the new findings presented here of DET overlap between ASD^{GI} and IBD (Crohn's and ulcerative colitis) provides further evidence in support of a novel ASD-associated enterocolitis. Perhaps more importantly, although there were significant numbers of overlapping DETs in each of the two tissues for ASD^{GI}, Crohn's disease, and ulcerative colitis, the pair-wise comparisons between ASD^{GI} and controls resulted in the largest number of DETs unique to those comparisons (1409 in terminal ileum; 1189 in colonic tissue). This provides important molecular evidence that, while similar to Crohn's disease and ulcerative colitis, gene expression profiles in ASD^{GI} tissue remain significantly distinct not only from those of known IBD conditions but also from those of non-inflamed tissue as well. It remains to be seen specifically how these molecular (gene expression) differences in Crohn's disease, ulcerative colitis and ASD^{GI} are expressed phenotypically.

In the terminal ileum mucosal tissue, gene expression analysis revealed that for ASD^{GI}, Crohn's disease, and ulcerative colitis, a large majority of DETs (59–73%) were down-regulated compared to non-inflamed control tissue. In the pair-wise comparisons for Crohn's disease and for ASD^{GI}, the disease categories that were most significantly represented were: (a) gastrointestinal disease and, (b) inflammatory response/disease. In contrast, for ulcerative colitis, disease categories including cardiovascular disease and connective tissue disorders were significantly represented. All of the categories identified within these comparisons were accompanied by highly significant p values, indicating that in all of these tissues there was a strong association with a pathologic gastrointestinal phenotype. The pathway involvement, while demonstrating some common themes across comparisons (e.g. cell signaling and metabolic processes), was somewhat different for each of the three conditions, highlighting variation in the associated underlying biology that distinguishes them.

In the colonic mucosal tissue, gene expression analysis revealed that in CD and UC a majority of the DEGs were up-regulated (65–68%) whereas in ASD^{GI} the majority of transcripts (69%) were down-regulated. The disease categories significantly represented in ASD^{GI} were gastrointestinal disease and neurologic disease. In the CD samples there was a highly significant association with gene ontologies representing inflammatory disease and immunological disease, as well as gastrointestinal disease. The ulcerative colitis profiles were correlated strongly with organismal injury and nutritional disease. The pathways that showed significant involvement in each of the three comparisons again varied somewhat but, as in the terminal ileal mucosa, generally involved cell signaling and metabolic processes.

All of the terminal ileal ASD^{GI} samples displayed lymphoid nodular hyperplasia (LNH) but only a portion of them also had inflammation (ileitis). To determine the additional impact of ileitis on gene expression in ASD^{GI} cases, an analysis was performed between ASD^{GI} TI samples with (8) and without (17) ileitis. Interestingly, the disease categories most significantly represented by these DEGs unique to the LNH + ileitis samples were inflammatory response, immunologic disease and dermatological diseases and conditions. The biological pathways that were found to be significantly regulated in this comparison are largely involved in immune-mediated signaling. This data set adds the additional significant observations that: (1) although the absence of cellular infiltrate does not preclude the presence of a unique molecular signature, the presence of cellular infiltrate (i.e. ileitis) results in further refining the discerning nature of the signature to specific DEGs and, (2) the presence of LNH without ileitis in the ASD^{GI} group is associated with unique DETs, suggesting that LNH in the setting of ASD, chronic gastrointestinal symptoms, and cellular infiltrate (anywhere in the bowel) is part of the disease process.

In summary, the overall gene expression patterns from comparisons of inflamed and non-inflamed tissue in CD, UC and ASD^{GI} exhibited unique DETs as well as some degree of overlap. The dendogram in Figure 3 displays these relationships for each of the two tissues. The Kruskal-Wallis test results lend further support to the findings in the individual pair-wise comparisons; i.e. DETs in IBD conditions (CD and UC) are more similar to each other than to ASD^{GI}, and all three groups are more similar to each other than to the non-inflamed controls.

Several aspects of the data are reassuring from a methodological perspective: first, the relatively tight clustering of gene expression profiles from the typically developing non-inflamed group depicted in the PCA for both ileal and colonic mucosa – a clustering that excluded the great majority of those with mucosal inflammation and, second, aberrant gene expression profiles in IBD cases that are in accord with independent reports from other groups [24–27]. Abnormal gene expression in ASD^{GI} tissues is consistent with previous reports of cellular and structural changes within the mucosa [11–13,15,16] accompanied by pro-inflammatory bias in mucosal $CD3^{+}$ lymphocyte cytokine profiles [10,31], and a more recent report of abnormal mucosal mRNA profiles in other ASD children who, while suffering GI symptoms, did not appear to have associated mucosal inflammation [20]. In the only published study that reports gene expression results in ileal mucosal tissue derived from ASD^{GI} cases compared to controls, Williams et al measured the mRNA levels of three disaccharidases (SI, MGAM and LCT), two glucose transporters (SGLT1 and GLUT2), an enterocyte marker (villin), and a master transcriptional regulator in the intestine (CDX2) [20]. With the exception of villin mRNA (no change), all other transcripts were significantly down-regulated in ASD^{GI} samples compared to controls. Moreover, the ileal expression of the master regulator, CDX2, was a significant predictor of mRNA expression of the three disaccharidases and two transport molecules in ASD^{GI} and $Control^{GI}$ children, based on linear regression models. Data in the present study correlate well with these findings. In the present study, expression of CDX2 was significantly down-regulated in the ASD^{GI} ileum (2.1 fold) as were 2 of the three enzymes (SI and MGAM), both transporters, and villin. These interesting findings may broaden the GI disease repertoire in ASD to include not only mucosal inflammation, as defined by abnormal cellular infiltrate seen during routine light microscopy, but also molecular abnormalities occurring in the absence of obvious light microscopic changes.

One of the study's limitations was the relatively small and unequal sample numbers, especially in the IBD groups, although the pattern of aberrant gene expression was consistent with that described previously for these disease groups. The original goal of this preliminary study was to describe the molecular phenotype(s) for the ASD^{GI} group – the IBD cases were included for comparison. Despite the differences in group sizes, highly significant differences emerged, particularly between ASD^{GI} cases and non-inflamed controls.

Additional factors known to influence human intestinal mucosal gene expression include, but are not limited to, age, gender, ethnicity, prescription medications, diet, and dietary supplements. Insofar as this is a retrospective study designed primarily to explore the relationship between the ASD^{GI} phenotype and inflammatory bowel disease, these potential confounding factors could not be adequately controlled for. The variety of diets, medications, and nutritional supplements in the ASD-GI group is depicted in Table **S1**. For the most part ASD-GI children were on a diet that restricted ingestion of both gluten and casein, and in some instances also soy, whereas individuals in the control groups were not on restrictive diets. In addition, food auto-restriction, a common feature in autism, serves to further limit the variety of foods to which the bowel mucosa is exposed and could potentially impact mucosal gene expression. None of the ASD^{GI} cases in this study were receiving medications known to impact inflammatory processes of the intestinal mucosa for at least four weeks prior to obtaining the biopsies. This includes NSAIDS, H2 blockers, proton pump inhibitors, corticosteroids, antibiotics, probiotics, and immune-suppressants. Well-designed prospective studies that would control for additional mitigating factors such as these are both important and necessary.

Because the cellular composition of biopsy material would be expected to influence gene expression, it is theoretically possible that greater levels of lymphoid tissue present in the younger ASD^{GI} patients in the study group may have contributed to differences between them and the older patients in the other three groups. Although this may have been a factor in the terminal ileal gene expression (all of which demonstrated the histologic presence of LNH), this cannot be the case in the colonic analyses as only two of the colonic specimens contained histologic LNH. It therefore seems likely that LNH, by itself, does not contribute to DET variation in this study.

Lastly, not all study participants were diagnosed with ASD using the same standardized diagnostic tools and by the same clinicians. The variety of diagnostic methods used for participants of this study included the Autism Diagnostic Observation Schedule (ADOS), the Autism Diagnostic Interview-Revised (ADIR), or having met the DSM-IV criteria based on standardized non ASD-specific developmental scales such as the Bayley Scale of Infant and Toddler Development, the Mullen scale of Early Learning, and the Vineland Adaptive Behavior Scales, among others. Some patients were determined to have met DSM-IV criteria without use of a quantitative score on standardized testing.

The relatively broad distribution of gene expression profiles in the ASD^{GI} samples represented in the PCA analysis may be attributable to a number of different factors. First, the larger number of cases in this group, relative to the IBD groups, may account for some of this effect. Heterogeneity in the underlying inflammatory process, its severity and location, as well as the average age of individuals within this group, is among the variables that may influence this distribution. It is also possible that the heterogeneity in gene expression profiles in the ASD^{GI} group is reflective of a disease in various stages of evolution. We may therefore speculate that the broad distribution of DETs in ASD^{GI} is reflective of a dynamic process in which the repertoire of DETs is evolving over time, perhaps towards those of other established IBDs. Longitudinal studies currently underway are designed specifically to address this question.

An important consideration when examining between-group differences in gene expression reported here is the disparity in mean age between the ASD^{GI} group (5 years) and the non-ASD groups (12.5 years). Although this factor represents a limitation to this study, we are not aware of any gene expression studies that have reported a significant age-related pattern of expression in pediatric gastrointestinal tissue. In the absence of these data, we are making the assumption that, while there may be *some* differences in gastrointestinal tissue gene expression in children as they age from 5 to 13, these differences would not significantly skew the overall transcriptome profile. A second important limitation in the design of this study is the lack of gender-matched samples. Given the increased risk of ASD in boys, the ASD cases tend to be mostly male, whereas the non-ASD patients are more evenly distributed between male and female. Once again, although we are not aware of any report suggesting significant gender-related differences in gene expression in pediatric gastrointestinal tissue, we acknowledge that they may exist and if so, could confound the interpretation of these results. Importantly, the largest source of variation found via principal component analysis of gene expression in these 53 biopsy samples was *disease state*, i.e. the presence or absence of light microscopic histopathologic findings.

The IBD patients included in this study represent a spectrum ranging from those presenting at initial diagnosis (not currently on medications) to patients with a flare of symptoms due to previously identified IBD. In many cases, the latter group was maintained on some level of treatment for their IBD. However, in both cases, subjects demonstrated active symptoms justifying the need for endoscopic assessment. Thus, despite the difference regarding immune suppression agents, the vast majority of cases in both patient groups had active disease at the time of endoscopy. The authors acknowledge that the use of medications in IBD patients at the time of procedure represents a limitation of this retrospective study. Future prospective studies will be designed to account for this variability.

Taken as a whole, the picture that emerges is one in which GI symptomatic children with ASD in whom cellular infiltrate is present in the ileum and colon have a distinct molecular signature that is consistent with the larger disease categories of gastrointestinal disease, and more specifically, overlaps with Crohn's disease, ulcerative colitis, and autoimmunity. The shared uniquely expressed DETs seen in both the ileum and colon suggest that intestinal mucosal inflammatory infiltrates in the setting of GI symptomatic patients with ASD reflect a single unifying autoimmune process at play in both the small and large bowel. Future studies are necessary to determine whether these markers can be extended to the larger, non-ileocolitic cohort of ASD children.

Materials and Methods

This study examined gene expression in histologically inflamed colonic and ileal intestinal mucosal tissue from consecutive GI symptomatic children undergoing diagnostic ileocolonoscopy and biopsy for active GI symptoms. Subjects included children with a diagnosis of ASD (ASD^{GI}; n = 25, mean age 5.08±2.06 years; 23 male and 2 female) and three typically-developing groups including: (1) children who underwent diagnostic ileocolonoscopy for chronic GI symptoms in which no histopathology was found (n = 15, mean age 12.2±3.07 years; 6 male and 9 female), (2) children with a diagnosis of Crohn's disease (n = 8, mean age 12.97±3.07 years; 3 male and 5 female), (3) and children with a diagnosis of ulcerative colitis (n = 5, mean age 12.0±4.0 years; all female).

Case selection and Biopsy Procurement

Most patients of the ASD-GI group (Table 1; Table **S1**) were referred for gastrointestinal evaluation by their primary care provider though some patients were self referred. All were patients of a single pediatric gastroenterologist (AK) and were selected based upon a history of normal development for at least 12 months followed by developmental regression and onset of GI symptoms (Table 2). For all individuals in this group, this was their first diagnostic ileocolonoscopy and no patients were taking medication thought to alter the histologic appearance of the GI mucosa. All cases had ileal lymphoid nodular hyperplasia (LNH) and all had histologically-confirmed colitis and/or ileitis in at least one of 8–10 collected and archived ileocolonic biopsies. 25 consecutive patients meeting these criteria were selected.

All patients were assigned a diagnosis of ASD (Autism, Asperger's or PDD-NOS; 16 had a diagnosis of *autism*; 9 had a diagnosis of *autism spectrum disorder*) by one or more practitioners from the following specialties: pediatric neurology, developmental pediatrics, pediatric psychiatry or psychology. Of the twenty five ASD individuals included in this study, there were 22 Caucasians, one black, one Caucasian/Hispanic, and one whose ethnicity was not recorded. A detailed history of GI symptoms was documented (Table 2). Patients who met clinical criteria for diagnostic ileocolonoscopy and biopsy and whose parents agreed to participate in this IRB-approved study (Copernicus Group Independent Review Board) were provided with a study description and informed written consent from the next of kin, carers or guardians on the behalf of all the minors/children participants involved in all studies was obtained.

Specimens were obtained using a standard disposable forceps biopsy device, in accordance with routine diagnostic biopsy protocol. Immediately upon procurement of biopsy tissue, a specimen from each of seven anatomic locations (from the terminal ileum to rectum) was processed for paraffin embedding and subsequent routine histopathology. Biopsies for microarray analysis were obtained from the divided mucosal specimen at each anatomic location. These tissues were placed directly into RNAlater (Qiagen Inc; Valecia, CA) and stored at −80°C prior to processing.

Control biopsy procurement. Prospective controls (Table 1; Table **S2**), recruited through an IRB approved protocol (Wake Forest University Health Sciences Institutional Review Board) from the Pediatric Gastroenterology Clinic at the Wake Forest University Health Sciences, included children who presented with symptoms and laboratory testing suggesting possible intestinal disease (Crohn's disease, ulcerative colitis, celiac disease) or food allergy. Non-IBD Control subjects were further defined as those who, following colonoscopy, were without endoscopic or pathologic findings explaining their symptoms. However, the initial indication for colonoscopy was presence of unexplained GI symptoms ranging from abdominal pain, diarrhea, malnutrition, blood observed in the stools, etc. Failure to diagnose the etiology of observed symptoms by endoscopy was subsequently followed by clinical reassessment or additional diagnostic testing.

No concerns regarding developmental delays for any participant in any of the control groups were reported by parents, relatives, caretakers, or teachers and none were noted by physicians at the Wake Forest Pediatric GI Clinic.

For the twenty eight children in the control groups there were 22 Caucasian, 1 black, and 1 Hispanic. The ethnicities for the other four were not recorded. Tissues for microarray analysis were collected, processed and stored in identical fashion to those from children with ASD. Informed written consent from the next of kin, carers or guardians on the behalf of all the minors/children participants involved in all studies was obtained.

All specimens (cases and controls) were collected and stored in identical fashion (e.g. pinch cold biopsy forceps, immediate placement in RNA later, and freezing at −80 degrees within 24–48 hours), cases were collected at a single location with controls collected at a second location, and both cases and controls were collected using identical specimen collection protocols as outlined in the SOP submissions to the respective IRB's.

Microarray and Data Analysis

Sample preparation. Total RNA was isolated from mucosal biopsies that had been stored in RNAlater by sonicating the tissue in the presence of TriReagent (Molecular Research Center, Inc., Cincinnati, Ohio) according to the method of Chomcynski and Sacchi [32]. Total RNA was purified using RNeasy Minelute Plus columns (includes an on-column DNAse step) and reagents (Qiagen, Valencia, CA) and eluted in nuclease-free water. RNA concentration and quality were determined using a Nanodrop ND-1000 (Nanodrop Technologies, Wilmington, DE) and Agilent Bioanalyzer, respectively. A single biopsy specimen was typically 3–5 mg of tissue and yielded from 3–10 µg of high quality (e.g. RIN ≥ 7) total RNA.

Microarray. For microarray hybridizations, 500 ng of total RNA from each biopsy was labeled with fluorescent dye (Cy3; Amersham Biosciences Corp, Piscataway, NJ) using the Low RNA Input Linear Amplification Labeling kit (Agilent Technologies, Palo Alto, CA) following the manufacturer's protocol. The amount

Table 6. Comparison of microarray results with qPCR results from 12 representative transcripts differentially-regulated in both terminal ileum and colon, exclusively in ASD^{GI} samples.

TERMINAL ILEUM							
		microarray data			PCR data		
Gene Symbol	Gene Identifier	Ratio	Direction	adj. p-value	Ratio	Direction	p-value
AMPD1	NM_000036	3.7	↓	4.47E-07	4.29	↓	4.92E-01
IL2RA	NM_000417	2.63	↑	2.94E-06	4.93	↑	4.10E-05
TXLNG2P	NM_001005852	8.5	↑	2.62E-02	97.67	↑↑	3.41E-04
RPS4Y1	NM_001008	43.3	↑↑	5.89E-03	132.11	↑↑	1.46E-03
RPS4Y2	NM_001039567	29.65	↑↑	8.41E-03	25.71	↑↑	1.02E-03
SCGB2A1	NM_002407	5.25	↓	3.64E-07	5.9	↓	2.50E-01
ZFY	NM_003411	5.08	↑	3.27E-02	1.42	↑	1.77E-02
INSL5	NM_005478	2.2	↓	2.25E-02	1.27	↓	5.27E-01
NTS	NM_006183	5.71	↓	7.84E-07	10.33	↓↓	3.27E-02
IGF2BP1	NM_006546	4.28	↑	1.65E-06	7.13	↑	1.22E-01
TNFRSF12A	NM_016639	2.07	↓	4.58E-05	1.83	↓	9.00E-03
KCTD4	NM_198404	3.58	↓	5.23E-06	1.96	↑	2.13E-01
COLONIC BIOPSY							
		microarray data			PCR data		
Gene Symbol	Gene Identifier	Ratio	Direction	adj. p-value	Ratio	Direction	p-value
AMPD1	NM_000036	3.85	↓	1.62E-04	14.07	↓↓	4.37E-04
IL2RA	NM_000417	4.58	↑	9.01E-07	3.45	↑	1.11E-02
TXLNG2P	NM_001005852	9.71	↑	2.60E-02	97.35	↑↑	4.18E-02
RPS4Y1	NM_001008	56.76	↑↑	1.68E-02	121.79	↑↑	1.38E-01
RPS4Y2	NM_001039567	42.65	↑↑	1.84E-02	16.05	↑↑	3.13E-02
SCGB2A1	NM_002407	4.34	↓	6.32E-07	6.4	↓	3.18E-03
ZFY	NM_003411	5.45	↑	1.84E-02	1.02	↓	6.56E-01
INSL5	NM_005478	28.45	↓↓	2.15E-04	14.17	↓↓	2.20E-01
NTS	NM_006183	2.05	↓	2.66E-03	16.92	↓↓	5.63E-04
IGF2BP1	NM_006546	14.18	↑↑	1.29E-07	7.55	↑	1.03E-01
TNFRSF12A	NM_016639	2.94	↑	2.11E-03	2.88	↑	9.65E-02
KCTD4	NM_198404	4.1	↓	2.46E-05	1.4	↓	2.20E-01

and quality of the fluorescently labeled cRNA was assessed using a NanoDrop ND-1000 spectrophotometer and an Agilent Bioanalyzer. According to manufacturer's specifications, 1.6 μg of Cy3-labeled cRNA was hybridized to the Agilent Human Whole Genome Oligo Microarray (Agilent Technologies, Inc., Palo Alto, CA) for 17 hrs, prior to washing and scanning. Data were extracted from scanned images using Agilent's Feature Extraction Software (Agilent Technologies, Inc., Palo Alto, CA).

Quantitative Real-time PCR (qPCR). Quantitative real-time PCR was used to validate representative transcripts that showed differential expression, by microarray, from terminal ileum and colonic tissue in ASD^{GI} tissues compared to control tissues. For these assays, six paired RNAs (one TI and one colonic RNA sample) from ASD^{GI} cases and six paired RNAs from the control individuals were used as representative samples for PCR. Twelve differentially-expressed transcripts were chosen from the 178 DETs listed in Table **S3** for validation. Of these twelve transcripts, six (IL2RA, TXLNG2P, RPS4Y1, RPS4Y2, ZFY, and IGF2BP1) were up-regulated in both the TI and colon, five (AMPD1, SCGB2A1, INSL5, NTS, and KCTD4) were down-regulated in both tissues and one transcript (TNFRSF12A) was up-regulated in colonic tissue and down-regulated in the terminal ileum.

The qPCR analyses were performed using the RT^2 SYBR Green ROX qPCR Mastermix (Qiagen) with cDNA samples generated from 0.5 ug total RNA using RT^2 First Strand Kit (Qiagen) following the manufacturer's instructions. Custom-made 96 well plates (SABiosciences) contained primers for each of the 12 transcripts of interest, two reference genes (ACTB and GAPDH) and two positive controls, aligned in two adjacent columns on the plate. Each 96 well plate was used to assay six individual cDNAs. Following the qPCR run on a StepOnePlus Real-time PCR system (Applied Biosystems), using the custom plate manufacuturer's recommendations, the raw data from each 96 well plate (4 total) were uploaded to the SABiosciences web-based analysis software to determine differential expression parameters (fold change and p value). The software automatically performs all $\Delta\Delta C_t$ based fold-change calculations from the uploaded raw quantification cycle data. The results from these assays, compared to the corresponding microarray results, can be found in Table 6.

Data Analysis

Pair-wise analysis to determine differentially-expressed transcripts. Gene expression data were uploaded into the GeneSifter® Analysis Edition (Geospiza, Inc, Seattle, WA) software suite. For all pair-wise comparisons the data were first normalized by global normalization using the median intensity and transformed (log base 2) prior to running the non-parametric Wilcoxon Rank-Sum Test, with Benjamini-Hochberg FDR correction, to generate lists of differentially-expressed transcripts (DETs). The fold-change threshold was set at 2.0 and the data were considered significant if the comparison had an associated log ratio adjusted p-value less than 0.05. The list of differentially-expressed transcripts from a given pair-wise comparison was then imported into Ingenuity Pathway Analysis software for determination of biologically relevant functional categories and canonical pathway involvement. This analysis was performed for each of the eight individual pair-wise comparisons.

Principal component analysis. In order to determine the overall similarity between samples, ratio data were subjected to Principal Components Analysis (PCA) and two-way agglomerative cluster analysis using Ward's minimum variance as heuristic criteria and Pearson correlation as the distance metric for *experiments*, and average linkage as heuristic and Pearson correlation distance as the distance metric for *genes* to determine the overall similarity between samples and within groups (Rosetta Resolver version 7.2.2.0). No filtering was applied to the profile level data prior to PCA.

Hierarchial clustering analysis. The non-parametric Kruskal-Wallis test, with Benjamini and Hochberg FDR correction, was performed on all 102 microarray datasets (@ fold change ≥ 2; adjusted $p \leq 0.001$) representing the eight experimental groups (four conditions; two tissues).

Supporting Information

Table S1 Demographic and medical history data for ASD^{GI} cases.

Table S2 Demographic and medical history data for non-ASD controls.

Table S3 Gene list for 178 transcripts that were differentially-regulated in both terminal ileum and colon, exclusively in ASD^{GI} samples.

Table S4 Gene list for 41 transcripts that were differentially-regulated in a comparison of ASD^{GI} samples with LNH + ileitis.

Acknowledgments

First and foremost we acknowledge and thank the families who agreed to participate in this study. Without their support these studies would not have been possible.

Author Contributions

Conceived and designed the experiments: AK SJW. Performed the experiments: SJW. Analyzed the data: AK LGG SJW. Wrote the paper: AK SJW. Provided clinical samples: AK JF. Created Figures and Tables: AK LGG SJW. Supervised research: AK SJW.

References

1. Valicenti-McDermott M, McVicar K, Rapin I, Wershil BK, Cohen H, et al. (2006) Frequency of gastrointestinal symptoms in children with autistic spectrum disorders and association with family history of autoimmune disease. J Dev Behav Pediatr 27(2 Suppl): S128–136.
2. Ming X, Brimacombe M, Chaaban J, Zimmerman-Bier B, Wagner GC (2008) Autism spectrum disorders: concurrent clinical disorders. J Child Neurol 23: 6–13.
3. Buie T, Campbell DB, Fuchs GJ 3rd, Furuta GT, Levy J, et al. (2010) Evaluation, diagnosis, and treatment of gastrointestinal disorders in individuals with ASDs: a consensus report. Pediatrics 125 Suppl 1: S1–18.
4. Bauman ML (2010) Medical comorbidities in autism: challenges to diagnosis and treatment. Neurotherapeutics 7(3): 320–327.
5. Horvath K, Perman JA (2002) Autistic disorder and gastrointestinal disease. Current Opinion in Ped 14: 583–587.
6. Levy SE (2007) Relationship of dietary intake to gastrointestinal symptoms in children with autistic spectrum disorders. Biol Psychiatry 61: 492–497.
7. Jarocka-Cyrta E, Wasilewska J, Kaczmarski MG (2011) Eosinophilic esophagitis as a cause of feeding problems in an autistic boy. J Autism Dev Disord 41(3): 372–374.
8. Black C, Kaye JA, Jick H (2002) Relation of shildhood gastrointestinal disorders to autism: nested case-control study using data from UK General Practice Research Database. BMJ 325(24): 419–421.

9. Horvath K, Papadimitriou JC, Rabsztyn A, Drachenberg C, Tildon JT (1999) Gastrointestinal abnormalities in children with autistic disorder. J Pediatr 135: 559–563.
10. Ashwood P, Anthony A, Torrente F, Wakefield AJ (2004) Spontaneous mucosal lymphocyte cytokine profiles in children with autism and gastrointestinal symptoms: mucosal immune activation and reduced counter regulatory interleukin-10. J Clin Immunol 24: 664–673.
11. Gonzalez L, López C, Navarro D, Negron L, Flores L, et al. (2005) Endoscopic and histological characteristics of the digestive mucosa in autistic children with gastro-intestinal symptoms. Arch Venez Pueric Pediat 69: 19–25.
12. Krigsman A, Boris M, Goldblatt A, Stott C (2010) Clinical presentation and histologic findings at ileocolonoscopy in children with autistic spectrum disorder and chronic gastrointestinal symptoms. Autism Insights 1: 1–11.
13. Torrente F, Anthony A, Herushkel RB, Thompson MA, Ashwood P, et al. (2004) Focal-enhanced gastritis in regressive autism with features distinct from Crohn's and helicobacter pylori gastritis. Am J Gastroenterol 4: 598–605.
14. Torrente F, Ashwood P, Day R, Machado N, Furlano RI, et al. (2002) Small intestinal enteropathy with epithelial IgG and complement deposition in children with regressive autism. Mol Psychiatry 7: 375–382.
15. Balzola F, Barbon V, Repici A, Rizzetto M, Clauser D, et al. (2005) Panenteric IBD-like disease in a patient with regressive autism shown for the first time by wireless capsule enteroscopy: another piece in the jig-saw of the gut-brain syndrome? Am J Gastroenterol 100: 979–981.
16. Furlano RI, Anthony A, Day R, Brown A, McGarvey L, et al. (2001) Colonic CD8 and gamma delta T-cell infiltration with epithelial damage in children with autism. J Pediatr 138: 366-372. D'Eufemia P, Celli M, Finnochiaro R, Pacifico L, Viozzi L, et al. (1996) Abnormal intestinal permeability in children with autism. J Pediatr 38: 366–372.
17. D'Eufemia P, Celli M, Finnochiaro R, Pacifico L, Viozzi L, et al. (1996) Abnormal intestinal permeability in children with autism. Acta Paediatr 85: 1076–1079.
18. De Magistris L, Familiari V, Pascotto A, Sapone A, Frolli A, et al. (2010) Alterations of the intestinal barrier in patients with autism spectrum disorders and in their first-degree relatives. J Pediatr Gastroenterol Nutr 51: 418–424.
19. Finegold SM, Molitoris D, Song Y, Liu C, Vaisanen ML, et al. (2002) Gastrointestinal microflora studies in late-onset autism. Clin Infect Dis (Suppl 1): S6–S16.
20. Williams BL, Hornig M, Buie T, Bauman ML, Cho Paik M, et al. (2011) Impaired carbohydrate digestion and transport and mucosal dysbiosis in the intestines of children with autism and gastrointestinal disturbances. PLoS One 6(9): e24585. Epub 2011 Sep 16.
21. Jyonouchi H, Sun S, Le H (2001) Proinflammatory and regulatory cytokine production associated with innate and adaptive immune responses in children with autism spectrum disorders and developmental regression. J Neuroimmunol 120(1–2): 170–179.
22. Jyonouchi H, Geng L, Ruby A, Zimmerman-Bier B (2005) Dysregulated innate immune responses in young children with autism spectrum disorders: their relationship to gastrointestinal symptoms and dietary intervention. Neuropsychobiology 51(2): 77–85.
23. Vargas DL, Nascimbene C, Krishnan C, Zimmerman AW, Pardo CA (2005) Neuroglial activation and neuroinflammation in the brain of patients with autism. Ann Neurol 57(1): 67–81. Erratum in: Ann Neurol. 2005;57(2): 304.
24. Wu F, Dassopoulos T, Cope L, Maitra A, Brant SR (2007) Genome-wide gene expression differences in Crohn's disease and ulcerative colitis from endoscopic pinch biopsies: insights into distinctive pathogenesis. Inflamm Bowel Dis 13(7): 807–821.
25. Galamb O, Sipos F, Dinya E, Spisak S, Tulassay Z, et al. (2006) mRNA expression, functional profiling and multivariate classification of colon biopsy specimen by cDNA overall glass microarray. http://www.ncbi.nlm.nih.gov/pubmed?term = mRNA%20expression%2C%20functional%20profiling%20and%20multivariate%20classification%20of%20colon%20biopsy%20specimen%20by%20cDNA%20overall%20glass%20microarray World J Gastroenterol 12(43): 6998–7006.
26. Costello CM, Mah N, Hasler R, Rosentiel P, Waetzig GH, et al. (2005) Dissection of the inflammatory bowel disease transcriptome using genome-wide cDNA microarrays. PLoS Med 2(8): e199.
27. Lawrance IC, Fiocchi C, Chakravarti S (2001) Ulcerative colitis and Crohn's disease: distinctive gene expression profiles and novel susceptibility candidate genes. Hum Mol Genet 10(5): 445–456.
28. von Stein P, Lofberg R, Kuznetsov NV, Gielen AW, Persson JO, et al. (2008) Multigene analysis can discriminate between ulcerative colitis, Crohn's disease, and irritable bowel syndrome. Gastroenterology 134(7): 1869–1881.
29. Galiatsatos P, Gologan A, Lamoureux E (2009) Autistic enterocolitis: fact or fiction. Can J Gastroenterol 23: 95–98.
30. Wright N (2010) Does autistic enterocolitis exist? BMJ 340: c1807.
31. Ashwood P, Wakefield AJ (2006) Immune activation of peripheral blood and mucosal CD3+ lymphocyte cytokine profiles in children with autism and gastrointestinal symptoms. J Neuroimmunol 173: 126–134.
32. Chomcynski P, Sacchi N (1987) Single-step method of RNA isolation by acid guanidinium thiocyanate-phenol-chloroform extraction. Anal Biochem 162(1): 156–159.

13

Genome-Wide Maps of Circulating miRNA Biomarkers for Ulcerative Colitis

Radha Duttagupta[1], Sharon DiRienzo[3], Rong Jiang[1], Jessica Bowers[2], Jeremy Gollub[1], Jessica Kao[1], Keith Kearney[4], David Rudolph[4], Noor B. Dawany[5], Michael K. Showe[5], Tom Stamato[3], Robert C. Getts[2], Keith W. Jones[1]*

1 Applied Reasearch Group, Affymetrix Inc, Santa Clara, California, United States of America, **2** Research and Development, Genisphere LLC, Hatfield, Pennsylvania, United States of America, **3** Lankenau Institute for Medical Research, Wynnewood, Pennsylvania, United States of America, **4** Division of Gastroenterology, Lankenau Medical Center, Wynnewood, Pennsylvania, United States of America, **5** The Wistar Institute, Philadelphia, Pennsylvania, United States of America

Abstract

Inflammatory Bowel Disease – comprised of Crohn's Disease and Ulcerative Colitis (UC) - is a complex, multi-factorial inflammatory disorder of the gastrointestinal tract. In this study we have explored the utility of naturally occurring circulating miRNAs as potential blood-based biomarkers for non invasive prediction of UC incidences. Whole genome maps of circulating miRNAs in micro-vesicles, Peripheral Blood Mononuclear Cells and platelets have been constructed from a cohort of 20 UC patients and 20 normal individuals. Through Significance Analysis of Microarrays, a signature of 31 differentially expressed platelet-derived miRNAs has been identified and biomarker performance estimated through a non-probabilistic binary linear classification using Support Vector Machines. Through this approach, classifier measurements reveal a predictive score of 92.8% accuracy, 96.2% specificity and 89.5% sensitivity in distinguishing UC patients from normal individuals. Additionally, the platelet-derived biomarker signature can be validated at 88% accuracy through qPCR assays, and a majority of the miRNAs in this panel can be demonstrated to sub-stratify into 4 highly correlated intensity based clusters. Analysis of predicted targets of these biomarkers reveal an enrichment of pathways associated with cytoskeleton assembly, transport, membrane permeability and regulation of transcription factors engaged in a variety of regulatory cascades that are consistent with a cell-mediated immune response model of intestinal inflammation. Interestingly, comparison of the miRNA biomarker panel and genetic loci implicated in IBD through genome-wide association studies identifies a physical linkage between hsa-miR-941 and a UC susceptibility loci located on Chr 20. Taken together, analysis of these expression maps outlines a promising catalog of novel platelet-derived miRNA biomarkers of clinical utility and provides insight into the potential biological function of these candidates in disease pathogenesis.

Editor: Philippe Rouet, I2MC INSERM UMR U1048, France

Funding: Support for this work was provided by Sharpe-Strumia Research Foundation of Bryn Mawr Hospital. The funder had no role in study design, data collection and analysis, decision to publish, or preparation of the manuscript. No additional external funding received for this study.

Competing Interests: The authors RD, RJ, JG, JK and KWJ are employees of Affymetrix. Inc. RCG and JB are employees of Genisphere, LLC. TS, SD, KK and DR are employees of LIMR. ND and MKS are employees of The Wistar Institute.

* E-mail: Keith_Jones@affymetrix.com

Introduction

Inflammatory Bowel Disease (IBD) represents - a chronic relapsing disorder of the gastrointestinal (GI) tract affecting over 6.6 million individuals in the US and Europe [1]. A significant risk factor for colorectal cancer, IBD is stratifiable into two disorders: Crohn's Disease (CD) and Ulcerative Colitis (UC) [2]. Both these subtypes are characterized by inflammation of the digestive tract, with CD involving widespread inflammation of all layers of the GI tract while UC is characterized by localized inflammation of the colon. Current modalities for the diagnosis of both the subtypes involve a combination of invasive endoscopic procedures and diverse clinical indices that provide only relative measures of disease severity and outcome. In the absence of well-established diagnostic gold standards for IBD, there is a collective interest in the identification of novel clinical biomarkers that are cost-effective, afford rapid turnover and provide needed insight into disease complexity and biology [3,4].

The accessibility of nucleic acids in circulation and their emerging value in correlating disease burden to clinical outcomes provides an important paradigm for disease surveillance and therapeutic management [5]. Described first in 1948 in human blood [6], extra-cellular nucleic acids exist abundantly as both DNA and RNA species. Despite enigmatic biological functions, global characterization of their distributions, size and genomic origins have established them as discriminating indicators of a range of tumor associated genomic, epigenetic and transcriptional change [5,7]. Within the various classes of cell-free circulating nucleic acids, a significant fraction of the genomic content is composed of miRNAs [8]. Representing a highly stable and conserved class of ~22 nt long endogenous non-coding transcripts, miRNAs represent approximately 1–2% known genes in eukaryotes [9] and function to negatively regulate gene expression through base-pairing to target mRNAs [10]. Currently over 1000 mature miRNAs are annotated in the human genome [11,12] with the potential to post-transcriptionally regulate about 30% of all protein coding genes [13]. This interleaved regulatory organization encompasses a vast array of cellular and developmental cascades with an increasing number of miRNAs being correlated to deregulation of these processes [14]. The oncogenic and tumor suppressive functions of miRNAs are now well-established with mechanisms ranging from copy number changes, epigenetic silencing and modification of transcriptional control of miRNA loci [15]. Specific examples encompass cancers of both hematopoietic and non-hematopoietic origin – thus making this species a promising and tractable candidate for diagnostic screening [7,8]. Biologically, circulating miRNAs survive the extracellular catalytic environment through sequestration within sub-cellular particles such as micro-vesicles and exosomes [7]. Current models for their functionality involve trafficking through circulation to facilitate long–range communication between different inter-cellular sites.

A key component of the biology of inflammatory bowel disease (IBD) involves a deregulated immune response against intra-luminal bacterial antigens leading to intestinal tissue injury. In recent years, a collection of expression profiling studies have provided compelling evidence for the role of miRNAs in modulating crucial steps of the immune response [16]. Specific examples include varied roles of miR-16, miR-17~92 and the miR-146 family in modulating different aspects of innate and adaptive immunity. Additionally, evidence from auto-immune disorders such as rheumatoid arthritis, psoriasis and systemic lupus erythematosus further endorse the diversity of miRNA functions in various immune cascades [16]. Although the specific role of miRNAs in intestinal diseases are poorly understood, loss of intestinal miRNAs in mouse models are known to result in impaired epithelial barrier function resulting in acute inflammation [17]. Taken together, this evidence suggests that the fundamental physiological role of miRNAs in inflammatory disorders, such as IBD, is to maintain normal intestinal homeostasis.

Given that the pathology of IBD involves a complex interplay of immune and non-immune cells, it is of interest to understand the impact of different classes of blood-derived miRNAs as indicators of disease physiology [18]. Importantly, platelets, representing an abundant class of circulating non-immune cells classically engaged in blood hemostasis are now increasingly recognized as critical drivers of cell-mediated enteric immune response that lead to the infiltration of inflammatory cells into the intestinal lumen [18,19,20]. As a first step towards understanding the contribution of circulating miRNAs of specific lineages in IBD, we have explored through microarray analysis, miRNA expression levels in micro-vesicle, PBMC and platelet fractions from a cohort of 20 normal and 20 affected individuals diagnosed with Ulcerative Colitis. Using a Significance Analysis of Microarrays approach [21,22] we can identify profiles of differentially expressed miRNAs in each fraction. Furthermore, through a non-probabilistic binary linear classification using Support Vector Machines (SVM) [23], we can segment the dataset to delineate a 31 marker platelet-derived miRNA signature that has 92.8% accuracy, 96.2% specificity and 89.5% sensitivity in stratifying UC patients from normal individuals. This panel can be validated successfully through qPCR assays. Additionally, correlation analysis of intensity levels across the patient-control strata reveal subgroups of tightly clustered miRNAs – suggestive of potential functional relationships through coordinate regulation of miRNA expression. Taken together, this data suggests that platelet-derived biomarkers are compelling clinical predictors of disease outcome; consistent with the emerging role of platelets as critical players in the pathology of UC. Examination of biological pathways targeted by these miRNAs reveal enrichment of genes involved in modulation of cellular architecture and regulatory cascades implicated in cell-mediated immune response. These global expression maps thus provide a necessary and critical resource for biomarker development and begin to provide needed perspective into the extensive regulatory networks influencing the clinical expression of this disease.

Results

Biomarker Derivation from circulating miRNA profiles in different hematological fractions

Given that miRNAs have been shown to reliably classify disease from normal population and are important mediators in the IBD mediated inflammatory response, we chose to investigate the changes in blood-derived miRNA spectrum in a cohort of Ulcerative Colitis patients. Blood samples from 20 patients and 20 normal individuals, characterized in Table 1 were collected with informed consent. The case versus control cohorts did not significantly differ by ethnicity, age, gender or familial cancer incidences. A statistically significant disposition to Gastrointestinal (GI) disorders (i.e., Gastritis, IBD, Crohn's Disease, Colitis) was found in the patient cohort (8 versus 0 individuals, $P = 0.0016$ by one-sided Fisher's Exact Test) while the control patients demonstrated a greater incidence of non-GI disorders such as diabetes, coronary diseases, thyroid disorders, hypertension (6 versus 0 individuals, $P = 0.01$ by one-sided Fisher's Exact Test) (Table 1). To enable identification of inflammation-mediated changes the samples were specifically sub-fractionated into PBMC (Peripheral Blood Mononuclear Cells) and platelets. The purity of the isolated fractions were verified by quantitative PCR amplification of either the leukocytic mRNA CD45 or platelet specific gene product Glycoprotein IIB [24] and show a statistically significant and clear separation of the two fractions (data not shown). Additionally, micro-vesicular sub-fractions were isolated to identify markers that were detected free in circulation. Total mRNA from all three sub-fractions (PBMC, micro-vesicles and platelets) were extracted and independently profiled on the Affymetrix miRNA arrays containing 847 human miRNAs. For derivation of miRNA biomarkers that were differentially expressed (DE) each individual hematopoietic fraction was initially analyzed independently. For each analysis, the datasets were split 90:10 with 18 individuals randomly

Table 1. Demographics of individuals recruited for this study.

		Control	Patient
Total		20	20
Ethnicity	Caucasian	15/20 (75%)	13/20 (65%)
	Others	5/20 (25%)	4/20 (20%)
	Unknown	none	3/20 (15%)
Gender	F	13/20 (65%)	14/20 (70%)
	M	7/20 (35%)	6/20 (30%)
Age (yrs)		42.7±12.9	49.5±11.9
Average age at diagnosis (yrs)		N/A	35.5±11.9
Family Medical History	Cancer	3/20 (15%)	4/20 (20%)
	others (non GI)	6/20 (30%)	none
	others (GI)	none	8/20 (40%)
Medical History	Cancer	2/20 (10%)	none
	Ulcerative Colitis	none	20/20 (100%)
	CD	none	none

Gender is designated as either M (Male) or F (Female). Disorders are designated as GI (Gastro-intestinal) or CD (Crohn's Disease).

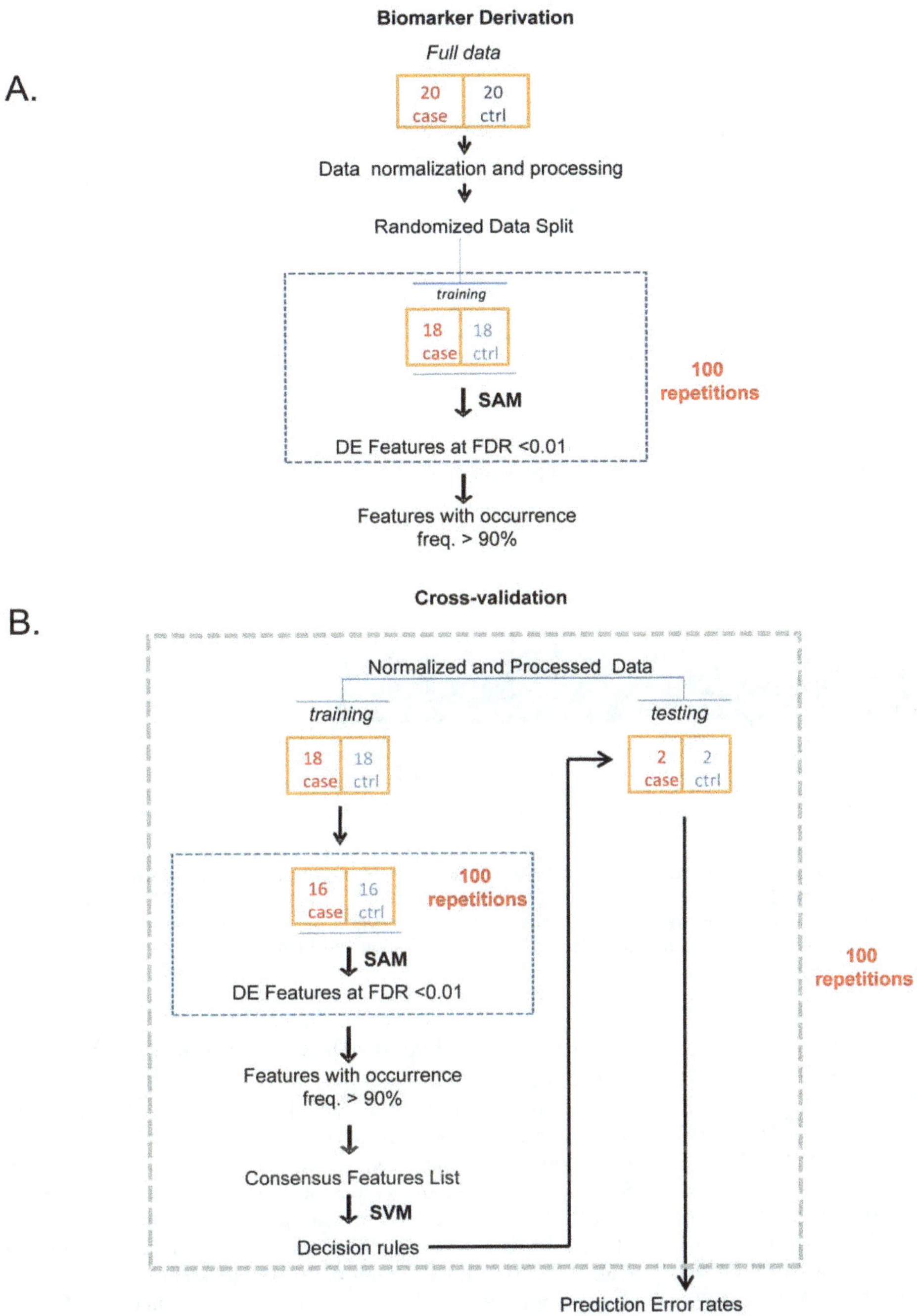

Figure 1. Workflow for biomarker derivation and computation of predictive estimates. (A) Differentially expressed miRNAs were first derived by SAM and those exhibiting a FDR of <1% and frequency of occurrence >90% in 100 iterations, were selected as biomarkers. (B) The decision rules were obtained by SVM classification and the predictive estimates of the selected biomarkers determined by 10-fold cross-validation.

selected from each arm of the study and control cohorts (Fig. 1A). Quantile normalized and processed data from all three fractions (Fig S1) were analyzed using Significance Analysis of Microarrays (SAM) and Differentially Expressed (DE) features selected at a False Discovery Rate (FDR) threshold of 1% (Fig. 1A and Fig S2). A total of 6, 11 and 52 miRNAs were identified as differentially expressed from a single iteration of SAM across the PBMC, micro-vesicular and platelet fractions, respectively (Table S1). We find that the majority of these signatures to be dominated by profiles of up-regulated miRNAs, with 92% and 100% of miRNAs demonstrating increased expression in the platelet and micro-vesicular fractions, respectively. Interestingly, we find all miRNAs derived from the PBMC isolates to display down-regulated expression suggesting distinct biology of each of these isolated miRNA populations. In order to select miRNAs useful for stratifying patients from controls, the derivation procedure was repeated 100 times with random re-sampling of the data to minimize the dependency on a single dataset. Finally, the occurrence of the DE features obtained from this iterative process was counted and features demonstrating a frequency no less than 90% selected as potential biomarkers (Fig. 1A and Fig. 2A). A signature of 31 platelet-derived, 6 microvesicle-derived and 0 PBMC miRNAs

A. B.

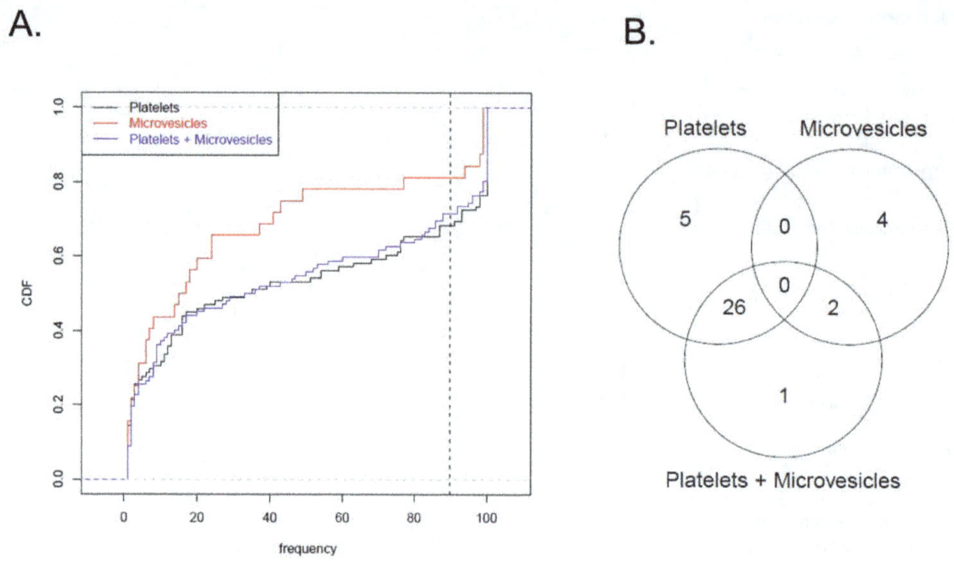

C.

Fraction	Frequency threshold (%)	Accuracy	Specificity	Sensitivity
Platelets	90%	92.8	96.2	89.5
Microvesicles	90%	62.5	84.8	40.3
Platelets + Microvesicles	90%	92.3	96.8	87.8

Figure 2. Characteristics and performance measures of biomarkers derived from Platelets, Micro-vesicles or Platelet/Micro-vesicle combined fraction. (A) Cumulative distribution frequency (CDF) plots of biomarkers derived from the different fractions. The dotted line represents the 90% cut-off frequency across the study population (B) Counts and overlaps of miRNA biomarkers derived from the platelet, micro-vesicular and combined fraction (C) Performance measures of biomarkers from each fraction selected at the 90% frequency threshold.

were obtained through this process (Fig. 2B and Tables S2 and S3). In order to determine if a combination of the fractions led to a more discriminative signature the entire derivation process was re-run using a union of platelet and micro-vesicle fractions. PBMC were excluded since there were no differentially expressed miRNAs within that fraction alone. We isolated a list of 29 biomarkers from this concatenated group and mapped the overlap between the different lists (Fig. 2B and Fig S2D). We find that 89.6% (26/29) miRNAs obtained from the combined fraction (derived from platelet and micro-vesicle) overlap with biomarkers derived from the platelet fraction only (Fig. 2B, Tables S2 and S4). A subset of only 6 miRNAs are found to be unique between these two datasets with hsa-miR-423-3p exclusive to the platelet-micro-vesicle combined fraction and hsa-let-7i-star, hsa-miR-1271, hsa-miR-1296, hsa-miR-31 and hsa-miR-345 identified from the platelet derived fraction only. Additionally, we can also co-identify 33% (2/6) miRNAs (hsa-miR-202 and hsa-miR-1263) between the independent micro-vesicle and the micro-vesicle/platelet combined fractions. The remaining set of 4 miRNAs representing 66% (4/6) of the dataset and comprised of hsa-miR-628-5p, hsa-miR-603, hsa-miR-221-star and has-miR-455-3p are unique only to the group of micro-vesicular miRNAs derived from independent analysis of this fraction (Fig. 2B, Tables S3 and S4). Taken together, this data characterizes two major signatures of differentially expressed miRNA biomarkers of hematopoetic origins in Ulcerative Colitis – those that are principally derived from the platelet fraction and a minority subset of micro-vesicular ancestry.

Development and validation of recurrent miRNA predictors

To estimate the predictive capability of these signatures, each of the biomarker categories were subjected to non-probabilistic binary linear classification using Support Vector Machines (SVM) (Fig. 1B). Measurement of classifier success was assessed through a 10-fold cross-validation method. A cohort of randomly selected 18 case-control subjects were chosen as the training set while 2 individuals each from the two enrollment categories were reserved for testing. The training set was further stratified to randomly sub-select 16 case-control individuals that were subject to the same feature selection process using SAM, originally used in biomarker derivation (Fig. 1B). The prediction error rates were then estimated based on application of the SVM classifier to the test set (Fig. 2C and Fig S3). Through an iterative cycle of 100 repetitions the performance measures (confusion matrix of true positives, true negatives, false positives and false negatives) were computed and recorded for the three principal classes (platelets, micro-vesicle and their union). The aggregated summary statistics for these 3 fractions demonstrate that the best classifier performance is obtained from the 31 miRNAs derived from the platelet fractions that can classify patient from control individuals with 92.8% accuracy, 96.2% specificity and 89.5% sensitivity (Fig. 2C). The platelet and micro-vesicle derived class comprising of 29 miRNA biomarkers similarly significantly predicted disease outcome with 92.3% accuracy, 96.8% specificity and 87.8% sensitivity (Fig. 2C). The performance measures of micro-vesicle biomarkers in contrast had the least predictive powers (62.5% accuracy, 84.8% specificity and 40.3% sensitivity) (Fig. 2C). None of these performance estimates were significantly correlated to independent biometric variables such as age, gender, height or weight though regression analysis (data not shown). Misclassification estimates of the training data by the final classifier reveal that only 4 diseased individuals in the micro-vesicle derived category (p14, p15, p18, p21) were anomalously categorized as normal. In contrast these estimates were much more conservative in the platelet-derived or platelet-micro-vesicle combined classes with respectively only 1 (p3) and 0 individuals, being inaccurately classified, respectively (Fig S4). These categorization and performance measures thus indicate that the principal statistical power in classification of disease versus normal individuals is driven by the platelet-derived miRNA biomarker class. This category of biomarkers therefore represents the most discriminating candidates with the best diagnostic potential.

Independent validation of levels of specific circulating miRNA biomarkers

We next sought to gain an improved understanding of the biological levels and validity of the platelet-derived biomarker panel derived from classifier analysis. The differentially expressed profiles of the 31 platelet-derived miRNAs (Fig. 3 and Fig S5A) demonstrating the highest predictive performance was analyzed through unsupervised hierarchical clustering. The expression map of the 31 candidate miRNAs displayed a clear separation of the patient versus control groups (Fig. 3) with 3 patients (p3, p19 and p21) being misclassified by the clustering algorithm. The relatively higher proportion of misclassified individuals obtained through this analysis compared to classifier estimates obtained by SVM (3 vs 1 individual) indicate that unsupervised hierarchical clustering does not separate the samples as well as the SVM algorithm. The majority of miRNAs in this panel displayed an average $\log_2$ signal intensity magnitude of >6 with only 23% (7/31) target miRNAs demonstrating lower abundance processed $\log_2$ signal intensity <6 (Fig S5A). Similarly, the major proportion of biomarkers derived from the platelet and micro-vesicular combined fraction (72% or 21/29 miRNAs) display comparable $\log_2$ intensity distributions of 6 or greater. Both the micro-vesicle specific miRNAs in this biomarker panel are low abundant with an average $\log_2$ signal intensity of 4.8 for hsa-miR-202 and $\log_2 <= 6$ for hsa-miR-1263 (Fig S5B). These differences are visualized through unsupervised hierarchical clustering of the data which also identify misclassification of the same 3 individuals (p3, p19 and p21) as was observed in the group of platelet-derived miRNAs (Fig S6). In order to

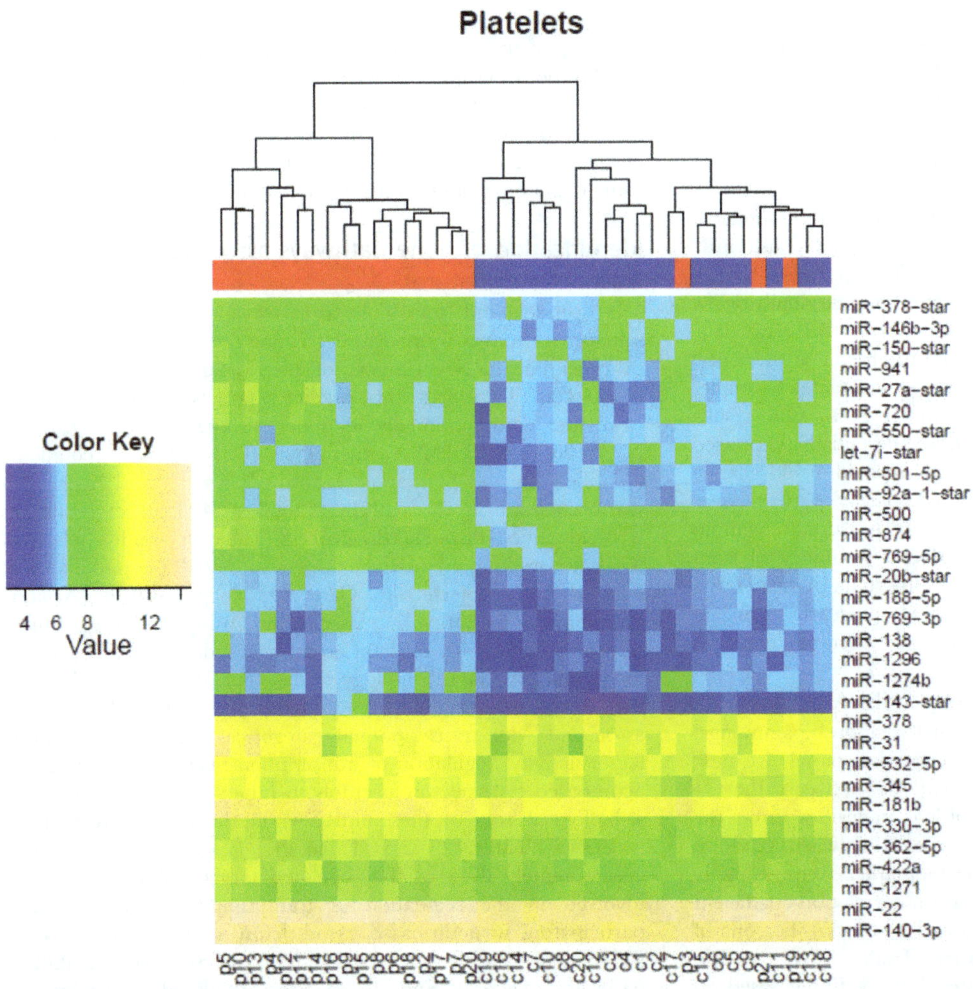

Figure 3. Comparison of expression levels of the platelet-derived miRNA biomarkers in the patient and control cohorts. Unsupervised hierarchical clustering of samples (controls in blue: C1–C20 and patients in red: P2–P21) based on summarized intensity values from the 31 differentially expressed miRNA biomarkers. The $\log_2$ intensity values are shown in the Color Key bar scale.

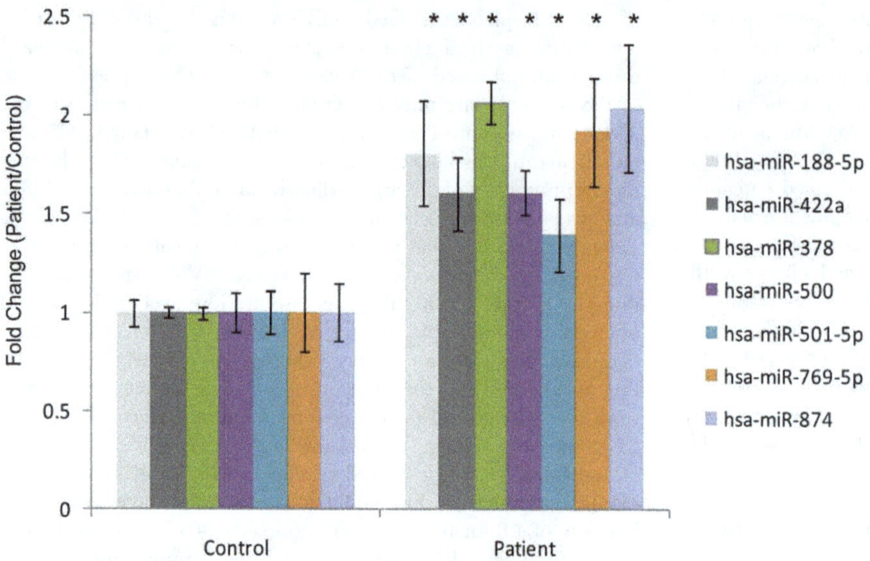

Figure 4. Validation of expression levels of miRNA biomarkers derived from the platelet fraction. miRNA expression levels of 7 biomarkers (n = 4, *P values<0.001) were validated by qPCR. The p values are calculated based on a Student's t-test of the replicate 2^ (−ΔCt) values for each miRNA in the control group (normal individuals) and test groups (patients).

independently validate specific candidate biomarkers, we selected sub categories of miRNAs from the platelet-derived biomarker panel for verification by quanititative PCR (qPCR) assays. First, 24 of the 31 marker panel were identified based on 100% representation in the cross-validation iterations. These were divided into 4 quartiles based on p-values, mean intensity and fold changes. A union of all of these categories were taken and eight representative candidate biomarkers (hsa-miR-188-5p, hsa-miR-22, hsa-miR-422a, hsa-miR-378, hsa-miR-500, hsa-miR-501-5p, hsa-miR-769-5p, hsa-miR-874), with distributions ranging from marginally below the mean to the maximum intensity measurable on the array ($\log_2$ intensity values ranging from 7.6 to 13.6 for this frequency measure) were randomly chosen for validation in pooled platelet samples derived from patient and control cohorts (Fig. 4). Our results demonstrate that 88% (7/8) of all the differentially expressed candidates validated successfully and demonstrated a fold change difference ranging from 1.4–2.04 on comparing patients over controls (Fig. 4). These estimates match the array estimates with no significant difference between the two platforms (p-value of 0.6 from paired Student's t-test). Taken together this data indicates the capability of the selected biomarker panel to clearly delineate patient and control samples with a high degree of confidence.

Segregation of biomarker panel into miRNA clusters

In order to examine possible functional relationships amongst the miRNA members of the platelet biomarker panel, we next analyzed correlation of expression patterns between the 31 selected species through comparison of $\log_2$ intensities across the patient and control strata. Our results revealed a clear separation of 90% of the data or 28/31 of the biomarkers into 4 highly correlated clusters with an average Pearson correlation coefficient of 0.75 and p-value<3.95E-05 (Fig. 5 and Table S5). For one of the largest clusters (Cluster 1) (Fig. 5 and Table S5) we can also additionally identify miRNA candidates that co-cluster based on genomic location (i.e. hsa-miR-500 and has-miR-501-5p that reside closely on Chr. X and hsa-miR-27a-star and hsa-miR-150-star originating from Chr. 19). Co-localization is observed for two additional candidate miRNAs in Cluster 3 that are processed products of the same pre-miRNA: hsa-mir-769-5p and hsa-mir-769-3p; both localized on Chr. 19. Positional concordance is not observed for any of the remaining markers (Table S5). This analysis therefore identifies subsets of miRNAs that demonstrate correlated expression across the samples, with additional chromosome-dependent physical association seen for some selected pairs.

Identification of gene pathways associated with miRNA biomarker signatures

To understand the biological relevance of the diagnostic signatures we next wanted to determine the spectra and response of potential mRNAs targets of the identified platelet-derived biomarkers. To address this, predicted targets of the 31 miRNAs were first computationally identified through Target Scan 5.0 [13,25,26] and DIANA microT v3.0. No targets could be identified for the biomarker hsa-miR-92a-star– and hence this was excluded from the analysis. A total of 5493 conserved targets were identified through this process (Table S6) and a subset of 3304 non-redundant mRNA targets of 30/31 biomarkers were selected and subjected to Gene Ontology (GO) or Ariadne Ontology and pathway classification using Pathway Studio software. Biologically relevant groups were identified by analyzing for significant shared ontology terms. Our analysis revealed that the biomarker targets were significantly enriched in genes associated with transcriptional categories such as transcription factor activity, regulation of transcription nucleotide binding and actin-based cytoskeleton assembly (p-value$<1.33\times10^{-8}$) implying a biological role of these miRNAs in the regulation of these processes (Table 2 and Table S7). Significantly, we find approximately 27% of the regulated targets (526 genes) to be involved in the regulation of transcription, 32% (65 genes) participating in actin-based cytoskeleton assembly and between 9–14% (15–54) of genes engaged in diverse lipid metabolism pathways (Table 2 and Table S7). Additionally, through the analysis of annotated signaling pathways we also find enrichment of signaling pathways that participate in both cytoskeleton regulation and immune-mediated inflammatory response. Specifically we observe between 24–58% overlap of miRNA targets with

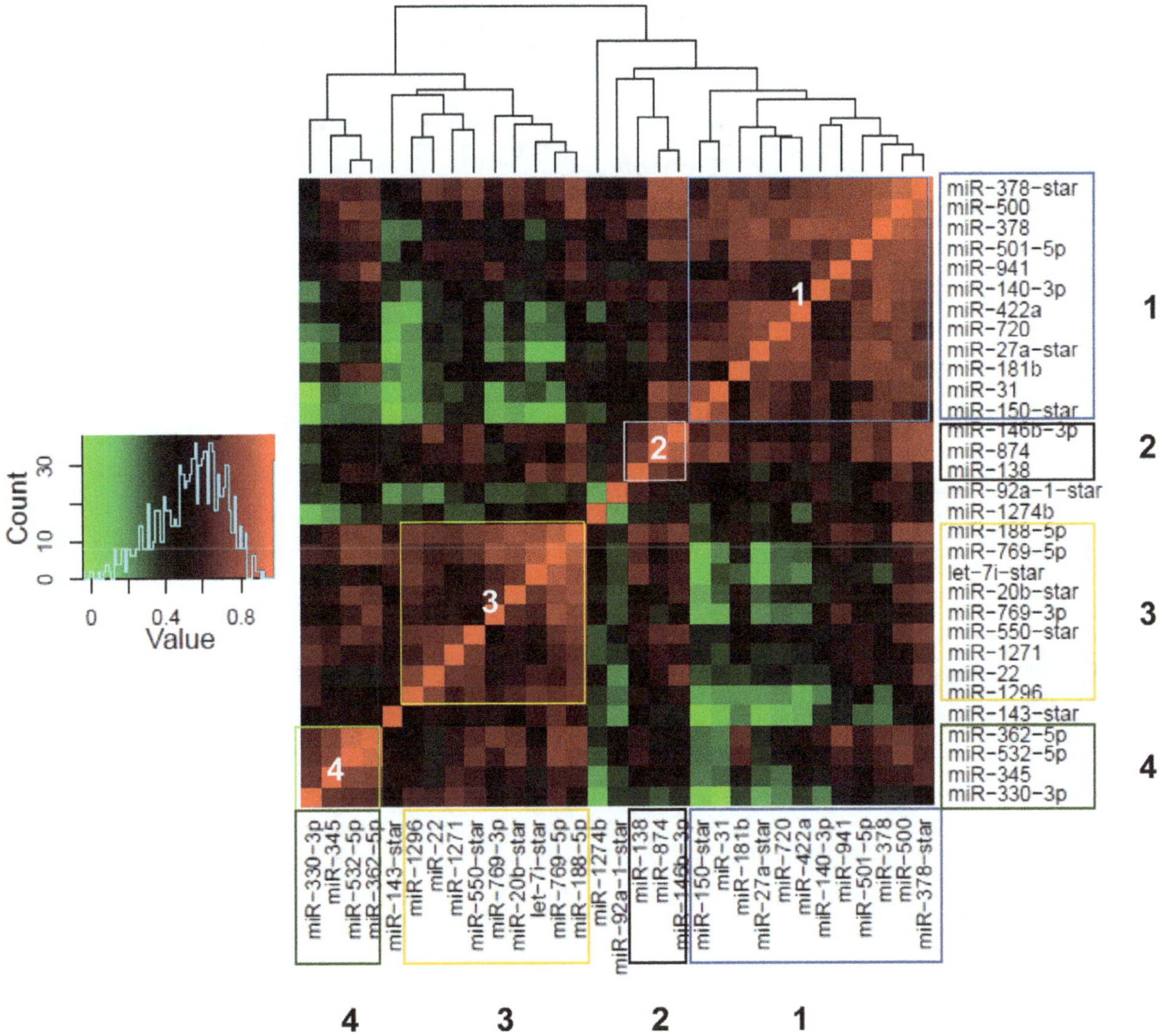

Figure 5. Sub-clusters of platelet-derived miRNA biomarkers. Unsupervised hierarchical clustering of miRNA biomarkers based on the Pearson correlation coefficients among the miRNA expression profiles from 20 patients and 20 controls. The coefficient values are shown in the bar scale. Each of the 4 main clusters with significant correlation values are indicated in boxes.

signalling cascades such as TNF-α or T-cell activation pathways known to be involved in triggering the innate immune response (Table 2 and Table S7). Taken together this data indicates that genic targets of diagnostic miRNA biomarkers of Ulcerative Colitis are selectively enriched in candidate genes that engage in aspects of the pro-inflammatory response observed in the pathophysiology of this disease.

Discussion

Diagnostic assessment and therapeutic management of IBD spectrum disorders currently derives from a combination of clinical examination, laboratory indices and invasive procedures [27]. Given the emerging association of circulating miRNA species with a spectrum of physiological and disease conditions [7] we have systematically explored the utility of secretory miRNAs isolated from different hematological fractions as non-invasive predictors of Ulcerative Colitis.

To address this question, we have investigated broadly across distinct whole blood fractions comprising both cellular (platelets, PBMC) and acellular compartments (exosomal/micro-vesicular) that are known to express and shuttle miRNA cargo through circulation. A set of distinct, differentially expressed maps of annotated miRNAs have been constructed from a cohort of 20 diseased versus 20 normal individuals through hybridization to miRNA arrays. Fraction-specific differentially expressed miRNA signatures have been interrogated through SAM [21] at a 1% FDR [22] that identify primarily up-regulated miRNA candidates in the full dataset with only a minority of miRNAs displaying down-regulation of expression. Through molecular classifiers derived from a Support Vector Machine model and a multiple random sub-sampling strategy, our results (Fig. 2C) have isolated a distinct diagnostic signature of 31 miRNAs with increased expression that derive specifically from the platelet fraction and can stratify UC patients from normal individuals with 92.8% accuracy, 96.2% specificity and 89.5% sensitivity. Given the low number of differentially expressed miRNAs from the PBMC and micro-vesicular fractions, no predictive miRNA species could be identified from the PBMC isolates and only a poorly performing minority 6-marker panel derived from independent analysis of the

Table 2. Gene ontology (GO) classification and pathway analysis of predicted mRNA targets of the 31 platelet-derived biomarkers.

Annotation	Term	Genome annotation	Overlap#	% Overlap	p-value
Actin-based cytoskeleton assembly	Ariadne Ontology	202	65	32	2.74E-10
Transcription factors		955	203	21	1.33E-08
Vesicular secretory pathway		93	33	35	5.69E-07
TGFBR		16	9	56	0.000143
Regulation of transcription	Biological Process	1937	526	27	2.41E-125
Transcription		2282	517	22	5.18E-90
Nucleotide binding	Molecular Function	2265	462	20	1.50E-43
Transcription factor activity		1215	297	24	1.53E-42
DNA binding		2430	476	19	4.89E-40
Kinase activity		783	207	26	1.09E-34
Transferase activity		1547	325	21	1.40E-32
Actin binding		375	86	22	2.18E-11
Actin Cytoskeleton Regulation	Signaling Pathways	548	176	32	3.10E-16
NTRK→AP-1/CREB/ELK-SRF/MYC/SMAD3/TP53		95	45	47	7.75E-11
Gonadotrope Cell Activation		722	197	27	2.24E-10
FGFR→AP-1/CREB/CREBBP/ELK-SRF/MYC		98	44	44	1.09E-09
EGFR→AP-1/CREB/ELK-SRF/MYC		93	42	45	2.11E-09
ThrombopoietinR→AP-1/CREB/ELK-SRF/MYC		85	39	45	4.57E-09
ThrombinR→AP-1/CREB/ELK-SRF/SP1		110	46	41	7.58E-09
VEGFR→AP-1/CREB/MYC		87	39	44	1.03E-08
FibronectinR→AP-1/ELK-SRF/SREBF		104	44	42	1.05E-08
EphrinR→actin		216	74	34	1.12E-08
PDGFR→AP-1/MYC		77	35	45	3.83E-08
EGFR/ERBB3→MEF/MYOD/NFATC/MYOG		130	50	38	4.63E-08
Focal Adhesion Regulation		322	98	30	5.07E-08
EGFR→AP-1/ATF2		82	36	43	7.40E-08
TNFRSF1A→AP-1/ATF/TP53		36	21	58	1.01E-07
T Cell Activation		951	233	24	1.78E-07
EGFR/ERBB2→TP53		81	35	43	1.82E-07
IGF1R→MEF/MYOD/MYOG		62	29	46	2.65E-07
VasopressinR2→MEF/MYOD/NFATC/MYOG		123	46	37	4.20E-07
ErythropoietinR→AP-1/CREB/MYC		80	34	42	4.39E-07
VasopressinR2→CREB/ELK-SRF/AP-1/EGR		128	47	36	5.88E-07
Glycerophospholipids and ether lipids metabolism	Metabolic Pathways	372	54	14	2.65E-09
Sphingolipid metabolism		206	25	12	0.001593
Metabolism of triacylglycerols		103	15	14	0.002504
Glycosylphosphatidylinositol-anchor biosynthesis		136	18	13	0.002855
Pterine biosynthesis		227	22	9	0.038294

Overlap# refers to the number of gene annotations intersecting with genome annotations. The top ranking GO terms, % overlaps and the counts of overlapping entities ranked by the most significant p-values are listed.

micro-vesicular fraction. Additionally, no added benefit is obtained from combination of the platelet and micro-vesicular strata which generate a 29 marker panel consisting 27 platelet-derived and 2 micro-vesicular markers with comparative predictive performance in distinguishing case from control (92.3% accuracy, 96.8% specificity and 87.8% sensitivity). Given the significant overlap observed between the platelet-derived and platelet+micro-vesicle-derived profiles (Fig. 2B) and the poor performance metrics of the non-platelet miRNAs we conclude that the origin of the majority of disease-specific predictors in UC map back to the anucleate platelet fraction. Additionally, since classifier analysis did not identify any down- regulated miRNA biomarkers, this data also suggests that the primary physiological response in Ulcerative Colitis is to enhance expression of miRNA subsets. The divergence of platelet vs. micro-vesicular signatures is interesting and indicates distinct sub-cellular addresses for these miRNA species. Taken together, this supports the hypotheses that the isolated micro-vesicle fraction mapped in this study either do not originate from platelet progenitors or very selectively sort platelet derived miRNA cargo into classes destined for trafficking through the hematopoietic circuit. Given the significant overlaps observed in previous studies between platelet and micro-vesicular signatures [28], this disparity may be indicative of disease specific characteristics of Ulcerative Colitis. The validity of the identified platelet-derived class can be additionally verified with 88% success through qPCR assays run on pooled patient and control samples (Fig. 4) – thus providing independent confirmation of the differential regulation of this panel. Furthermore, these markers segregate into 4 highly correlated intensity clusters, often containing specific pairs of miRNAs that share proximity of sub-chromosomal location (Table S5). Cumulatively these results suggest distinct sets of biomarkers that may be coordinately regulated or share functional regulatory sub-networks closely synchronized under the given physiological conditions.

The biology of IBD spectrum disorder is known to encompass a complex interplay of innate and adaptive immunity that ultimately regulates a regional intestinal inflammation response [29]. Circulating blood platelets representing non-immune cells and engaged classically in the hemostatic function of surveying vessel integrity are emergent mediators of active inflammation modulating local intestinal tissue injury [19,20]. Enriched in a small but diverse transcriptome [30], platelets contain a large proportion of mature miRNA that can potentially engage in the regulation of gene expression. In order to understand the diversity of our identified miRNA biomarker panel, we have assessed the overlap between our maps and miRNA profiles from normal or disease-specific signatures surveyed across different studies. These analyses identify between 6% (2/31) to 29% (9/31) overlap between the 31-platelet-derived biomarker panel with miRNAs derived from platelet populations of normal individuals [24,28,31] and no overlap with UC specific miRNAs profiled from peripheral blood [32]. Additionally comparison to miRNA maps of non-platelet origin involved in a broad spectrum of inflammatory disorders [16] reveal only two overlapping miRNAs: hsa-miR-140 and hsa-miR-146b with the majority of the 31 marker panel thus being exclusive to our study. Taken together, these comparative analyses clearly delineate that members of the platelet-derived 31 biomarkers are (a) enriched in miRNA species that are typically not detected in the normal platelet transcriptome, (b) are highly compartment specific and detectable only on enrichment of the platelet fraction and (c) display specificity of expression restricted to Ulcerative Colitis compared to other inflammatory disorders.

Given that miRNAs are known to be collective regulators of approximately 30% of human genes [13] understanding of the mechanism of gene regulation mediated through the 31-miRNA biomarker panel is of importance. The prevalence of biological functional processes was evaluated through analysis of GO terms on 3304 non-redundant predicted mRNA targets representing approximately 13% of the estimated number of protein coding genes in the human genome [33]. Stratification of the top canonical groups and pathways reveal enrichment of genes engaged in actin-cytoskeleton assembly, vesicular secretary pathway, biosynthesis and metabolism of diverse lipids such as glycerol phospholipds, pterin and tri-acylglycerol, implicated in a variety of cell-regulatory and immune stimulation roles (Table 2). Specific examples include (a) regulation of the members of the Rho-ROCK pathway involved in cytoskeletal reorganization/cell adhesion response to wound healing ([34] and references therein), (b) involvement of sphingolipids as modulators of growth factor receptors and second messengers of known agonists of the inflammatory response such as tumor necrosis factor-α, interleukin-1β [35], (c) regulation of Pterin metabolism- in response to IFN-γ stimulation [36], (d) genes involved in ionic transport and regulation of calcium homeostasis that may influence membrane permeability and (e) modulators of classic inflammatory regulators such as TNF-α. The predicted mRNA target spectrum is also dominated by transcription factors/mediators such as PI3K, KLF5, etc. that we hypothesize play a role in modulation of key genes involved in the regulation of the other diverse functions of metabolism, biosynthesis, transport, etc. [37]. Additionally, we also find that a subset of the biomarkers (i.e., hsa-miR-1271, hsa-miR-874, hsa-let-7i-star and hsa-miR-20b-star) can target ATGs16L, a gene necessary for autophagy and implicated in IBD susceptibility [38,39]. Therefore, comparison of these targets to published studies [34,37,40,41] reveal a high degree of concordance in functional groups but often limited overlaps in terms of specific gene targets – suggesting that the landscape of physiologically relevant mRNAs in IBD is far from being saturated. Therefore, this study complements our current understanding of the UC transcriptome and provides interesting insight into the expression divergence of this disorder.

In principal, the platelet derived miRNAs could contribute to the pathophysiology of UC through regulation of the platelet transcriptome, consequently influencing downstream interaction with the intestinal mucosa. Adhesion of platelets to the mucosal endothelium is known to occur though a CD40/CD40L contact-dependent process resulting in platelet activation [19,20] and a chemokine mediated immune response. The ultimate outcome of this trigger is the recruitment of leucocytes to the endothelium which results in a focal inflammatory response. These mechanisms are consistent with the functional classes of mRNA target genes identified in this study and implicated in the modulation of cellular architecture and inflammation. Taken together, these results support a hypothesis which offers a direct role for miRNAs in influencing platelet activation and cell-cell mediated immune response in gut inflammation.

Given that micro-vesicles are known mediators of cell-cell communication [42] it is intriguing to speculate if the miRNA content of platelets can potentially be transferred to endothelial cells through vesicular fusion. In this model, the epithelial transcriptome would be directly targeted by the identified platelet miRNA regulators. Analysis of differentially expressed miRNA profiles from colonic epithelial tissues from UC patients can isolate 34% (30 out of 89) significantly down-regulated mRNAs [37] corresponding to representative targets of 57% (17 out of 30) miRNAs from our biomarker panel. Comparison of fold change densities of these anti-correlated target mRNAs against all down-regulated transcripts on the array, reveal a statistically significant difference (p-value of 0.011 by Binomial test and 0.007 by Fisher Exact Test) between the two groups (Fig S7). This suggests that the platelet miRNAs could possibly be a significant factor in the down-regulation of endothelial gene expression in the context of IBD.

Given the prevalence and increasing disease-specific role of miRNAs, it is of interest to catalogue the association of these sequences with naturally occurring polymorphisms in polygenic disorders [43]. Mechanistically, single nucleotide changes can have significant functional impact through either impeding miRNA biogenesis, or through inhibition of binding to target miRNA sequences. Examples of such functional polymorphisms are numerous [44] (http://www.patrocles.org/Patrocles_miRNAs.htm) and has been demonstrated to impact a variety of disease states [45,46,47,48]. We can map polymorphisms in the mature miRNA sequence of 35% of the miRNAs (11 of 31) in our biomarker signature and 20% (673 out of 3304) of their computationally predicted mRNA targets (http://compbio.uthsc.edu/miRSNP/). It is intriguing to speculate whether the patient who is misclassified by the platelet-derived miRNA signature is impacted by this type of variation. A link between polymorphisms and miRNAs were also explored by examining possible associations of the 31-biomarker prognostic panel with IBD susceptibility loci identified through genome-wide association studies. We can identify a close physical link (220 Kb) between hsa-miR-941 and rs2297441, a SNP mapping to the 20q telomere that is associated with high confidence to UC [49]. As more evidence demonstrating the significance of polymorphisms affecting miRNA synthesis, binding, stability or functional activity accumulates, it will become important to investigate these changes in the context of disease associations and diagnostic accuracy of miRNA biomarkers.

The abundance and stability of miRNAs in circulation holds the promise of easy and rapidly accessible biomarkers. Given the prognostic and diagnostic utility of this class in cancer and the inherently vast regulatory potential of miRNA molecules, we have assessed the ability of fraction-specific miRNAs in delineating incidences of Ulcerative Colitis. To our knowledge the current results outline for the first time platelet-specific miRNA signatures for an inflammatory disorder, with exceedingly high predictive measures. The potential of these biomarkers to influence gene expression in context of modulating intestinal homeostasis is explored and the spectrum of putative physiological targets evaluated for their regulatory potential. In summary, results obtained from this study support a model where expression and coordinate control of various polygenic components of UC pathogenesis may be mediated by the interplay of circulating miRNA species and their physiological targets. As universally applicable tests are developed a combinatorial use of these indicators would perhaps provide the most rational strategy for disease determination and clinical therapy.

Materials and Methods

Ethics statement

The study cohort consisted of 20 anonymized patients recruited from the office of Main Line Gastroenterology. Additionally, 20 normal samples were obtained from the volunteer staff of the Lankanau Institute of Medical Research and Lankenau Hospital. Written informed consent was obtained from all patients prior to obtaining samples and medical history. The Main Line Hospital's Institutional Review Board approved of this study.

Fractionation of whole blood into Micro-vesicle, PBMC and Platelet fractions and isolation of RNA

Whole blood (7 to 9 ml) was collected from patient and control individuals in BECTON-DICKINSON 16×100 mm 10.0 mL BD Vacutainer® plastic EDTA blood collection Tubes (Becton & Dickinson, Franklin Lakes, NJ). To protect against RNA degradation samples were treated with Baker's yeast RNA (Sigma R6750) within 5 minutes of draw to give a final concentration of 1.25 mg/ml and then diluted with equal volume of PBS. Samples were separated into the different hematopoietic fractions by density gradient centrifugation. Briefly, the diluted blood samples were layered over Ficoll-Paque™ plus (GE Healthcare) at a 3:4 ratio by volume and centrifuged at 400 g for 30 to 40 minutes at 25°C. This process resulted in a fractionation of the sample into plasma (upper layer), PBMCs and platelets (narrow central band), and a band of erythrocytes and granulocytes at the bottom of the tube. The upper plasma layer was removed, centrifuged at 100,000 g for 1 hr at 4°C using a Beckman Ti50 rotor and the pellet isolated to generate the **micro-vesicular fraction**. This fraction consists of microparticles, exosomes, and other cellular debris. To fractionate the PBMC from Platelets, the Ficoll-Paque layer containing these cellular populations was removed, and 3 volumes of 1 × PBS added to the layer and the mixture centrifuged at 65 g for 15 min at room temperature. The supernatant fraction was saved and the pellet re-suspended in 10 ml PBS and re-centrifuged under the same conditions. The resulting pellet was isolated to represent the high density **PBMC population**. The supernatant fractions from the first and second washes were pooled and centrifuged at 450 g for 20 min at room temperature to isolate the pellet representing the **platelet fraction**. All three pellet fractions were mixed with 1 ml of Trizol-LS reagent and total RNA extracted according to the Trizol procedure.

Labeling and hybridization of platelet, micro-vesicle and PBMC samples to the Affymetrix miRNA Arrays

Total RNA ranging in concentration from 1 ug–3 ug was labeled using the Genisphere HSR labeling kit (P/N HSR30FTA) and hybridized overnight to the Affymetrix Genechip miRNA array (P/N 901326). The arrays were washed and stained using standard Affymetrix protocols and scanned using the Affymetrix GCS 3000 7G Scanner. Feature intensities were extracted using the miRNA_1-0_2xgain library files.

Quantitative RT-PCR

Assays to quantify differential expression of miRNAs in patients vs. healthy controls were performed using the ABI 7300 real-time PCR instrument and miScript quantitative PCR System (Qiagen). Pooled Patient (P2–P21) and Control (C1–C18 and C20) samples were used in duplicate Reverse Transcription (RT) reactions. Approximately 10 ng of cDNA was used in duplicate PCR assays for each RT. The normalizers used for this analysis were: Hs_RNU6B_3, Hs_miR-320b_2, Hs_miR-543_1and Hs_miR-654-3p_2. For analysis of the purity of the platelet fraction, patient and control pools from each of the plasma-derived classes of platelets and PBMCs were similarly tested using 66.6 ng of total RNA and QuantiFast™ SYBR® Green RT-PCR system (Qiagen). The platelet specific gene ITGA2B (Glycoprotein IIB) and the leukocyte specific CD45-common antigen marker PTPRC were used as target mRNAs and 18S (RRN18S) and Actin (ACTB) used as normalizers. All oligonucleotide sets were purchased from Qiagen.

Datasets

The datasets described in this manuscript are MIAME compliant and have been deposited in NCBI's Gene Expression Omnibus Database (http://www.ncbi.nlm.nih.gov/geo/).

The data series is accessible through GEO Series accession number GSE32273:http://www.ncbi.nlm.nih.gov/geo/query/acc.cgi?acc = GSE32273.

Analysis of the miRNA data

Data Preprocessing: Data preprocessing was performed via Affymetrix miRNA QC Tool, which consisted of extraction of raw intensities for each individual feature followed by background subtraction based on GC content of anti-genomic probes, transformation of values through addition of a small constant (value 16), quantile normalization and finally median summarization of all probe sets for each feature. The intensity data used in all analysis are $\log_2$ transformed. Triplicates available for one case (p7) and one control (c9) for each of the fractions under study were analyzed by utilizing the mean intensity values.

Software Packages: All statistical analysis was performed under the R programming language environment (www.r-project.org). The R "samr" package was used for Significance Analysis for Microarray (SAM) and the R "e1071" package was used for Support Vector Machine (SVM) with the non-linear radial basis function as the kernel. The unsupervised Hierarchical clustering algorithm was implemented in the R "hclust" function and generated using Euclidean distance matrix and complete-linkage agglomeration. All heat maps were generated using the R "gplots" package.

miRNA Biomarker Selection: Biomarker selection was based on 100 iterative cycles of SAM run on re-sampling of the full 20 patient and 20 control sample set through a randomized 9:1 data split (i.e., a 'training set' of 18 cases and 18 control individuals per iteration). Each individual fraction (platelet, micro-vesicle or PBMCs), or the combination of all three fractions were separately analyzed. Differentially expressed (DE) miRNA features were identified at a False Discovery Rate of 1% and features occurring at a frequency greater than 90% (consensus features) selected as potential biomarkers.

Cross-Validation to Estimate Prediction Error Rates: Support Vector Machines (SVM) was used for classifying the IBD cases from controls. To assess the prediction error rates a 10-fold cross-validation procedure was applied (Fig. 1). Briefly, the full data set of 20 cases/controls was randomly sampled to generate a training set of 18 cases/controls and a testing set of 2 cases/controls. The training set was further split into a random subset of 16 cases/controls and the biomarker derivation process run iteratively through SAM to select the consensus features followed by SVM classification. The decision function obtained by SVM classification was applied to the testing set and the confusion matrix (e.g., counts of false positives and false negatives) recorded. The entire procedure was repeated 100 times and the prediction error rates estimated from the aggregated confusion matrix.

Inter-feature correlation analysis among the 31 Biomarkers: The correlation structure among the 31 platelet-derived biomarkers was examined by calculating the Pearson's correlation coefficients among the 31 miRNAs based on their normalized expression profiles across all cases and control individuals. Clusters were defined as subgroups exhibiting minimal correlation coefficients >0.6 and were identified by visualizing the heat map plotted by unsupervised hierarchical clustering.

Prediction of miRNA targets and enrichment analysis: For prediction of mRNA targets, the 31 platelet derived biomarkers were first separated into two categories based on the star designation. Targets were determined using either DIANA-microT 3.0 algorithm for the star miRNA sequences (http://diana.cslab.ece.ntua.gr/) or TargetScan Human v5.0 (http://www.targetscan.org/cgi-bin/targetscan/data_download.cgi?db=vert_50) for the non-star miRNA sequences. Targets were selected based on conservation of families/sites from Target Scan and a precision score greater than 0.4 from DIANA. A total of 5493 mRNA targets were identified out of which 3304 unique mRNAs were selected after removing redundancies and subjected to pathway exploration using Pathway Studio software from Ariadne Genomics (http://www.ariadnegenomics.com/). Using this software and its accompanying Gene Ontology and Interaction databases, incidence of predicted miRNA targets were matched against the target collection and the top-ranking pathways and Gene Ontology groups selected. The statistical enrichment for each of these pathways/groups was computed by the similarity score or p-value calculated as a ratio of a number of common objects between two pathways to the total number of objects in them.

Correlation Analysis of miRNA and mRNA Expressions: To identify expression changes in putative target tissue mRNAs, genome-wide mRNA expression data from colonic pinch biopsies of Ulcerative Colitis patients were analyzed [37]. The pre-processed raw intensities for 12,258 probes (excluding the control probes from the array) were extracted from patient-control cohorts (4 normal individuals and 5 affected Ulcerative Colitis patients). Differentially expressed mRNAs were identified by SAM at an FDR <0.1% and genes exhibiting a fold change >2 selected for further analysis. The numbers of differentially expressed genes were counted for both the whole array and the miRNA targets and enrichment of down-regulated target mRNAs assessed by either the Binomial test or the Fisher's Exact test. The null hypothesis for this analysis tests that the proportion of down-regulated miRNA target genes is equivalent to the fraction of down-regulated genes predicted not to be miRNA targets. The alternative hypothesis tests that the proportion of down-regulated miRNA target genes is larger than the non-target miRNA genes.

Supporting Information

Figure S1 Box plot of $\log_2$ signal intensity distribution of human miRNAs (white) and background probes (red) for 20 patients and 20 controls for each fraction (A) Platelets (B) Micro-vesicles (C) PBMC after background subtraction, quantile normalization and median summarization. The black bar represents the median of each distribution and the dashed lines represent the box–plot range set by the whiskers.

Figure S2 Analysis of differentially expressed miRNA biomarkers from (A) Platelets (B) PBMC (C) Micro-vesicular and (D) Combined Platelet and Micro-vesicle fractions. Comparison of observed vs. the expected scores obtained by performing Significance analysis of microarrays on all 847 miRNAs from 20 patients and 20 controls. Each miRNA is represented by a point (open circle), and the differentially expressed miRNAs represented as red (for up-regulated) or green (for down-regulated) points in the graph. The dashed line represents a FDR threshold of 1%.

Figure S3 Performance estimates for the different fractions isolated in this study at a frequency cutoff of 90%. The Combined fraction denoted by asterisk is representative of the union of all the 3 different fractions of PBMC, micro-vesicles and platelets. The different error rate calculations are given by FPR (False Positive Rate), FNR (False Negative Rate), PPV (Positive Prediction Value) and NPV (Negative Prediction Value).

Figure S4 Table of predicted and observed values from each analyzed fraction based on Confusion Matrix derived from SVM on the full data comprising 20 cases and 20 controls.

Figure S5 miRNA expression levels in patient and control cohorts. (A) Box plot of processed $\log_2$ intensity distributions of 31 miRNA biomarkers from Platelet fraction or (B) 29 miRNAs from the Platelet/Micro-vesicle combined fraction. The black bar represents the median of each distribution and the dashed lines the box-plot ranges. The open circles represent the outliers. The patient samples are denoted by red (cases) and normal samples by blue (controls). The platelet-derived miRNAs are denoted with the prefix 'pl' and the micro-vesicular miRNAs are designated as 'mv'.

Figure S6 Comparison of expression levels of miRNAs biomarkers in the patient and control cohorts derived

from the combination of platelet and microvescicle fractions. Unsupervised hierarchical clustering of samples (controls in blue: C1–C20 and patients in red: P2–P21) based on processed $\log_2$ intensity values from 29 biomarkers. The $\log_2$ intensity values are shown in the Color Key bar scale. The platelet-derived miRNAs are denoted with the prefix 'pl' and the micro-vesicular miRNAs are designated as 'mv'.

Figure S7 Correlation of platelet-derived miRNA and mRNA targets. Relationship between the fold change densities of miRNA targets and all transcripts measured from expression profiling of endothelial pinch biopsies from UC vs normal individuals. The p-values denote significant differences in the population of down-regulated genes between miRNA targets and all transcripts by either Bionomial test (*) or by Fisher's Exact Test (**).

Table S1 Lists of differentially expressed miRNAs identified by SAM from the entire dataset of platelets, PBMC and micro-vesicular fractions at an FDR of 1%. The "Score" represents the modified t-test statistics calculated by SAM. The "Fold Change" denotes the ratios of the mean intensity in patient samples over control samples. The q-value represents an *estimate* of FDR. This number is typically greater than 0. In our dataset due to the limiting sample size (20 cases and 20 controls) we observe for some features the test statistic to be more extreme than all observed in permutations. Therefore the *estimated* FDR for declaring that feature to be significant is set to 0.

Table S2 List of 31 biomarkers derived from the platelet fraction.

Table S3 List of 6 biomarkers derived from the micro-vesicle fractions.

Table S4 List of 29 biomarkers derived from a combination of platelets and micro-vesicular fraction.

Table S5 List of 4 principle miRNA clusters derived from the platelet biomarker panel showing correlated expression profiles and genomic coordinates of the miRNAs.

Table S6 List of predicted mRNA targets of the 31 biomarkers identified by TargetScan and DIANA.

Table S7 List of enriched GO and Pathway analysis terms and mRNA targets in each significant category. The percentage of overlap and the overlapping entities of the top groups/pathways ranked by the most significant p-values are shown.

Acknowledgments

We thank Barrett Eynon and John Burrill of Affymetrix for thoughtful discussions during various parts of the project.

Author Contributions

Conceived and designed the experiments: RD TS RCG KWJ. Performed the experiments: RD JB SD. Analyzed the data: RD RJ. Contributed reagents/materials/analysis tools: RCG JG TS KK DR. Wrote the paper: RD KWJ. Analysis review: ND MKS. Technical guidance: JK. Intellectual guidance: RCG KWJ.

References

1. Loftus EV, Jr. (2004) Clinical epidemiology of inflammatory bowel disease: Incidence, prevalence, and environmental influences. Gastroenterology 126: 1504–1517.
2. Nikolaus S, Schreiber S (2007) Diagnostics of Inflammatory Bowel Disease. Gastroenterology 133: 1670–1689.
3. Beniwal P, Harrell L (2010) The status of diagnostic markers for inflammatory bowel disease. Current Gastroenterology Reports 12: 479–484.
4. Roda G, Caponi A, Benevento M, Nanni P, Mezzanotte L, et al. (2010) New proteomic approaches for biomarker discovery in inflammatory bowel disease. Inflammatory Bowel Diseases 16: 1239–1246.
5. Fleischhacker M, Schmidt B (2007) Circulating nucleic acids (CNAs) and cancer-A survey. Biochimica et Biophysica Acta - Reviews on Cancer 1775: 181–232.
6. Mandel P, Metais P (1948) Les acides nucleiques du plasma sanguin chez l'homme. CR Acad SciParis 142: 241–243.
7. Kosaka N, Iguchi H, Ochiya T (2010) Circulating microRNA in body fluid: A new potential biomarker for cancer diagnosis and prognosis. Cancer Science 101: 2087–2092.
8. Reid G, Kirschner MB, van Zandwijk N (2010) Circulating microRNAs: Association with disease and potential use as biomarkers. Critical Reviews in Oncology/Hematology.
9. John B, Enright AJ, Aravin A, Tuschl T, Sander C, et al. (2004) Human MicroRNA targets. PLoS Biol 2: e363.
10. Bartel DP (2004) MicroRNAs: Genomics, Biogenesis, Mechanism, and Function. Cell 116: 281–297.
11. Griffiths-Jones S (2004) The microRNA Registry. Nucleic Acids Res 32: D109–111.
12. Griffiths-Jones S (2010) miRBase: microRNA sequences and annotation. Current protocols in bioinformatics/editoral board, Andreas D Baxevanis [et al] Chapter 12: Unit 12.19.11–10.
13. Lewis BP, Burge CB, Bartel DP (2005) Conserved seed pairing, often flanked by adenosines, indicates that thousands of human genes are microRNA targets. Cell 120: 15–20.
14. Bartel DP (2009) MicroRNAs: Target Recognition and Regulatory Functions. Cell 136: 215–233.
15. Garzon R, Calin GA, Croce CM (2009) MicroRNAs in Cancer. Annu Rev Med 60: 167–179.
16. Pekow JR, Kwon JH (2011) MicroRNAs in inflammatory bowel disease. Inflammatory Bowel Diseases.
17. McKenna LB, Schug J, Vourekas A, McKenna JB, Bramswig NC, et al. (2010) MicroRNAs control intestinal epithelial differentiation, architecture, and barrier function. Gastroenterology 139: 1654–1664, 1664 e1651.
18. Danese S (2011) Immune and nonimmune components orchestrate the pathogenesis of inflammatory bowel disease. American Journal of Physiology - Gastrointestinal and Liver Physiology 300: G716–G722.
19. Danese S, De La Motte C, Fiocchi C (2004) Platelets in inflammatory bowel disease: Clinical, pathogenic, and therapeutic implications. American Journal of Gastroenterology 99: 938–945.
20. Danese S, Scaldaferri F, Papa A, Pola R, Sans M, et al. (2004) Platelets: new players in the mucosal scenario of inflammatory bowel disease. Eur Rev Med Pharmacol Sci 8: 193–198.
21. Tusher VG, Tibshirani R, Chu G (2001) Significance analysis of microarrays applied to the ionizing radiation response. Proc Natl Acad Sci U S A 98: 5116–5121.
22. Benjamini YYD (2001) The control of the false discovery rate in multiple testing under dependency. Annals of Statistics 29: 1165–1188.
23. Cortes CVV (1995) Support-Vector Networks. Machine Learning 20: 273–297.
24. Landry P, Plante I, Ouellet DL, Perron MP, Rousseau G, et al. (2009) Existence of a microRNA pathway in anucleate platelets. Nature Structural and Molecular Biology.
25. Friedman RC, Farh KK, Burge CB, Bartel DP (2009) Most mammalian mRNAs are conserved targets of microRNAs. Genome Res 19: 92–105.
26. Grimson A, Farh KK, Johnston WK, Garrett-Engele P, Lim LP, et al. (2007) MicroRNA targeting specificity in mammals: determinants beyond seed pairing. Mol Cell 27: 91–105.
27. Vermeire S, Van Assche G, Rutgeerts P (2006) Laboratory markers in IBD: Useful, magic, or unnecessary toys? Gut 55: 426–431.
28. Hunter MP, Ismail N, Zhang X, Aguda BD, Lee EJ, et al. (2008) Detection of microRNA expression in human peripheral blood microvesicles. PLoS One 3: e3694.
29. Bamias G, Cominelli F (2007) Immunopathogenesis of inflammatory bowel disease: Current concepts. Current Opinion in Gastroenterology 23: 365–369.
30. Gnatenko DV, Dunn JJ, McCorkle SR, Weissmann D, Perrotta PL, et al. (2003) Transcript profiling of human platelets using microarray and serial analysis of gene expression. Blood 101: 2285–2293.

31. Nagalla S, Shaw C, Kong X, Kondkar AA, Edelstein LC, et al. (2011) Platelet microRNA-mRNA coexpression profiles correlate with platelet reactivity. Blood 117: 5189–5197.
32. Wu F, Guo NJ, Tian H, Marohn M, Gearhart S, et al. (2011) Peripheral blood MicroRNAs distinguish active ulcerative colitis and Crohn's disease. Inflammatory Bowel Diseases 17: 241–250.
33. Clamp M, Fry B, Kamal M, Xie X, Cuff J, et al. (2007) Distinguishing protein-coding and noncoding genes in the human genome. Proc Natl Acad Sci U S A 104: 19428–19433.
34. Costello CM, Mah N, Häsler R, Rosenstiel P, Waetzig GH, et al. (2005) Dissection of the inflammatory bowel disease transcriptome using genome-wide cDNA microarrays. PLoS Medicine 2: 0771–0787.
35. Merrill AH, Jr., Schmelz EM, Wang E, Dillehay DL, Rice LG, et al. (1997) Importance of sphingolipids and inhibitors of sphingolipid metabolism as components of animal diets. J Nutr 127: 830S–833S.
36. Schoedon G, Troppmair J, Adolf G, Huber C, Niederwieser A (1986) Interferon-gamma enhances biosynthesis of pterins in peripheral blood mononuclear cells by induction of GTP-cyclohydrolase I activity. J Interferon Res 6: 697–703.
37. Wu F, Dassopoulos T, Cope L, Maitra A, Brant SR, et al. (2007) Genome-wide gene expression differences in Crohn's disease and ulcerative colitis from endoscopic pinch biopsies: Insights into distinctive pathogenesis. Inflammatory Bowel Diseases 13: 807–821.
38. Saitoh T, Fujita N, Jang MH, Uematsu S, Yang BG, et al. (2008) Loss of the autophagy protein Atg16L1 enhances endotoxin-induced IL-1beta production. Nature 456: 264–268.
39. Cadwell K, Liu JY, Brown SL, Miyoshi H, Loh J, et al. (2008) A key role for autophagy and the autophagy gene Atg16l1 in mouse and human intestinal Paneth cells. Nature 456: 259–263.
40. Lawrance IC, Fiocchi C, Chakravarti S (2001) Ulcerative colitis and Crohn's disease: distinctive gene expression profiles and novel susceptibility candidate genes. Hum Mol Genet 10: 445–456.
41. Rybaczyk L, Rozmiarek A, Circle K, Grants I, Needleman B, et al. (2009) New bioinformatics approach to analyze gene expressions and signaling pathways reveals unique purine gene dysregulation profiles that distinguish between CD and UC. Inflammatory Bowel Diseases 15: 971–984.
42. Skog J, Wurdinger T, van Rijn S, Meijer DH, Gainche L, et al. (2008) Glioblastoma microvesicles transport RNA and proteins that promote tumour growth and provide diagnostic biomarkers. Nat Cell Biol 10: 1470–1476.
43. Saunders MA, Liang H, Li WH (2007) Human polymorphism at microRNAs and microRNA target sites. Proc Natl Acad Sci U S A 104: 3300–3305.
44. Bao L, Zhou M, Wu L, Lu L, Goldowitz D, et al. (2007) PolymiRTS Database: Linking polymorphisms in microRNA target sites with complex traits. Nucleic Acids Research 35: D51–D54.
45. Boni V, Zarate R, Villa JC, Bandrés E, Gomez MA, et al. (2011) Role of primary miRNA polymorphic variants in metastatic colon cancer patients treated with 5-fluorouracil and irinotecan. Pharmacogenomics Journal 11: 429–436.
46. Borel C, Antonarakis SE (2008) Functional genetic variation of human miRNAs and phenotypic consequences. Mammalian Genome 19: 503–509.
47. Liu Z, Wei S, Ma H, Zhao M, Myers JN, et al. (2011) A functional variant at the miR-184 binding site in TNFAIP2 and risk of squamous cell carcinoma of the head and neck. Carcinogenesis 32: 1668–1674.
48. Mishra PJ, Banerjee D, Bertino JR (2008) MiRSNPs or MiR-polymorphisms, new players in microRNA mediated regulation of the cell: Introducing microRNA pharmacogenomics. Cell Cycle 7: 853–858.
49. Hindorff LA, Sethupathy P, Junkins HA, Ramos EM, Mehta JP, et al. (2009) Potential etiologic and functional implications of genome-wide association loci for human diseases and traits. Proc Natl Acad Sci U S A 106: 9362–9367.

Gene Expression Changes Associated with Resistance to Intravenous Corticosteroid Therapy in Children with Severe Ulcerative Colitis

Boyko Kabakchiev[1,10]*⁹, Dan Turner[9⁹], Jeffrey Hyams[5], David Mack[4], Neal Leleiko[7], Wallace Crandall[8], James Markowitz[6], Anthony R. Otley[3], Wei Xu[10], Pingzhao Hu[2], Anne M. Griffiths[2], Mark S. Silverberg[1,10]

1 Mount Sinai Hospital, Toronto, Ontario, Canada, **2** The Hospital for Sick Children, Toronto, Ontario, Canada, **3** Izaak Walton Killam Hospital, Halifax, Nova Scotia, Canada, **4** Children's Hospital of Eastern Ontario, Ottawa, Ontario, Canada, **5** Connecticut Children's Medical Center, Hartford, Connecticut, United States of America, **6** Schneider's Children's Hospital, New Hyde Park, New York, United States of America, **7** Brown University, Providence, Rhode Island, United States of America, **8** Columbus Children's Hospital, Columbus, Ohio, United States of America, **9** Shaare Zedek Medical Center, Jerusalem, Israel, **10** University of Toronto, Toronto, Ontario, Canada

Abstract

Background and Aims: Microarray analysis of RNA expression allows gross examination of pathways operative in inflammation. We aimed to determine whether genes expressed in whole blood early following initiation of intravenous corticosteroid treatment can be associated with response.

Methods: From a prospectively accrued cohort of 128 pediatric patients hospitalized for intravenous corticosteroid treatment of severe UC, we selected for analysis 20 corticosteroid responsive (hospital discharge or PUCAI ≤45 by day 5) and 20 corticosteroid resistant patients (need for second line medical therapy or colectomy, or PUCAI >45 by day 5). Total RNA was extracted from blood samples collected on day 3 of intravenous corticosteroid therapy. The eluted transcriptomes were quantified on Affymetrix Human Gene 1.0 ST arrays. The data was analysed by the local-pooled error method for discovery of differential gene expression and false discovery rate correction was applied to adjust for multiple comparisons.

Results: A total of 41 genes differentially expressed between responders and non-responders were detected with statistical significance. Two of these genes, *CEACAM1* and *MMP8*, possibly inhibited by methylprednisolone through *IL8*, were both found to be over-expressed in non-responsive patients. *ABCC4* (*MRP4*) as a member of the multi-drug resistance superfamily was a novel candidate gene for corticosteroid resistance. The expression pattern of a cluster of 10 genes selected from the 41 significant hits were able to classify the patients with 80% sensitivity and 80% specificity.

Conclusions: Elevated expression of several genes involved in inflammatory pathways was associated with resistance to intravenous corticosteroid therapy early in the course of treatment. Gene expression profiles may be useful to classify resistance to intravenous corticosteroids in children with severe UC and assist with clinical management decisions.

Editor: Guillaume Dalmasso, Emory University, United States of America

Funding: This investigator-initiated study was funded by Schering-Plough Canada Inc. (http://www.schering-plough.ca/), the Crohn's and Colitis Foundation of Canada (http://www.ccfc.ca/), and the National Institutes of Health (http://www.nih.gov/). The funders had no role in study design, data collection and analysis, decision to publish, or preparation of the manuscript.

Competing Interests: Study participants were aware of the following potential conflicts of interest: Dan Turner: Proctor and Gamble - consultant; Medici medical - consultant, research support; Jeffrey Hyams: Centocor Ortho Biotech - research support, consultant, speaker's bureau; Abbott - research support, consultant; UCB - research support, consultant; Astra Zeneca - research support; Anne M Griffiths: Proctor and Gamble - consultant; Centocor Ortho Biotech - research support, consultant; UCB - consultant; Abbott - consultant; James Markowitz: Centocor Ortho Biotech - research support, consultant; Abbott - research support; UCB - research support, consultant; Astra Zeneca - research support; Prometheus Laboratories - research support, consultant, honorarium; Abbott Nutritionals - speaker's bureau, honoraria; Wallace Crandall: Centocor Ortho Biotech - consultant, research support; Abbott - research support; Neal LeLeiko: Centocor - research support; Astra Zeneca - research support; Proctor and Gamble - research support; Anthony Otley: Abbott - research support, consultant, speaker's bureau; UCB - research support; Schering - research support; Proctor and Gamble - research support; David Mack: Axcan Pharma - consultant; Schering-Plough - speaker's bureau, consultant; Abbott - speaker, research support; AstraZeneca - speaker; Merck-Frosst - speaker; Proctor and Gamble - research support; Novartis - consultant; Bristol-Myers Squibb - consultant, speaker; all others have nothing to declare.

* E-mail: kabakchiev@lunenfeld.ca

⁹ These authors contributed equally to this work.

Introduction

Although corticosteroids remain a mainstay of therapy for UC, a meta-regression of cohort studies in acute severe ulcerative colitis (UC) showed that 29% of patients fail corticosteroid therapy and require escalation of medical management or colectomy [1]. Evidence suggests that the dose of the administered corticosteroid and its bioavailability do not account for response or failure to therapy [1,2]. Although some case series suggest that prolongation of corticosteroid therapy is effective in achieving remission in some refractory cases [3], this approach is associated with increased toxicity, discomfort, and cost. Several studies have attempted to identify predictors of corticosteroid response and allow for escalation of medical therapy or colectomy early during admission [1]. In adults, number of daily stools and C-reactive protein have good predictive ability on the third day of treatment [4,5]. Albumin and bowel luminal width have been also associated with response to corticosteroid therapy [6]. In children, a predictive rule based on the Pediatric UC Activity Index (PUCAI) at days three and five of corticosteroid therapy has been shown to be superior to the adult scores [7]. A PUCAI value greater than 70 points should prompt initiation of second line therapy as was recently validated in a prospective cohort of children with severe UC, yielding positive predictive value (PPV) of 100% and negative predictive value (NPV) of 79% [8]. Although fecal calprotectin and pyruvate kinase have a fair predictive role, they do not add significantly to the clinical PUCAI score [9].

The expression of various proteins and genetic sequence alterations may contribute to corticosteroid resistance in asthma, rheumatic disease, and inflammatory bowel disease [10,11,12,13]. For example, high expression levels of Multi Drug Resistance-1 (MDR-1) were found in UC patients who required colectomy [14]. MDR-1 may be involved in corticosteroid resistance by transporting the drug out across the cell membrane. Additionally, *in vitro* corticosteroid resistance of T-cells obtained from corticosteroid refractory UC patients no longer showed similar findings 3-months after discharge [15]. No differences in glucocorticoid receptor expression were observed in leukocytes obtained from previously corticosteroid responsive and resistant UC patients currently in remission [16].

RNA microarrays on 6 asthma patients revealed 9 genes, primarily involved in macrophage activation, to be differentially expressed between responders and non-responders to corticosteroids [17]. A different study by Hakonarson and colleagues identified over 900 transcripts which were differentially regulated between corticosteroid responsive and non-responsive asthma patients [18]. 15 of these transcripts could separate responders from non-responders with 84% accuracy [19]. No similar studies exist in UC. The aim of this prospective, multicenter study was to compare gene expression among children who responded to or failed intravenous corticosteroid therapy in acute, severe UC.

Methods

Study design

The evaluated patient population was from a nested case-control study of the *outcome of intravenous steroid therapy in ulcerative colitis individuals* (OSCI) study [20]. The OSCI study was a multicenter, prospective cohort study involving children, 2–18 years of age, hospitalized for intravenous corticosteroid therapy for acute UC. A diagnosis of UC was established by the presence of accepted clinical, radiologic, endoscopic and histological criteria [21]. The research ethics boards of the Hospital for Sick Children, Mount Sinai Hospital, Izaak Walton Killam Hospital, Children's Hospital of Eastern Ontario, and the institutional review boards of Connecticut Children's Medical Center, Schneider's Children's Hospital, the Children's Hospital of Philadelphia, Columbus Children's Hospital, and the Hasbro Children's Hospital approved this study. Informed, written consent and age-appropriate assent were obtained from participants and their caregiver, according to the local policy.

Pre-defined clinical, laboratory and radiographic data were collected on standardized case report forms at admission, on Day 3 and Day 5 of corticosteroid treatment, upon introduction of second line medical therapy (infliximab or calcineurin inhibitors) or colectomy (if applicable), and at hospital discharge. Disease activity was measured at each visit by the PUCAI [22] which is a non-invasive, 6-item index, ranging from 0 to 85, intended to measure disease activity in children with UC. This index was previously developed and validated by some of the authors using prospective cohorts and combined mathematical and judgmental strategies [7,23,24,25]. As part of the OSCI study, in addition to clinical data, blood was collected for RNA extraction from all patients on Day 3 of corticosteroid treatment.

Patient selection

The OSCI cohort consisted of 128 children and adolescents hospitalized for intravenous corticosteroid treatment of acute severe ulcerative colitis. Of these, 20 corticosteroid-responsive patients and 20 corticosteroid-refractory patients were selected for analysis of mRNA expression. All selected patients had been treated with methylprednisolone. Two batches of 20 patients, each composed of 10 non-responders and 10 responders, underwent microarray analysis (Table 1). Selection of subjects among the eligible non-responders (see below) was random for each batch. Responders of similar age and matching gender were selected in order to minimize potential confounding effects. To avoid selection bias, the inclusion of patients in the two groups was performed before the RNA assay was carried out and thus investigators were blinded to the expression results. Response was defined as no requirement for second line medical intervention or surgery by discharge and a PUCAI score less than or equal to 45 points by day 5 of therapy. Conversely, patients were categorized as non-responsive if they required second line medical

Table 1. Basic characteristics of included patients.

		Response to IVCS		
		Yes	No	p-value
Batch 1	N	10	10	-
	Male/Female	5/5	5/5	1.0000
	Age	14.4±2.2	14.6±2.2	0.852
	Disease Duration (mon.)	9±19	12±17	0.7372
	PUCAI Day 1	77±9	75±13	0.6986
	PUCAI Day 3	44±23	71±10	0.0033
	PUCAI Day 5	36±8	67±13	0.0012
Batch 2	N	10	10	-
	Male/Female	7/3	7/3	1.0000
	Age	12.7±2.6	14.6±2.4	0.1134
	Disease Duration (mon.)	18±39	20±35	0.8825
	PUCAI Day 1	66±11	73±8	0.1524
	PUCAI Day 3	34±13	61±14	0.0003
	PUCAI Day 5	19±11	54±16	0.0014
Combined	N	20	20	-
	Male/Female	12/8	12/8	1.0000
	Age	13.6±2.5	14.6±2.3	0.1831
	Disease Duration (mon.)	14±30	16±28	0.7778
	PUCAI Day 1	71±12	74±11	0.5217
	PUCAI Day 3	39±19	66±13	<0.0001
	PUCAI Day 5	27±13	61±16	<0.0001

N - Number of patients.
IVCS - Intravenous corticosteroids.

therapy or surgery, or presented with a PUCAI score greater than 45 on day 5.

Blood sample handling and RNA extraction

Blood samples were collected on Day 3 of intravenous corticosteroid therapy in *PAXgene* tubes (*PreAnalytiX, QIAGEN*) and stored at −80°C within 24 hours of collection for a period of less than 1 year. Total RNA was extracted with *PAXgene Blood RNA Kits* (*QIAGEN*) and the obtained elutes were stored at −80°C. The integrity of all RNA elutes was assessed with Bioanalyzer 2100 (*Agilent Technologies*) and only samples with RNA Integrity Number (RIN) greater than 5.5 were used for further analysis [26].

Microarray analysis

Total RNA samples were hybridized to GeneChip Human Gene 1.0 ST Arrays (*Affymetrix*), with whole-transcript coverage of 28,869 genes and open reading frames (ORFs). GeneChip Whole Transcript (WT) Sense Target Labeling Assays with included quality control GeneChip Hybridization Control Kits (*Affymetrix*) were used for sample preparation. The chips were scanned and raw expression values were obtained with GeneChip Scanner 3000 (*Affymetrix*). (NCBI Gene Expression Omnibus series record - GSE21231).

RT-PCR

The reliability of the microarray measurements was assessed through reverse-transcription real-time polymerase chain reaction (RT-PCR) measurements of the relative messenger RNA levels of 7 genes. These were selected based on their apparent importance to IBD disease mechanism. 6 pairs of specific primers were used to amplify exonic sequences in *OLFM4, MMP8, BPI, HP, CD177, DEFA1* and *DEFA3*. (Table S1) Due to the high homology between the sequences of *DEFA1* and *DEFA3* (99%), GeneChip Human Gene 1.0 ST Array probes measured the combined expression of the messenger RNA molecules. Likewise, RT-PCR primers were chosen to amplify a common segment between the two genes. The hypoxanthine phosphoribosyltransferase 1 (*HPRT1*) gene was used as an internal RT-PCR control. 300–600 ηg of total RNA were used with iScrip cDNA Synthesis Kits (*Bio-Rad*) to obtain complementary DNA. RT-PCR was performed with SYBR Green Supermix With ROX (*Bio-Rad*) and 15–30 ηg of template in a total reaction volume of 25 μL on 96-well plates.

Data analysis

Probesets lacking annotation information were removed from further analysis. Raw data were background corrected, log transformed, and quantile normalized using a robust multi-array average (RMA) algorithm [27]. Within each batch, 21,176 genes and ORFs were correlated with a binary intravenous-corticosteroid therapy response variable across all samples using the local-pooled error (LPE) method for detection of significance [28]. Gene variance was estimated by pooling variance estimates of genes with similar expression from biological replicas across the response groups. Raw p-values were adjusted for multiple comparisons by the step-up FDR method [29]. A Monte Carlo simulation was used to estimate the expected overlap between the results from the two batches [30]. Only the most differentially expressed genes in each batch were considered for this analysis – 1059 (5% of total) genes with lowest p-values. Pearson's chi-squared test was used to compare the expected to the observed proportion of overlap. All 40 samples were first normalized separately, then scaled using the R function "scale" (http://www.r-project.org/), and finally pooled together into a single LPE analysis while controlling for batch effects.

Pharmacogenomic and gene-gene interaction data mining was accomplished via the Search Tool for Interactions of Chemicals (STITCH) [31]. Various aspects of molecular interaction were considered, including: activation, inhibition, binding, phenotypic similarity, catalysis, and co-expression.

The predictive value of genes correlated significantly with corticosteroid resistance was assessed by prediction analysis for microarrays (PAM). This approach utilizes the shrunken centroid method to identify genes which best characterize each response group [32]. The procedure was carried out in a 10-fold cross-validation fashion whereby the complete sample set was randomly divided into 10 subsets of equal size. Each of the 10 subsets was consecutively used for validating a classifier which was trained on the remaining 9 subsets. A classification score for each sample was determined based on the distance to the nearest shrunken centroid. The performance of the classifier was then averaged over the 10 validation events (folds). This cross-validation approach is very robust and preferred for analyzing fewer than 50 samples due to its high data utilization efficiency [33].

Results

After screening the entire OSCI study cohort, 40 patients were included according to the predefined criteria as described in Table 1. Separate LPE analyses of each batch of samples produced very similar results. When ranked by p-value, an overlap of 341 genes was found between the 5% (1059 genes) of genes with lowest p-values in both batches. (Figure S1) In other words, the observed overlap between the results from the two separate analyses was 32.2%. A Monte Carlo simulation indicated that the mean expected overlap, assuming no correlation between the two batches, was 52.963±0.007 genes with a median of 53 genes (5%). A chi-squared test showed that there was a very significant difference between the observed and expected proportion of overlap ($p = 4.18 \times 10^{-57}$).

After correction for multiple testing, 41 genes expressed differentially between responders and non-responders to therapy were detected with statistical significance in the pooled analysis. (Table 2) Some of the most significant genes were Olfactomedin 4 (*OLFM4*), Matrix Metallopeptidase 8 (*MMP8*), RAP1 GTPase Activating Protein (*RAP1GAP*), 6-phosphofructo-2-kinase (*PFKFB2*), Bactericidal Permeability-increasing Protein (*BPI*), and N-terminal EF-hand Calcium Binding Protein 1 (*NECAB1*). The expression of all significant genes was elevated in patients who had no response to the administered therapy.

RT-PCR was used to confirm the relative expression obtained from the microarray experiment. The transcripts of *OLFM4, MMP8, BPI, HP, CD177, DEFA1* and *DEFA3* were successfully measured in real-time using the primers listed in Table S1. We demonstrated that the RT-PCR and microarray expression values were highly correlated confirming the validity of the microarray results. (Figure S2)

Intriguing information on the interconnectivity of some of the 41 significant genes was obtained through network analysis. A diagrammatic representation of the immediate interactome of methylprednisolone indicated an inhibitory action on *K60*, also known as *IL8* (Figure 1) [34]. In turn, *IL8* is a known inducer of *CEACAM1* and *MMP8* [35,36,37], and it also interacts with *BPI, LCN2* and *PPBP* [36,38,39,40]. All of these partners of *IL8* were expressed significantly higher in our patients who had no response to intravenous corticosteroid therapy. A study by Matsuda *et al.* showed that *IL8* mRNA levels are high during active disease and low during quiescent disease in UC patients [41]. However, 4% elevation of *IL8* expression levels in our cohort of corticosteroid

Table 2. List of genes significantly associated with response to intravenous corticosteroid therapy.

FDR Adjusted P-value	Fold Change	Gene Symbol	Description	Immune System Associated
<0.0001	1.8	**OLFM4**	Olfactomedin 4	Yes
<0.0001	1.9	**MMP8**	Matrix Metallopeptidase 8 (Neutrophil Collagenase)	Yes
<0.0001	1.6	**RAP1GAP**	RAP1 GTPase Activating Protein	Yes
<0.0001	1.3	**PFKFB2**	6-phosphofructo-2-kinase	-
<0.0001	1.3	**BPI**	Bactericidal Permeability-increasing Protein	Yes
<0.0001	1.7	**NECAB1**	N-terminal EF-hand Calcium Binding Protein 1	-
<0.0001	2.5	**CLC**	Charcot-Leyden Crystal Protein	Yes
<0.0001	1.8	**TSTA3**	Tissue Specific Transplantation Antigen P35B	Yes
<0.0001	1.8	**GPR84**	G Protein-coupled Receptor 84	-
<0.0001	1.3	**RPS26P2**	Ribosomal Protein S26 Pseudogene 2	-
<0.0001	1.6	**HP**	Haptoglobin	Yes
0.0001	1.2	**MS4A3**	Membrane-spanning 4-domains	Yes
0.0001	1.4	**SERPINB10**	Serpin Peptidase Inhibitor	Yes
0.0001	1.4	**TDRD9**	Tudor Domain Containing 9	-
0.0003	1.3	**LCN2**	Lipocalin 2	Yes
0.0012	2.0	**CD177**	CD177 Molecule	Yes
0.0012	1.3	**RPS26P15**	Ribosomal Protein S26 Pseudogene 15	-
0.0013	1.5	**GMPR**	Guanosine Monophosphate Reductase	-
0.0017	1.4	**CLIC2**	Chloride Intracellular Channel 2	-
0.0027	1.5	**PROS1**	Protein S (Alpha)	Yes
0.0063	1.6	**TCN1**	Transcobalamin I (Vitamin B12 Binding Protein)	Yes
0.0072	1.5	**CEACAM1**	Carcinoembryonic Antigen-related Cell Adhesion Molecule 1	Yes
0.0073	1.5	**HEPACAM2**	HEPACAM family member 2	Yes
0.0073	1.5	**ATP9A**	ATPase	-
0.0082	1.2	**RPS26L**	40S Ribosomal Protein S26-like	-
0.0128	1.2	**DEFA1/DEFA3**	Defensin	Yes
0.0129	1.3	**MBNL3**	Muscleblind-like 3 (Drosophila)	-
0.0155	1.4	**PPBP**	Pro-platelet Basic Protein	Yes
0.0221	1.6	**ITGB3**	Integrin	Yes
0.0244	1.2	**CLEC4C**	C-type Lectin Domain Family 4	Yes
0.0257	1.5	**GYPC**	Glycophorin C (Gerbich blood group)	-
0.0257	1.3	**CA1**	Carbonic Anhydrase I	-
0.0284	1.6	**ENTPD7**	Ectonucleoside Triphosphate Diphosphohydrolase 7	-
0.0284	1.3	**VSTM1**	V-set and Transmembrane Domain Containing 1	-
0.0361	1.2	**SUCNR1**	Succinate Receptor 1	-
0.0445	1.6	**ELOVL7**	ELOVL Family Member 7	-
0.0445	1.2	**PSTPIP2**	Proline-serine-threonine Phosphatase Interacting Protein 2	-
0.0459	2.2	**RNF182**	Ring Finger Protein 182	-
0.0459	1.3	**ABCC4**	ATP-binding Cassette	Yes
0.0459	1.8	**GPR146**	G Protein-coupled Receptor 146	-

Genes with statistically significant association to intravenous corticosteroid therapy response after correction for multiple testing (FDR-adjusted p-values$<$0.05). The average fold increase in expression in non-responsive compared to responsive patients, official gene symbol, a short description, and prior evidence of immune pathway involvement are listed for each gene.

non-responsive individuals was not statistically significant (FDR $p = 1$).

Finally, the predictive value of the total and various subsets of the 41 differentially-expressed genes was assessed. (Table 3) Using all 41 genes, it was possible to classify the 40 tested samples as belonging to either corticosteroid resistant or responsive patients with 80% sensitivity and 70% specificity. Subgroups including the top 40, 35, 30, 25, 20, 15, 10, or 5 of differentially expressed genes performed similarly as classifiers. While the specificity and sensitivity decreased with the number of tested genes, neither value dropped below 60%. Interestingly, the 10 best classifiers of corticosteroid resistance – *RAP1GAP, CD177, ELOVL7, CLIC2,*

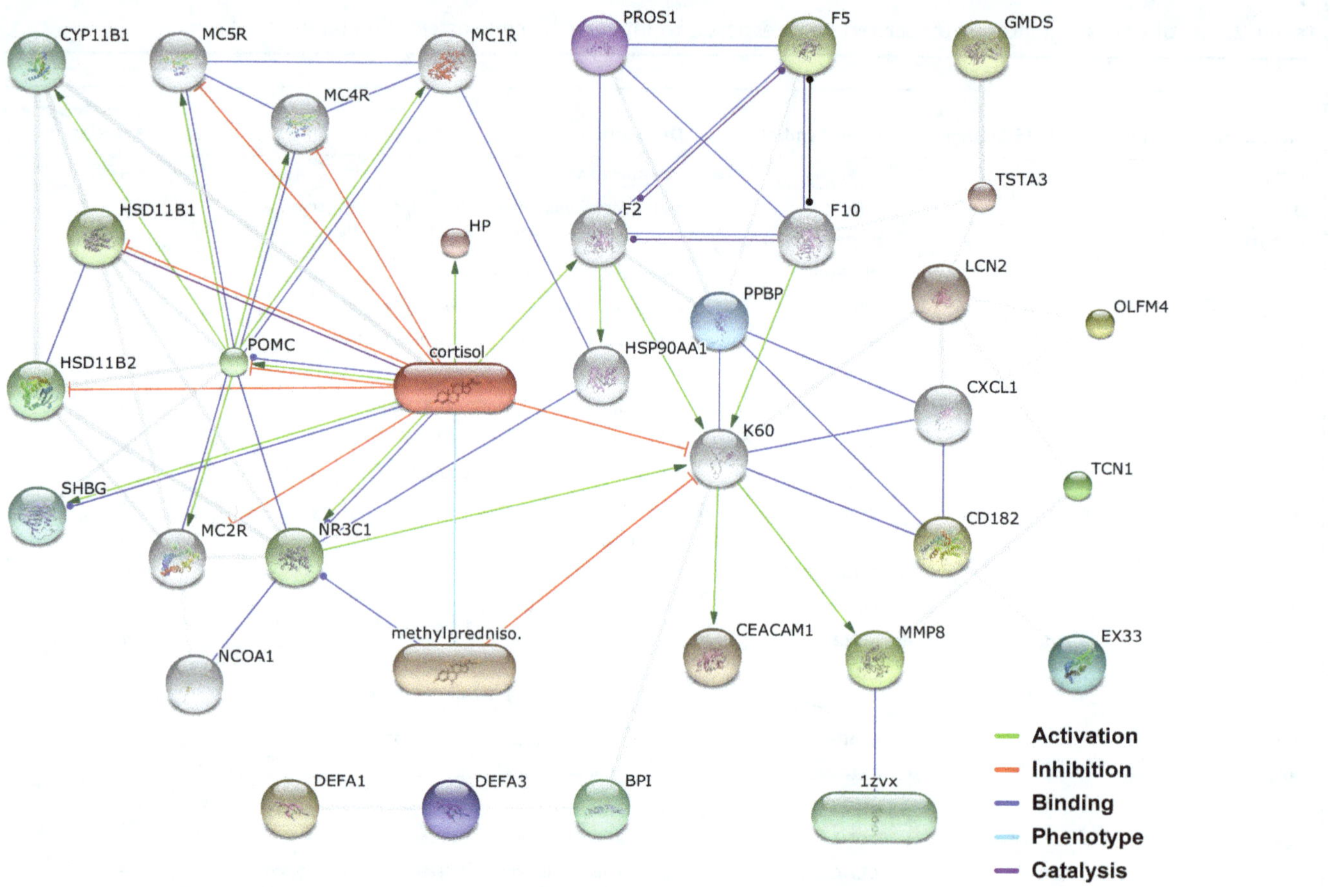

Figure 1. Immediate interactome of methylprednisolone. Point and block arrows indicate activation or inhibition, respectively. Grey lines represent interactions of undetermined nature, while coloured lines indicate evidence for specific interactions.

TSTA3, *HP*, *MMP8*, *NECAB1*, *PROS1* and *ITGB3* – were 80% specific and 80% sensitive. (Table 4) In a completely unbiased PAM analysis, 9 out of these 10 classifier genes remained within the 46 best classifiers out of all 21, 176 tested genes. In this analysis, the most accurate classification was achieved by the use of 662 genes (data not shown) with specificity and sensitivity of 75%.

Table 3. Class prediction analysis for microarrays using nearest shrunken centroid method.

Most Significant Genes (N)	Specificity	Sensitivity	Accuracy
41	80%	70%	75%
40	75%	75%	75%
35	80%	70%	75%
30	70%	70%	70%
25	75%	65%	70%
20	75%	70%	73%
15	70%	60%	65%
10	75%	70%	73%
5	65%	65%	65%

Assessment of the specificity, sensitivity and accuracy for the N most significant genes (where N equals 41 through 5 in decreasing increments of 5). Accuracy % = 100 * (True Positives+True Negatives)/Total.

Discussion

Whole-genome expression analysis of patients receiving intravenous corticosteroid revealed 41 genes with expression levels significantly associated with resistance to the therapy. A substantial proportion of these genes are known to be involved in the inflammatory response. Furthermore, mining molecular interaction databases provided a basis for interpreting how these expression results fit the paradigm of corticosteroid resistance. Of potential clinical relevance was a set of 10 genes which classified the treated patients with 80% sensitivity and specificity. Conceivably, measurement of the expression levels of these genes could be developed into a practical tool to help identify individuals who are likely to fail such intravenous corticosteroid therapy and improve their medication course.

While gene expression changes that occur during treatment may help elucidate the mechanism of corticosteroid resistance, it is essential to further investigate the various molecular interactions alluded to in this study. All genes found to be good classifiers of corticosteroid resistance must necessarily be validated in a large, prospective study. Gene expression changes observed on the third day of therapy are likely to highlight pathways relevant to corticosteroid metabolism and may be temporal. Conversely, sampling patients prior to the initiation of therapy would establish

Table 4. Specificity, sensitivity and accuracy of the 10 best indicators of corticosteroid resistance.

10 Best Indicators of Corticosteroid Resistance	Specificity	Sensitivity	Accuracy
RAP1GAP, CD177, ELOVL7, CLIC2, TSTA3, HP, MMP8, NECAB1, PROS1, ITGB3	80%	80%	80%

whether the discovered pathways are intrinsic to the individual's disease behaviour.

Network analysis revealed that IL-8 function provides a possible explanation for the observed overexpression of *CEACAM1* and *MMP8* in non-responsive patients [35,36,37]. Corticosteroid resistance could result in reduced inhibition of *IL8* by methylprednisolone and thus affect its downstream interactions [34]. *IL8* expression was not significantly different between responders and non-responders in this study despite a previous report of elevated *IL8* mRNA levels in active UC [41]. However, methylprednisolone appears to inhibit IL-8 by preventing its release rather than by affecting its gene expression [34]. Indeed, this claim is partially supported by evidence that IL-8 can be stored in Weibel-Palade bodies for rapid release [42] and its protein levels could remain briefly stable after changes in its gene expression.

A number of the significant genes identified in this study are of specific interest due to their prior association with IBD or pathways implicated in IBD. Olfactomedin 4 (*OLFM4*) is a gene encoding a member of the olfactomedin-related protein family. Selective over-expression of *OLFM4* has been reported in inflamed colonic crypt epithelium in ulcerative colitis patients [43]. The exact function of the protein, however, is not known. A study by Zhang *et al.* indicates that *OLFM4* is an anti-apoptotic factor which attenuates the ability of *GRIM19* to facilitate retinoic acid-IFN-β-mediated apoptosis and the expression of apoptotic genes [44]. Barnich *et al.* report that *GRIM19* interacts with nucleotide oligomerization domain 2 (*NOD2*) and is required for the activation of *NF-κB* [45]. Interestingly, Liu *et al.* recently demonstrated that *OLFM4* down-regulates the innate immune response by influencing NOD1 and NOD2 mediated NF-κB activation in a mouse model of *Helicobacter pylori* infection [46]. Other reports implicate *OLFM4* expression in tumour growth and, more specifically, in colon cancer [47,48]. *OLFM4* has also been shown to bind cell-surface lectins and cadherin [49].

Matrix metalloproteinase 8 (*MMP8*), a collagenase secreted by neutrophils, was also expressed more highly in patients who were not responding to intravenous corticosteroids. This proteinase can degrade type I, II and III collagen and thus affect the extracellular matrix. A study by Schaaf et al. shows elevated activity of MMP8 in hospitalized patients in the presence of bacteria compared to controls [50]. Alpha defensin 1 (*DEFA1*) and 3 (*DEFA3*) as well as bactericidal/permeability-increasing protein (*BPI*) are peptides secreted by neutrophils in response to bacterial antigens. Elevated levels of all three proteins have been associated with inflammatory activity in rheumatoid arthritis [51]. *DEFA1* and *DEFA3* have also been implicated in lung epithelial wound repair [52].

HP encodes both the alpha and beta chains of the haptoglobin tetramer, a protein responsible for the clearance of free plasma haemoglobin and a mediator of the inflammatory response. *HP* is an inducer of IL-6 and plays a role in the balance of Th1 and Th2 cell populations [53,54]. Polymorphisms in this gene have been associated with Crohn's disease, disease behaviour and extraintestinal manifestations [55]. *CD177* is a glycoprotein selectively expressed by neutrophils and found on their surface. Although its exact function is not known, it has been identified as a binding partner of platelet endothelial cell adhesion molecule-1 (*PECAM-1*) and it may play a crucial role in the extravasation of neutrophils into tissues [56]. *CD177* expression is increased in individuals with severe bacterial infections and polycythaemia vera, but not rheumatoid arthritis [57]. In our study, expression of *CD177* was increased two-fold in patients who did not respond to intravenous corticosteroid therapy compared to those who did well.

ATP-binding cassette, sub-family C, member 4 (*ABCC4*) is a gene that may directly influence corticosteroid response. *ABCC4* is also known as multi-drug resistance protein 4 (*MRP4*) and is part of the same superfamily as *MDR1*. ABCC4 is an ATP-dependent transporter and it has been associated with resistance to multiple drugs. More specifically, it has been shown to actively transport prostaglandins, methotrexate and steroid- and bile acid-conjugates [58,59,60].

The results of this study demonstrate that significant gene expression differences exist between patients who respond to intravenous corticosteroid therapy and those who are resistant. It also validates the use of RNA expression analysis as a useful approach toward improving the understanding of disease processes and response to medical therapy. Clinically meaningful tools may also be developed that would allow for the early stratification of patients into prognostic categories that would individualize care approaches.

Web Resources

NCBI Gene Expression Omnibus (GEO) - http://www.ncbi.nlm.nih.gov/geo/

R function "scale" - http://www.r-project.org/

Search Tool for Interactions of Chemicals - http://stitch.embl.de/

Supporting Information

Figure S1 Graphical representation of the analysis used to compare the results from batch 1 and batch2. The expected overlap under the null hypothesis was obtained by a Monte Carlo simulation.

Figure S2 Scatterplots illustrate data for genes in each batch as well as a combined analysis, including R2 values.

Table S1 Forward and reverse primers and corresponding length of RT-PCR products are listed for each of the 7 amplified genes.

Acknowledgments

The authors would like to acknowledge the contribution of Krista Uusoue (The Hospital for Sick Children, main OSCI coordinator), Joanne Stempak and Lucy Zhang (Mount Sinai Hospital, sample coordination and processing) as well as each of the coordinators at the OSCI sites for their efforts in patient recruitment, data and sample collection. M.S.

Silverberg holds the Gale and Graham Wright Research Chair in Digestive Diseases at Mount Sinai Hospital.

Author Contributions

Conceived and designed the experiments: BK DT JH DM NL WC JM ARO AMG MSS. Performed the experiments: BK DT JH DM NL WC JM ARO AMG MSS. Analyzed the data: BK DT WX PH. Contributed reagents/materials/analysis tools: BK DT JH DM NL WC JM ARO WX PH AMG MSS. Wrote the paper: BK DT JH DM NL WC JM ARO WX PH AMG MSS.

References

1. Turner D, Walsh CM, Steinhart AH, Griffiths AM (2007) Response to corticosteroids in severe ulcerative colitis: a systematic review of the literature and a meta-regression. Clin Gastroenterol Hepatol 5: 103–110.
2. Turner D, Kolho KL, Mack DR, Raivio T, Leleiko N, et al. (2009) Glucocorticoid bioactivity does not predict response to steroid therapy in severe pediatric ulcerative colitis. Inflamm Bowel Dis.
3. Gold DM, Levine JJ, Weinstein TA, Kessler B, Pettei MJ (1995) Prolonged medical therapy for severe pediatric ulcerative colitis. Am J Gastroenterol 90: 732–735.
4. Lindgren SC, Flood LM, Kilander AF, Lofberg R, Persson TB, et al. (1998) Early predictors of glucocorticosteroid treatment failure in severe and moderately severe attacks of ulcerative colitis. Eur J Gastroenterol Hepatol 10: 831–835.
5. Travis SP, Farrant JM, Ricketts C, Nolan DJ, Mortensen NM, et al. (1996) Predicting outcome in severe ulcerative colitis. Gut 38: 905–910.
6. Ho GT, Mowat C, Goddard CJ, Fennell JM, Shah NB, et al. (2004) Predicting the outcome of severe ulcerative colitis: development of a novel risk score to aid early selection of patients for second-line medical therapy or surgery. Aliment Pharmacol Ther 19: 1079–1087.
7. Turner D, Walsh CM, Benchimol EI, Mann EH, Thomas KE, et al. (2008) Severe paediatric ulcerative colitis: incidence, outcomes and optimal timing for second-line therapy. Gut 57: 331–338.
8. Turner D, Mack D, Leleiko N, Walters TD, Uusoue K, et al. (2010) Severe pediatric ulcerative colitis: a prospective multicenter study of outcomes and predictors of response. Gastroenterology 138: 2282–2291.
9. Ho GT, Lee HM, Brydon G, Ting T, Hare N, et al. (2009) Fecal calprotectin predicts the clinical course of acute severe ulcerative colitis. Am J Gastroenterol 104: 673–678.
10. Bray PJ, Cotton RG (2003) Variations of the human glucocorticoid receptor gene (NR3C1): pathological and in vitro mutations and polymorphisms. Hum Mutat 21: 557–568.
11. Leung DY, Martin RJ, Szefler SJ, Sher ER, Ying S, et al. (1995) Dysregulation of interleukin 4, interleukin 5, and interferon gamma gene expression in steroid-resistant asthma. J Exp Med 181: 33–40.
12. Ito K, Chung KF, Adcock IM (2006) Update on glucocorticoid action and resistance. J Allergy Clin Immunol 117: 522–543.
13. Tantisira KG, Lake S, Silverman ES, Palmer LJ, Lazarus R, et al. (2004) Corticosteroid pharmacogenetics: association of sequence variants in CRHR1 with improved lung function in asthmatics treated with inhaled corticosteroids. Hum Mol Genet 13: 1353–1359.
14. Farrell RJ, Murphy A, Long A, Donnelly S, Cherikuri A, et al. (2000) High multidrug resistance (P-glycoprotein 170) expression in inflammatory bowel disease patients who fail medical therapy. Gastroenterology 118: 279–288.
15. Hearing SD, Norman M, Probert CS, Haslam N, Dayan CM (1999) Predicting therapeutic outcome in severe ulcerative colitis by measuring in vitro steroid sensitivity of proliferating peripheral blood lymphocytes. Gut 45: 382–388.
16. Flood L, Lofberg R, Stierna P, Wikstrom AC (2001) Glucocorticoid receptor mRNA in patients with ulcerative colitis: a study of responders and nonresponders to glucocorticosteroid therapy. Inflamm Bowel Dis 7: 202–209.
17. Goleva E, Hauk PJ, Hall CF, Liu AH, Riches DW, et al. (2008) Corticosteroid-resistant asthma is associated with classical antimicrobial activation of airway macrophages. J Allergy Clin Immunol 122: 550–559 e553.
18. Hakonarson H, Bjornsdottir US, Halapi E, Bradfield J, Zink F, et al. (2005) Profiling of genes expressed in peripheral blood mononuclear cells predicts glucocorticoid sensitivity in asthma patients. Proc Natl Acad Sci U S A 102: 14789–14794.
19. Donn R, Berry A, Stevens A, Farrow S, Betts J, et al. (2007) Use of gene expression profiling to identify a novel glucocorticoid sensitivity determining gene, BMPRII. FASEB J 21: 402–414.
20. Turner D, R. Mack D, Uusoue K, Jeffrey SH, Neal L, et al. (2009) T1745 A Prospective Multicenter Study of Outcomes and Predictors of Response in Severe Pediatric Ulcerative Colitis. Gastroenterology 136: A-571.
21. Bousvaros A, Antonioli DA, Colletti RB, Dubinsky MC, Glickman JN, et al. (2007) Differentiating ulcerative colitis from Crohn disease in children and young adults: report of a working group of the North American Society for Pediatric Gastroenterology, Hepatology, and Nutrition and the Crohn's and Colitis Foundation of America. J Pediatr Gastroenterol Nutr 44: 653–674.
22. Turner D, Otley AR, Mack D, Hyams J, de Bruijne J, et al. (2007) Development, validation, and evaluation of a pediatric ulcerative colitis activity index: a prospective multicenter study. Gastroenterology 133: 423–432.
23. Turner D, Hyams J, Markowitz J, Lerer T, Mack DR, et al. (2009) Appraisal of the pediatric ulcerative colitis activity index (PUCAI). Inflamm Bowel Dis 15: 1218–1223.
24. Turner D, Griffiths AM, Steinhart AH, Otley AR, Beaton DE (2009) Mathematical weighting of a clinimetric index (Pediatric Ulcerative Colitis Activity Index) was superior to the judgmental approach. J Clin Epidemiol 62: 738–744.
25. Turner D, Seow CH, Greenberg GR, Griffiths AM, Silverberg MS, et al. (2009) A systematic prospective comparison of noninvasive disease activity indices in ulcerative colitis. Clin Gastroenterol Hepatol 7: 1081–1088.
26. Schroeder A, Mueller O, Stocker S, Salowsky R, Leiber M, et al. (2006) The RIN: an RNA integrity number for assigning integrity values to RNA measurements. BMC Mol Biol 7: 3.
27. Irizarry RA, Bolstad BM, Collin F, Cope LM, Hobbs B, et al. (2003) Summaries of Affymetrix GeneChip probe level data. Nucleic Acids Res 31: e15.
28. Jain N, Thatte J, Braciale T, Ley K, O'Connell M, et al. (2003) Local-pooled-error test for identifying differentially expressed genes with a small number of replicated microarrays. Bioinformatics 19: 1945–1951.
29. Benjamini Y, Hochberg Y (1995) Controlling the False Discovery Rate: A Practical and Powerful Approach to Multiple Testing. Journal of the Royal Statistical Society Series B (Methodological) 57: 289–300.
30. Metropolis N, Ulam S (1949) The Monte Carlo Method. Journal of the American Statistical Association 44: 335–341.
31. Kuhn M, Szklarczyk D, Franceschini A, Campillos M, von Mering C, et al. STITCH 2: an interaction network database for small molecules and proteins. Nucleic Acids Res 38: D552–556.
32. Tibshirani R, Hastie T, Narasimhan B, Chu G (2002) Diagnosis of multiple cancer types by shrunken centroids of gene expression. Proc Natl Acad Sci U S A 99: 6567–6572.
33. Simon R, Radmacher MD, Dobbin K, McShane LM (2003) Pitfalls in the use of DNA microarray data for diagnostic and prognostic classification. J Natl Cancer Inst 95: 14–18.
34. Celik JB, Gormus N, Okesli S, Gormus ZI, Solak H (2004) Methylprednisolone prevents inflammatory reaction occurring during cardiopulmonary bypass: effects on TNF-alpha, IL-6, IL-8, IL-10. Perfusion 19: 185–191.
35. Azuz-Lieberman N, Markel G, Mizrahi S, Gazit R, Hanna J, et al. (2005) The involvement of NK cells in ankylosing spondylitis. Int Immunol 17: 837–845.
36. Thirumangalakudi L, Yin L, Rao HV, Grammas P (2007) IL-8 induces expression of matrix metalloproteinases, cell cycle and pro-apoptotic proteins, and cell death in cultured neurons. J Alzheimers Dis 11: 305–311.
37. Kelly RW (2002) Inflammatory mediators and cervical ripening. J Reprod Immunol 57: 217–224.
38. Dentener MA, Francot GJ, Hiemstra PS, Tool AT, Verhoeven AJ, et al. (1997) Bactericidal/permeability-increasing protein release in whole blood ex vivo: strong induction by lipopolysaccharide and tumor necrosis factor-alpha. J Infect Dis 175: 108–117.
39. Yan L, Borregaard N, Kjeldsen L, Moses MA (2001) The high molecular weight urinary matrix metalloproteinase (MMP) activity is a complex of gelatinase B/MMP-9 and neutrophil gelatinase-associated lipocalin (NGAL). Modulation of MMP-9 activity by NGAL. J Biol Chem 276: 37258–37265.
40. Petersen F, Van Damme J, Flad HD, Brandt E (1991) Neutrophil-activating polypeptides IL-8 and NAP-2 induce identical signal transduction pathways in the regulation of lysosomal enzyme release. Lymphokine Cytokine Res 10: 35–41.
41. Matsuda R, Koide T, Tokoro C, Yamamoto T, Godai T, et al. (2009) Quantitive cytokine mRNA expression profiles in the colonic mucosa of patients with steroid naive ulcerative colitis during active and quiescent disease. Inflamm Bowel Dis 15: 328–334.
42. Utgaard JO, Jahnsen FL, Bakka A, Brandtzaeg P, Haraldsen G (1998) Rapid secretion of prestored interleukin 8 from Weibel-Palade bodies of microvascular endothelial cells. J Exp Med 188: 1751–1756.
43. Shinozaki S, Nakamura T, Iimura M, Kato Y, Iizuka B, et al. (2001) Upregulation of Reg 1alpha and GW112 in the epithelium of inflamed colonic mucosa. Gut 48: 623–629.
44. Zhang X, Huang Q, Yang Z, Li Y, Li CY (2004) GW112, a novel antiapoptotic protein that promotes tumor growth. Cancer Res 64: 2474–2481.
45. Barnich N, Hisamatsu T, Aguirre JE, Xavier R, Reinecker HC, et al. (2005) GRIM-19 interacts with nucleotide oligomerization domain 2 and serves as downstream effector of anti-bacterial function in intestinal epithelial cells. J Biol Chem 280: 19021–19026.
46. Liu W, Yan M, Liu Y, Wang R, Li C, et al. Olfactomedin 4 down-regulates innate immunity against Helicobacter pylori infection. Proc Natl Acad Sci U S A 107: 11056–11061.
47. Liu W, Liu Y, Zhu J, Wright E, Ding I, et al. (2008) Reduced hGC-1 protein expression is associated with malignant progression of colon carcinoma. Clin Cancer Res 14: 1041–1049.

48. Conrotto P, Roesli C, Rybak J, Kischel P, Waltregny D, et al. (2008) Identification of new accessible tumor antigens in human colon cancer by ex vivo protein biotinylation and comparative mass spectrometry analysis. Int J Cancer 123: 2856–2864.
49. Liu W, Chen L, Zhu J, Rodgers GP (2006) The glycoprotein hGC-1 binds to cadherin and lectins. Exp Cell Res 312: 1785–1797.
50. Schaaf B, Liebau C, Kurowski V, Droemann D, Dalhoff K (2008) Hospital acquired pneumonia with high-risk bacteria is associated with increased pulmonary matrix metalloproteinase activity. BMC Pulm Med 8: 12.
51. Bokarewa MI, Jin T, Tarkowski A (2003) Intraarticular release and accumulation of defensins and bactericidal/permeability-increasing protein in patients with rheumatoid arthritis. J Rheumatol 30: 1719–1724.
52. Aarbiou J, Verhoosel RM, Van Wetering S, De Boer WI, Van Krieken JH, et al. (2004) Neutrophil defensins enhance lung epithelial wound closure and mucin gene expression in vitro. Am J Respir Cell Mol Biol 30: 193–201.
53. Sharpe-Timms KL, Zimmer RL, Ricke EA, Piva M, Horowitz GM (2002) Endometriotic haptoglobin binds to peritoneal macrophages and alters their function in women with endometriosis. Fertil Steril 78: 810–819.
54. Arredouani M, Matthys P, Kasran A, Baumann H, Ceuppen JL (2001) Haptoglobin and the Th1/Th2 balance: hints from in vitro and in vivo studies. Redox Rep 6: 369–371.
55. Papp M, Lakatos PL, Palatka K, Foldi I, Udvardy M, et al. (2007) Haptoglobin polymorphisms are associated with Crohn's disease, disease behavior, and extraintestinal manifestations in Hungarian patients. Dig Dis Sci 52: 1279–1284.
56. Sachs UJ, Andrei-Selmer CL, Maniar A, Weiss T, Paddock C, et al. (2007) The neutrophil-specific antigen CD177 is a counter-receptor for platelet endothelial cell adhesion molecule-1 (CD31). J Biol Chem 282: 23603–23612.
57. Gohring K, Wolff J, Doppl W, Schmidt KL, Fenchel K, et al. (2004) Neutrophil CD177 (NB1 gp, HNA-2a) expression is increased in severe bacterial infections and polycythaemia vera. Br J Haematol 126: 252–254.
58. Reid G, Wielinga P, Zelcer N, van der Heijden I, Kuil A, et al. (2003) The human multidrug resistance protein MRP4 functions as a prostaglandin efflux transporter and is inhibited by nonsteroidal antiinflammatory drugs. Proc Natl Acad Sci U S A 100: 9244–9249.
59. Chen ZS, Lee K, Walther S, Raftogianis RB, Kuwano M, et al. (2002) Analysis of methotrexate and folate transport by multidrug resistance protein 4 (ABCC4): MRP4 is a component of the methotrexate efflux system. Cancer Res 62: 3144–3150.
60. Zelcer N, Reid G, Wielinga P, Kuil A, van der Heijden I, et al. (2003) Steroid and bile acid conjugates are substrates of human multidrug-resistance protein (MRP) 4 (ATP-binding cassette C4). Biochem J 371: 361–367.

15

An Investigation of Genome-Wide Studies Reported Susceptibility Loci for Ulcerative Colitis Shows Limited Replication in North Indians

Garima Juyal[1], Pushplata Prasad[1], Sabyasachi Senapati[1], Vandana Midha[2], Ajit Sood[2], Devendra Amre[3,4], Ramesh C. Juyal[5], Thelma BK[1]*

1 Department of Genetics, University of Delhi, South Campus, New Delhi, India, 2 Dayanand Medical College and Hospital, Ludhiana, Punjab, India, 3 Department of Pediatrics, University of Montreal, Montreal, Canada, 4 Research Center, Sainte-Justine Hospital, Montreal, Canada, 5 National Institute of Immunology, New Delhi, India

Abstract

Genome-Wide Association studies (GWAS) of both Crohn's Disease (CD) and Ulcerative Colitis (UC) have unearthed over 40 risk conferring variants. Recently, a meta-analysis on UC revealed several loci, most of which were either previously associated with UC or CD susceptibility in populations of European origin. In this study, we attempted to replicate these findings in an ethnically distinct north Indian UC cohort. 648 UC cases and 850 controls were genotyped using Infinium Human 660W-quad. Out of 59 meta-analysis index SNPs, six were not in the SNP array used in the study. Of the remaining 53 SNPs, four were found monomorphic. Association ($p<0.05$) at 25 SNPs was observed, of which 15 were CD specific. Only five SNPs namely rs2395185 (*HLA-DRA*), rs3024505 (*IL10*), rs6426833 (*RNF186*), rs3763313 (*BTNL2*) and rs2066843 (*NOD2*) retained significance after Bonferroni correction. These results (i) reveal limited replication of Caucasian based meta-analysis results; (ii) reiterate overlapping molecular mechanism(s) in UC and CD; (iii) indicate differences in genetic architecture between populations; and (iv) suggest that resources such as HapMap need to be extended to cover diverse ethnic populations. They also suggest a systematic GWAS in this terrain may be insightful for identifying population specific IBD risk conferring loci and thus enable cross-ethnicity fine mapping of disease loci.

Editor: Amanda Toland, Ohio State University Medical Center, United States of America

Funding: Research grant # BT/01/COE/07/UDSC from Dept. of Biotechnology, New Delhi, India is gratefully acknowledged. The funders had no role in study design, data collection and analysis, decision to publish, or preparation of the manuscript.

Competing Interests: The authors have declared that no competing interests exist.

* E-mail: thelmabk@gmail.com

Introduction

Ulcerative colitis (UC) and Crohn's disease (CD), the two sub-phenotypes of inflammatory bowel diseases (IBDs), are polygenic conditions that are suspected to result from dysregulated activation of immune mechansism to commensal microbes in genetically predisposed individuals. Considered to be a disease of the developed populations, there is growing evidence that the incidence of the disease may be high in developing countries as well. This is more so for ethnically heterogeneous populations such as the north Indian population, where we have recently shown that the incidence of disease in particular for UC is comparable to that reported in Western countries [1].

It is well established that genetic factors contribute to susceptibility for both CD and UC. Recently Genome wide association studies (GWAS) together with meta-analysis of GWAS findings involving UC [2–7] and CD [8–12] unearthed several risk conferring loci. Although some loci showed specific association with CD (*ATG16L1*) [10] or UC (*IL10*, *ECM1*, *HERC2*) [13], a substantial overlap in genetic risk factors between the phenotypes have also been observed with genes such as *IL23R* at the forefront [6,14–15]. Discovery of these susceptibility genes, common as well as unique, has provided valuable insights into the link between the innate and adaptive immunity vis-à-vis risk for IBD.

Most candidate gene studies and recent GWAS have confirmed absence of associations with susceptibility variants in NOD2 gene and UC in Caucasians. However, we have previously reported notable allelic heterogeneity in this gene in a UC cohort from north India wherein the three frequently CD associated variants namely rs2066844, rs2066845 and rs2066847 were either absent or rarely present. Upon re-sequencing the gene in control subjects, only two reported polymorphisms, rs2066842 (Pro268Ser) and rs2067085 (Ser178Ser) were found. Of these, Pro268Ser that is common in Caucasians but associated with CD only in the presence of SNP13 was significantly associated with UC in our cohort. Analyzing the tag SNP profile for *NOD2* locus in this population revealed that the LD structure around Pro268Ser in the north Indians differs from that among Caucasians. These novel findings suggest population specific genetic profiles for UC in the north Indian population [16] warranting replication of other promising candidate genes.

With this background, we investigated whether the UC/CD genes/loci reported in the recent meta-analyses [6] were associated with UC in the ethnically distinct north Indian population.

Results

Six of the 59 meta-analysis index SNPs were not present in the Infinium Human 660W-quad array used in this study (Table 1).

Of the remaining 53 tested, four SNPs namely rs11465804 and rs11209026 (*IL23R*); rs2476601 (*PTPN22*) and rs4613763 (LOC730002) were monomorphic and therefore additional SNPs from these genes/loci were tested. Barring *IL23R*, both *PTPN22* and LOC730002 were not significant ($p>0.05$) in our cohort. The associated *IL23R* SNPs are shown in Table 2.

Of the remaining 49 index SNPs, associations were replicated with 25 SNPs ($p<0.05$) with 15 of them previously identified as CD specific (including rs2188962 located in IBD5 locus) (Table 1). Among these, five SNPs namely rs6426833 (*RNF186*, $p=0.0004$), rs3024505 (IL10, $p=0.001$), rs3763313 (*BTNL2*, $p=2.415e^{-}05$), rs2395185 (*HLA-DRA*, $p=2.038e^{-}06$) and rs2066843 (NOD2, $p=0.0002$) withstood Bonferroni correction (Table 1, Fig. 1). It is noteworthy to mention here that we previously reported association of Pro268Ser in *NOD2*, a famous CD specific gene, [16] which is in complete LD ($r^2=1$) with aforementioned SNP rs2066843.

While loci harbouring *ITLN1* and *CCL2*, both reported as CD specific genes showed borderline significance $p=0.07$ and 0.06 respectively, other notable functional genes/ loci such as *CARD9*, *IL26*, *IL12B*, CEP72, *PUS10*, *FCGR2A*, *KIF21B*, *CDKAL1* and MAP3K7IP2 otherwise replicated in Caucasians were not significantly associated with UC in north Indians (Table 1). Interestingly, another promising CD associated candidate, *ATG16L1*, also showed modest association ($p=0.05$) in our sample. With about 650 cases/850 controls and after accounting for 49 comparisons (alpha set at 0.001), the study had sufficient power (80% using QUANTO http://hydra.usc.edu) to detect associations with odds ratios 1.3 or higher (or 0.77 or lower) for allele frequencies between 20%~30%, odds ratios 1.4 or higher (0.71 or lower) for allele frequencies between 10%–20% & odds ratios 1.6 or higher for allele frequencies of 5~10% assuming a log-additive model of inheritance.

Discussion

Recent GWAS have identified >30 susceptibility genes/loci that predispose populations of European origin to IBD. The credibility and relevance of these genetic association studies is indicated by the success of replication attempts in diverse ethnic groups. Thus, in this study we investigated the contribution of these IBD specific loci in our ethnically heterogeneous north Indian UC cohort in order to define its genetic architecture more conclusively.

Our study showed that SNPs from *IL23R*, *PTPN22* and LOC730002/*PTGER4* were largely monomorphic in our cohort. Though additional SNPs from in and around *PTPN22* and LOC730002 did not show any association with UC, findings from *IL23R* locus (Table 2) warrant discussion. *IL23R* is considered as a genuine "generic" IBD susceptibility gene and has attained genome-wide significance with both UC [4,9,18–20] and CD [9,19,21–22] in various GWAS and independent replication studies. Interestingly, the non-synonymous SNP (rs11209026), the most widely replicated marker, with a potential protective role in Caucasians [9,19,23] and rs11465804 were almost monomorphic in both UC cases and controls. However, significant association ($p<0.05$) of additional SNPs selected from both within and around this gene (Table 2) is strongly suggestive of *IL23R* being a potential susceptibility gene and therapeutic target for UC in the north Indian population as well. However, the strength of association of this gene may vary in different populations. It may be mentioned here that resequencing of the complete *IL23R* exonic regions in 30 north Indian population based controls did not reveal any exonic SNPs in this gene. Thus, the suggestive association of SNPs around this gene (Table 2) may indicate the role of regulatory variants in *IL23R* in UC etiology in our cohort. Alternatively, the associated SNP may be in linkage disequilibrium with another yet undetected causal variant. These results also demonstrate the importance of normative allelic data for populations under investigation while selecting SNPs for replication of association findings in them. Absence of *IL23R* SNPs (rs11465804 and rs11209026) has also been reported in Japanese, Korean and Chinese cohorts [7,24–26]. Such a fluctuation in allele frequencies across geographic regions could be attributed to different environmental conditions leading to apparent genetic/ allelic heterogeneity of disease between Asians and Caucasians.

An enticing highlight of this study is that we could replicate a few previously acknowledged UC specific SNPs in or near genes/ loci such as RNF186, IL10, DLD, and NKX2-3 with HLA-DRA leading the list (Table 1). The anti-inflammatory cytokine IL10 has long been proposed to limit intestinal inflammation, and genetically engineered IL-10 deficient mice develop spontaneous colitis suggesting it might serve as a therapeutic target for UC [27]. NKX2-3, association of which has previously been shown with CD, is a transcription factor gene found to be associated with UC among Caucasians [6] seems to be a generic IBD gene in our sample also. Reassessment of such potential regions in both Caucasian and north Indian populations, who are ethnically related to Caucasian stock [28] may illuminate the common key pathogenic pathways underlying UC.

It has been reported that there exists an excess clustering of both CD and UC in families, which underscores the concept that the genetic architecture of these two disorders are overlapping. Of the 49 informative index SNPs tested in our UC cohort, 17 have been previously reported to be CD specific (Table 1). Of these, observed association of functionally relevant CD loci such as JAK2, IL18RAP, LYRM4, TRIB1, TNFSF15, ZPBP2 with BTNL2 and NOD2 at the forefront is noteworthy (Table 1). Recent investigation has shown an association between BTNL2 gene and UC in population of European and Asian descent [29–30]. Both in our previous [16] and this study we observed association of *NOD2* with UC in the north Indian cohort suggesting the ethnic-specificity of this gene. Further, to investigate its possible contribution to CD, extensive resequencing in our CD cohort ($N=50$) was carried out. Similar to UC, absence of SNPs 8, 12 and 13 and occurrence of Pro268Ser indicated that allelic heterogeneity with regards to *NOD2* may be at play for CD as well. It has been reported that SNPs 8, 12 and 13 represent 82% of the NOD2-mutated chromosomes, [31] and that these polymorphisms account for about 18% of the genetic risk of CD in the Caucasian population [32]. Thus, our findings reiterate population specific genetic susceptibilities underlying complex disorders such as IBD which is a pathogen driven condition. These observations were corroborated by *ATG16L1* ($p=0.05$) (Table 1) further support that population specific disease susceptibility genes exist for IBD. Additionally, *FCGR2A-FCGR2C* region which reached genome-wide significance in both Japanese and Caucasian cohorts [6–7] was not significant in our population (Table 1). Similar findings have also been reported for TNFSF-15 wherein the variants strongly associated with Caucasian UC cohort were not significant in Japanese UC samples [33].

To summarize, our replication attempt of meta-analysis findings clearly reveal (a) partial concordance of Caucasian based meta-analysis results; and (b) apparent genetic/ allelic heterogeneity at UC/CD loci. It is likely that some SNPs that did not pass correction may be associated with UC in north Indians but the study did not have sufficient power to detect these associations. In conclusion, the observed disparity in the allele frequency of GWAS hits in our cohort confirms differences in genetic architecture between populations. These results also suggest that

Table 1. Association status of 59 GWAS reported UC/CD specific susceptibility loci in a north Indian UC cohort.

Meta-analysis Index SNPs[a]	Chr	Gene/Locus of interest	Previously identified phenotype in caucasians	P-value	Allele	OR
rs1317209	1	RNF186	UC	0.62		
rs3806308	1	RNF186	UC	0.008*	A	0.80
rs6426833	1	RNF186	UC	0.0004**	G	0.74
rs2201841	1	IL23R	UC	0.044*	A	0.85
rs11465804[b]	1	IL23R	CD	-		
rs11209026[b]	1	IL23R	UC	-		
rs2476601[b]	1	PTPN22	CD	-		
rs2274910	1	ITLN1	CD	0.08		
rs10800309	1	FCGR2A	UC	0.40		
rs9286879	1	LOC441915	CD	0.15		
rs3024505	1	IL10	UC	0.001**	A	1.41
rs11584383	1	KIF21B	CD	0.41		
rs780094	2	GCKR	CD	0.027*	A	1.21
rs6706689	2	PUS10	UC	0.33		
rs13003464	2	PUS10	IBD	0.68		
rs917997	2	IL18RAP	CD	0.006*	A	1.23
rs3828309	2	ATG16L1	CD	0.06		
rs3197999	3	MST1	IBD	0.027*	A	1.21
rs4957048	5	CEP72	UC	0.65		
rs4613763[b]	5	LOC730002	CD	-		
rs2188962	5	LOC441108	CD	0.028*	A	1.27
rs10045431	5	IL12B	CD	0.33		
rs13361189[c]	5	IRGM	CD	-		
rs12529198	6	LYRM4	CD	0.020*	G	0.80
rs6908425	6	CDKAL1	CD	0.90		
rs3763313	6	BTNL2	CD	0.00002**	C	0.56
rs2395185	6	HLA-DRA	UC	0.000002**	A	0.63
rs7758080	6	MAP3K7IP2	CD	0.32		
rs2301436	6	FGFR1OP	CD	0.047*	A	1.17
rs7746082	6	PRDM1	CD	0.019*	A	1.24
rs17309827[c]	6	SLC22A23	CD	-		
rs1456893	7	ZPBP	CD	0.12		
rs4598195	7	DLD	UC	0.005*	C	0.78
rs1551398	8	TRIB1	CD	0.004*	A	1.24
rs10758669	9	JAK2	CD	0.008*	C	1.22
rs4077515	9	CARD9	UC	0.16		
rs4263839	9	TNFSF15	CD	0.019*	A	0.81
rs11190140	10	NKX2-3	IBD	0.006*	A	1.23
rs17582416	10	CUL2	CD	0.14		
rs10995271	10	ZNF365	CD	0.43		
rs7927894	11	C11orf29	CD	0.09		
rs1558744	12	LOC341333	UC	0.31		
rs971545	12	IL26	UC	0.73		
rs11175593[c]	12	LRRK2,MUC19	CD	-		
rs3764147	13	C13orf31	CD	0.282		
rs2066843	16	NOD2	CD	0.0002**	A	1.46
rs2066844[c]	16	CARD15	CD	-		
rs2066845[c]	16	CARD15	CD	-		

Table 1. Cont.

Meta-analysis Index SNPs[a]	Chr	Gene/Locus of interest	Previously identified phenotype in caucasians	P-value	Allele	OR
rs2066847[c]	16	CARD15	CD	-		
rs2872507	17	ZPBP2	CD	0.009*	A	1.22
rs2305480	17	GSDML	UC	0.011*	A	1.21
rs744166	17	STAT3	CD	0.047*	G	0.86
rs991804	17	CCL2	CD	0.06		
rs8098673	18	LOC728473	CD	0.038*	C	0.85
rs2542151	18	PTPN2	CD	0.041*	G	1.21
rs4807569	19	SBNO2	CD	0.53		
rs2836878	21	LOC391282	UC	0.011*	A	0.79
rs762421	21	ICOSLG	CD	0.09		
rs1736135	21	LOC388814	CD	0.85		

[a]Mc Govern, et al., Genome-wide association identifies multiple ulcerative colitis susceptibility loci (2010) Nat Genet.; 42(4):332-7.
[b]Monomorphic.
[c]SNPs not in the Illumina Human600W-Quad used in this study.
*p<0.05.
**Significant after Bonferroni correction.

resources such as HapMap need to be extended to cover diverse ethnic populations within the Indian subcontinent in order to enhance their utility for the conduct of association studies within these heterogeneous populations. Further, as the current study was limited to a selection of SNPs identified as susceptibility markers from the recent UC specific meta-analysis, a systematic GWAS in this terrain may not only be insightful for identifying population specific IBD risk conferring loci but also enable cross-ethnicity fine mapping of disease loci. Collectively, these data may help define the genetic relationship between CD and UC and thus unravel common, as well as disease-specific mechanisms of pathogenesis in diverse populations.

Table 2. List of significant (p<0.05) SNPs in and around IL23R gene.

SNP	Allele	P-value	OR (95% Confidence Intervals)
rs10889657	G	0.005	0.79 (0.67–0.95)
rs1884444	C	0.01	0.83 (0.70–0.96)
rs2064689	A	0.01	0.81 (0.69–0.97)
rs10489630	C	0.02	0.83 (0.71–0.98)
rs1004819	G	0.04	0.86 (0.72–0.97)
rs7517847	C	0.004	0.79 (0.67–0.94)
rs6682033	G	0.01	0.76 (0.62–0.96)
rs1343151	A	0.01	0.77 (0.61–0.93)
rs11209032	G	0.02	0.84 (0.70–0.94)
rs1495965	A	0.03	0.85 (0.71–0.96)
rs3790562	G	0.02	0.69 (0.51–0.95)
rs3790565	G	0.01	0.76 (0.63–0.99)
rs4297265	G	0.04	0.86 (0.75–1.02)
rs2270614	A	0.04	0.86 (0.75–1.02)
rs7555183	A	0.02	0.84 (0.75–1.03)

Materials and Methods

Ethics Statement

Ethical approval for this study was given by the respective institutional ethical committees (IEC, DMCH and IEC, UDSC) and informed written consent was acquired from the participants.

UC and control subjects

A case-control study was carried out in subjects recruited from a tertiary hospital in Punjab, India. In brief, the diagnosis of UC was based on standard criteria that included clinical, endoscopic, radiologic and histopathological criteria. Patients with infectious colitis and indeterminate colitis were excluded. Controls were individuals recruited from the same study hospital and included blood donors and patients diagnosed with other ailments not related to IBD. Controls were selected such that they were ethnically similar to the cases and whose age range (±10 years) was within that of the cases.

DNA extraction and Genotyping

DNA was collected from peripheral blood samples of UC patients and control samples using conventional phenol-chloroform method. For replicating meta-analysis based associations, 648 cases and 850 controls were genotyped using Infinium Human 660W-quad. Quality control steps were applied before the SNP genotypes were included in the final analysis. The average genotyping success rate was 99% and no marker deviated significantly (P<0.0001) from Hardy–Weinberg equilibrium in controls. In addition, SNPs with a minor allele frequency (MAF)<0.05 and missingness rate >0.05 were excluded. SNPs were tested for association with UC by Chi-square test implemented in PLINK [16] and Bonferroni correction was also applied.

Resequencing

Exonic and exon-intron boundary regions of both *NOD2* and *IL23R* were amplified by PCR and sequenced on an ABI 3730

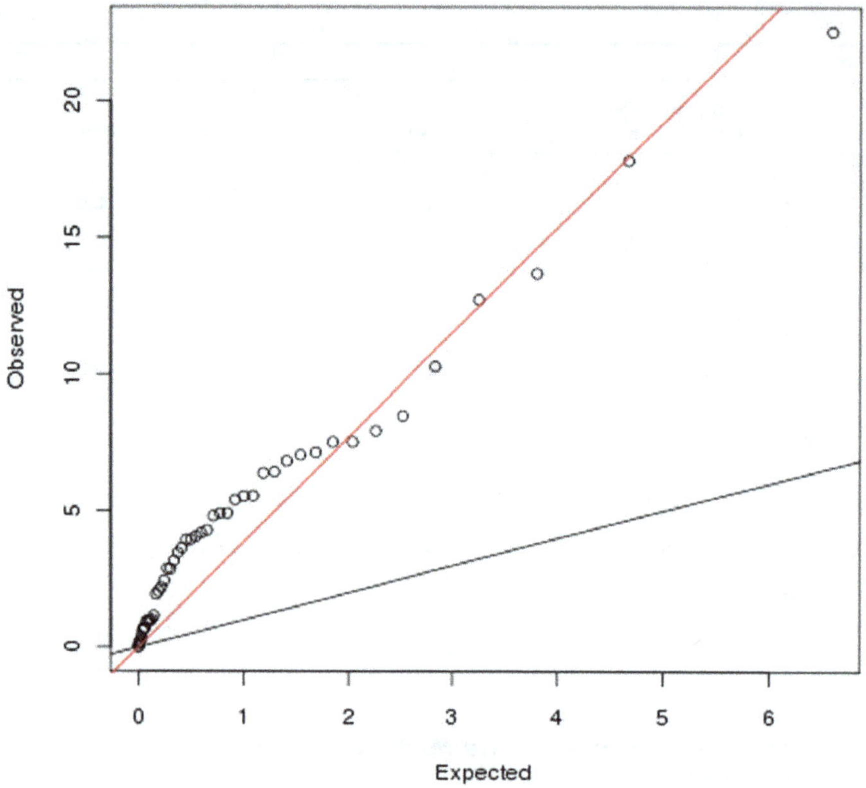

Figure 1. Quantile-Quantile plot of chi-square test of association p-values of 49 SNPs.

genetic analyzer. Details of primers used for amplification of all the exons are available on request.

Acknowledgments

We thank Prof. Cisca Wijmenga, Dept. of Human Genetics, University of Groningen, The Netherlands for her critical inputs. We gratefully acknowledge the Central Instrumentation, Facility, University of Delhi South Campus, for the sequencing work.

Author Contributions

Conceived and designed the experiments: TBK RCJ AS VM DA GJ. Performed the experiments: GJ PP. Analyzed the data: GJ PP SS. Contributed reagents/materials/analysis tools: TBK VM AS. Wrote the paper: GJ. Candidate gene associations and resequencing: GJ MS. Editing: GJ PP SS VM AS DA RCJ TBK.

References

1. Sood A, Midha V, Sood N, Bhatia AS, Avasthi G (2003) Incidence and prevalence of ulcerative colitis in Punjab, North India. Gut 52(11): 1587–90.
2. Fisher SA, Tremelling M, Anderson CA, Gwilliam R, Bumpstead S, et al. (2008) Genetic determinants of ulcerative colitis include the ECM1 locus and five loci implicated in Crohn's disease. Nat Genet 40(6): 710–712.
3. Franke A, Balschun T, Karlsen TH, Sventoraityte J, Nikolaus S, et al. (2008) Sequence variants in IL10, ARPC2 and multiple other loci contribute to ulcerative colitis susceptibility. Nat Genet 40(11): 1319–23.
4. Silverberg MS, Cho JH, Rioux JD, McGovern DP, Wu J, Annese V, et al. (2009) Ulcerative colitis-risk loci on chromosomes 1p36 and 12q15 found by genome-wide association study. Nat Genet 2009; 41(2): 216–20.
5. Franke A, Balschun T, Sina C, Ellinghaus D, Häsler R, et al. (2010) Genome-wide association study for ulcerative colitis identifies risk loci at 7q22and 22q13 (IL17REL). Nat Genet 2010; 42(4): 292–4.
6. McGovern DP, Gardet A, Törkvist L, Goyette P, Essers J, et al. (2010) Genome-wide association identifies multiple ulcerative colitis susceptibility loci. Nat Genet 42(4): 332–7.
7. Asano K, Matsuhita T, Umeno J, Hosono N, Takahashi A, et al. (2009) A genome-wide association study identifies three new susceptibility loci for ulcerative colitis in the Japanese population. Nature Genetics 41: 1325–1329.
8. Yamazaki K, McGovern D, Ragoussis J, Paolucci M, Butler H, et al. (2005) Single nucleotide polymorphisms in TNFSF15 confer susceptibility to Crohn's disease. Hum Mol Genet 15; 14(22): 3499–506.
9. Duerr RH, Taylor KD, Brant SR, Rioux JD, Silverberg MS, et al. (2006) A genome-wide association study identifies IL23R as an inflammatory bowel disease gene. Science 314(5804): 1461–3.
10. Hampe J, Franke A, Rosenstiel P, Till A, Teuber M, et al. (2007) A genome-wide association scan of nonsynonymous SNPs identifies a susceptibility variant for Crohn disease in ATG16L1. Nat Genet 39(2): 207–11.
11. Barrett JC, Hansoul S, Nicolae DL, Cho JH, Duerr RH, et al. (2008) Genome-wide association defines more than 30 distinct susceptibility loci for Crohn's disease. Nat Genet 40(8): 955–62.
12. The Wellcome Trust Case Control Consortium (2007) Genome-wide association study of 14,000 cases of seven common diseases and 3,000 shared controls. Nature 447: 661–678.
13. Franke A, Balschun T, Karlsen TH, Hedderich J, May S, et al. (2008) Replication of signals from recent studies of Crohn's disease identifies previously unknown disease loci for ulcerative colitis. Nat Genet 40(6): 713–5.
14. Zhernakova A, van Diemen CC, Wijmenga C (2009) Detecting shared pathogenesis from the shared genetics of immune-related diseases. Nat Rev Genet 10(1): 43–55.
15. Budarf ML, Labbe C, David G, Rioux JD (2009) GWA studies: rewriting the story of IBD. Trends Genet 25: 137–46.
16. Juyal G, Amre D, Midha V, Sood A, Seidman E, et al. (2007) Evidence of allelic heterogeneity for associations between the NOD2/CARD15 gene and ulcerative colitis among North Indians. Aliment Pharmacol Ther 26(10): 1325–32.
17. Purcell S, Neale B, Todd-Brown K, Thomas L, Ferreira MA, et al. (2007) PLINK: a tool set for whole-genome association and population-based linkage analyses. Am J Hum Genet 81(3): 559–75.
18. Weersma RK, Zhernakova A, Nolte IM, Lefebvre C, Rioux JD, et al. (2008) ATG16L1 and IL23R are associated with inflammatory bowel diseases but not with celiac disease in the Netherlands. Am J Gastroenterol 103(3): 621–7.

19. Tremelling M, Cummings F, Fisher SA, Mansfield J, Gwilliam R, et al. (2007) IL23R variation determines susceptibility but not disease phenotype in inflammatory bowel disease. Gastroenterology 132(5): 1657–64.
20. UK IBD Genetics Consortium, Barrett JC, Lee JC, Lees CW, Prescott NJ, et al. (2009) Genome-wide association study of ulcerative colitis identifies three new susceptibility loci, including the HNF4A region. Nat Genet 41(12): 1330–4.
21. Raelson JV, Little RD, Ruether A, Fournier H, Paquin B, et al. (2007) Genome-wide association study for Crohn's disease in the Quebec Founder Population identifies multiple validated disease loci. Proc Natl Acad Sci 104(37): 14747–52.
22. Roberts RL, Gearry RB, Hollis-Moffatt JE, Miller AL, Reid J, et al. (2007) IL23R R381Q and ATG16L1 T300A are strongly associated with Crohn's disease in a study of New Zealand Caucasians with inflammatory bowel disease. Am J Gastroenterol 102(12): 2754–61.
23. Büning C, Schmidt HH, Molnar T, De Jong DJ, Fiedler T, et al. (2007) Heterozygosity for IL23R p.Arg381Gln confers a protective effect not only against Crohn's disease but also ulcerative colitis. Aliment Pharmacol Ther 26(7): 1025–33.
24. Yang SK, Park M, Lim J, Park SH, Ye BD, et al. (2009) Contribution of IL23R but not ATG16L1 to Crohn's disease susceptibility in Koreans. Inflamm Bowel Dis 15(9): 1385–90.
25. Yamazaki K, Onouchi Y, Takazoe M, Kubo M, Nakamura Y, et al. (2007) Association analysis of genetic variants in IL23R, ATG16L1 and 5p13.1 loci with Crohn's disease in Japanese patients. J Hum Genet 52(7): 575–83.
26. Bin C, Zhirong Z, Xiaoqin W, Minhu C, Mei L, et al. (2009) Contribution of rs11465788 in IL23R gene to Crohn's disease susceptibility and phenotype in Chinese population. J Genet 88(2): 191–6.
27. Madsen KL, Doyle JS, Tavernini MM, Jewell LD, Rennie RP, et al. (2000) Antibiotic therapy attenuates colitis in interleukin 10 gene-deficient mice. Gastroenterology 118: 1094–1105.
28. Rajkumar R, Kashyap VK (2004) Genetic structure of four socio-culturally diversified caste populations of southwest India and their affinity with related Indian and global groups. BMC Genetics 5: 23.
29. Mochida A, Kinouchi Y, Negoro K, Takahashi S, Takagi S, et al. (2007) Butyrophilin-like 2 gene is associated with ulcerative colitis in the Japanese under strong linkage disequilibrium with HLA-DRB1*1502. Tissue Antigens 70: 128–35.
30. Fisher SA, Tremelling M, Anderson CA, Gwilliam R, Bumpstead S, et al. (2008) Genetic determinants of ulcerative colitis include the ECM1 locus and five loci implicated in Crohn's disease. Nat Genet 40: 710–2.
31. Hugot JP, Zaccaria I, Cavanaugh J, Yang H, Vermeire S, et al. (2007) Prevalence of CARD15 /NOD2 mutations in Caucasian healthy people. Am J Gastroenterol 102: 1259–67.
32. Mathew CG, Lewis CM (2004) Genetics of inflammatory bowel disease: progress and prospects. Hum Mol Genet 13: 161–8.
33. Kakuta Y, Kinouchi Y, Negoro K, Takahashi S, Shimosegawa T (2006) Association study of TNFSF15 polymorphisms in Japanese patients with inflammatory bowel disease. Gut 55(10): 1527–8).

Long-Term Alteration of Intestinal Microbiota in Patients with Ulcerative Colitis by Antibiotic Combination Therapy

Shigeo Koido[1], Toshifumi Ohkusa[1]*, Takayuki Kajiura[2,3], Junko Shinozaki[2,3], Manabu Suzuki[3], Keisuke Saito[1], Kazuki Takakura[1], Shintaro Tsukinaga[1], Shunichi Odahara[1], Toyokazu Yukawa[1], Jimi Mitobe[1], Mikio Kajihara[1], Kan Uchiyama[1], Hiroshi Arakawa[1], Hisao Tajiri[1]

1 Division of Gastroenterology and Hepatology, Department of Internal Medicine, The Jikei University School of Medicine, Tokyo, Japan, **2** Frontier Research Laboratories, Institute for Innovation, Ajinomoto Co., Inc., Kawasaki, Japan, **3** Pharmaceutical Laboratories, Ajinomoto Co., Inc., Kawasaki, Japan

Abstract

Previous work has demonstrated that intestinal bacteria, such as *Fusobacterium varium* (*F. varium*), contribute to the clinical activity in ulcerative colitis (UC); thus, an antibiotic combination therapy (amoxicillin, tetracycline, and metronidazole (ATM)) against *F. varium* can induce and maintain UC remission. Therefore, we investigated whether ATM therapy induces a long-term alteration of intestinal microbiota in patients with UC. Patients with UC were enrolled in a multicenter, randomized, double-blind, placebo-controlled study. Biopsy samples at the beginning of the trial and again at 3 months after treatment completion were randomly obtained from 20 patients. The terminal restriction fragment length polymorphism (T-RFLP) in mucosa-associated bacterial components was examined to assess the alteration of the intestinal microbiota. Profile changes of T-RFLP in mucosa-associated bacterial components were found in 10 of 12 patients in the treatment group and in none of 8 in the placebo group. Dice similarity coefficients using the unweighted pair group method with arithmetic averages (Dice-UPGMA) confirmed that the similarity of mucosal microbiota from the descending colon was significantly decreased after the ATM therapy, and this change was maintained for at least 3 months. Moreover, at 3 months after treatment completion, the *F. varium*/β-actin ratio, examined by real-time PCR using nested PCR products from biopsy samples, was reduced less than 40% in 8 of 12 treated patients, which was higher, but not significantly, than in 4 of 8 patients in the placebo group. Together, these results suggest that ATM therapy induces long-term alterations in the intestinal microbiota of patients with UC, which may be associated, at least in part, with clinical effects of the therapy.

Editor: Fabio Cominelli, CWRU/UH Digestive Health Institute, United States of America

Funding: This work was supported by Grants-in-Aid for Scientific Research (C) from the Ministry of Education, Culture, Sports, Science and Technology of Japan. The funders had no role in study design, data collection and analysis, decision to publish, or preparation of the manuscript.

Competing Interests: The authors have the following interests. Takayuki Kajiura and Junko Shinozaki are employed by Frontier Research Laboratories, Institute for Innovation, Ajinomoto Co., Inc. Kawasaki, Japan & Pharmaceutical Laboratories, Ajinomoto Co., Inc. Kawasaki, Japan and Manabu Suzuki is employed by Pharmaceutical Laboratories, Ajinomoto Co., Inc. There are no patents, products in development or marketed products to declare.

* E-mail: ohkusa@jikei.ac.jp

Introduction

The etiology of ulcerative colitis (UC) is still unknown; however, increasing evidence suggests that the intestinal microbiota play important roles in the pathogenesis of inflammatory bowel disease (IBD), including: a) intestinal microbiota adhere to the crypt epithelium via Toll-like receptors (TLR)2 and TLR4 and then invade the epithelium, resulting in inflammatory cytokine production; b) intestinal microbiota are necessary for the development of spontaneous colitis and immune system activation in IL-2- and IL-10-deficient mice; and c) an overly aggressive cell-mediated immune response to endogenous intestinal bacterial constituents in genetically susceptible patients results in intestinal inflammation [1–4]. Although the immune cells in the intestinal lamina propria balance the requirements for immune tolerance of microbiota with defense against microbial pathogens [5], IBD is described as a state of excessive inflammation in response to bacterial microbiota antigens leading to impaired function of the intestinal barrier [6–8]. Moreover, the intestinal microbiota profile varies considerably between active UC patients and healthy controls [2]. Therefore, appropriate antibiotic therapy against microbial pathogens could alter the intestinal microbiota in patients with UC, resulting in the improvement and remission of active UC.

Previously, we have reported that *Fusobacterium varium* (*F. varium*) was present in the colonic mucosa of a high proportion (84%) of UC patients [9] and that butyric acid, a product of *F. varium* culture supernatants, caused UC-like lesions in mice [10]. Therefore, we recently conducted a double-blind placebo-controlled multicenter trial to determine whether an antibiotic combination regimen (amoxicillin, tetracycline, and metronidazole (ATM) for 2 weeks) against the microbial pathogens of UC, including *F. varium*, induces and/or maintains remission of active UC [11]. The ATM therapy produced an improvement of endoscopic and Mayo scores, remission, and steroid withdrawal in active UC more effectively than a placebo. Moreover, among the patients positive for *F. varium* antibodies, the clinical response rate was significantly higher in the ATM group than in the placebo group vs. the placebo group [11]. That study indicated that *F. varium*, at least in part, is associated with the UC condition. In this study to assess the alteration of intestinal microbiota by the ATM therapy, biopsy samples that were randomly obtained from the clinical trial were analyzed.

We show that the profile of the terminal restriction fragment length polymorphism (T-RFLP) in the mucosa-associated bacterial components is significantly changed at 3 months after the ATM therapy. Dice similarity coefficients using the unweighted pair group method with arithmetic averages (Dice-UPGMA) cluster analysis confirms the alteration of the intestinal microbiota after the ATM treatment. While the *F. varium*/β-actin ratio in the intestinal microbiota, as analyzed by real-time PCR from nested PCR products, is reduced after the ATM treatment, the reduction is not significant compared with the placebo group.

Materials and Methods

Study subjects

A multicenter, randomized, double-blind, placebo-controlled study was conducted between January 2004 and July 2006 at 11 hospitals in Japan [11]. This trial was registered at http://www.umin.ac.jp/ctr/index-j.htm:UMIN000000078 (Newly developed antibiotic combination therapy for ulcerative colitis: a double-blind placebo-controlled multicenter trial). All eligible patients had an established diagnosis of UC. Study subjects were selected from among patients with chronic relapsing UC (at least one relapse per year) with more than 1 year of follow-up and regular visits to outpatient clinics. The eligibility criteria for study entry were mild-to-severe disease with a colonoscopy score of at least 1 (erythema, decreased vascular pattern, and mild friability) based on a scale of 0 (normal or inactive) to 3 (spontaneous bleeding and ulceration), and/or watery diarrhea at least 5 times/day, with visible blood in stools. Patients with toxic megacolon or a penicillin allergy, and those who were pregnant, had serious liver or renal disease or any psychological illness, were excluded. Patients who had taken antibiotics within 4 weeks before study entry or had *Clostridium difficile* or other stool pathogens (*Salmonellae*, pathogenic *Escherichia coli*, *Campylobacter jejuni*, *Shigellae*, etc.) at entry were also excluded.

Study design

We recruited 210 patients and randomly assigned them to either the ATM or the control placebo group in the clinical trial [11]. The ATM treatment group (oral amoxicillin 1500 mg/day, tetracycline 1500 mg/day, and metronidazole 750 mg/day) and the placebo group each had 105 subjects. Each group was treated for 2 weeks and were then followed up. Twenty subjects in these clinical trials were randomly selected for this study. The study used central randomization with a treatment allocation produced by a computer-generated randomization list. Among the 20 patients, 12 patients were in the antibiotic treatment group and 8 were in the placebo group. Therapy was started after initial endoscopy at entry. The follow-up endoscopy was carried out 3 months after treatment to determine whether the antibiotic combination therapy induces and/or maintains the remission of active UC. Biopsy samples were taken from the cecum, ascending colon, and descending colon at the beginning of the trial and again at 3 months after treatment completion. The biopsy samples were immediately placed in formalin for histopathological assessment or in liquid nitrogen for storage at −80°C until the subsequent isolation of DNA. All histopathology, clinical evaluations, and endoscopies were carried out by physicians who were blinded to the patients' therapy. Clinical assessments were evaluated by the symptom score of Lichtiger et al. [12]. Endoscopic-and histological scores were graded according to the Matts score [13]. Histological scores were the sum of the scores of the cecum, ascending colon, transverse colon, and descending colon. The study protocol was reviewed and approved by the ethics committee of the Juntendo institutional review board, Juntendo University School of Medicine, as well as the clinical study committee of the Juntendo University Hospital (No. 2003-016). All subjects gave written informed consent. All authors had access to the study data and have reviewed and approved the final manuscript.

Isolation of DNA

DNA from each biopsy sample (the cecum, ascending colon, and descending colon) was extracted using the UltraClean Soil DNA Isolation Kit (Mo Bio Laboratories, Solana Beach, CA, USA) with some modifications [14]. Briefly, each biopsy sample was washed by gently shaking in sterile water to remove loosely adherent fecal material and mucus. The samples were placed in 2 mL Bead Solution tubes containing 550 μL Bead Solution and mixed by vortexing on a FastPrep instrument (Bio 101, Vista, CA, USA) for 10 s at 4 m/s, followed by the addition of lysozyme (final concentration of 1 mg/mL) and N-acetylmuramidase (final concentration of 20 μg/mL) and incubation at 37°C for 1 h. After incubation, 60 μL of Solution S1 and 200 μL of Solution IRS (inhibitor removal solution) were added and the samples were vortexed on a FastPrep for 10 s at 4 m/s. The supernatant was collected by centrifugation at 12,000 g for 5 min, mixed with Solution S2, vortexed gently, and placed on ice for 5 min. The mixture was centrifuged at 13,000 rpm for 1 min and the supernatant was transferred to a clean microcentrifuge tube. After the addition of 900 μL of Solution S3, the sample was gently vortexed. The mixture was loaded onto a spin filter tube and centrifuged at 12,000 g for 1 min. The flow-through solution was discarded, 300 μL Solution S4 was added, and the spin filter was centrifuged at 13,000 rpm for 1 min. The flow-through solution was discarded and the spin filter was placed in a new tube. Approximately 50 μL of Solution S5 was added, and after the sample was centrifuged at 13,000 rpm for 1 min, the spin filter was discarded and the DNA was collected in the tube.

Nested-PCR

The primers used for PCR amplification of 16S ribosomal DNA (rDNA) sequences were 27F (5′-AGAGTTTGATCCTGGCT-CAG-3′) and 1492R (5′-GGTTACCTTGTTACGACTT-3′) [15,16]. The secondary primers were 529F (5′-ACGTGCCAG-CAGCCGCCG-3′) and 1492R. Primer 529F was labeled at the 5′-end with 6′-carboxyfluorescein (6-FAM), which was synthesized by Sigma-Aldrich Japan K.K. (Tokyo, Japan). Amplification reactions were performed in a total volume of 50 μL containing 5 μL dissolved DNA (100 ng), 1.25 U TaKaRa Ex Taq (Takara Shuzo, Shiga, Japan), 5 μL of 10X Ex Taq buffer, 4 μL dNTP mixture (2.5 mM each), and 10 pmol of each primer. The 16S rDNAs were amplified in a thermal cycler (Gene Amp PCR System 9700; Applied Biosystems, Foster City, CA, USA) using the following program: 95°C for 3 min, followed by 30 cycles consisting of 95°C for 30 s, 50°C for 30 s, and 72°C for 1.5 min, with a final extension period at 72°C for 10 min. The PCR reaction mixture and the PCR cycling conditions in the second round of nested-PCR were the same. Amplified DNA was verified by electrophoresis of aliquots of PCR mixtures (2 μL) on 1.5% agarose gels in 1× TAE buffer. The PCR products were purified using the polyethylene glycol (PEG) precipitation method [17],

Table 1. Clinical characterization of patients with ulcerative colitis in antibiotics and placebo groups.

Characteristics	Antibiotic group (n = 12)	Placebo group (n = 8)	*p*-value
Mean age, year (range)	39.75 (27–69)	44.0 (18–62)	*P*>0.2
Gender (male/female)	7/5	7/1	*P*>0.2
Mean duration of disease, year (range)	7.1 (1–20)	6.4 (1–21)	*P*>0.2
Current activity (mild/moderate/severe)	5/7/0	4/3/1	*P*>0.2
Extent of disease, number of patients (%)			*P*>0.2
Pan colitis	3 (25)	2 (25)	
Left-sided colitis	6 (50)	4 (50)	
Proctitis	3 (25)	2 (25)	
Concomitant medications during study			
Number of patients (%)			*P*>0.2
Sulfasalazine	8 (66.7)	5 (62.5)	
5-ASA	4 (33.3)	3 (37.5)	
Glucocorticoid	3 (25.0)	2 (25.0)	

5-ASA, mesalazine.

with some modifications. A 50 µL aliquot of the 16S rDNA solution was mixed with 30 µL of PEG solution (40% PEG 6000 and 10 mM $MgCl_2$) and 12 µL of 3 M sodium acetate and then centrifuged at 15,000 rpm for 15 min. The supernatant was carefully removed by pipetting, and then the precipitated DNA was washed twice with 70% ethanol and was redissolved in 20 µL sterile distilled water. Negative controls for PCR consisted of sterile water used in place of the DNA template, and they were used in parallel for every round of PCR preparation.

Terminal restriction fragment length polymorphism (T-RFLP) analysis from nested-PCR products

The purified nested-PCR products (2 µL) were digested with 20 U of *Hha*I (Takara Shuzo) in a total volume of 10 µL at 37°C for 3 h. The restriction digestion product (1 µL) was mixed with 12 µL of deionized formamide and 1 µL of DNA fragment length standard. The standard size marker was a 1:1 mixture of the size standard GS 500 ROX (including 35, 50, 75, 100, 139, 150, 160, 200, 300, 350, 400, 450, 490 and 500 bp) and GS 1000 ROX

Table 2. Symptom score, endoscopic finding score, histological score, and inflammatory markers in antibiotics and placebo groups.

Variable	Antibiotic group (n = 12)	Placebo group (n = 8)	*P*-value
Mean symptom score (range)			
at entry	5.8 (4–13)	6.3 (2–13)	*P*>0.2
at 3 months	3.3 (0–8)	4.1 (1–12)	*P*>0.2
Mean endoscopic finding score (range)			
at entry	2.2 (1–3)	1.9 (1–3)	*P*>0.2
at 3 months	1.6 (0–3)	1.6 (1–3)	*P*>0.2
Mean histological score (range)			
at entry	3.2 (2–4)	2.9 (2–4)	*P*>0.2
at 3 months	2.6 (1–3)	2.6 (2–4)	*P*>0.2
ESR (range)			
at entry	19.2 (1–57)	11.8 (1–19)	*P*>0.2
at 3 months	10.6 (1–30)	10.86 (1–26)	*P*>0.2
CRP (range)			
at entry	0.4 (0.1–1.6)	0.4 (0.1–1.5)	*P*>0.2
at 3 months	0.1 (0–0.3)	0.2 (0.1–0.6)	*P* = 0.072
WBC (range)			
at entry	5850 (3200–9700)	5863 (3100–11600)	*P*>0.2
at 3 months	5517 (3100–9000)	6213 (3700–9200)	*P*>0.2

Symptom grades were scored according to Lichtiger et al.'s symptom score. Endoscopic and histological findings were scored according to Matts's grading score. ESR: erythrocyte sedimentation rate (mm). CRP: C-reactive protein (mg/dl). WBC: white blood cell (count/µl).

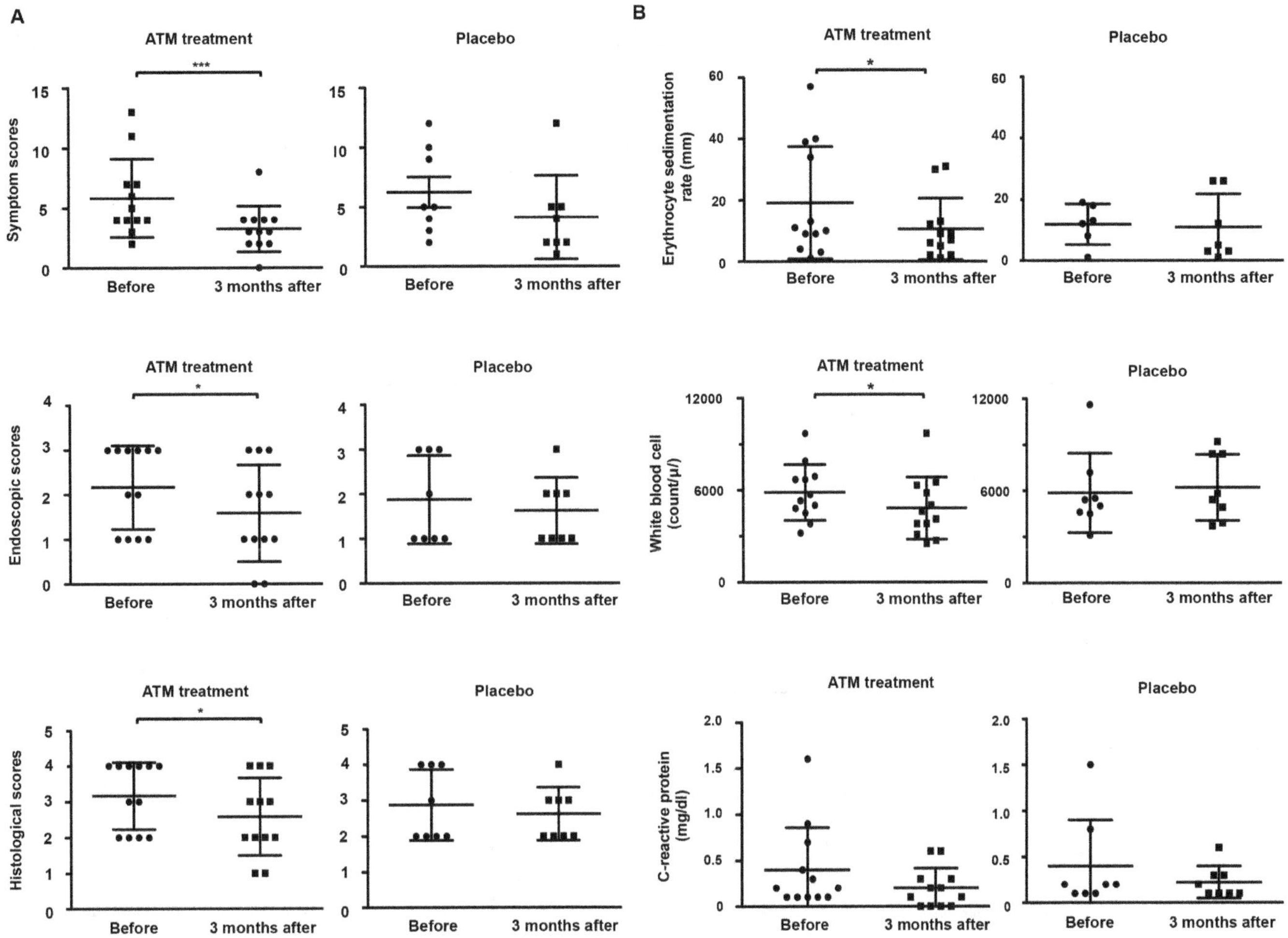

Figure 1. Characterization of the patients with UC. Patients with UC were treated with the ATM therapy (n = 12) or placebo (n = 8) for 2 weeks. (A) The symptom score (upper panel), endoscopic score (middle panel), and histological score (lower panel) at 3 months after the ATM treatment or placebo were compared with the trial start. (B) Inflammatory markers such as the erythrocyte sedimentation rate (upper panel), white blood cell count (middle panel), and C-reactive protein (CRP) (lower panel) at 3 months after the ATM treatment or placebo were compared with the trial start. The results are expressed as the mean ± SD. ***$P<0.001$; **$P<0.01$; *$P<0.05$.

(including 29, 33, 37, 64, 67, 75, 81, 108, 118, 244, 275, 299, 421, 539, 674, 677 and 926 bp) (Applied Biosystems). Each sample was denatured at 95°C for 2 min and then immediately placed on ice. The length of the TRF was determined on an ABI PRISM 3130 genetic analyzer (Applied Biosystems) in GeneMapper mode (15 kV, 8 mA and 60°C for 48 min for each sample). Fragment sizes were estimated using the Local Southern Method in Genescan 3.1 software (Applied Biosystems).

Cluster analysis of T-RFLP profiles

Mucosal microbiota from the ATM treatment group and the placebo group were collected at the beginning of the trial and again at 3 months after treatment completion. Cluster analysis of mucosal microbiota from the descending colon was performed by Dice similarity coefficients using the unweighted pair group method with arithmetic averages (Dice-UPGMA) [18].

Real-time PCR for quantification of *F. varium* DNA

Nested-PCR products were used to quantify *F. varium* DNA because the sample amounts were extremely small. The primer sets for *F. varium* were designed as previously reported [19,20]. The primer sets for *F. varium* were designed by aligning their 16S rDNA gene sequences (obtained from GenBank database) with those from closely related bacteria using the ClustalW program [20]. First, 16S rDNA was amplified using the 27F and 1492R primers [15,16], and then the DNA was amplified using the primer sets specific for 16S rDNA sequences in *F. varium*. The primer sets for 16S rDNA sequences in *F. varium* were (5′-CCGTTGCTTA-TATGGGGTTG-3′) and (5′-CCTCGCAGATTCACACAGAA-3′). The primer set for human β-actin was purchased from Maxim Biotech Inc. (South San Francisco, CA, USA). The primer set sequences for human β-actin were (5′-GCCAACCGCGAGAA-GATGACC-3′) and (5′-CTTTAGCACGCACTGTAATT-CCTC-3′). DNA isolated from biopsy samples (the cecum, ascending colon, and descending colon) was amplified with species-specific primers and the primer set for human β-actin. PCR was performed in a 50 μL volume containing 2.5 μL of the DNA sample, 25 μL of SYBR Green PCR Master Mix (Applied Biosystems) and 15 pmol of each primer. Amplification and detection were performed with a sequence detection system (ABI PRISM 7900HT; Applied Biosystems). The protocol for *F. varium* was 50°C for 2 min, 95°C for 10 min, and then 50 cycles at 95°C for 15 s and 60°C for 1 min. The protocol for human β-actin was

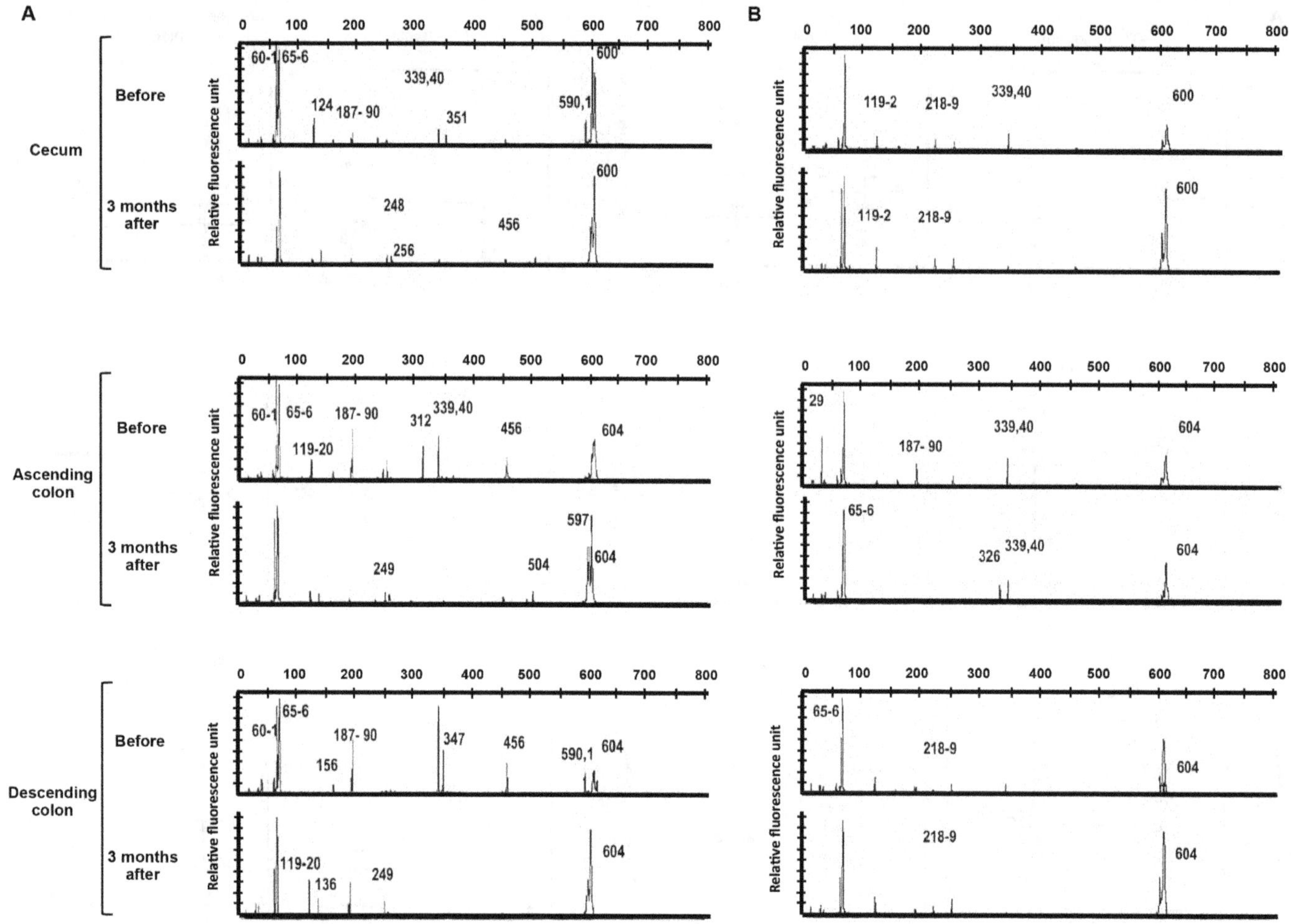

Figure 2. Representative T-RFLP patterns of 16S rDNAs from mucosal bacteria. (A) There were no characteristic peak patterns in the ATM treatment groups. At 3 months after treatment completion, the peak heights of the restriction enzyme *HhaI* were changed in the ATM therapy group (A) but not changed in the placebo group (B).

50°C for 2 min, 95°C for 10 min, and then 50 cycles at 95°C for 30 s and 60°C for 1 min. The number of bacterial cells or human β-actin gene copies in tissue samples was estimated with a standard curve for each species or for the human β-actin gene. The standard curves were drawn using the results from five concentrations of bacterial cells (10^7, 10^6, 10^5, 10^4 and 10^3 cells/μL) or the human β-actin gene (10^6, 10^5, 10^4, 10^3 and 10^2 copies/μL). Finally, the results of real-time PCR for each sample were expressed as the number of bacterial cells per 10^6 copies of the human β-actin gene.

Statistical analysis

Statistical analysis was performed using Student's *t*-test and Fisher's exact test for statistical comparison of clinical, histological, and endoscopic grades, and the number of bacterial cells at the trial start and 3 months after treatment completion. STAT VIEW software, version J 5.1 (SAS Institute, Inc., Cary, NC, USA) was used for all analyses. $P<0.05$ was considered significant.

Ethical considerations

This study, UMIN000000078, was registered at http://www.umin.ac.jp/ctr/index-j.htm. The institutional review board or ethics committee approved the protocol.

Results

Characterization of enrolled patients with UC

Biopsy samples (the cecum, ascending colon, and descending colon) were obtained from 20 patients with UC in the randomized clinical study that had demonstrated the significant clinical effects of the ATM therapy (n = 105) compared with placebo (n = 105) ($P=0.0011$) [11]. The 20 patients included 12 patients from the ATM treatment group and 8 patients from the placebo group. There were no differences in age, gender, mean duration of disease, current activity, extent of disease, or concomitant medications between the ATM treatment and placebo groups (Table 1). Before the treatment, there were also no differences in the symptom [12], endoscopic, and histological scores between the ATM treatment and placebo groups [13] (Table 2). The symptom, endoscopic and histological scores at 3 months after the ATM treatment were significantly improved compared with study entry ($P=0.0033$, 0.0463 and 0.0463, respectively) (Fig. 1A). Moreover, at 3 months after the ATM treatment, inflammatory markers, such as the ESR and WBC, were significantly decreased compared with study entry ($P=0.0226$ and 0.0495, respectively) (Fig. 1B). C-reactive protein (CRP) was also reduced at 3 months after the ATM treatment, but not significantly, compared with study entry ($P=0.0580$). At 3 months after the ATM treatment, the symptom,

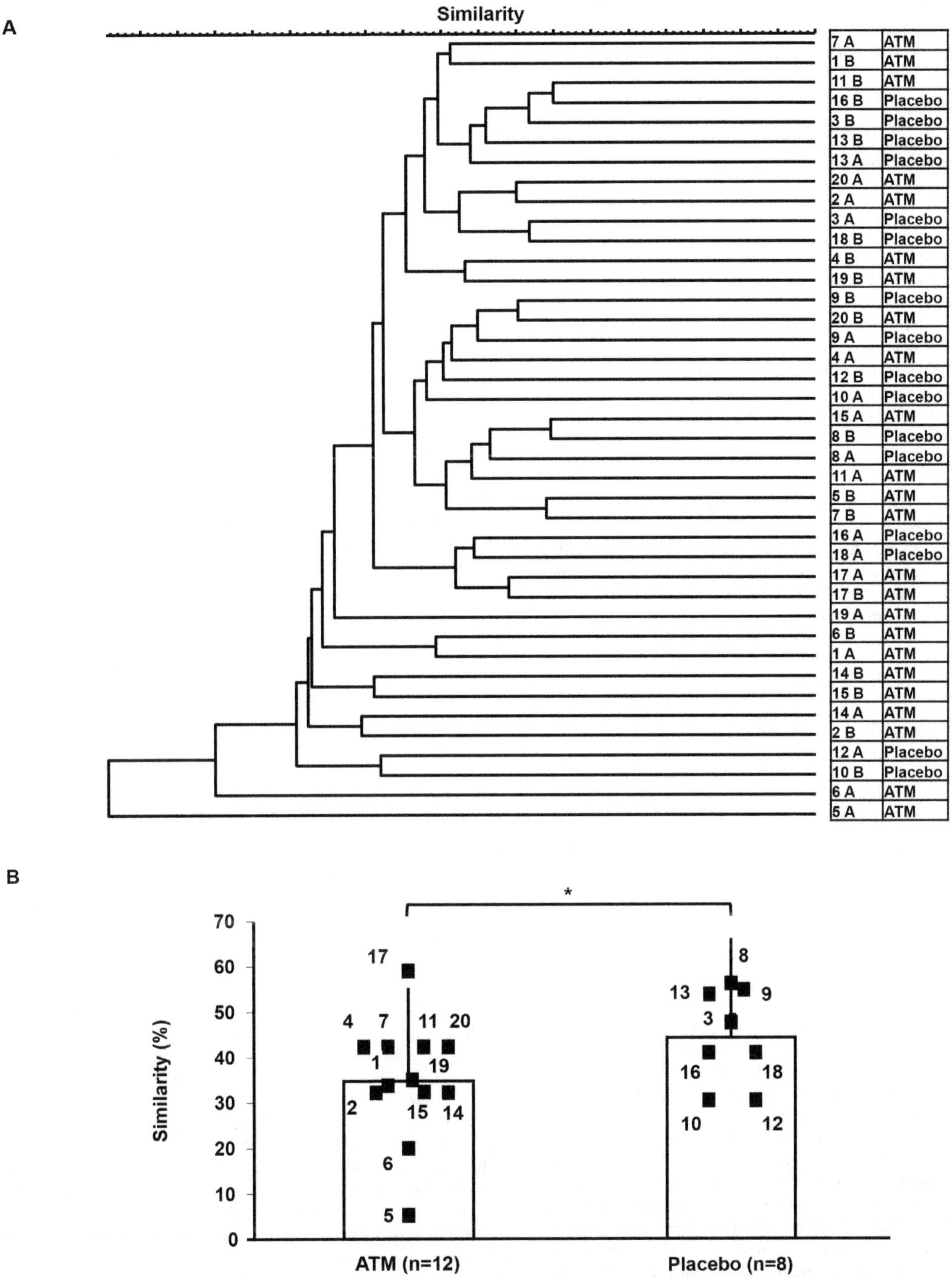

Figure 3. Dendrogram of T-RFLP profiles before and after the ATM therapy. (A) The similarity dendrogram was constructed using a binary coefficient dendrogram (Dice-UPGMA). The numbers indicate the subject code number in the ATM and placebo groups. A; after therapy, B; before therapy. (B) Similarity values from the dendrogram at trial start and again at 3 months after treatment completion (ATM or placebo) were analyzed. The results are expressed as the mean ± SD. *$P<0.05$.

endoscopic, and histological scores were also improved in 25% (3/12), 50% (6/6), 41.7% (5/12) of the patients, respectively, which was higher, but not significantly, than the placebo group (12.5% (1/8), 25% (2/8), 12.5% (1/8), respectively). However, among the 20 patients randomly enrolled in this study, there were no significant differences in the symptom, endoscopic, histological scores or the inflammatory markers at 3 months after treatment completion between the ATM group and the placebo group (Table 2). In addition, no serious drug-related toxicity was observed during the trial (data not shown).

T-RFLP analysis

The 16S ribosomal RNA (rRNA) gene is highly conserved between different species of bacteria and archaea. Therefore, the 16SrRNA gene has been used as the standard for classification and identification of microbes. The genes coding for it are referred to as 16S rDNA. Thus, to avoid contamination by human mucosal DNA, the 16S rDNA was amplified by PCR in all 20 patients. T-RFLP analysis of the PCR amplified product was used to characterize the differences in mucosal flora from UC patients in the antibiotic treatment group (n = 12) and the placebo group (n = 8). The peaks of each T-RF length (bp) show the relative quantity of 16S rDNA fragments for each T-RF length. There were no characteristic peak patterns in UC between the antibiotic treatment group (Fig. 2A) and the placebo group (Fig. 2B). Interestingly, a sub-set of the fragments for the restriction enzyme *Hha*I changed after treatment in 10 of 12 patients (83.3%) in the antibiotic treatment group, but no changes were observed in the placebo group ($P = 0.0007$). These results indicate bacteria whose 16S rDNA fragments change length after restriction by *Hha*I were reduced by antibiotic treatment.

Cluster analysis of T-RFLP profiles

Three months after treatment, the similarity of mucosal microbiota was significantly decreased in the ATM group (35.0%) compared to the placebo group (44.5%) by Dice-UPGMA cluster analysis ($P = 0.0454$) (Fig. 3A and B). This result indicates that ATM therapy can induce and maintain significant alterations of intestinal microbiota in patients with UC at least 3 months after the treatment.

Quantitative analysis of *F. varium*

To analyze *F. varium* quantitatively in the mucosal flora after ATM treatment, real-time PCR from nested-PCR products was used, as clinically obtained biopsy sample amounts were usually extremely small. In the clinically obtained biopsy samples, there are the variations in biopsy size, and DNA extracts of the biopsies have a preponderance of human nucleic acid relative to bacterial nucleic acid. The human β-actin gene has frequently been used as an internal control gene to normalize the expression of the target mRNA levels between different samples measured by real-time PCR. Therefore, we standardized comparison of the numbers of bacteria associated with biopsies by determining the ratio of *F. varium* equivalents to the number of human β-actin equivalents. In this study, the numbers of *F. varium* in each sample (the cecum, ascending colon, and descending colon) per 10^6 copies of the human β-actin gene were examined. Based on this method, the total number of the *F. varium*/β-actin ratio in each sample (the cecum, ascending colon, and descending colon) was 40% reduced after treatment in 8 of 12 patients (66.7%) in the ATM group, which was higher, but not significantly, than 4 out of 8 patients (50.0%) in the placebo group ($P > 0.05$) (Table S1).

Discussion

The data presented here show that the 2-week triple-antibiotic therapy produced a long-term alternation of the intestinal microbiota that persisted at least 3 months compared to a placebo in a multicenter, randomized, double-blind, placebo-controlled study.

To analyze the alteration of mucosa-associated bacteria after the ATM therapy, we first used T-RFLP analysis. In this study, significant profile changes of the T-RFLP in the mucosa-associated bacterial components were found in 10 of 12 patients in the ATM treatment group, compared with none of 8 patients in the placebo group; therefore, ATM therapy is strongly associated with the alteration of mucosa-associated bacteria in patients with UC. UPGMA analysis also confirmed the significant alteration of mucosal microbiota at least 3 months after the ATM therapy. Importantly, an alteration of the intestinal microbiota may cause a breakdown of the barrier function, such as an abnormal immune response to normal flora, and result in UC [21–26]. Therefore, long-term alterations in the intestinal microbiota produced by ATM therapy may be associated with improvements in UC. However, among the 20 patients with UC analyzed in this study, there were no differences in the symptom, endoscopic and histological scores or in the inflammatory markers at 3 months after treatment completion between ATM and placebo groups. The small sample size used in this study may be associated with this contradiction. Indeed, our 20 subjects were from a randomized clinical trial that demonstrated significant clinical effects of the ATM therapy (n = 105) compared with a placebo (n = 105) [11].

Our previous research demonstrated that *F. varium* was one of the causative agents in UC [9,10]. Therefore, we also analyzed *F. varium* quantitatively in the mucosal flora of UC patients treated with ATM. In this study, samples were taken from the cecum, ascending colon, and descending colon at the beginning of the trial and again at 3 months after treatment completion. Because extremely small amounts were obtained in the clinical trial; we tried to quantify *F. varium* by real-time PCR from nested-PCR products in the mucosal flora. We demonstrated that the *F. varium*/β-actin ratio in the ATM treatment group tended to decrease, but not significantly, compared with the placebo group. In contrast, a decreased number of *F. varium* in UC patients treated by the ATM therapy was reported in a previous study [24]. However, the decreased number of *F. varium* in that study was analyzed by real-time PCR using samples taken from the appendix, caecum, ascending colon, transverse colon, descending colon, sigmoid colon, and rectum. Therefore, analysis using the nested PCR products from small amounts of biopsy specimens may not be suitable for quantifying *F. varium* in UC patients. Other pathogens besides *F. varium* may also be associated with the pathogenesis of UC. As these three antibiotics used for the ATM therapy are lethal to many bacterial species, unidentified pathogens could be more significantly decreased by the ATM therapy.

In conclusion, the mucosa-associated bacterial components analyzed by T-RFLP are useful to assess the alteration of the intestinal microbiota in UC after ATM therapy. The ATM antibiotic combination regimen significantly altered intestinal microbiota in UC patients compared to the placebo group. Our study supports the association of microbial agents with the pathogenesis of UC. A limitation of our study is the relatively small sample size. Further studies are needed to evaluate the clinical significance of long-term alteration of intestinal microbiota in UC patients treated with ATM.

Author Contributions

Conceived and designed the experiments: SK TO TK JS MS HT. Performed the experiments: SK TO TK JS MS. Analyzed the data: SK TO TK JS MS. Contributed reagents/materials/analysis tools: SK TO TK JS MS KT ST SO TY JM MK KU HA. Wrote the manuscript: SK TO TK.

References

1. Bell AJ, Nicholls RJ, Forbes A, Ellis HJ, Ciclitira PJ (2004) Human lymphocyte stimulation with pouchitis flora is greater than with flora from a healthy pouch but is suppressed by metronidazole. Gut 53: 1801–1805.
2. Ohkusa T, Yoshida T, Sato N, Watanabe S, Tajiri H, et al. (2009) Commensal bacteria can enter colonic epithelial cells and induce proinflammatory cytokine secretion: a possible pathogenic mechanism of ulcerative colitis. J Med Microbiol 58: 535–545.
3. Furrie E, Macfarlane S, Cummings JH, Macfarlane GT (2004) Systemic antibodies towards mucosal bacteria in ulcerative colitis and Crohn's disease differentially activate the innate immune response. Gut 53: 91–98.
4. Okayasu I (2012) Development of ulcerative colitis and its associated colorectal neoplasia as a model of the organ-specific chronic inflammation-carcinoma sequence. Pathol Int 62: 368–380.
5. Neuman MG (2007) Immune dysfunction in inflammatory bowel disease. Transl Res 149: 173–186.
6. Oliva-Hemker M, Fiocchi C (2002) Etiopathogenesis of inflammatory bowel disease: the importance of the pediatric perspective. Inflamm Bowel Dis 8: 112–128.
7. Danese S, Fiocchi C (2006) Etiopathogenesis of inflammatory bowel diseases. World J Gastroenterol 12: 4807–4812.
8. Feillet H, Bach JF (2004) Increased incidence of inflammatory bowel disease: the price of the decline of infectious burden? Curr Opin Gastroenterol 20: 560–564.
9. Ohkusa T, Sato N, Ogihara T, Morita K, Ogawa M, et al. (2002) Fusobacterium varium localized in the colonic mucosa of patients with ulcerative colitis stimulates species-specific antibody. J Gastroenterol Hepatol 17: 849–853.
10. Ohkusa T, Okayasu I, Ogihara T, Morita K, Ogawa M, et al. (2003) Induction of experimental ulcerative colitis by Fusobacterium varium isolated from colonic mucosa of patients with ulcerative colitis. Gut 52: 79–83.
11. Ohkusa T, Kato K, Terao S, Chiba T, Mabe K, et al. (2010) Newly developed antibiotic combination therapy for ulcerative colitis: a double-blind placebo-controlled multicenter trial. Am J Gastroenterol 105: 1820–1829.
12. Lichtiger S, Present DH, Kornbluth A, Gelernt I, Bauer J, et al. (1994) Cyclosporine in severe ulcerative colitis refractory to steroid therapy. N Engl J Med 330: 1841–1845.
13. Matts SG (1961) The value of rectal biopsy in the diagnosis of ulcerative colitis. Q J Med 30: 393–407.
14. Clement BG, Kitts CL (2000) Isolating PCR-quality DNA from human feces with a soil DNA kit. Biotechniques 28: 640–642, 644, 646.
15. Collins MD, Wallbanks S, Lane DJ, Shah J, Nietupski R, et al. (1991) Phylogenetic analysis of the genus Listeria based on reverse transcriptase sequencing of 16S rRNA. Int J Syst Bacteriol 41: 240–246.
16. Scheidegger EM, Fracalanzza SA, Teixeira LM, Cardarelli-Leite P (2009) RFLP analysis of a PCR-amplified fragment of the 16S rRNA gene as a tool to identify Enterococcus strains. Mem Inst Oswaldo Cruz 104: 1003–1008.
17. Hayashi H, Sakamoto M, Benno Y (2002) Phylogenetic analysis of the human gut microbiota using 16S rDNA clone libraries and strictly anaerobic culture-based methods. Microbiol Immunol 46: 535–548.
18. Sneath PH, Sokal RR (1962) Numerical taxonomy. Nature 193: 855–860.
19. Wang RF, Cao WW, Cerniglia CE (1996) PCR detection and quantitation of predominant anaerobic bacteria in human and animal fecal samples. Appl Environ Microbiol 62: 1242–1247.
20. Thompson JD, Higgins DG, Gibson TJ (1994) CLUSTAL W: improving the sensitivity of progressive multiple sequence alignment through sequence weighting, position-specific gap penalties and weight matrix choice. Nucleic Acids Res 22: 4673–4680.
21. Sartor RB (2001) Intestinal microflora in human and experimental inflammatory bowel disease. Curr Opin Gastroenterol 17: 324–330.
22. Neish AS (2009) Microbes in gastrointestinal health and disease. Gastroenterology 136: 65–80.
23. Zoetendal EG, Akkermans AD, De Vos WM (1998) Temperature gradient gel electrophoresis analysis of 16S rRNA from human fecal samples reveals stable and host-specific communities of active bacteria. Appl Environ Microbiol 64: 3854–3859.
24. Nomura T, Ohkusa T, Okayasu I, Yoshida T, Sakamoto M, et al. (2005) Mucosa-associated bacteria in ulcerative colitis before and after antibiotic combination therapy. Aliment Pharmacol Ther 21: 1017–1027.
25. Imler JL, Hoffmann JA (2000) Toll and Toll-like proteins: an ancient family of receptors signaling infection. Rev Immunogenet 2: 294–304.
26. Szebeni B, Veres G, Dezsofi A, Rusai K, Vannay A, et al. (2008) Increased expression of Toll-like receptor (TLR) 2 and TLR4 in the colonic mucosa of children with inflammatory bowel disease. Clin Exp Immunol 151: 34–41.

17

Haplotype Analyses of DNA Repair Gene Polymorphisms and their Role in Ulcerative Colitis

Avinash Bardia[1], Santosh K. Tiwari[1], Sandeep K. Vishwakarma[1], Md. Aejaz Habeeb[1], Pratibha Nallari[2], Shaik A. Sultana[3], Shaik A. Pasha[3], Yugandhar P. Reddy[4], Aleem A. Khan[1]*

1 Centre for Liver Research and Diagnostics, Deccan College of Medical Sciences, Kanchanbagh, Hyderabad, Andhra Pradesh, India, **2** Department of Genetics, Osmania University, Hyderabad, Andhra Pradesh, India, **3** College of Applied Medical Sciences, King Saud University, Riyadh, Kingdom of Saudi Arabia, **4** Neurobiology lab, Department of Zoology, University College of Sciences, Osmania University, Hyderabad, Andhra Pradesh, India

Abstract

Ulcerative colitis (UC) is a major clinical form of inflammatory bowel disease. UC is characterized by mucosal inflammation limited to the colon, always involving the rectum and a variable extent of the more proximal colon in a continuous manner. Genetic variations in DNA repair genes may influence the extent of repair functions, DNA damage, and thus the manifestations of UC. This study thus evaluated the role of polymorphisms of the genes involved in DNA repair mechanisms. A total of 171 patients and 213 controls were included. Genotyping was carried out by ARMS PCR and PCR-RFLP analyses for *RAD51*, *XRCC3* and *hMSH2* gene polymorphisms. Allelic and genotypic frequencies were computed in both control & patient groups and data was analyzed using appropriate statistical tests. The frequency of 'A' allele of *hMSH2* in the UC group caused statistically significant increased risk for UC compared to controls (OR 1.64, 95% CI 1.16–2.31, $p = 0.004$). Similarly, the CT genotype of *XRCC3* gene was predominant in the UC group and increased the risk for UC by 1.75 fold compared to controls (OR 1.75, 95% CI 1.15–2.67, $p = 0.03$), further confirming the risk of 'T' allele in UC. The GC genotype frequency of *RAD*51 gene was significantly increased ($p = 0.02$) in the UC group (50.3%) compared to controls (38%). The GC genotype significantly increased the risk for UC compared to GG genotype by 1.73 fold (OR 1.73, 95% CI 1.14–2.62, $p = 0.02$) confirming the strong association of 'C' allele with UC. Among the controls, the SNP loci combination of *hMSH2*:*XRCC3* were in perfect linkage. The GTC and ACC haplotypes were found to be predominant in UC than controls with a 2.28 and 2.93 fold significant increase risk of UC.

Editor: Javier S. Castresana, University of Navarra, Spain

Funding: The authors have no support or funding to report.

Competing Interests: The authors have declared that no competing interests exist.

* Email: aleem_a_khan@rediffmail.com

Introduction

The repair of damaged DNA forms an integral part of cell rejuvenation and is known to protect against different diseases [1]. Approximately four major DNA repair pathways viz., nucleotide excision repair (NER), base excision repair (BER), double strand break repair (DBR) and mismatch repair (MMR) [3–5] operate on specific types of damaged DNA [2]. A deficiency in DNA repair capacity due to gene mutations can lead to genomic instability and disease susceptibility [6].

The mismatch repair human mutS homolog 2 (*hMSH2*) genes are integral components of the DNA mismatch repair pathway. The *hMSH2* gene is located on chromosome 2p21, an area initially identified as an important candidate region for genes involved in hereditary nonpolyposis colorectal cancer (HNPCC) [9]. *hMSH2* can form a heterodimer with one of the two other mismatch repair proteins, *hMSH6* or *hMSH3* [10]. An amino acid substitution at codon 322 (*Gly*322*Asp*) of *hMSH*2 may affect the heterodimer formation with other proteins. Other investigators have demonstrated that genotypes in this gene have an increased risk for colorectal cancer [9]. The *XRCC3* and *RAD*51 gene encodes protein involved in homologous recombinational repair (HRR) of double strand DNA [11]. The *XRCC*3 gene has a sequence variation in exon 7 (C18067T), which result in an amino acid substitution at codon 241 (*Thr*241*Met*). This substitution may affect its interaction with other proteins involved in DNA damage and repair [12]. Several study demonstrated that *XRCC*3 polymorphisms are implicated in breast cancer [13], lung cancer [14]. Among several polymorphisms in *RAD*51 gene, a functional SNP at position 135 in 5′ UTR, changing a guanine to cytosine, was reported. Recently, two important meta-analyses [15–16], covering tens of other studies and thousands of subjects, were unanimous to state that the variant allele of *RAD51* G135C may contribute to increased breast cancer susceptibility, which is in accordance with biological function study, which showed a more aggressive and poor prognosis phenotype [17].

UC is complex disease with a strong genetic component [7]. It is presumed to be a multifactorial interplay between host genetics

Table 1. Allele frequency distributions of *hMSH2 XRCC3 RAD51* (G135C) in UC and healthy controls.

	Controls (213)		Patients (171)			
Allele	**N**	**Freq**	**N**	**Freq**	**OR 95% CI**	***p*- value**
hMSH2						
G	348	0.82	250	0.73	0.60 (0.43–0.85)	0.004
A	78	0.18	92	0.27	**1.64 (1.16–2.31)**	0.004
XRCC3						
C	345	0.81	256	0.75	0.69 (0.49–0.98)	0.041
T	81	0.19	86	0.25	**1.43 (1.01–2.01)**	0.041
RAD51 (G135C)						
G	335	0.79	242	0.71	0.65 (0.47–0.91)	0.012
C	91	0.21	100	0.29	**1.52 (1.09–2.11)**	0.012

and environmental factors, leading to an aberrant inflammatory response [8]. The present study explored the impact of polymorphisms in important DNA repair genes (*hMSH2*, *XRCC3*, *RAD51*) in UC. The role of polymorphisms in these genes and their relation in UC needs to be elucidated to understand the pathogenesis of UC.

Materials and Methods

Patients and study design

A total of 171 patients (104 males and 67 females) with UC and 213 (131 males and 82 females) healthy volunteers were included. Healthy controls were selected without any prior history of GI presentations, autoimmune diseases and infections. There was no history of malignancy in the control group or in the UC patient group. The patients were selected from the symptomatic subjects who underwent colonoscopy at the Department of Gastroenterology, Deccan College of Medical Sciences, Hyderabad, India. To avoid selection bias, extensive care was taken not to include any patient with concomitant chronic inflammatory diseases such as arthritis, upper GI disorder etc. All the patients were asked to provide maximum information about their symptoms, disease, duration, and history of any disease that could affect the study outcome. The study protocol was approved by the Institutional Ethics Committee, Deccan College of Medical Sciences, Hyderabad, India. All study participants were asked to provide their written and signed consent to be part of this study protocol.

Genotyping

Five milliliter (5 mL) of peripheral venous blood was collected by venipuncture from all the subjects. DNA was isolated from 200 μL whole blood using a commercially available kit (Bioserve Biotechnology Pvt. Ltd., Hyderabad, India). Polymorphisms at *Thr241Met* in the *XRCC3* gene were screened by polymerase chain reaction (PCR) with specific primers as described elsewhere [18]. Polymorphisms at Gly322Asp in the *hMSH2* gene and G135C in the *RAD51* gene were determined by PCR-restriction fragment length polymorphism as described previously [19]. The 252 bp PCR product was digested at 37°C for 1 hour with 5 U of the restriction enzyme *HinfI*. The *Asp* allele was identified by a 70 and 182 bp fragments and the *Gln* allele as 252 bp. For *RAD51* gene the 157 bp PCR product was digested at 37°C for 1 hour with 5 U of the restriction enzyme *MvaI*. G allele was identified as 157 bp and C allele was identified by 86 and 71 bp fragments.

Statistical Analysis

The sample size was determined by using the openEPi statistics and 95% of confidence was used to detect the results with 90% of sample power. Odds ratios, with 95% confidence intervals were calculated to compare allele and genotype frequencies. The extent of linkage disequilibrium (LD) was expressed in terms of the maximum likelihood estimate of disequilibrium, D′. For each of the SNPs, the covariates such as age and gender were adjusted. A Bonferroni test was performed for multiple testing because this

Table 2. *hMSH2* genotypic distribution in UC compared to healthy controls.

	Genotype	Controls	Patients	OR (95% CI)	*p*-value
Co-dominant	G/G	136 (63.9%)	83 (48.5%)	1.00	
	G/A	76 (35.7%)	84 (49.1%)	**1.81 (1.20–2.74)**	0.0048
	A/A	1 (0.5%)	4 (2.3%)	6.55 (0.72–59.64)	0.095
Dominant	G/G	136 (63.9%)	83 (48.5%)	1.00	0.0026
	G/A-A/A	77 (36.1%)	88 (51.5%)	**1.87 (1.24–2.82)**	
Recessive	G/G-G/A	212 (99.5%)	167 (97.7%)	1.00	0.1
	A/A	1 (0.5%)	4 (2.3%)	5.08 (0.56–45.81)	
Over-dominant	G/G-A/A	137 (64.3%)	87 (50.9%)	1.00	0.0079
	G/A	76 (35.7%)	84 (49.1%)	**1.74 (1.15–2.62)**	

Table 3. *XRCC3* genotypic distribution in patients with UC and healthy controls.

	Genotype	Controls	Patients	OR (95% CI)	*p*-value
Co-dominant	C/C	138 (64.8%)	89 (52%)	1.00	
	C/T	69 (32.4%)	78 (45.6%)	**1.75 (1.15–2.67)**	0.03
	T/T	6 (2.8%)	4 (2.3%)	1.03 (0.28–3.77)	0.95
Dominant	C/C	138 (64.8%)	89 (52%)	1.00	0.012
	C/T-T/T	75 (35.2%)	82 (48%)	**1.70 (1.12–2.56)**	
Recessive	C/C-C/T	207 (97.2%)	167 (97.7%)	1.00	0.77
	T/T	6 (2.8%)	4 (2.3%)	0.83 (0.23–2.98)	
Over-dominant	C/C-T/T	144 (67.6%)	93 (54.4%)	1.00	0.0081
	C/T	69 (32.4%)	78 (45.6%)	**1.75 (1.15–2.65)**	

method is valid for equal and unequal sample sizes and it can be used to correct any set of P values for multiple comparisons. Statistical analysis was carried out using SNPstats software, available online (www.bioinfo.iconcologia.net/SNPstats) and Haploview software. For all tests, significance level was set as $p<0.05$.

Results

Distribution of allelic and genotypic frequency of G322A polymorphisms in *hMSH2* gene

The frequency of **'A'** allele was found to be predominant in UC group compared to controls (27% vs 18% respectively), with a 1.64 folds increased risk for UC (OR 1.64, 95% CI 1.16–2.31, $p=0.004$) **(Table 1)**. Heterozygotes (GA) were found to be predominant in the UC group compared to controls (49.1%, 35.7% respectively, $p=0.004$) with 1.81 folds increased risk for UC, which was statistically significant (OR 1.81, 95% CI 1.20–2.74, $p=0.004$). Based on the dominant model, combination of GA+AA genotypes was also observed to be associated with high risk for UC (OR 1.87, 95% CI 1.24–2.82, $p=0.002$). In recessive model no such variation was observed (compared with GG+GA) (OR 5.08, 95% CI 0.56–45.81, $p=0.1$) **(Table 1)**. Whereas in the overdominant model, GA (Compared with GG+AA genotype) genotype found to be associated with a 1.74 folds increased risk for UC (OR 1.74, 95% CI 1.15–2.62, $p=0.007$), further confirming the risk of **'A'** allele in UC **(Table 2)**.

Distribution of allelic and genotypic frequency of C241T polymorphisms in *XRCC3* gene

The frequency of **'T'** allele was found to be predominant in UC group compared to controls (25% vs 19% respectively), with a 1.43 folds increased risk for UC (OR 1.43, 95% CI 1.01–2.01, $p=0.041$) **(Table 3)**.

CT genotype were found to be predominant in the UC group compared to controls (45.6%, 32.4% respectively, $p=0.03$) with 1.75 folds increased risk for UC, which was statistically significant (OR 1.75, 95% CI 1.15–2.67, $p=0.03$) **(Table 3)**. Based on the dominant model, combination of CT+TT genotypes were also observed are at high risk for UC (OR 1.70, 95% CI 1.12–2.56, $p=0.012$) **(Table 3)**. Whereas in the recessive model, TT genotype (compared with CC+CT genotype) was insignificant in UC compare to control (OR 0.83, 95% CI 0.23–2.98, $p=0.77$) but the overdominant model, CT genotype (compared with CC+TT genotype) is a risk genotype for UC (OR 1.75, 95% CI 1.15–2.65, $p=0.0082$), further confirming the risk of **'T'** allele in UC **(Table 3)**.

Distribution of allelic and genotypic frequency of G135C polymorphisms in *RAD*51 gene

The *RAD*51 gene encodes protein involved in homologous recombinational repair (HRR) of double strand DNA (Cui *et al.*, 1999). The *RAD51* protein is responsible for the central activity of the HRR pathway, in which it catalyses the invasion of the broken ends of the DSB into the intact sister chromatid.

Table 4. *RAD*51 genotypic distribution in patients with UC compared to healthy controls.

Model	Genotype	Controls	Patients	OR (95% CI)	*p*-value
Co-dominant	G/G	127 (59.6%)	78 (45.6%)	1.00	
	G/C	81 (38%)	86 (50.3%)	**1.73 (1.14–2.62)**	0.021
	C/C	5 (2.4%)	7 (4.1%)	2.28 (0.70–7.43)	0.171
Dominant	G/G	127 (59.6%)	78 (45.6%)	1.00	0.0062
	G/C-C/C	86 (40.4%)	93 (54.4%)	**1.76 (1.17–2.64)**	
Recessive	G/G-G/C	208 (97.7%)	164 (95.9%)	1.00	0.33
	C/C	5 (2.4%)	7 (4.1%)	1.78 (0.55–5.70)	
Over-dominant	G/G-C/C	132 (62%)	85 (49.7%)	1.00	0.016
	G/C	81 (38%)	86 (50.3%)	**1.65 (1.10–2.48)**	

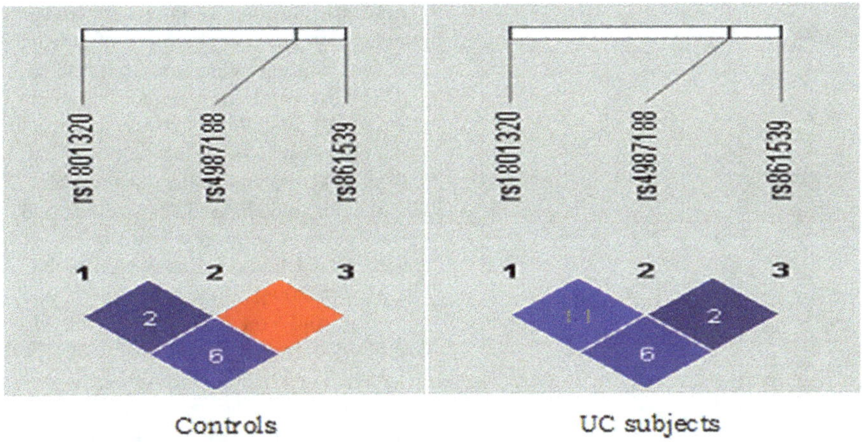

Figure 1. Linkage disequilibrium observed in control and ulcerative colitis groups.

The **'C'** allele frequency was found to be predominant in UC group (29%) compared to the control group (21%) **(Table 4)**.

GC genotypic frequency was found to be predominant in UC group (50.3%) compared to controls (38%) with the difference being statistically significant (p = 0.02). The GC genotype was found to be associated with 1.73 folds increased risk for UC compared to GG genotype (OR 1.73, 95% CI 1.14–2.62, p = 0.02) **(Table 4)**. Based on the dominant model, combination of GC+CC genotypes were also observed to be associated with high risk for UC (OR 1.76, 95% CI 1.17–2.64, p = 0.006). Based on the recessive model CC genotype did not show any statistical significant compare with the combination of GG+GC genotype (OR 1.78, 95% CI 0.55–5.70, p = 0.33) **(Table 4)**. Whereas overdominant model GC (Compared with GG+CC genotype) genotype were also observed to be associated with high risk for UC (OR 1.65, 95% CI 1.10–2.48, p = 0.016), further strengthening the association of **'C'** allele with UC manifestation **(Table 4)**.

Linkage Disequilibrium

In present study, pairwise LD estimates were obtained for the case and control group separately for the *hMSH*2, *XRCC*3 and *RAD*51 gene polymorphisms. The analysis revealed that most of the SNP marker combinations exhibited low LD scores, with the exception of few combinations that showed differential pattern of high LD scores in each of the analysis groups (cases and controls).

While in the control group, the SNP loci combination of *hMSH*2: *XRCC*3 were in perfect LD. In contrast to this, the cases did not show any SNP loci combination with a perfect LD score **(Figure 1)**. Pairwise LD score were also calculated for the three polymorphisms studied **(Table 5)**.

Haplotype Analysis

Haplotype analysis is believed to be more informative approach in strengthening the genetic influence on disease manifestation than testing for individual genotypes, hence haplotypes were constructed based on the four polymorphisms and analyzed for the possible association with UC.

Of the all haplotypes obtained **(Table 6)**, one haplotypes carrying the recessive allele of *XRCC*3 and *RAD*51 polymorphism, **GTC** were found to be significantly predominant in the disease group. The **GTC** haplotype was found to be predominant in UC than controls with a **2.28** fold significant increase, (OR 2.28, 95% CI 1.08–4.83, p = 0.032). Another haplotypes carries the recessive allele of *hMSH*2 and *RAD*51 gene, **ACC** haplotype were found to be significant in UC when compared with control (OR 2.93, 95% CI 1.18–7.28, p = 0.021). Whereas the other haplotype did not shown any statistically significant. Hence these two haplotypes could be the risk haplotype for UC.

Discussion

UC is a chronic inflammatory bowel disease (IBD) of unknown aetiology. The pathophysiology of UC relates to a dysregulated

Table 5. Pairwise Linkage Disequilibrium estimates in controls and Ulcerative colitis group.

	D′	LOD	r^2
Controls			
*RAD*51: *hMSH*2	0.027	0.0	0.0
*RAD*51:*XRCC*3	0.065	0.14	0.004
*hMSH*2: *XRCC*3	1.0	1.67	0.053
Ulcerative colitis			
*RAD*51: *hMSH*2	**0.11**	**0.04**	**0.002**
*RAD*51:*XRCC*3	**0.068**	**0.09**	**0.004**
*hMSH*2: *XRCC*3	**0.021**	**0.01**	**0.0**

Table 6. Haplotype association with response.

Haplotype association with response (n = 384, crude analysis)

	hMSH2	*XRCC3*	*RAD51*	Freq	Control	Patient	OR (95% CI)	P-value
1	G	C	G	0.4695	0.5006	0.43	1.00	—
2	A	C	G	0.1335	0.1462	0.1182	1.10 (0.56–2.18)	0.78
3	G	C	C	0.1246	0.1267	0.1242	1.42 (0.73–2.77)	0.31
4	G	T	G	0.1163	0.1396	0.0847	0.88 (0.45–1.72)	0.71
5	**G**	**T**	**C**	**0.0683**	**0.05**	**0.0921**	**2.28 (1.08–4.83)**	**0.032**
6	**A**	**C**	**C**	**0.055**	**0.0364**	**0.0761**	**2.93 (1.18–7.28)**	**0.021**

mucosal immune response to antigenic stimulation from gut microbiota on a background of genetic susceptibility [20].

Our findings elucidate that the GA genotypic frequency of *hMSH2* was relatively higher in patients than in control (OR 1.81, 95% CI 1.20–2.74, $p = 0.004$) which is in absolute conformity with data of Poplawski *et al.*, (2006) [21] Significant association of *Gly322Asp* polymorphism of the *hMSH2* gene with breast cancer and colorectal cancer [22] was reported. The frequency of A allele was found to be predominant in UC group compared to controls, with a 1.64 folds increased risk for UC (OR 1.64, 95% CI 1.16–2.31, $p = 0.004$).

Our study on genotype CT of *XRCC3* gene polymorphisms showed statistical significance with an OR of 1.75 and 95% CI of 1.15–2.67, $p = 0.03$. Interestingly, similar result was observed in melanoma and bladder cancer [18,12]. Improta *et al.*, (2008) [23] demonstrated a significant association between the *XRCC3* Thr241Met polymorphism and colorectal and lung cancer. This *XRCC3* codon 241 polymorphism was shown to have a significant association with colorectal [24] and lung [14] cancer risk; hence, our findings are in agreement with those reported by Mort *et al.*, (2003) [24]. But no association was found between this polymorphism and squamous cell carcinoma of the head and neck [6], gastric cancer [25] or basal cell carcinoma [26]. The heterozyte (CT) and homozygote variant (TT) genotypes were associated with a decreased risk of bladder cancer but these results were not significant [27]. The study of Shen *et al.* (2003) [28] was the first and the only one to suggest a protective role of *XRCC3* codon 241 polymorphism against bladder cancer risk. The frequency of T allele was found to be high in UC group when compared to controls with a 1.43 folds increased risk for UC (OR 1.43, 95% CI 1.01–2.01, $p = 0.041$).

In *RAD51*, GC genotypic frequency was found to be predominant in UC group (50.3%) compared to controls (38%) with the difference being statistically significant ($p = 0.02$). We found that the SNP in the *RAD51* gene GC genotype (OR 1.73, 95% CI 1.14–2.62, $p = 0.02$) may be an important predictive determinant for UC. Hosseini *et al.*, (2013) [29] also demonstrated that there was a significant association of breast cancer risk with *RAD51* polymorphism. Wang *et al.*, (2001) [30] identified a *RAD51* SNP that may be associated with an increased risk of breast cancer and a lower risk of ovarian cancer. Krupa *et al.*, (2011) [31] found that CC genotype decreased the risk of colorectal cancer in the Polish population. Other data has shown that GC heterozygote of the *RAD51* polymorphism may be associated with the increased risk of colorectal cancer development [32]. Makowska *et al.*, (2012) [33] demonstrated that the variant genotypes of the CC RAD51 polymorphism may be positively associated with colorectal carcinoma in the Polish population. The homozygote variant (CC) genotypes was not associated in UC cohort (OR 2.28, 95% CI 0.70–7.43, $p = 0.17$). However C allele frequency was found to be high in UC group (29%) when compared to the control group (21%). GC genotypic frequency was found to be predominant in UC group (50.3%) when compared to controls (38%) with the difference being statistically significant ($p = 0.02$).

In the control group, the SNP loci combination of *XRCC3:hMSH2* were in perfect LD, there was one other combination that demonstrated a moderate LD effect, i.e XRCC3: RAD51 (D′ = 60). In contrast to this, the cases did not show any SNP loci combination with a perfect LD score. In a recent report, it was found that the 399Gln allele of *XRCC1* was in complete linkage disequilibrium (LD) with the 280His allele of same gene (D′ = 1.0) and the 280His allele was in complete LD with the 194Arg allele in *XRCC1* gene (D′ = 1.0) in both whites and African Americans [21] in cutaneous melanoma. **GTC and ACC** haplotypes could be the risk haplotypes for UC. T′ and 'C' alleles of *XRCC3* and *RAD51* respectively contribution being significant in risk stratification of UC. Sant et al., (2011) [34] identified that the CTC haplotype in BRCA1 gene was significantly associated with decreased mean number of breaks per cell (MBPC).

Further studies on the epistatic interactions are warranted to elucidate their possible underlying mechanisms. Since different populations have distinct genetic backgrounds, it is necessary to validate or replicate such associations with independent samples collected from other ethnic groups/populations.

Acknowledgments

The authors thank the staff and administration of Centre for Liver Research and Diagnostics, Deccan College of Medical Sciences, Hyderabad, India and the Department of Genetics, Osmania University, Hyderabad, India for their support and cooperation through-out the study. Thanks are due to the patients and volunteers who participated in this study.

Author Contributions

Conceived and designed the experiments: AB SKT SKV MAH PN SAS SAP YRP AAK. Performed the experiments: AB SKV MAH. Analyzed the data: AB SKT SKV MAH PN SAS SAP YRP AAK. Contributed reagents/materials/analysis tools: PN AAK. Contributed to the writing of the manuscript: AB SKT SKV MAH PN SAS SAP YRP AAK.

References

1. Friedberg EC (2003) DNA damage and repair. Nature 421: 436–440.
2. Goode EL, Ulrich CM, Potter JD (2002) Polymorphisms in DNA repairs genes and associations with cancer risk. Cancer Epidemiol Biomarker Preven 11:1513–1530.
3. Friedberg EC (2001) How nucleotide excision repair protects against cancer. Nature Reviews Cancer 1: 22–33.
4. Tauchi H, Kobayashi J, Morishima K (2002) Nbs1 is essential for DNA repair by homologous recombination in higher vertebrate cells. Nature 420: 93–98.
5. Wood RD, Mitchell M, Sgouros J, Lindahl T (2001) Human DNA repair genes. Science 291: 1284–1289.
6. Benhamou S, Sarasin A (2000) Variability in nucleotide excision repair and cancer risk: a review. Mutation Res 462: 149–158.
7. Abreu MT, Sparrow MP (2006) Translational research in inflammatory bowel disease. The Mount Sinai Journal of Medicine 73: 1067–1073.
8. Furusho JKY, Podolsky DK (2007) Innate immunity in inflammatory bowel disease. W J Gastroenterol 13: 5577–5580.
9. Leach FS, Nicolaides NC, Papadopoulos N (1993) Mutations of a mutS homolog in hereditary nonpolyposis colorectal cancer. Cell 75: 1215–1225.
10. Mitchell RJ, Farrington SM, Dunlop MG, Campbell H (2002) Mismatch repair genes *hMLH1* and *hMSH2* and colorectal cancer: A HuGE Review. Ameri J Epidemiol 56: 885–902.
11. Cui X, Brenneman M, Meyne J, Oshimura M, Goodwin EH, et al (1999) The XRCC2 and XRCC3 repair genes are required for chromosome stability in mammalian cells. Mutation Rese 434: 75–88.
12. Matullo GG, Carturan S (2001) DNA repair gene polymorphisms, bulky DNA adducts in white blood cells and bladder cancer in a case-control study. Internat J Cancer 92: 562–567.
13. Kuschel B, Auranen A, McBride S, Novik KL, Antoniou A, et al (2002) Variants in DNA double-strand break repair genes and breast cancer susceptibility. Human Molecular Genetics 11: 1399–1407.
14. Jacobsen NR, Raaschou-Nielsen O, Nexo B, Wallin H, Overvad K, et al (2004) XRCC3 polymorphisms and risk of lung cancer. Cancer Let 213: 67–72.
15. Gao LB, Pan XM, Li LJ (2011) RAD51 135G/C polymorphism and breast cancer risk: a metaanalysis from 21 studies. Breast Cancer Res Treat 125: 827–835.
16. Sun H, Bai J, Chen F (2011) RAD51 G135C polymorphism is associated with breast cancer susceptibility: a meta-analysis involving 22,399 subjects. Breast Cancer Res Treat 125: 157–161.
17. Costa S, Pinto D, Pereira D (2008) XRCC1 Arg399Gln and RAD51 5′UTR G135C polymorphisms and their outcome in tumor aggressiveness and survival of Portuguese breast cancer patients. Breast Cancer Res Treat 109: 183–185.
18. Winsey SL, Haldar NA, Marsh HP, Bunce M, Marshall SE, et al (2000) A variant within the DNA repair gene *XRCC3* is associated with the development of melanoma skin cancer. Cancer Research 60: 5612–5616.
19. Poplawski T, Zadrozny M, Kolacinska A, Rykala J, Morawiec Z, et al (2005) Polymorphisms of the DNA mismatch repair gene HMSH2 in breast cancer occurence and progression. Bre Can Res Treat 94: 199–204.
20. Danese S, Fiocchi C (2006) Etiopathogenesis of inflammatory bowel diseases. W J Gastroenterol 12: 4807–4812.
21. Pachkowski BF, Winkel S, Kubota Y (2006) XRCC1 genotype and breast cancer: functional studies and epidemiologic data show interactions between XRCC1 codon 280 His and smoking. Cancer Res 66: 2860–2868.
22. Chio YH, Cotterchio M, Eyssen GM, Neerav (2009) Penetrance of colorectal cancer among *MLH1/MSH2* carriers participating in the colorectal cancer familial registry in Ontario. Hereditary Cancer Clin Prac 7: 1–11.
23. Improta G, Sgambato A, Bianchino G (2008) Polymorphisms of the DNA repair genes *XRCC1* and *XRCC3* and risk of lung and colorectal cancer: a case-control study in a southern italian population. Anticancer Res 28: 2941–2946.
24. Mort R, Mo L, McEwan C (2003) Lack of involvement of nucleotide excision repair gene polymorphisms in colorectal cancer. Br J Cancer 89: 333–337.
25. Shen H, Wang X, Hu (2004) Polymorphisms of DNA repair gene XRCC3 Thr241Met and risk of gastric cancer in a Chinese population. Cancer Lett 206: 51–58.
26. Jacobsen NR, Nexo B, Olsen(2003) No association between the DNA repair gene XRCC3 T241M polymorphism and risk of skin cancer and breast cancer. Cancer Epidemio Biomar Preven 12: 584–585.
27. Fontana L, Bosviel R, Delort L (2008) DNA repair gene *ERCC2, XPC, XRCC1, XRCC3* polymorphisms and associations with bladder cancer risk in a french cohort. Anticancer Res 28: 1853–1856.
28. Shen M, Hung RJ, Brennan P (2003) Polymorphisms of the DNA repair genes XRCC1, XRCC3, XPD, interaction with environmental exposures, and bladder cancer risk in a case control study in northern Italy. Cancer Epidemiol Biomarkers Pre 1:1234–1240.
29. Hosseini M, Houshmand M, Ebrahimi A (2013) RAD51 polymorphisms and breast cancer risk. Mol Biol Rep 40: 665–668.
30. Wang WW, Spurdle AB, Kolachana P (2001) A single nucleotide polymorphism in the 5_ untranslated region of *RAD51* and risk of cancer among *BRCA1/2* mutation carriers. Cancer Epidemiol Biomark Prevent 10: 955–960.
31. Krupa R, Sliwinski T, Jarosinska M (2011) Polymorphisms in RAD51, XRCC2 and XRCC3 genes of the homologous recombination repair in colorectal cancer – a case control study. Mol Biol Rep 38: 2849–2854.
32. Jarosińska MW, Sliwińfski T, Krupa R (2009) The role of RAD 51 gene polymorphism in patients with colorectal cancer in the Polish subpopulation. Pol Merkur Lekarski 26: 455–457.
33. Makowska HR, Samulak D, Michalska M (2012) *RAD51* gene polymorphisms and sporadic colorectal cancer risk in poland. Pol J Pathol 3: 193–198.
34. Sant L, Sucheston LE, Yang Y (2011) Association of Rad51 polymorphism with DNA repair in BRCA1 mutation carriers and sporadic breast cancer risk. BMC Cancer 11: 1471–1477.

Heat Shock Factor 2 Levels are Associated with the Severity of Ulcerative Colitis

Jiarong Miao[1], Junkun Niu[1], Kunhua Wang[2], Yuliang Xiao[1], Yan Du[3], Lifeng Zhou[1], Liping Duan[1], Shuan Li[1], Gang Yang[1], Lifang Chen[1], Mingxia Tong[1], Yinglei Miao[1]*

1 Department of Gastroenterology, The First Affiliated Hospital of Kunming Medical University, Kunming, P. R. China, **2** Department of General Surgery, The First Affiliated Hospital of Kunming Medical University, Kunming, P. R. China, **3** Department of Clinical Laboratory, The First Affiliated Hospital of Kunming Medical University, Kunming, P. R. China

Abstract

Background and Aims: The morbidity of ulcerative colitis (UC) is increasing in China every year. In addition, there is a lack of accurate diagnostic indices with which to evaluate the activity of the disease. The aim of this study was to identify UC-associated proteins as biomarkers for the diagnosis, and objective assessment of disease activity.

Methods: Differential expression of serum proteins from UC patients compared to normal controls was analyzed by two-dimensional electrophoresis (2-DE) and matrix-assisted laser desorption/ionization-time-of-flight mass spectrometry (MALDI-TOF-MS). The expression of heat shock factor 2(HSF2)in colonic mucosa in Crohn's disease, Behcet's disease, ulcerative colitis, intestinal tuberculosis, infective enteritis, intestinal lymphoma, and normal controls was investigated by immunohistochemistry (IHC). The expression of the HSF2 in colonic mucosa of UC subjects with varying severity of disease was measured by real time-PCR and Western Blots. The expression of HSF2 was inhibited by HSF2 small interfering RNA (siRNA) transfection in Caco-2 cells. The concentrations of HSF2, IL-1β, and TNF-α in serum and IL-1β, and TNF-α in the supernatants of transfected Caco-2 cells were determined by ELISA.

Results: HSF2 was differentially expressed in UC patients compared to normal controls. HSF2 expression was significantly higher in the intestinal mucosa of UC patients compared to other six groups. The results of immunohistochemistry, real time-PCR, Western Blots, and ELISA showed that the expression of HSF2 increased in parallel with the severity of UC. The serum concentration of HSF2 also positively correlated with levels of IL-1β and TNF-α. After down-regulation expression of HSF2 in Caco-2 cells by RNA interference, the productions of IL-1β and TNF-α stimulated by lipopolysaccharide (LPS) increased dramatically.

Conclusions: HSF2 appears to be a potential novel molecular marker for UC activity, and may provide a basis for studies on the pathogenesis and novel therapeutic targets for UC.

Editor: Emiko Mizoguchi, Massachusetts General Hospital, United States of America

Funding: This work was supported by National Natural Science Foundation of China (81260074/H0310, 81160055/H0310), Confederative Special Foundation of Science & Technology Department of Yunnan Province and Kunming Medical College (2011FB183, 2007C0010R), Medical academic leader of Yunnan Provincial Bureau of Health (D-201215) and Social development of science and technology projects of Yunnan Province (2013CA021). No additional external funding received for this study. The funders had no role in study design, data collection and analysis, decision to publish, or preparation of the manuscript.

Competing Interests: The authors have declared that no competing interests exist.

* E-mail: myldu@sina.com

These authors contributed equally to this work.

Introduction

Ulcerative colitis (UC) is an inflammatory bowel disease (IBD) characterized by chronic inflammation of the colonic mucosa, often resulting in intermittent bloody diarrhea and abdominal pain [1]. In China, approximately 140,000 cases of UC have been diagnosed during past 15 years, with an 8.5-fold increase during the last 5 years [2]. Although genetic [3,4], infectious [5], and immunological [6] factors have been postulated to be involved in the pathogenesis of UC, the precise cause of the disease remains unclear. UC is currently diagnosed by clinical, radiologic, endoscopic and histopathological findings. Fecal markers such as calprotectin and lactoferrin have been studied for their ability to identify patients with IBD, assess disease activity, and predict relapse [7]. Serum biomarkers such as C-reactive protein and erythrocyte sedimentation rate have been used to assess inflammatory processes and predict the course of IBD progression [8]. Unfortunately, reliable biomarkers for monitoring disease activity have not been clinically established for use in UC. Therefore, more sensitive and specific biomarkers for UC are needed. Proteomics have been applied to search biomarkers in various diseases [9,10]. The aim of this study was to analyze protein expression profiles in human serum from patients with UC and normal control subjects using 2-DE and MALDI-TOF MS analysis.

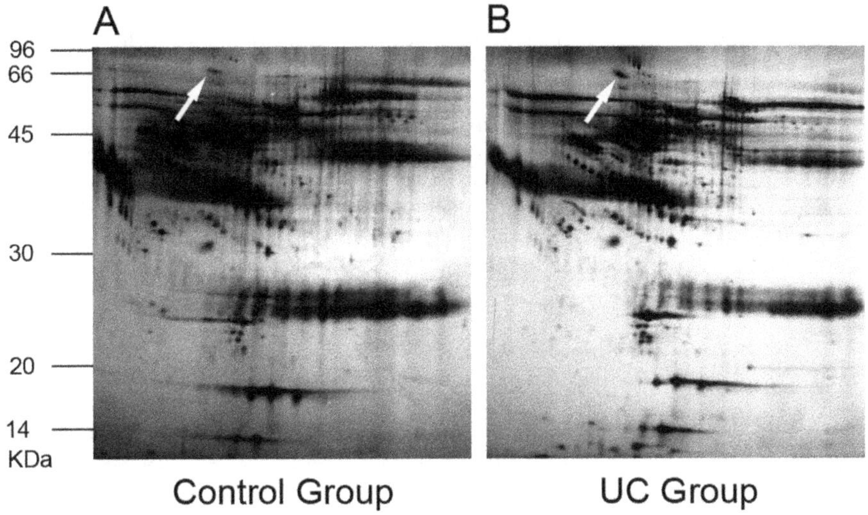

Figure 1. Total proteins from serum of normal control subjects and UC patients were analyzed by 2-DE. The proteins were separated by IEF (pH 3–10) and 10% SDS-PAGE and subsequently processed with silver staining. The spot marked with white arrow represented HSF2. **A**: Total proteins from serum of normal controls that were analyzed by 2-DE. **B**: Total proteins from serum of UC patients that were analyzed by 2-DE.

Materials and Methods

Patients and samples preparation

Patients were confirmed as UC by endoscopy and pathological examination. All blood samples were drawn under limosis condition at the next morning after diagnosis. All UC patients recruited for this study did not take any medications (or herbal remedies), especially the drugs recommend for UC, such as 5-aminosalicylate, glucocorticosteroid and other immunosuppressive agents. The occurrence of medication was excluded in all patients selected for blood samples collection. Serum and colonic mucosal tissue samples were taken from 40 patients (female to male ratio: 1/1, mean age(years): 36.5, rang from 18–60) with mild to severe UC. Disease activity was assessed using the Mayo Score system from 0 to 12, as described previously [11], in which mild, moderate and severe disease activity were defined by scores of 3–5, 6–10 and 11–12. All samples were collected at the time of diagnosis and stored at −80°C. A sample from each specimen was fixed in formalin for immunohistochemical staining. In addition, serum samples of 40 voluntary healthy controls (female to male ratio: 1/1, mean age(years): 34.5, rang from 18–56) were taken under the same conditions as patients' blood, and colon mucosal tissue samples of 10 people (female to male ratio: 1/1, mean age(years): 36, rang from 22–50) who were suspected to have UC, but then were determined to have Irritable Bowel Syndrome (IBS) instead, were chosen as normal controls. To compare the expression of HSF2 in UC with other diseases, paraffin-embedded intestinal tissue samples on-file at the Department of Pathology were obtained: intestinal tuberculosis (31 cases), Crohn's disease (29 cases), intestinal lymphoma (32 cases), Behcet's disease (28 cases), infective enteritis (32 cases). Written informed consent was obtained from all patients at the time samples were taken, and the study was approved by the Ethics Committee of The First Affiliated Hospital of Kunming Medical University, Kunming, China.

Table1. Protein spot identification by MALDI-TOF MS in conjunction with PMF with SWISS-PROT and NCBI non-redundant protein database searching.

Protein Total Spot Score	Protein Identified	Accession Number	Protein Score
Spot1 (181)	Haptoglobin	gi|3337390	208
Spot2 (43)	Aldehyde reductase	gi|225939	60
Spot3 (53)	Receptor tyrosine kinase	gi|225939	62
Spot4 (45)	Pericentriole material 1	gi|450277	55
Spot5 (50)	Heat shock factor 2	gi|13529107	66
Spot6 (39)	Tropomyosin 3	gi|55665776	56
Spot7 (49)	Filamin A interacting protein 1	gi|31542634	62
Spot8 (83)	Apolipoprotein C-III	IPI00657670	97
Spot9 (56)	Keratin 1	IPI00220327	114

Nine protein spots were excised from the 250 mg protein-loaded gel and analyzed by MALDI-TOF MS. A local MASCOT PMF search was performed with its MOWSE-based score (significance threshold score >51, P<0.05). Each EST sequence hit was submitted to a BLASTp search against the entire NCBI nr protein database. The accession number and protein name of nine protein spots are listed.

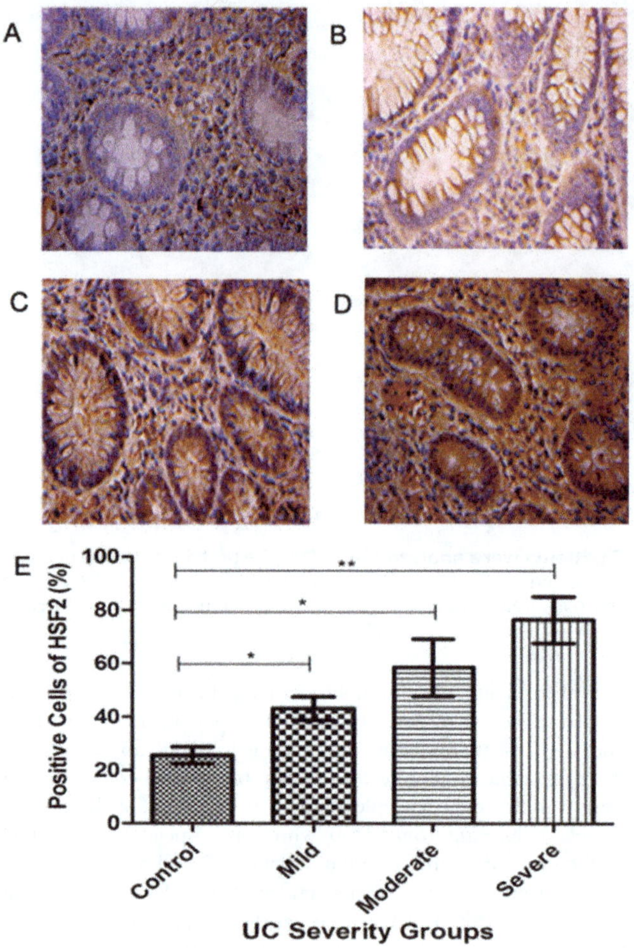

Figure 2. Expression of HSF2 in colonic mucosa tissues of normal control and UC was examined by IHC. A: Representative normal colonic mucosa tissue was negatively stained with anti-HSF2 antibody; **B**, **C** and **D**: Representative UC colonic mucosal tissues of mild, moderate and severe group were positively stained with anti-HSF2 antibody, respectively (magnification, ×400); **E**: Positive cell expression of HSF2 was compared. All IHC results were read automatic image analyzer, measured by HPIAS-2000 analytic software. *, $p<0.05$; **, $p<0.01$.

Two-dimensional electrophoresis (2-DE)

Fasting blood, 5 ml, was drawn from the patients, and centrifuged at 2,000 rpm for 20 min. Non-hemolyzed serum was collected, and 300 µl from 10 cases were mixed. Highly abundant albumin and IgG were removed with an albumin/IgG removal kit (Calbiochem, CA, USA) according to the manufacturer's instructions. Total protein concentrations of serum samples were determined by a Dye Reagent protein assay kit (Bio-Rad, CA, USA). Aliquots were kept at −80°C for two dimensional gel electrophoresis which was performed using an Ettan IP Gphor Isoelectric Focusing System according to the method of Boguth et al [12]. In brief, samples containing about 250 µg of treated serum proteins were dissolved in rehydration buffer, and isoelectrically focused at 250 V for 30 min, 1000 V for 2 h, 10 000 V for 5 h, and 10 000 V for a total of 60 000 Vh/gel. After isoelectric focusing (IEF), each immobilized pH gradient (IPG) strip was soaked in equilibration solution containing dithiothreitol (DTT) and iodoacetamide, and then placed on in contact with the top surface of SDS-PAGE and sealed with agarose. Separation in the second dimension gel was performed using a Tris-glycine running buffer, at a power setting of 5 mA/gel for 0.5 h and 30 mA/gel for 2 h, thereafter at a temperature of 17°C. The protein spots were visualized by silver staining and scanned on Umax Powerlook 1100 scanner. Target gels were analyzed with PDQuest 7.1.0 software including spot detection, background subtraction, and matching. Each assay was replicated three times, and protein spots for comparative analyses were detected on all the gels. Only the spots present in all three replicate gels and qualitatively consistent in size and shape in the replicate gels were considered.

In-gel Digestion

Spots from 2-DE were excised and digested with modified trypsin (Roche, Mannheim, Germany) as previously described by Millares et al [13]. In brief, gel particles were washed and dehydrated with acetonitrile. Proteins were reduced with DTT, and S-alkylated with iodoacetamide. Gel particles were washed with NH_4HCO_3 and then dried under vacuum rehydrated with the digestion solution. After incubation for 30 min at 4°C, supernatants were replaced by NH_4HCO_3, and gel particles were incubated overnight at 37°C. Trifluoroacetic acid, 2%, was added to end the digestion.

MALDI-TOF MS analysis for protein identification

Samples were mixed (1:1) with a saturated matrix solution (α-cyano-4-hydroxycinnamic acid prepared in 60% acetonitrile/ 0.1% trifluoroacetic acid). Matrix-assisted laser desorption ionization time of flight (MALDI-TOF) mass spectra were recorded on a BIFLEXIV mass spectrometer [14]. All spectra were collected in a positive ion reflector mode with a delayed extraction mass accuracy of about 100 ppm. The specific parameters were as follows: the ion acceleration voltage 19 kV, and nitrogen laser operating at a wavelength 337 nm. MS spectra were obtained in the mass range between 2000 and 3000 Da. The singly charged peaks were analyzed using an interpretation method present in instrument software. The nine most intense peaks were selected, and MS/MS spectra were generated automatically, excluding those from the matrix, due to trypsin autolysis peaks. Spectra were processed and analyzed by the Matrix science web which uses internal Mascot 2.1 software to search for peptide mass fingerprints and MS/MS data. Searches were performed against the SWISS-PROT and NCBI non-redundant (nr) protein database.

Immunohistochemistry (IHC) analysis

Colonic mucosal tissues were cut into three sections (5 µm each) with freezing microtome, and put them on the same slide. After fixation, we performed immunohistochemical staining of HSF2 in all cohorts. The HSF2 (1:50, Santa Cruz, TX, USA) primary antibodies were used for antigen detection. HRP-Polymer anti-mouse/rabbit IHC Kit and DAB (3, 3′-diaminobenzidine) substrate kit were used as detecting reagents according to the manufacturer's recommendations (Maxim Biotech, Fuzhou, CHN). The slides were counterstained with hematoxylin, fixed by Scott's solution, and dehydrated with various concentrations of ethanol.

Slides were mounted with permount mounting medium and observed under a light microscope, randomly selecting four visual fields on each slide.

Semi-quantitative analysis of staining intensity for the HSF2 protein was performed using the HPIAS-2000 image analysis software (Tongji Qianping Imaging Inc., Wuhan, China) according to Chen [15] and Wang et al. [16]. In brief, four highly magnified visual fields (10×40 magnification) (with no overlap)

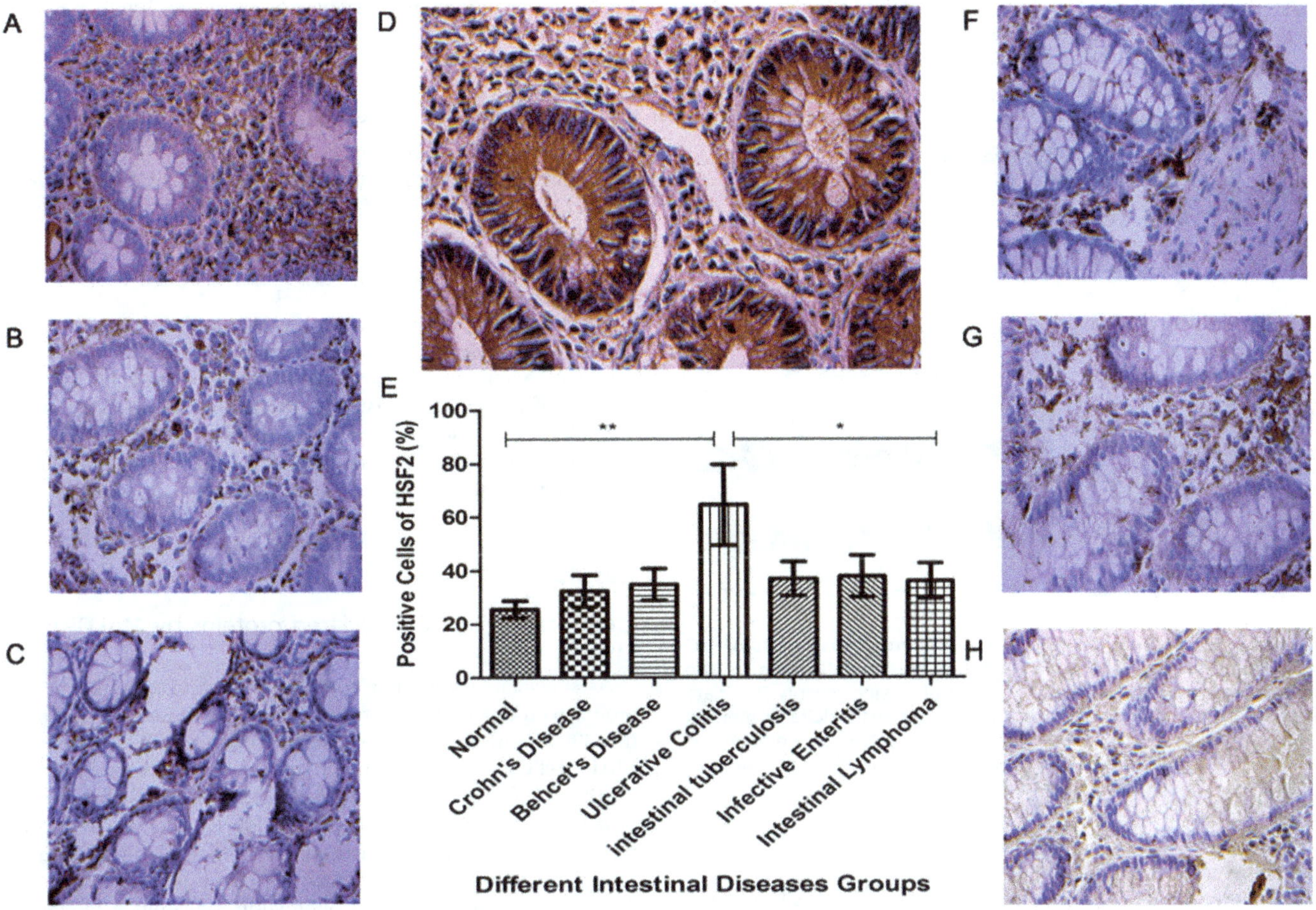

Figure 3. Expression of HSF2 in colonic mucosa tissues was examined by IHC. A: Representative normal colonic mucosa tissue was stained with anti-HSF2 antibody; B, **C**, **D**, **F**, **G** and **H**: Representative colonic mucosa tissues of Crohn's disease, Behcet's disease, ulcerative colitis, intestinal tuberculosis, infective enteritis, and intestinal lymphoma were stained with anti-HSF2 antibody, respectively (magnification, ×400); **E**: Positive cell expression of HSF2 was compared. All IHC results were read automatic image analyzer, measured by HPIAS-2000 analytic software. *, $p<0.05$;**, $p<0.01$.

from each tissue section were randomly selected, and theirs digitalized images were submitted to the image analysis software. HSF2 positive cells defined as those having brown-yellow granules in the cytoplasm and/or nucleus. Integral optical density was automatically measured by the computer with image analysis software. The mean optical density represented the relative expression levels of HSF2 protein. Assessments were performed by two independent pathologists from The First Affiliated Hospital of Kunming Medical University, who were unaware of the HSF2 status.

Quantitative real-time PCR

Total RNA from the colonic mucosal tissue was extracted with TRIzol reagent (Invitrogen, CA, USA) according to the manufacturer's protocol. The first-strand cDNA synthesis was performed with a cDNA synthesis kit (TaKaRa, Dalian, China) according to the manufacturer's instructions. Quantitative real-time PCR was carried out using an SYBR Green real-time PCR kit (TaKaRa, Dalian, China) under the following conditions: initial denaturation at 95°C for 1 min, followed by 40 cycles at 95°C for 15 s, 60°C for 15 s, and 72°C for 20 s. The primer sequences were as follows: human HSF2 (139 bp): 5′-ATAAGTAGTGCTCAGAAGGTTCAGA-3′ (forward) and 5′-GAATAACTTGTTGCTGTTGTGCATG-3′ (reverse), GAPDH (107 bp): 5′-ATGGGGAAGGTGAAGGTCG-3′ (forward) and 5′-GGGGTCATTGATGGCAACAATA-3′ (reverse). Each sample was run three times. The data from the real-time PCR were analyzed with the delta–delta Ct method and normalized to the amount of GAPDH cDNA as an endogenous control.

Western blotting

Colonic mucosal tissue samples and Caco-2 cells were homogenized in immunoprecipitation assay buffer (Roche, Mannheim, Germany) with a protease inhibitor cocktail (Roche, Mannheim, Germany). Homogenates were centrifuged at 4°C, 12000 rpm for 10 min, and the supernatants were collected to determine protein concentration using the Dye Reagent protein assay kit (Bio-Rad, CA, USA). Samples containing 50 µg of protein were loaded on an SDS-polyacrylamide gel electrophoresis, and then electrotransferred onto a PVDF membrane (Millipore, MA, USA). The membrane was blocked with 3% BSA and then incubated with antibodies specific for HSF2 (1:1000, Santa Cruz, TX, USA), Monoclonal ANTI-FLAG M2 antibody (1:5000, Sigma Aldrich, MO, USA), and β-actin (1:5000, Santa Cruz, TX, USA) overnight at 4°C. Membranes were incubated with appropriate peroxidase-conjugated secondary

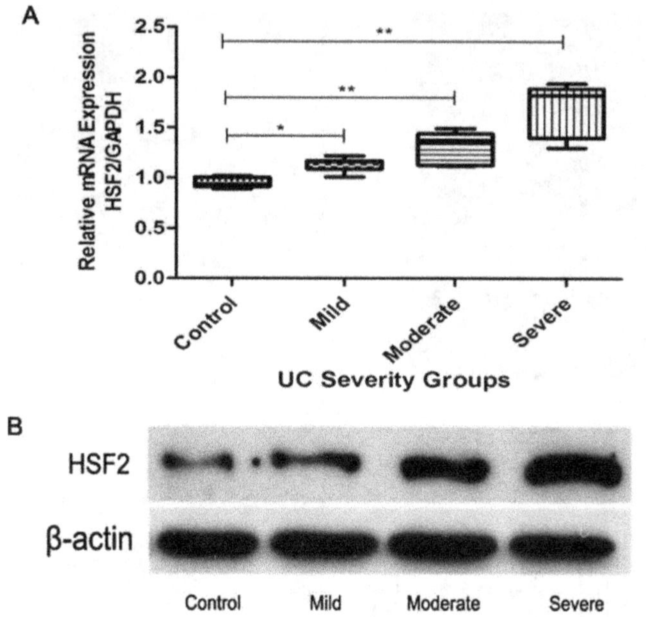

Figure 4. Expression of HSF2 in colonic mucosa tissues of UC was examined by real- time PCR and Western Blotting. A: the mRNA transcriptional levels of UC groups of varying severity. The data from the real-time PCR were analyzed with the delta–delta Ct method and normalized to the amount of GAPDH cDNA as an endogenous control. B: the protein expression levels of different UC severity groups, β-actin as an endogenous control. *, $p<0.05$; **, $p<0.01$.

antibodies (Santa Cruz, TX, USA). The blots were visualized using Super Signal West Pico reagent (Pierce, IL, USA) and the chemiluminescence signal was captured using a ChemiDoc XRS system (Bio-Rad, CA, USA).

Cell culture

Caco-2 cells, a human colon adenocarcinoma cell line that displays enterocyte-like features in culture, were obtained from Cell Bank of Type of Culture Collection of Kunming Institue of Zoology, Chinese Academy of Sciences. Cells were grown at 37°C in 5% CO_2 in Dulbecco's modified Eagle's medium (DMEM, HyClone, NY, USA) supplemented with 10% fetal bovine serum. Cells, between passages 5 and 25, were seeded at a density of 100,000 cells/ml onto 12-well tissue culture plates (Corning, NY, USA) and used at 40%–50%, 70%–80% confluence for RNA interference and plasmid transfection, respectively. After overnight transfection, the Caco-2 cells were treated with 50 ng/ml LPS (Sigma Aldrich, MO, USA) or equal physiological saline (as a normal cotrol) for 18 h, and the culture supernates were harvested for cytokine assays.

RNA interference and transfection

The sequences of HSF2 siRNA (Cat.No:SI04210598, Qiagen, Frankfurt, GER) were as follow: Target sequence:5′-CTGCG-CCGCGTTAACAATGAA-3′; Sense strand: 5′GCGCCGCGU-UAACAAUGAATT-3′; Antisense strand: 5′-UUCAUUGUUA-ACGCGGCGCAG-3′. A recombinant plasmid encoding HSF2 gene and containing an amino-terminal FLAG sequence (DYKDDDD), HSF2-FLAG, has been constructed as described by Chubet et al [17]. HSF2 siRNA and HSF2-FLAG recombinant plasmid were transfected into Caco-2 cells by Lipofectamine means according to manufacturer's protocols (Invitrogen, CA, USA).

ELISA assay

The concentrations of HSF2, IL-1β, and TNF-α in serum and IL-1β, and TNF-α in the supernatants of transfected Caco-2 cells were determined by ELISA kits according to manufacturer's protocols (HSF2, CUSABIO, Wuhan, China; IL-1β and TNF-α ELISA kits, Neobioscience, Beijing, China, respectively).

Statistical analysis

All data were presented as means ± standard deviation (SD). Statistical analyses were performed using SPSS17.0 statistical software. Multi-group data analyses were tested by one-way analysis of variance (ANOVA). Correlation analyses between the variables were assessed using the Pearson Test which gives a correlation coefficient (Pearson "r") and a "*p*" value. A *p* value of <0.05 was considered as the minimum level of significance in all cases.

Results

Identification of UC-associated proteins by MALDI-TOF MS

As shown in Figure 1, a total of 39 protein spots in the UC groups with differential expression levels were found on 2-DE. Of the 39 protein spots, 12 proteins were eventually identified by MALDI-TOF-MS, and 9 pieces of peptide mass fingerprinting (PMF) were obtained (Table 1). Among these identified proteins, 6 proteins were over-expressed: haptoglobin, aldehyde reductase, receptor tyrosine kinase, pericentriole material 1, heat shock factor 2 and apolipoprotein C-III. Three proteins were under-expressed in sera of patients with UC: tropomyosin 3, filamin A interacting protein 1 and keratin1. To clearly demonstrate the difference in expression of serum proteins between UC patients and normal controls, representative protein spots were picked up from 2-DE (Figure 1). These representative proteins had much higher expression in serum of patients with UC than that in normal controls.

Immunohistochemical staining of HSF 2 in colonic mucosa of UC

The expression profiles of HSF2 in colonic mucosa were examined by IHC (Figure 2). HSF2 was expressed in stromal cells and almost undetectable on the epithelial cells in normal intestinal mucosa (Figure 2A), but widely expressed in intestinal epithelial cells and stromal cells in UC group (Figure 2B, C and D), The expression level of HSF2 in mucosal tissues from the group with severe disease was the highest of these three groups ($p<0.01$), and HSF2 expression in the moderate group was higher than that in mild group($p<0.05$). The expression of HSF2 increased significantly with increasing severity of disease.

Immunohistochemical staining of HSF 2 in colonic mucosa of ulcerative colitis, Crohn's disease, Behcet's disease, intestinal tuberculosis, infective enteritis and intestinal lymphoma and normal controls

The results of IHC indicated that the expression of HSF2 in the intestinal mucosa of UC patients was significantly higher than that in other six groups (Figure 3), ($p<0.01$, for normal controls, Crohn's disease, Behcet's disease), ($p<0.05$ for intestinal tuberculosis, infective enteritis and intestinal lymphoma). However, there was no significant difference among six groups ($p>0.05$).

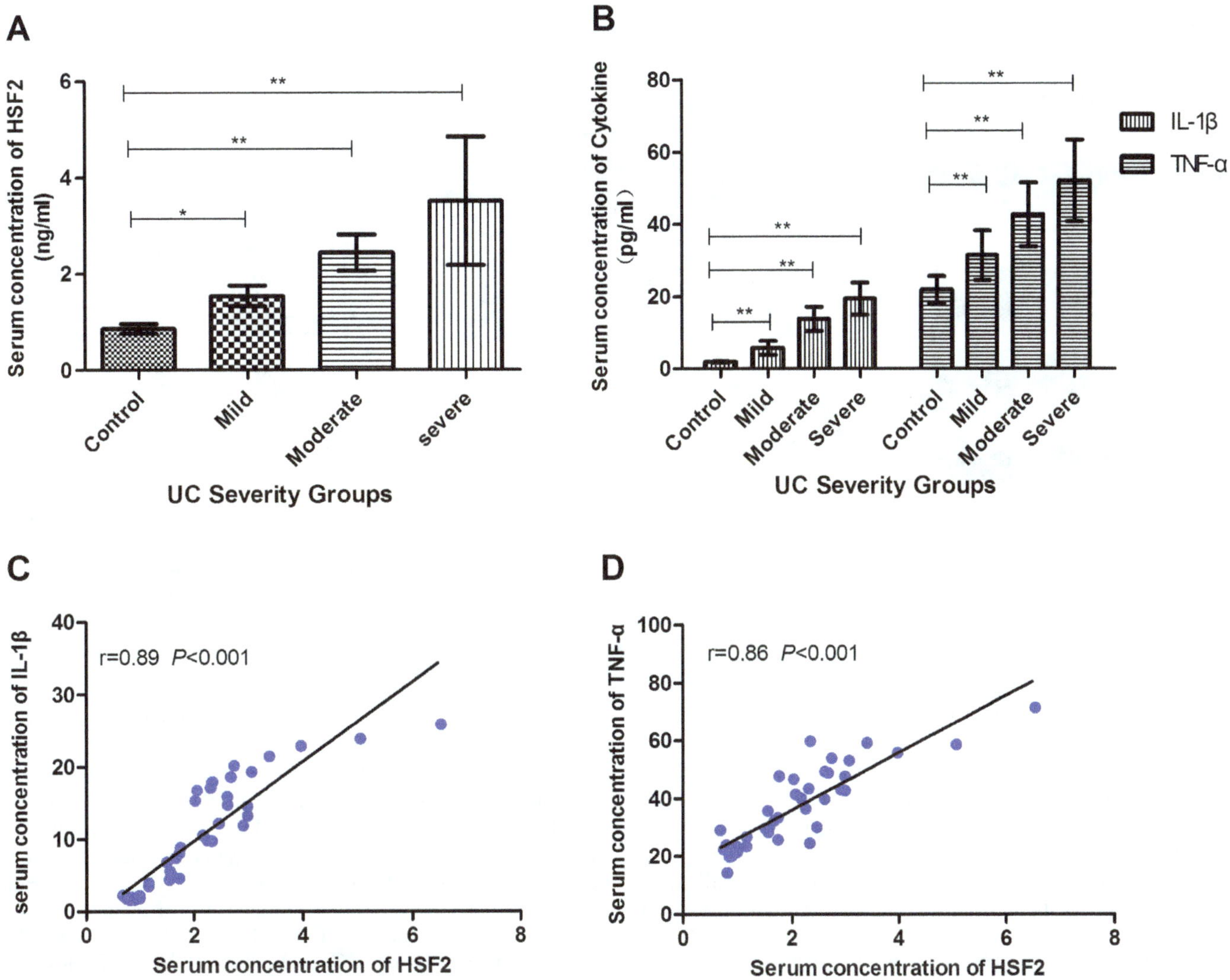

Figure 5. The concentration of HSF2, IL-1β and TNF-α in serum was determined by ELISA. A: serum concentration of HSF2 in patients with UC of varying severity. B: serum concentrations of IL-1β and TNF-α of different UC severity groups. C: Correlation analysis between the concentrations of HSF2 and IL-1β. D: Correlation analysis between the concentrations of HSF2 and TNF-α.Correlation analysis was assessed using the Pearson Test which gives a correlation coefficient (Pearson "r") and a "*p*" value. *, $p<0.05$; **, $p<0.01$.

Transcription and expression of HSF2 in colonic mucosa of UC

Real time-PCR results (Figure 4A) showed that the mRNA transcriptional level of HSF2 in colonic mucosa increased with disease severity. The mRNA levels of HSF2 in mucosal tissues from the severe group was the highest of the three groups ($p<0.01$), and that of the moderate group was higher than that in mild group and normal controls ($p<0.01$, for all). In addition, Western Blot results (Figure 4B) showed that the protein levels of HSF2 in colonic mucosa increased with increasing disease severity. There were significant differences among different UC severity groups.

Concentrations of HSF2, IL-1β, and TNF-α

As shown in Figure 5, the serum concentrations of HSF2, IL-1β and TNF-α increased with disease severity. In addition, the serum concentrations of HSF2 were positively correlated with IL-1β ($r = 0.89$, $p<0.001$), and with TNF-α ($r = 0.86$, $p<0.001$).

After down-regulation expression of HSF2 in Caco-2 cells by RNA interference (Figure 6A), the productions of IL-1β (Figure 6B) and TNF-α (Figure 6C) stimulated by LPS increased dramatically compared to the other four groups ($p<0.01$). Enhanced expression of HSF2 by plasmid transfection (Figure 6A) resulted in significantly decresased production of these two cytokines (Figure 6B and C) compared to other LPS-stimulated cell groups ($p<0.05$).

Discussion

Because of the dearth of molecular markers for UC, colonoscopy with colonic mucosal biopsy is currently routine for diagnostic evaluation for UC. Biomarkers have been considered to be objective, and non-invasive measurements of disease activity.

Alteration in the levels of some serum proteins have been shown to be early signs of altered physiology and may be indicative of disease [18]. In the present study, we identified 12 differential protein spots using MALDI-TOF-MS, and obtained nine pieces of PMF. PMFs were identified through searches of the SWISS-

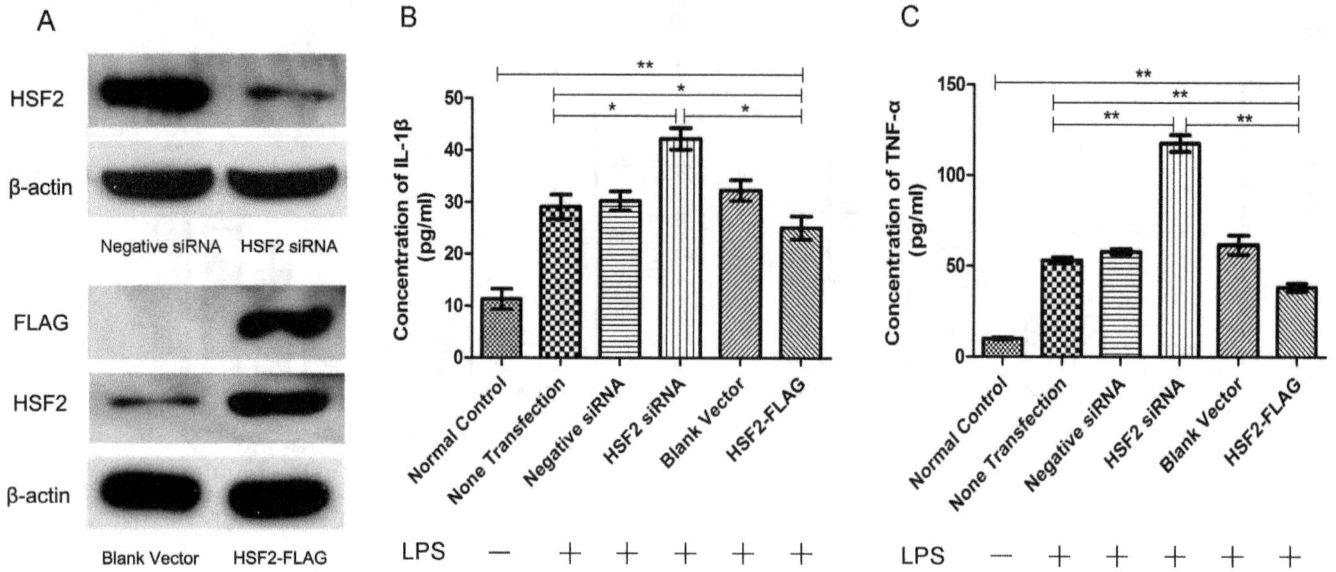

Figure 6. The secretion of IL-1β and TNF-α in Caco-2 cells after enhanced expression or siRNA of HSF2. A: The HSF2 expression levels after HSF2 RNA interferenc and HSF2-FLAG recombinant plasmid transfection, β-actin as an endogenous control. B: The productions of IL-1β in Caco-2 cells supernates stimulated or not by LPS (50 ng/ml). C: The productions of TNF-α in Caco-2 cells supernates stimulated or not by LPS (50 ng/ml). *, $p<0.05$;**, $p<0.01$.

PROT and NCBI nr databases. Among these identified proteins, six (heat shock factor protein 2, haptoglobin, apolipoprotein C-III, receptor tyrosine kinase, aldehyde reductase and pericentriolar material 1) were found to be up-regulated, and three (keratin 1, filamin A-interacting protein 1 and tropomyosin 3) were found to be down-regulated.

Over the last years evidence has accumulated that HSF1and HSPs are very important for the repair of colonic mucosa epithelium in inflammatory bowel disease and they suppress proinflammatory genes relevant to its pathogenesis [19–22], but little is known about the function of HSF2 in the pathogenesis of UC, most studies on HSF2 have been on protein misfolding diseases, delaying aging, development of embryo and sperm [23–25].

Based on the background facts and the findings of proteomic analysis, an up-regulated protein HSF2 was selected for further validation in the progression of UC. UC begins in the rectum and spreads variably to the proximal colon [26], and is characterized by continuous lesion, crypt abscess and abnormal branching [27]. Crypt abscesses are early lesions observed in inflammatory bowel disease, particularly in UC [28]. To some extent, crypt cells serves as a protective barrier between noxious stimuli and the sterile host environment. Exposure to such noxious stimuli may result in increased proliferation of crypt cells, secretion of enzymes, inflammatory cytokines and HSPs [29]. The results of the current study showed that the expression of HSF2 was up-regulated in the serum and intestinal mucosa of UC patients, suggesting that multiple stimuli might cause human stress responses, and high expression of HSF2 improves stress response. The expression of HSF2 in the intestinal mucosa of UC patients was significantly higher than that in normal controls, suggesting that HSF2 may be involved in the repair of colonic mucosa epithelium through activation of some protection proteins in response to intestinal mucosa membrane damage.

Recently, HSF1 has been shown to inhibit the expression of proinflammatory cytokines such as TNF-α and IL-1β by regulating the expression of the HSP, and suppressing key transcription factors of inflammatory signaling pathways, such as NF-κB and AP-1 [30]. The current data showed that serum concentrations of HSF2 were positively correlated with two proinflammatory factors, TNF-α and IL-1β. After down-regulation expression of HSF2 in Caco-2 cells by RNA interference, the secretions of these two cytokines stimulated by LPS increased dramatically, while enhanced expression of HSF2 by plasmid transfection resulted in significantly decresased production, suggesting that HSF2 might directly or indirectly affect inflammation-related transcription factors and down-regulates inflammatory cytokines to overcome inflammation.

It is important to understand the pathogenesis of UC and identify specific biomarkers and biological therapeutic targets [31,32]. Our results showed that HSF2 was over expressed in UC, and the increases paralleled the severity of disease. This suggests that HSF2 might be an endogenous protective factor against UC. This study will enable HSF2 as a potential novel molecular marker for UC and provide the basis for novel biological therapeutic targets.

Author Contributions

Conceived and designed the experiments: YM. Performed the experiments: JN JM. Analyzed the data: JN JM YM KW YX LC. Contributed reagents/materials/analysis tools: YD LZ LD SL GY MT. Wrote the paper: JN JM YM.

References

1. Braus NA, Elliott DE (2009) Advances in the pathogenesis and treatment of IBD. Clinical Immunology 132: 1–9.
2. Ouyang Q, Tandon R, Goh K-L, Ooi CJ, Ogata H, et al. (2005) The emergence of inflammatory bowel disease in the Asian Pacific region. Current opinion in gastroenterology 21: 408–413.

3. Thompson AI, Lees CW (2011) Genetics of ulcerative colitis. Inflammatory bowel diseases 17: 831–848.
4. Glas J, Seiderer J, Wagner j, Olszak T, Fries C, et al. (2012) Analysis of IL12B gene variants in inflammatory bowel disease. PLoS one 7(3):e34349.
5. Nell S, Suerbaum S, Josenhans C (2010) The impact of the microbiota on the pathogenesis of IBD: lessons from mouse infection models. Nature Reviews Microbiology 8: 564–577.
6. Koboziev I, Karlsson F, Grisham MB (2010) Gut-associated lymphoid tissue, T cell trafficking, and chronic intestinal inflammation. Annals of the New York Academy of Sciences 1207: E86–E93.
7. Judd TA, Day AS, Lemberg DA, Turner D, Leach ST (2011) Update of fecal markers of inflammation in inflammatory bowel disease. Journal of gastroenterology and hepatology 26: 1493–1499.
8. Lewis JD (2011) The utility of biomarkers in the diagnosis and therapy of inflammatory bowel disease. Gastroenterology 140: 1817–1826.
9. Calligaris D, Villard C, Lafitte D (2011) Advances in top-down proteomics for disease biomarker discovery. Journal of proteomics 74: 920–934.
10. Hatsugai M, Kurokawa MS, Kouro T, Nagai K, Arito M, et al. (2010) Protein profiles of peripheral blood mononuclear cells are useful for differential diagnosis of ulcerative colitis and Crohn's disease. Journal of gastroenterology 45: 488–500.
11. Lemmens B, Arijs I, Van Assche G, Sagaert X, Geboes K, et al. (2013) Correlation between the endoscopic and histologic score in assessing the activity of Ulcerative Colitis. Inflammatory bowel diseases 19: 1194–1201.
12. Boguth G, Harder A, Scheibe B, Wildgruber R, Weiss W (2000) The current state of two-dimensional electrophoresis with immobilized pH gradients. Electrophoresis 21: 1037–1053.
13. Millares P, LaCourse EJ, Perally S,Ward DA, Prescott MC, et al. (2012) Proteomic profiling and protein identification by MALDI-TOF mass spectrometry in unsequenced parasitic nematodes. PloS one 7(3): e33590.
14. Fan NJ, Gao CF, Zhao G, Wang XL, Liu QY (2012) Serum peptidome patterns of breast cancer based on magnetic bead separation and mass spectrometry analysis. Diagn Pathol 7: 45.
15. Chen Z, Brant S R, Li C, Shrestha UK, Jiang T, et al. (2010) CTLA4− 1661A/G and 3′ UTR long repeat polymorphisms are associated with ulcerative colitis and influence CTLA4 mRNA and protein expression. Genes and Immunity 11(7): 573–583.
16. Wang J, Huang H, Liu P, Tang F, Qin J, et al. (2006) Inhibition of phosphorylation of p38 MAPK involved in the protection of nephropathy by emodin in diabetic rats. European journal of pharmacology 553(1): 297–303.
17. Chubet RG, Brizzard BL (1996) Vectors for expression and secretion of FLAG epitope-tagged proteins in mammalian cells. Biotechniques 20(1): 136–141.
18. Iskandar HN, Ciorba MA (2012) Biomarkers in inflammatory bowel disease: current practices and recent advances. Translational Research 159: 313–325.
19. Tanaka K, Namba T, Arai Y, Fujimoto M, Adachi H, et al. (2007) Genetic evidence for a protective role for heat shock factor 1 and heat shock protein 70 against colitis. Journal of Biological Chemistry 282(32): 23240–23252.
20. Tomasello G, Sciumé C, Rappa F, Rodolico V, Zerilli M, et al. (2011) Hsp10, Hsp70, and Hsp90 immunohistochemical levels change in ulcerative colitis after therapy. European journal of histochemistry 55(4):e38.
21. Muhlig Nielsen M, Overgaard J, Sørensen JG, Holmstrup M, Justesen J, et al. (2005) Role of HSF activation for resistance to heat, cold and high-temperature knock-down. Journal of insect physiology 51: 1320–1329.
22. Arya R, Mallik M, Lakhotia SC (2007) Heat shock genes-integrating cell survival and death. Journal of biosciences 32: 595–610.
23. Åkerfelt M, Morimoto RI, Sistonen L (2010) Heat shock factors: integrators of cell stress, development and lifespan. Nature reviews Molecular cell biology 11: 545–555.
24. Calderwood SK, Murshid A, Prince T (2009) The shock of aging: molecular chaperones and the heat shock response in longevity and aging–a mini-review. Gerontology 55: 550–558.
25. Anckar J, Sistonen L (2011) Regulation of HSF1 function in the heat stress response: implications in aging and disease. Annual review of biochemistry 80: 1089–1115.
26. Geboes K (2008) What histologic features best differentiate Crohn's disease from ulcerative colitis? Inflammatory bowel diseases 14(S2): S168–S169.
27. Terada T (2013) Histopathologic study of the rectum in 1,438 consecutive rectal specimens in a single Japanese hospital: I. benign lesions. International journal of clinical and experimental pathology 6(3): 349–357.
28. Sokol H, Vasquez N, Hoyeau-Idrissi N, Seksik P, Beaugerie L, et al. (2010) Crypt abscess-associated microbiota in inflammatory bowel disease and acute self-limited colitis. World journal of gastroenterology 16(5): 583–587.
29. Malago JJ, Koninkx JF, van Dijk JE (2002) The heat shock response and cytoprotection of the intestinal epithelium. Cell stress & chaperones 7(2): 191–199.
30. Shimp SK 3rd, Parson CD, Regna NL, Thomas AN, Chafin CB, et al. (2012) HSP90 inhibition by 17-DMAG reduces inflammation in J774 macrophages through suppression of Akt and nuclear factor-κB pathways. Inflammation Research 61: 521–533.
31. Florholmen J, Fries W (2011) Candidate mucosal and surrogate biomarkers of inflammatory bowel disease in the era of new technology. Scandinavian journal of gastroenterology 46: 1407–1417.
32. Perrier C, Rutgeerts P (2011) Cytokine blockade in inflammatory bowel diseases. Immunotherapy 3: 1341–1352.

19

5-Aminosalicylates Reduce the Risk of Colorectal Neoplasia in Patients with Ulcerative Colitis

Li-Na Zhao, Jie-Yao Li, Tao Yu*, Guang-Cheng Chen, Yu-Hong Yuan, Qi-Kui Chen

Department of Gastroenterology, Sun Yat-Sen Memorial Hospital, Sun Yat-Sen University, Guangzhou, Guangdong, People's Republic of China

Abstract

Background: Although the chemopreventive effect of 5-aminosalicylates on patients with ulcerative colitis has been extensively studied, the results remain controversial. This updated review included more recent studies and evaluated the effectiveness of 5-aminosalicylates use on colorectal neoplasia prevention in patients with ulcerative colitis.

Methods: Up to July 2013, we searched Medline, Embase, Web of Science, Cochrane CENTRAL, and SinoMed of China for all relevant observational studies (case-control and cohort) about the effect of 5-aminosalicylates on the risk of colorectal neoplasia among patients with ulcerative colitis. The Newcastle-Ottawa Scale was used to assess the quality of studies. Adjusted odds ratios (ORs) were extracted from each study. A random-effects model was used to generate pooled ORs and 95% confidence intervals (95%CI). Publication bias and heterogeneity were assessed.

Results: Seventeen studies containing 1,508 cases of colorectal neoplasia and a total of 20,193 subjects published from 1994 to 2012 were analyzed. 5-aminosalicylates use was associated with a reduced risk of colorectal neoplasia in patients with ulcerative colitis (OR 0.63; 95%CI 0.48–0.84). Pooled OR of a higher average daily dose of 5-aminosalicylates (sulfasalazine ≥ 2.0 g/d, mesalamine ≥ 1.2 g/d) was 0.51 [0.35–0.75]. Pooled OR of 5-aminosalicylates use in patients with extensive ulcerative colitis was 1.00 [0.53–1.89].

Conclusion: Our pooled results indicated that 5-aminosalicylates use was associated with a reduced risk of colorectal neoplasia in patients with ulcerative colitis, especially in the cases with a higher average daily dose of 5-aminosalicylates use. However, the chemopreventive benefit of 5-aminosalicylates use in patients with extensive ulcerative colitis was limited.

Editor: Fabio Cominelli, CWRU/UH Digestive Health Institute, United States of America

Funding: This study was supported by the National Natural Science Foundation of China (No. 81270442 and No. 81000152) and the Youthful Teacher Foster Plan of Sun Yat-Sen University (No. 09ykpy10). The funders had no role in study design, data collection and analysis, decision to publish, or preparation of the manuscript.

Competing Interests: The authors have declared that no competing interests exist.

* E-mail: yutao2014@126.com

Introduction

Ulcerative colitis (UC) is associated with an increased risk of colorectal cancer (CRC). A recent meta-analysis encompassing 8 population-based cohort studies reported a 1.6% prevalence of CRC in patients with UC, <1.0% by 10 years, 0.4%–2.0% by 15 years, and 1.1%–5.3% by 20 years. The rate of CRC was 2.4-fold higher than that in the general population [1]. Because of the importance of prevention and early detection of CRC in patients with UC, they have been discussed in many studies. Colonoscopic surveillance at regular intervals with multiple biopsies is considered the most effective way to detect and manage CRC early in UC patients and has been recommended for patients with long-standing UC [2–3]. On the other hand, the effect of potential chemopreventive drugs, such as 5-aminosalicylates (5-ASA), thiopurines, and folic acid, on UC patients was also studied, but the results remain controversial.

5-ASA, a first-line agent for the treatment of mild to moderate UC, includes sulfasalazine and nonsulfasalazine (including mesalamine, balsalazide, and olsalazine). Since the meta-analysis by Velayos et al in 2005 demonstrated that 5-ASA could reduce the risk of CRC in patients with UC, this matter has been further discussed by a number of studies [4–9]. The recent meta-analysis based on population-based studies by Nguyen et al showed that 5-ASA was not effective to prevent CRC in patients with inflammatory bowel disease (IBD) [10]. However, a recent long-term population-based study by Jess et al did not show the increasing risk of CRC in patients with Crohn's disease (CD) [11]. Furthermore, chronic inflammation is presumed to be a key factor of CRC development in patients with IBD, but 5-ASA plays a limited role in inducing remission and maintenance of CD [12]. As a result, it is necessary to separately analyze the chemopreventive effect of 5-ASA in patients with UC.

The objective of this study is to identify and update the association between 5-ASA use and colorectal neoplasia (CRN),

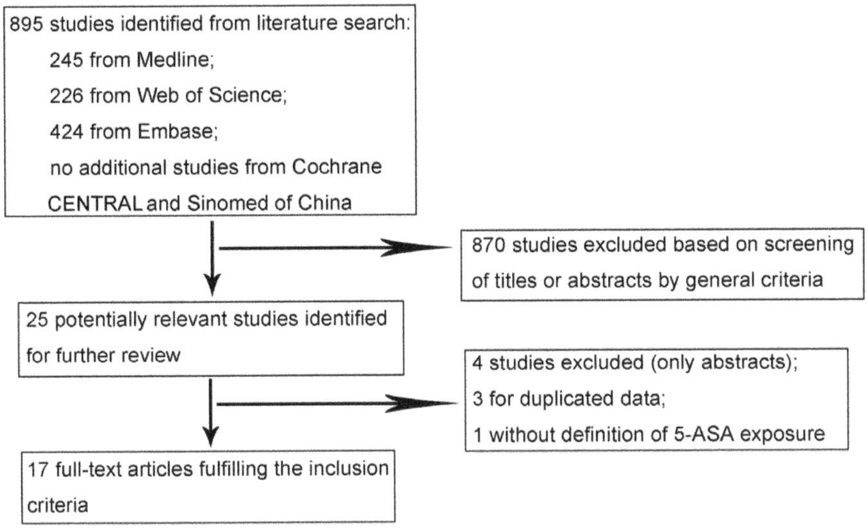

Figure 1. Flowchart of literature search for meta-analysis.

defined as low-grade dysplasia, high-grade dysplasia, and CRC, in patients with UC.

Methods

Search strategies

Up to July 2013, we searched Medline, Embase, Web of Science, Cochrane CENTRAL, and SinoMed of China for all relevant articles on the effect of 5-ASA use on the risk of CRN among patients with UC. Medical subject heading (MeSH) or key words used in the research included "Salicylazosulphapyridine", or "Salicylazosulfapyridine", or "Sulphasalazine", or "Sulfasalazine", or "Mesalazine", or "Mesalamine", or "5-aminosalicylic acid", or "5-aminosalicylate", or "Balsalazide", or "Olsalazine", with "colorectal cancer", or "colon cancer", or "dysplasia", or "carcinoma", or "neoplasia", or "advanced neoplasia", and "inflammatory bowel disease", or "ulcerative colitis". Reference lists of all included articles were scrutinized to disclose additional literature on this topic. All abstracts, review articles, commentaries, and book chapters were excluded. If an author published more than one articles using the same case series, we only used the article that reported the data with the largest number of cases and the most completed information.

Study selection

Two authors (LNZ and TY) selected target studies following a Proposal for Reporting Meta-analyses of Observational Studies in Epidemiology (MOOSE) guidelines [13]. Observational studies were included if they: 1) were case-control or cohort studies; 2) evaluated and clearly defined exposure to 5-ASA (sulfasalazine, mesalamine, balsalazide, and olsalazine) in patients with UC or IBD as a whole; 3) reported CRN outcomes; 4) reported odds ratios (ORs) or relative risks (RRs) with 95% confidence intervals (95%CIs), or provided data for their calculation; 5) were fully published.

Data extraction and Quality assessment

All data were abstracted onto a standard form and crosschecked by two reviewers independently. The data extracted from all the studies were as follows: the last names of first authors, years of publication, time periods of study, study designs, countries of origin, study settings (population-based or hospital-based), total numbers of cases in each group, distribution of IBD diagnosis (UC and CD), types of medications, durations, and average daily doses, outcomes reported, ORs, RRs or hazard ratios with and without adjustment for potential confounders, corresponding 95%CIs, and potential confounders used for adjustment. Disagreements were resolved by consensus including a third author.

The Newcastle-Ottawa Scale (NOS) was used to evaluate the quality of each study. This measure assesses aspects of methodology in observational studies related to study quality, including 8 items categorized into 3 major categories: selection (4 items, 1 star for each), comparability (1 item, up to two stars) and exposure/outcomes (3 items, 1 star for each) [14]. The ultimate score of 6 stars or more was regarded as high-quality.

Statistical analysis

We quantified the association between 5-ASA and CRN by using the Dersimonian and Laird random-effects model. Because the incidence of CRN was relatively low, the OR mathematically approximated the RR. All reported summary estimates were from studies with adjusted data, unless otherwise reported. When ORs were reported separately for different doses, types of 5-ASA (sulfasalazine or nonsulfasalazine) and durations of exposure, an overall estimate was calculated using the published individual adjusted ORs for each subgroup.

The Q and I^2 statistics were used to test statistical heterogeneity among studies. For the Q statistic, a P value of less than 0.1 is considered representative of statistically significant heterogeneity. I^2 is the proportion of total variation contributed by between-study variation. An I^2 index of around 25% is considered to demonstrate low levels of heterogeneity, 50% medium, and 75% high. Sensitivity analyses by reestimating pooled OR with omitting each study in turn were conducted to investigate the influence of each individual study on the overall meta-analysis summary estimate. Furthermore, subgroup analyses based on study designs (case-control or cohort), study settings (population-based or hospital-based), geographical regions, diseases (UC or IBD), and quality of studies were also performed to clarify the source of heterogeneity. In addition, cumulative meta-analysis was conducted to evaluate the change of the effect estimates over time. In the cumulative meta-analysis, studies were chronologically ordered by

Table 1. Characteristics of studies of 5-ASA and colorectal neoplasia in patients with ulcerative colitis.

Study	Study period	Study design	Country	Study setting	Cases/controls	CD%[&]	CRN
Pinczowski, 1994	1965–1983	Case-control	Sweden	Population	102/196	0	CRC
Moody, 1996	1972–1992	Cohort	UK	Population	10/158	0	CRC
Lashner, 1997	1986–1992	Cohort	USA	Hospital	29/69	0	CRN
Eaden, 2000	1972–1989	Case-control	UK	Hospital	102/102	0	CRC
Lindberg, 2001	1973–1993	Cohort	Sweden	Hospital	50/93	0	CRN
Rutter, 2004	1988–2002	Case-control	UK	Hospital	68/136	0	CRN
van Staa, 2005	1987–2001	Case-control	UK	Population	100/600	15	CRC
Rubin, 2006	1985–2000	Case-control	USA	Hospital	26/96	0	CRN
Velayos, 2006	1976–2002	Case-control	USA	Hospital	188/188	0	CRC
Terdiman, 2007	2001–2003	Case-control	USA	Population	364/1172	NR	CRC
Jess, 2007	1940–2002	Case-control	USA+Denmark	Population	43/102	26	CRN
Gupta, 2007	1996–2007	Cohort	USA	Hospital	65/353	0	CRN
Tang, 2010	1970–2005	Case-control	USA	Hospital	18/30	17	CRC
Baars, 2011	1990–2006	Case-control	Netherlands	Population	173/393	34	CRC
Bernstein, 2011*	1995–2008	Cohort	Canada	Population	108/8559	41	CRC
Gong W, 2012	1998–2009	Case-control	China	Hospital	34/3888	0	CRC
van Schaik, 2012	2001–2009	Cohort	Netherlands	Population	28/2550	NR	AN

Note: CD: Crohn's disease, NR: not reported, CRN: colorectal neoplasia, CRC: colorectal cancer, AN: advanced neoplasia.
*With effect estimates for ulcerative colitis and inflammatory bowel disease.
[&]Percentage of CD in inflammatory bowel disease with CRN.

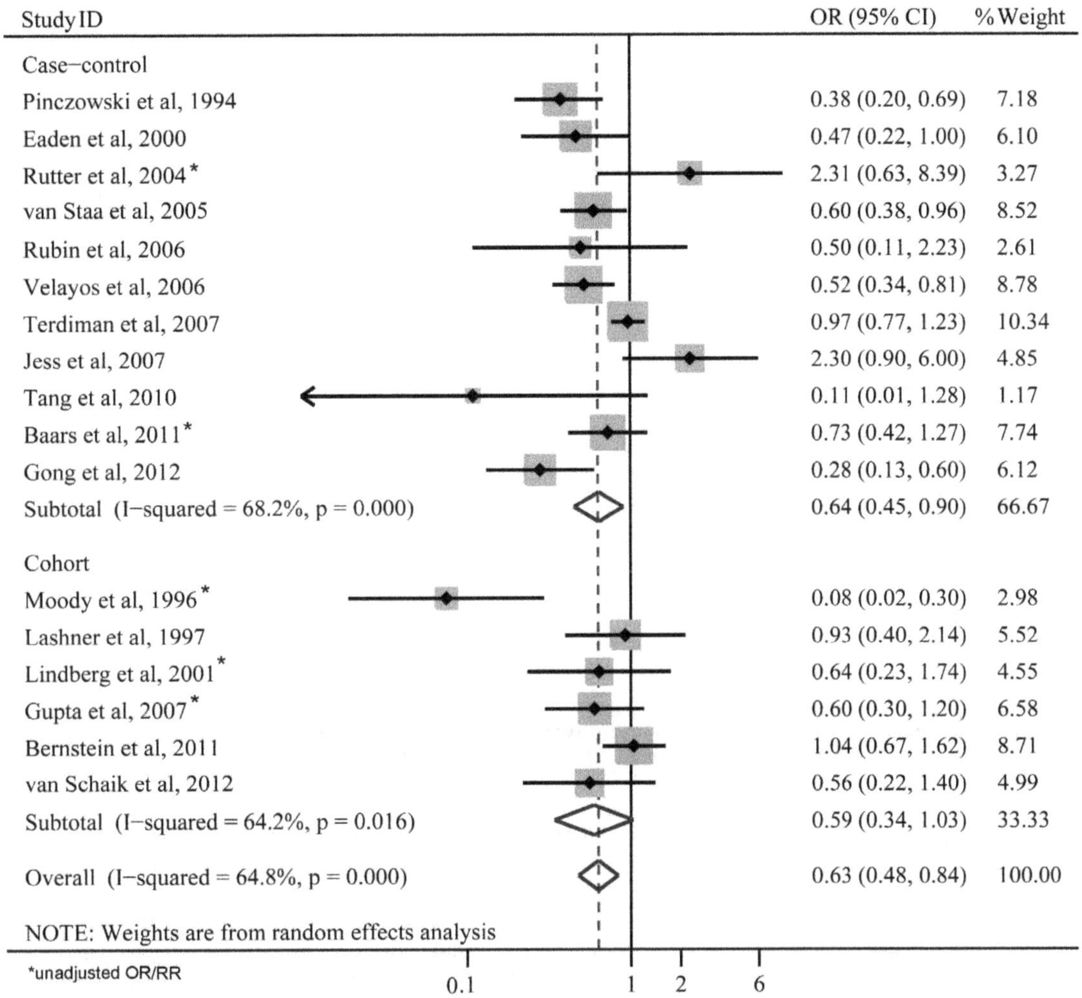

Figure 2. Forest plot (random-effects model) of 5-ASA use and colorectal neoplasia.

year of publication, and the pooled ORs were obtained at the end of each year.

Publication bias and small study effects were assessed by Begg's test and Egger's test, with $P<0.05$ considered to show significant publication bias. STATA (Version 12.0; STATA Corporation, College Station, TX, US) was used for all analyses.

Results

Literature search

We reviewed 245 titles and abstracts from Medline, 226 from Web of Science, 424 from Embase, and no additional studies from Cochrane CENTRAL and SinoMed of China, and eventually chose 25 studies for further review [5–9,11,15–33]. Four supplementary studies were identified, but only their abstracts from conference proceeding of scientific meetings had been published [15–18]. They were excluded from the pooled analysis because of lack of details on key study variables. Three studies were excluded for their duplicated data [19–21]. One study was excluded without the definition of 5-ASA exposure [11]. Finally, 17 full-text articles were identified in this meta-analysis (Figure 1) [5–9,22–33].

Seventeen studies containing 1,508 CRN cases, of which at least 75% were CRC cases, and a total of 20,193 subjects published from 1994 to 2012 were analyzed. Of the 17 studies, six were retrospective cohort studies and eleven case-control studies. Eight were population-based studies and nine hospital-based studies. Eight studies were conducted in Europe, seven in North America (six in USA, one in Canada), one in both Europe (Demark) and America, and one in Asia (China). Ten studies were exclusively based on UC patients; one study dealt with both UC and IBD patients; and six studies were based on IBD patients. The sample sizes ranged from 48 to 8,667 and the number of CRN cases varied from 10 to 364 (Table 1).

5-ASA and colorectal neoplasia

In a pooled analysis of all studies, 5-ASA use was associated with a reduced risk of CRN (OR 0.63; 95%CI 0.48–0.84; Figure 2). The protective effect remained significant with case-control studies (OR 0.64; 95%CI 0.45–0.90; Figure 2), and a trend towards reducing risk of CRN was also shown in retrospective cohort studies (OR 0.59; 95%CI 0.34–1.03; Figure 2). Although the pooled OR of cohort studies was lower than that of case-control studies, the range of 95%CI was wider and the difference was not statistically significant, indicating a lower power in cohort studies.

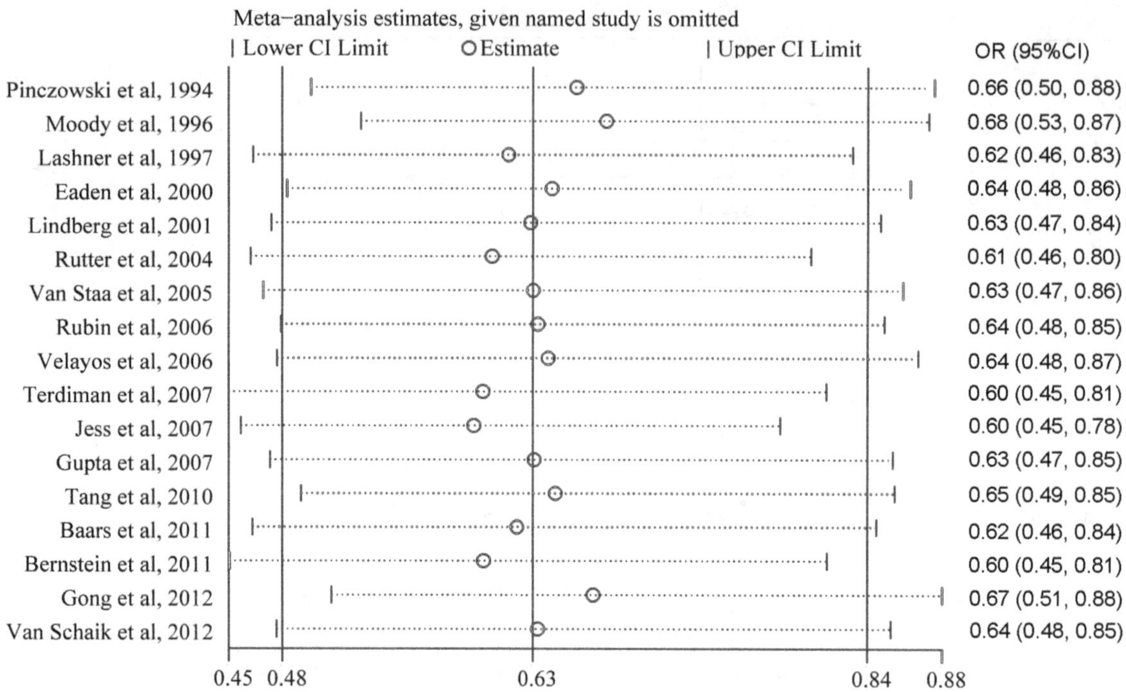

Figure 3. This diagram showed the influence of excluding each study in turn on the primary meta-analysis. The pooled ORs ranged from 0.60 to 0.68, with all showing statistically significant association between 5-ASA and colorectal neoplasia.

Methodological quality and risk of bias

There was significant heterogeneity across all studies ($I^2 = 64.8\%$, $P<0.001$; Figure 2). Sensitivity analyses by reestimating pooled OR with excluding each study in turn were conducted. Pooled ORs ranged from 0.60 to 0.68, with all showing statistically significant association between 5-ASA and CRN (Figure 3). No obvious publication bias was found by Begg's test (Figure 4A) and Egger's test (Figure 4B).

Subgroup analyses

Population-based and hospital-based. The protective effect of 5-ASA was significant in hospital-based studies (OR 0.56; 95%CI 0.40–0.78; Figure 5A), but not in population-based studies (OR 0.69; 95%CI 0.46–1.02; Figure 5A).

Geographical regions. The chemopreventive benefit was shown in Europe (OR 0.54; 95%CI 0.36–0.81; Figure 5B). However, no significant association was observed in North America (OR 0.77; 95%CI 0.57–1.03; Figure 5B). The OR of the study which included mixed patients in Europe (Demark) and America was 2.30 (95%CI 0.90–6.00). The OR of the study in Asia (China) was 0.28 (95%CI 0.13–0.60).

UC and IBD. 5-ASA use was associated with a reduced risk of CRN (OR 0.54; 95%CI 0.38–0.76; Figure 6A) in UC patients. No significant association was shown in IBD patients (OR 0.85; 95%CI 0.63–1.15; Figure 6A).

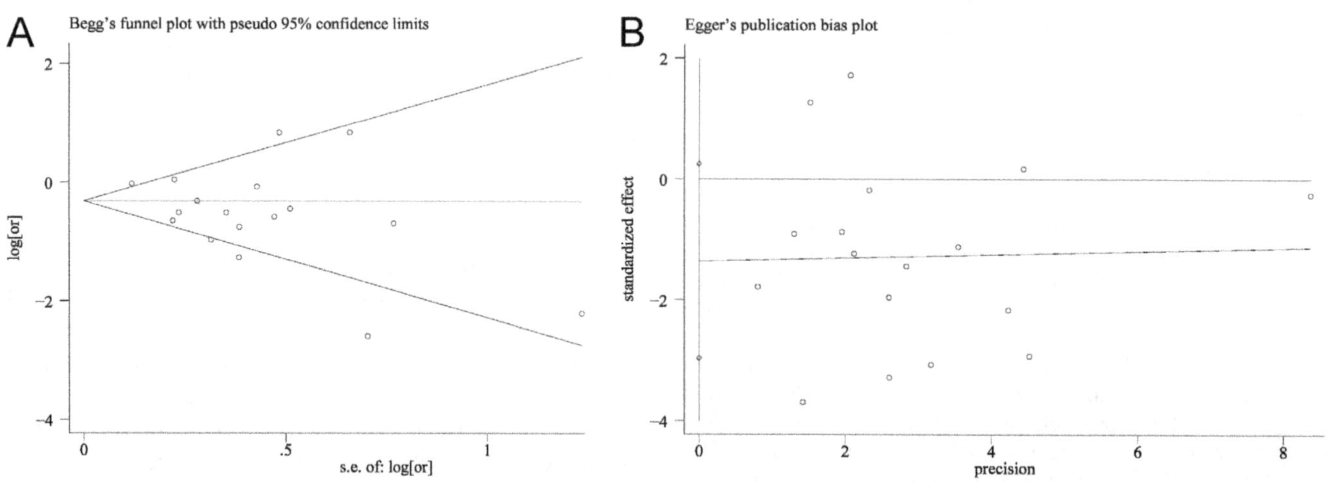

Figure 4. Begg's test and Egger's test. Begg's test and Egger's test identified no publication bias (Begg's test: Kendall's tau = −12, $P = 0.65$; Egger's test: bias = −1.36, $P = 0.092$).

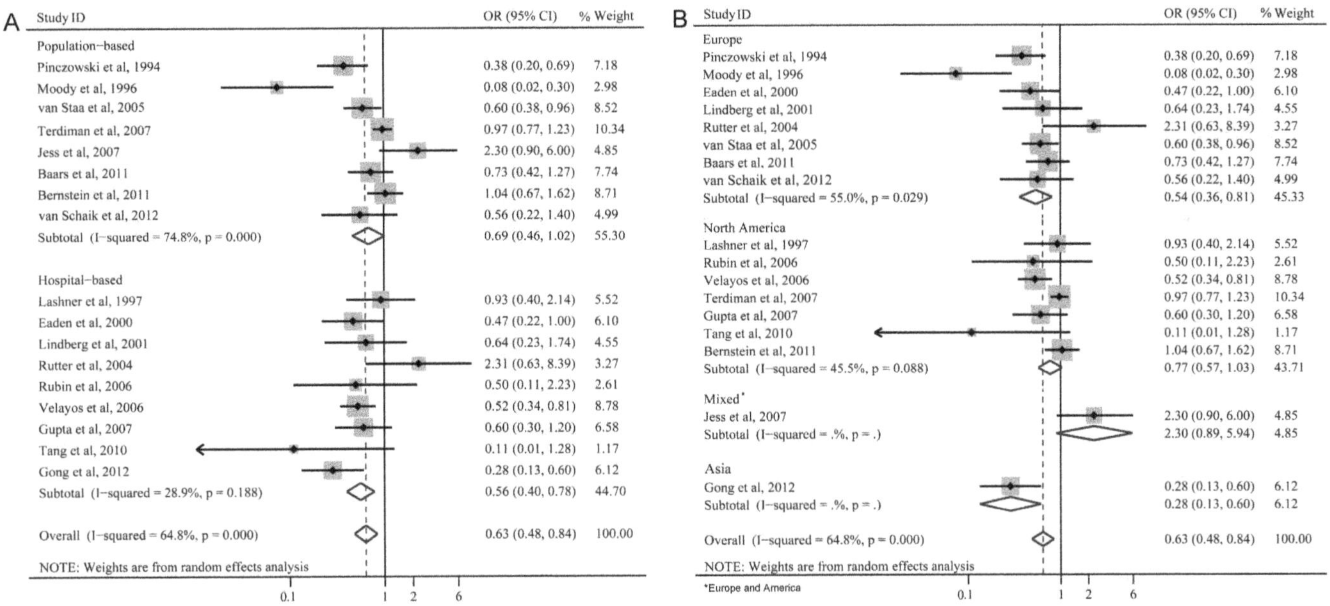

Figure 5. Forest plots of subanalyses of study settings (A) and geographical regions (B).

Average daily dose of 5-ASA use. Six studies were included for their higher average daily dose of 5-ASA use (sulfasalazine ≥ 2.0 g/d, mesalamine ≥ 1.2 g/d). The use of a higher average daily dose of 5-ASA was associated with a lower risk of CRN (OR 0.51; 95%CI 0.35–0.75; Figure 6B). Only two studies defined a lower average daily dose of 5-ASA use (sulfasalazine <2.0 g/d, mesalamine<1.2 g/d) and the OR was 0.64 (95%CI 0.30–1.36; Figure 6B).

5-ASA use in extensive UC. Three studies included patients with extensive UC (proximal to the splenic flexure). 5-ASA use in these patients was not associated with a lower risk of CRN (OR 1.00; 95%CI 0.53–1.89; Figure 6C).

Cumulative meta-analysis

A cumulative meta-analysis of the total 17 studies was conducted to evaluate the cumulative effect estimates over time. In 1994, Pinczowski first reported that 5-ASA was a protective factor for CRC in UC patients (OR 0.38; 95%CI 0.20–0.69). Between 1994 and 2006, nine studies were published, with a cumulative OR of 0.54 (95%CI 0.37–0.78; Figure 7). Between 2007 and 2012, eight more publications were added cumulatively, resulting in an overall effect estimate of 0.63 (95%CI 0.48–0.84; Figure 7).

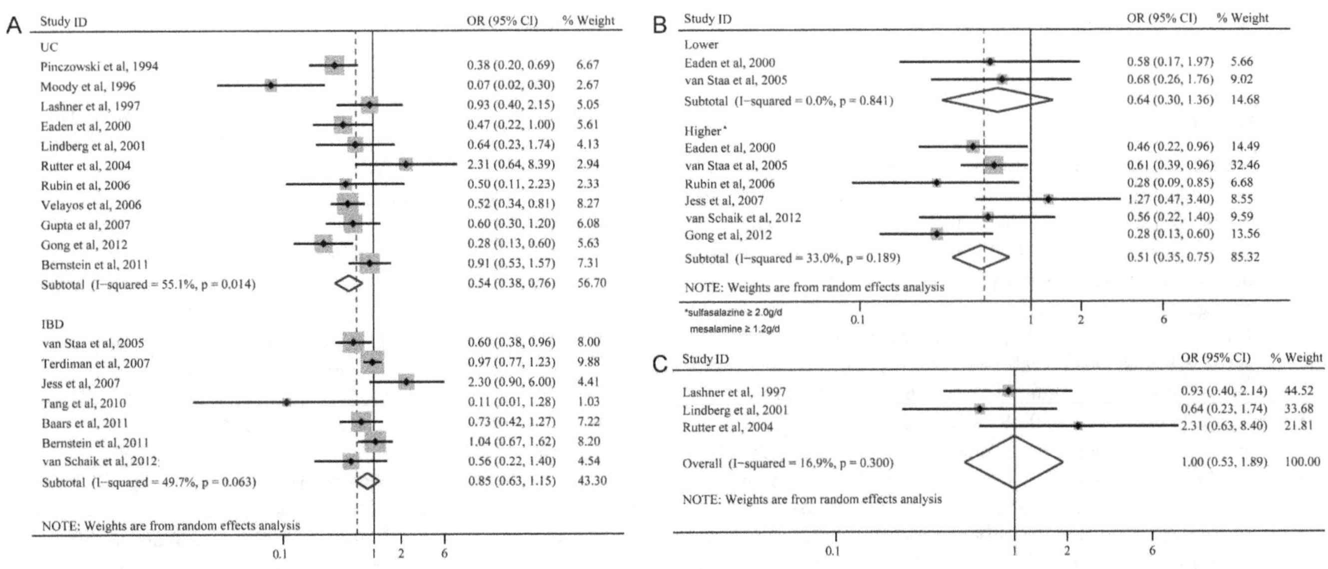

Figure 6. Forest plots of subanalyses of UC and IBD (A), average daily dose of 5-ASA use (B), and extensive UC (C).

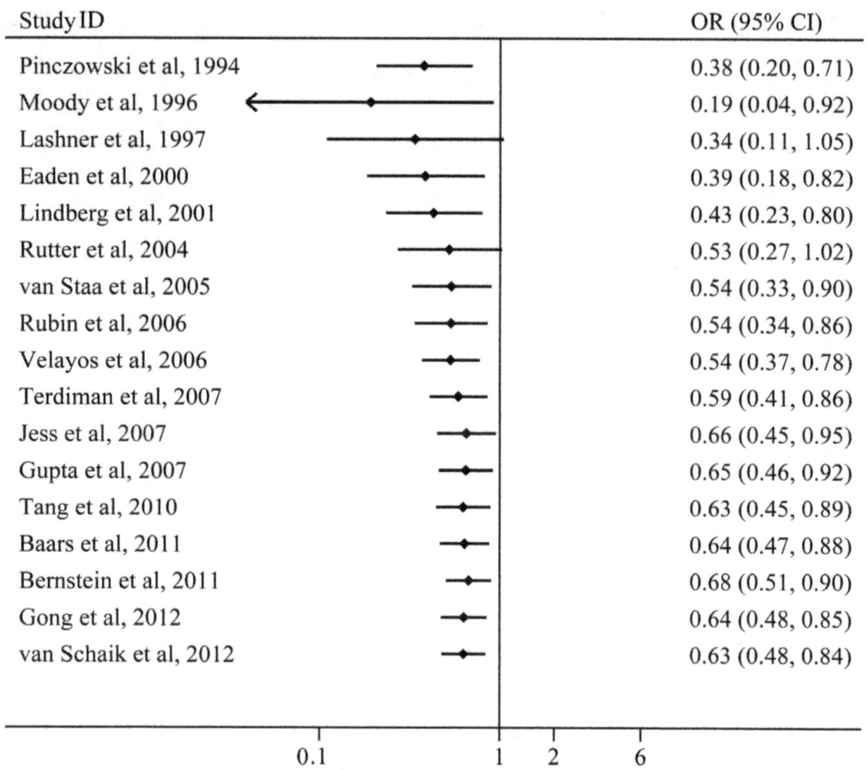

Figure 7. Forest plot of cumulative meta-analysis over time.

Quality assessment and Subanalyses of high-quality studies

The results of the quality assessment according to NOS for case-control and cohort studies were shown in Table 2. The scores of the included studies ranged from four to eight stars. Twelve studies (71%) scored six or more were defined as high-quality, indicating a moderate to good study quality.

The chemopreventive benefit was shown in high-quality studies (OR 0.70; 95%CI 0.54–0.92; $I^2 = 55.7\%$; Table 3). Significant association was also observed in hospital-based, Europe, and UC studies, but not in population-based, North America, and IBD studies (Table 3).

Discussion

Our pooled results from 17 studies indicated that the use of 5-ASA was associated with a reduced risk of CRN in patients with UC. The results also suggested that a higher average daily dose of 5-ASA use was more effective. The statistical analysis showed that there was significant heterogeneity across all studies ($I^2 = 64.8\%$, $P<0.001$; Figure 2). Therefore, sensitivity analyses by reestimating pooled OR with omitting each study in turn were conducted to investigate the influence of each individual study on the overall meta-analysis summary estimate. The results indicated that pooled ORs ranged from 0.60 to 0.68, with all showing statistically significant association between 5-ASA and CRN (Figure 3). The cumulative meta-analysis over time showed that the estimates gradually became consistent, and the corresponding CIs narrowed down with the increase in the number of included studies ordered by year of publication. In addition, the chemopreventive benefit remained significant in high-quality studies. Meanwhile, there was no obvious publication bias found by Begg's test and Egger's test (Figure 4). These analyses enhanced the reliability of this meta-analysis.

In general, hospital-based studies were more susceptible to selection bias than population-based studies. Our results demonstrated that population-based studies did not show a significantly protective effect on reducing the risk of CRN, while hospital-based studies did. This difference could be elucidated by the following two reasons. Firstly, hospital-based studies are prone to selecting more severe cases and have a higher risk of CRC compared with population-based studies. In addition, some population-based studies reported that patients with UC only had a modestly increasing risk of CRC, thus the benefit of 5-ASA for prevention of CRC in population-based studies might be inconspicuous [34–36]. Secondly, the compliance of the selected population in hospital-based studies was different from the general population, like avoiding unhealthy life style and taking 5-ASA more regularly. However, because of the significant heterogeneity among the population-based studies ($I^2 = 74.8\%$, $P<0.001$; Figure 5A), this result requires further investigations.

We found that the risk of CRN in Europe was significantly reduced, but it was not the case in North America. The reason for the difference is unclear. The differences in genetic susceptibility, culture, and lifestyle may explain part of the inconsistency of the results. Other confounders, such as the colectomy rates, the severity and extent of UC, and the selected population of UC and IBD, might also play an important role in the discrepancy.

The risk factors of CRC in patients with UC include: 1) duration/early onset age, severity and extent of UC; 2) degree of histological/endoscopic inflammatory activity; 3) family history; 4) primary sclerosing cholangitis [12]. The first two risk factors are related to inflammatory burden. And chronic mucosal inflammation is a putative predominant mechanism responsible for

Table 2. Results of quality assessment by Newcastle-Ottawa Scale.

Study	1	2	3	4	5A	5B	6	7	8	scores
Case-control										
Pinczowski, 1994	☆	☆	☆	☆	☆	☆	–	☆	–	7
Eaden, 2000	☆	☆	–	☆	☆	☆	–	☆	–	6
Rutter, 2004	☆	–	–	☆	☆	☆	–	☆	–	5
van Staa, 2005	☆	☆	☆	☆	☆	☆	☆	☆	–	8
Rubin, 2006	☆	☆	–	☆	☆	☆	–	☆	–	6
Velayos, 2006	☆	☆	–	☆	☆	☆	☆	☆	–	7
Terdiman, 2007	☆	☆	☆	☆	☆	☆	☆	☆	–	8
Jess, 2007	☆	☆	☆	☆	☆	☆	☆	☆	–	8
Tang, 2010	☆	☆	–	☆	☆	☆	–	☆	–	6
Baars, 2011	☆	☆	☆	–	☆	☆	–	☆	–	6
Gong, 2012	☆	☆	–	☆	–	☆	–	☆	–	5
Cohort										
Moody, 1996	☆	☆	–	–	–	–	☆	☆	☆	5
Lashner, 1997	–	☆	–	–	☆	☆	☆	☆	☆	6
Lindberg, 2001	–	☆	–	–	–	☆	☆	☆	–	4
Gupta, 2007	☆	☆	–	–	–	–	☆	☆	☆	5
Bernstein, 2011	☆	☆	☆	–	☆	☆	☆	☆	☆	8
van Schaik, 2012	☆	☆	☆	–	☆	☆	☆	☆	☆	8

Note: For case-control studies, 1 indicates adequate definition of cases; 2, cases are representative of population; 3, community controls; 4, controls have no history of colorectal neoplasia; 5A, study controls for age and gender; 5B, study controls for additional factor(s); 6, ascertainment of exposure by blinded interview or record; 7, same method of ascertainment used for cases and controls; and 8, nonresponse rate the same for cases and controls. For cohort studies, 1 indicates exposed cohort truly representative; 2, nonexposed cohort drawn from the same community; 3, ascertainment of exposure; 4, outcome of interest not present at start; 5A, cohorts comparable on basis of age and gender; 5B, cohorts comparable on other factor(s); 6, quality of outcome assessment; 7, follow-up long enough for outcomes to occur (at least 1 year); and 8, complete accounting for cohorts (>75% follow-up or description provided of those lost).

Table 3. Subanalyses of high-quality studies.

	Number of studies	OR	95%CI	I^2
Total	12	0.70	0.54–0.92	55.7%
Study setting				
Population-based	7	0.79	0.57–1.08	62.5%
Hospital-based	5	0.54	0.39–0.76	0
Region				
Europe	6	0.55	0.43–0.69	0
North America	5	0.96	0.78–1.17	0
Disease				
UC	6	0.59	0.43–0.79	18.8%
IBD	6	0.85	0.63–1.15	49.7%

Note: UC: ulcerative colitis, IBD: inflammatory bowel disease.

increased risk of CRC. 5-ASA, as an effective anti-inflammation drug for patients with UC, is reasonably considered as a chemopreventive drug for CRC. Furthermore, the molecular mechanisms of anticancer effects of 5-ASA are plausible. 5-ASA may inhibit cell-cycle progression by interfering with TGF-β, TNF-α, NF-κB pathway and Wnt/β-catenin signaling, improve DNA replication fidelity, and reduce free radicals as a scavenger of reactive oxygen species [37]. These support our findings that 5-ASA use could reduce the risk of CRN in patients with UC.

Consistent with the meta-analysis conducted by Velayos et al, the six studies with a higher average daily dose of 5-ASA (sulfasalazine ≥ 2.0 g/d, mesalamine ≥ 1.2 g/d) in our study also suggested a chemopreventive effect in patients with UC [4]. In our study, all of the three studies including patients with long-term and extensive UC illustrated that 5-ASA use was ineffective on CRN prevention [30,32,33]. Pooled OR of this subanalysis was 1.00 (95%CI 0.53–1.89; Figure 6C). One possible explanation is that the management and maintenance of remission of extensive UC is more difficult than that with distal colitis by 5-ASA use. Other long-term maintenance drugs (immunomodulators, like thiopurine and azathioprine, or biologics) are recommended to patients with extensive UC who have failed 5-ASA therapy, allowing such patients without 5-ASA use in quiescent disease [41]. Besides, it has been demonstrated that thiopurines can protect IBD patients against advanced neoplasia [27]. Accordingly, immunomodulators or biologics use in patients with extensive UC may exert significant bias on the effect of 5-ASA use in CRN prevention. Among the three studies, it was suggested that azathioprine showed no significant protective effect against CRN by Lasher and Rutter, but immunomodulators use was not reported by Linderberg [30,32,33]. Additionally, adherence and average daily dose of 5-ASA use, which have considerable influence on the effect of 5-ASA use on long-term maintenance therapy in patients with extensive UC, were not reported in all of the three studies [42]. Therefore, this result should be carefully interpreted and needs further investigations.

The included IBD studies (including CD patients) might result in a significant bias on the chemopreventive effect of 5-ASA on UC patients, because according to a recent Cochrane Database review and clinical guidelines, 5-ASA is not an effective drug to control CD and not highly recommended for the management of CD [38–40]. However, we included the six IBD studies and mixed them with the UC studies as the main analysis, considering that the six IBD studies were recently well-designed ones with large database and a majority of the subjects in these studies had UC. Nevertheless, we conducted a subgroup analysis of UC and IBD, demonstrating that the use of 5-ASA was associated with a reduced risk of CRN (OR 0.54; 95%CI 0.38–0.76; Figure 6A) in UC patients, but no significant association was shown in IBD patients (OR 0.85; 95%CI 0.63–1.15; Figure 6A).

There were several limitations in our study. Firstly, studies included in this meta-analysis were all observational studies (case-control and retrospective cohort studies). Therefore, the influence of confounding variables was inevitable in such long period studies. The main confounders, such as the colectomy rates and the severity and extent of UC, could not be obtained from all studies [8]. Secondly, most of these studies extracted data of 5-ASA exposure from medical records and might result in inaccuracy. Apart from that, most of them did not describe clearly the duration and average daily dose of 5-ASA use. Thirdly, there was significant heterogeneity among all the studies. Although we investigated the influence of each individual study on the overall estimate and conducted subgroup analyses according to different study settings, geographical regions, and average daily doses of 5-ASA use, the heterogeneity remained significant in some of the subgroup analyses and unable to be clearly classified.

In summary, our pooled results indicated that 5-ASA use was associated with a reduced risk of CRN in patients with UC, especially in the cases with a higher daily dose of 5-ASA use. However, the benefit of 5-ASA use in preventing CRN in patients with extensive UC was limited. Large population-based and well-designed studies are needed to confirm these results.

Author Contributions

Conceived and designed the experiments: TY QKC. Performed the experiments: LNZ JYL GCC. Analyzed the data: LNZ JYL GCC. Contributed reagents/materials/analysis tools: LNZ GCC YHY. Wrote the paper: LNZ JYL. Independent literature searching and data extraction: LNZ TY.

References

1. Jess T, Rungoe C, Peyrin-Biroulet L (2010) Risk of colorectal cancer in patients with ulcerative colitis: a meta-analysis of population-based cohort studies. Clin Gastroenterol Hepatol 10: 639–645.
2. Collins PD, Mpofu C, Watson AJ, Rhodes JM (2006) Strategies for detecting colon cancer and/or dysplasia in patients with inflammatory bowel disease. Cochrane Database Syst Rev 19: CD000279.
3. Subramanian V, Logan RF (2011) Chemoprevention of colorectal cancer in inflammatory bowel disease. Best Pract Res Clin Gastroenterol 25: 593–606.
4. Velayos FS, Terdiman JP, Walsh JM (2005) Effect of 5-aminosalicylate use on colorectal cancer and dysplasia risk: a systematic review and meta-analysis of observational studies. Am J Gastroenterol 100: 1345–1353.
5. Rubin DT, LoSavio A, Yadron N, Huo D, Hanauer SB (2006) Aminosalicylate therapy in the prevention of dysplasia and colorectal cancer in ulcerative colitis. Clin Gastroenterol Hepatol 4: 1346–1350.
6. Velayos FS, Loftus EV Jr, Jess T, Harmsen WS, Bida J, et al. (2006) Predictive and protective factors associated with colorectal cancer in ulcerative colitis: a case-control study. Gastroenterology 130: 1941–1949.
7. Gupta RB, Harpaz N, Itzkowitz S, Hossain S, Matula S, et al. (2007) Histologic inflammation is a risk factor for progression to colorectal neoplasia in ulcerative colitis: a cohort study. Gastroenterology 133: 1099–1105.
8. Bernstein CN, Nugent Z, Blanchard JF (2011) 5-aminosalicylate is not chemoprophylactic for colorectal cancer in IBD: a population based study. Am J Gastroenterol 106: 731–736.
9. Gong W, Lv N, Wang B, Chen Y, Huang Y, et al. (2012) Risk of ulcerative colitis-associated colorectal cancer in China: A multi-center retrospective study. Dig Dis Sci 57: 503–507.
10. Nguyen GC, Gulamhusein A, Bernstein CN (2012) 5-aminosalicylic acid is not protective against colorectal cancer in inflammatory bowel disease: a meta-analysis of non-referral populations. Am J Gastroenterol 107: 1298–1304.
11. Jess T, Simonsen J, Jørgensen KT, Pedersen BV, Nielsen NM, et al. (2012) Decreasing risk of colorectal cancer in patients with inflammatory bowel disease over 30 years. Gastroenterology 143: 375–381.
12. Andrews JM, Travis SP, Gibson PR, Gasche C (2008) Systematic review: does concurrent therapy with 5-ASA and immunomodulators in inflammatory bowel disease improve outcomes? Aliment Pharmacol Ther 29: 459–469.
13. Stroup DF, Berlin JA, Morton SC, Olkin I, Williamson GD, et al. (2000) Meta-analysis of observational studies in epidemiology: a proposal for reporting. Meta-analysis Of Observational Studies in Epidemiology (MOOSE) group. JAMA 283: 2008–2012.
14. Wells GA, Shea B, O'Connell D, Peterson'Connell J, Welch V, et al.The Newcastle-Ottawa Scale (NOS) for assessing the quality of nonrandomised studies in meta-analyses. Available: http://www.ohri.ca/programs/clinical_epidemiology/oxford.asp. Accessed 2103 Nov 9.
15. Georgescu EF, Ionescu RI, Niculescu M, Vancica L (2009) Systematic administration of 5-ASA derivatives during remissions for more than 9 months/year seems to protect patients with longstanding ulcerative colitis against colorectal cancer. Gastroenterology 136: A764.
16. Nourani S, Huo DZ, Strum W, Rubin DT (2008) 5-ASA therapy and a lower inflammatory score in chronic ulcerative colitis are associated with a decreased risk of dysplasia and colorectal cancer. Gastroenterology 134: A660.
17. Smith T, Swaroop P (2006) Mesalamine reduces the rate of colorectal dysplasia in patients with inflammatory bowel disease and primary sclerosing cholangitis who are on urosdeoxycholic acid. Gastroenterology 130: A653.
18. Carrat F, Seksik P, Bouvier AM, Brousse N, Carbonnel F, et al. (2010) Aminosalicylates, thiopurines and the risk of colorectal cancer in inflammatory bowel diseases: a case-control study nested in the CESAME cohort. Gastroenterology 138: S47.
19. Bernstein CN, Blanchard JF, Metge C, Yogendran M (2003) Does the use of 5-aminosalicylates in inflammatory bowel disease prevent the development of colorectal cancer? Am J Gastroenterol 98: 2784–2788.
20. Winther KV, Jess T, Langholz E, Munkholm P, Binder V (2004) Long-term risk of cancer in ulcerative colitis: a population-based cohort study from Copenhagen County. Clin Gastroenterol Hepatol 2: 1088–1095.
21. Ullman T, Croog V, Harpaz N, Hossain S, Kornbluth A, et al. (2008) Progression to colorectal neoplasia in ulcerative colitis: effect of mesalamine. Clin Gastroenterol Hepatol 6: 1225–1230.
22. van Staa TP, Card T, Logan RF, Leufkens HG (2005) 5-aminosalicylate use and colorectal cancer risk in inflammatory bowel disease: a large epidemiological study. Gut 54: 1573–1578.
23. Terdiman JP, Steinbuch M, Blumentals WA, Ullman TA, Rubin DT (2007) 5-aminosalicylic acid therapy and the risk of colorectal cancer among patients with inflammatory bowel disease. Inflamm Bowel Dis 13: 367–371.
24. Jess T, Loftus EV Jr, Velayos FS, Winther KV, Tremaine WJ, et al. (2007) Risk factors for colorectal neoplasia in inflammatory bowel disease: A nested case-control study from Copenhagen County, Denmark and Olmsted County, Minnesota. Am J Gastroenterol 102: 829–836.
25. Tang J, Sharif O, Pai C, Silverman AL (2010) Mesalamine protects against colorectal cancer in inflammatory bowel disease. Dig Dis Sci 55: 1696–1703.
26. Baars JE, Looman CW, Steyerberg EW, Beukers R, Tan AC, et al. (2011) The risk of inflammatory bowel disease-related colorectal carcinoma is limited: results from a nationwide nested case-control study. Am J Gastroenterol 106: 319–328.
27. van Schaik FD, van Oijen MG, Smeets HM, van der Heijden GJ, Siersema PD, et al. (2012) Thiopurines prevent advanced colorectal neoplasia in patients with inflammatory bowel disease. Gut 61: 235–240.
28. Pinczowski D, Ekbom A, Baron J, Yuen J, Adami HO (1994) Risk factors for colorectal cancer in patients with ulcerative colitis: a case-control study. Gastroenterology 107: 117–120.
29. Moody GA, Jayanthi V, Probert CS, Mac Kay H, Mayberry JF (1996) Long-term therapy with sulphasalazine protects against colorectal cancer in ulcerative colitis: A retrospective study of colorectal cancer risk and compliance with treatment in Leicestershire. Eur J Gastroenterol Hepatol 8: 1179–1183.
30. Lashner BA, Provencher KS, Seidner DL, Knesebeck A, Brzezinski A (1997) The effect of folic acid supplementation on the risk for cancer or dysplasia in ulcerative colitis. Gastroenterology 112: 29–32.
31. Eaden J, Abrams K, Ekbom A, Jackson E, Mayberry J (2000) Colorectal cancer prevention in ulcerative colitis: a case-control study. Aliment Pharmacol Ther 14: 145–153.
32. Lindberg BU, Broome U, Persson B (2001) Proximal colorectal dysplasia or cancer in ulcerative colitis. The impact of primary sclerosing cholangitis and sulfasalazine: Results from a 20-year surveillance study. Dis Colon Rectum 44: 77–85.
33. Rutter M, Saunders B, Wilkinson K, Rumbles S, Schofield G, et al. (2004) Severity of inflammation is a risk factor for colorectal neoplasia in ulcerative colitis. Gastroenterology 126: 451–459.
34. Winther KV, Jess T, Langholz E, Munkholm P, Binder V (2004) Long-term risk of cancer in ulcerative colitis: a population-based cohort study from Copenhagen County. Clin Gastroenterol Hepatol 2: 1088–1095.
35. Jess T, Loftus EV Jr, Velayos FS, Harmsen WS, Zinsmeister AR, et al. (2006) Risk of intestinal cancer in inflammatory bowel disease: a population-based study from olmsted county, Minnesota. Gastroenterology 130: 1039–1046.
36. Baars JE, Looman CW, Steyerberg EW, Beukers R, Tan AC, et al. (2011) The risk of inflammatory bowel disease-related colorectal carcinoma is limited: results from a nationwide nested case-control study. Am J Gastroenterol 106: 319–328.
37. Lyakhovich A, Gasche C (2010) Systematic review: molecular chemoprevention of colorectal malignancy by mesalazine. Aliment Pharmacol Ther 31: 202–209.
38. Lim WC, Hanauer S (2010) Aminosalicylates for induction of remission or response in Crohn's disease. Cochrane Database Syst Rev 12: CD008870.
39. Mowat C, Cole A, Windsor A, Ahmad T, Arnott I, et al; IBD Section of the British Society of Gastroenterology (2011) Guidelines for the management of inflammatory bowel disease in adults. Gut 60: 571–607.
40. Lichtenstein GR, Hanauer SB, Sandborn WJ; Practice Parameters Committee of American College of Gastroenterology (2009) Management of Crohn's disease in adults. Am J Gastroenterol 104: 465–483.
41. Kornbluth A, Sachar DB; Practice Parameters Committee of the American College of Gastroenterology (2010) Ulcerative colitis practice guidelines in adults: American College Of Gastroenterology, Practice Parameters Committee. Am J Gastroenterol 105: 501–523.
42. Feagan BG, Macdonald JK (2012) Oral 5-aminosalicylic acid for maintenance of remission in ulcerative colitis. Cochrane Database Syst Rev 10: CD000544.

DNA Methylation Status of Epithelial-Mesenchymal Transition (EMT) - Related Genes is Associated with Severe Clinical Phenotypes in Ulcerative Colitis (UC)

Tomomitsu Tahara[1]*, Tomoyuki Shibata[1], Masaaki Okubo[1], Takamitsu Ishizuka[1], Masakatsu Nakamura[2], Mitsuo Nagasaka[1], Yoshihito Nakagawa[1], Naoki Ohmiya[1], Tomiyasu Arisawa[2], Ichiro Hirata[1]

1 Department of Gastroenterology, Fujita Health University School of Medicine, Toyoake, Japan, **2** Department of Gastroenterology, Kanazawa Medical University, Ishikawa, Japan

Abstract

Background: Epithelial-to-mesenchymal transition (EMT) is a phenomenon that allows the conversion of adherent epithelial cells to a mesenchymal cell phenotype, which enhances migratory capacity and invasiveness. Recent studies have suggested that EMT contributes to the pathogenesis of ulcerative colitis (UC). We investigated the promoter DNA methylation status of EMT-related genes in the colonic mucosa in UC.

Methods: Colonic biopsies were obtained from the rectal inflammatory mucosa of 86 UC patients and the non-inflammatory proximal colonic mucosa of 10 paired patients. Bisulfite pyrosequencing was used to quantify the methylation of 5 candidate CpG island promoters (*NEUROG1*, *CDX1*, *miR-1247*, *CDH1*, and *CDH13*) and *LINE1*.

Results: Using an unsupervised hierarchical clustering analysis, inflamed rectal mucosa was well separated from mucosa that appeared normal. The *CDH1* and *CDH13* promoters were significantly associated with patient age ($p = 0.04$, 0.03, respectively). A similar trend was found between those genes and the duration of disease (*CDH1*: $p = 0.07$, *CDH13*: $p = 0.0002$, mean of both: $p < 0.00001$). Several positive associations were found between hypermethylation and severe clinical phenotypes (*CDX1* and *miR-1247* and a refractory phenotype: $p = 0.04$ and 0.006, respectively. *miR-1247* and *CDH1* hyper methylation and a more severe Mayo endoscopic subscore: *miR-1247*: $p = 0.0008$, *CDH1*: $p = 0.03$, mean of both: $p = 0.003$). When the severe clinical phenotype was defined as having any of five phenotypes (hospitalized more than twice, highest Mayo endoscopic subscore, steroid dependence, refractory, or a history of surgery) *miR-1247* hypermethylation was associated with the same phenotype ($p = 0.008$).

Conclusions: Our data suggest that variability in the methylation status of EMT-related genes is associated with more severe clinical phenotypes in UC.

Editor: Regine Schneider-Stock, Institute of Pathology, Germany

Funding: The authors have no support or funding to report.

Competing Interests: The authors have declared that no competing interests exist.

* Email: tomomiccyu@yahoo.co.jp

Introduction

Ulcerative colitis (UC) affects the colon and rectum and involves the innermost lining mucosa, manifesting as continuous areas of inflammation, with no segments of normal mucosa [1]. It is characterized by chronic and relapsing colonic inflammation of unknown etiology. UC is a multifactorial, heterogeneous, polygenic disease and is precipitated by a complex interaction of environmental, genetic, and immunological factors [2]. The factors explaining the heterogeneity of this disease have remained largely unidentified, and accurate biomarkers to predict disease severity are also limited.

DNA methylation, particularly promoter CpG island hypermethylation, contributes to carcinogenesis [3]. Subsequent studies have also revealed that CpG island hypermethylation also occurs in aged or inflamed tissue [3–5]. A high degree of CpG island hypermethylation is observed in both inflamed colonic tissues and dysplastic lesions, suggesting the potential usefulness of DNA methylation as a biomarker for predicting disease severity and cancer risk [6–8].

Epithelial-mesenchymal transition (EMT) is a biological phenomenon allowing polarized epithelial cells, which are normally bound to each other within an organized tissue, to transition into independent fibroblastic cells possessing migratory properties and the ability to invade the extracellular matrix [9–11]. It has been shown that EMT is involved in the initial step, that is, the acquisition of migratory and invasive capability, in carcinogenesis [12]. Recent studies have also suggested that EMT contributes to the pathogenesis of inflammatory bowel disease (IBD), based on a clinical analysis and animal experiments [13,14]. Indeed, *CDH1* encoding the epithelial cell marker E-cadherin is known to be reduced in areas of active ulcerative colitis [15]. Promoter hyper methylation of *CDH1* has been shown in inflamed colonic mucosa in UC [16]. A recent genome-wide association scan also identified *CDH1* as a susceptibility locus for UC [17]. Moreover, *CDH13*, encoding another cadherin protein H-cadherin has been shown to be methylated in colorectal cancer [18], an established complication of longstanding ulcerative colitis [19].

A recent genome-scale methylation analysis using an EMT model with ectopic expression of the transcription factor Twist1 in immortalized human mammary epithelial cells identified a number of methylated promoter CpG islands [20]. Because of the importance of DNA methylation and EMT in UC, we hypothesized that epigenetic modification of EMT-related genes may be a pathogenic mechanism in UC. To evaluate the importance of DNA methylation in EMT-related genes in UC, we investigated the promoter DNA methylation status of EMT-related genes in non-neoplastic rectal colonic mucosa of UC and assessed its relationship with various clinical phenotypes.

Methods

Ethics statement

This study was approved by the Human Research Ethics Committee of the Fujita Health University School of Medicine. Each participant provided written informed consent for the clinical and laboratory data to be used and published for research purposes. The study was conducted according to the principles outlined in the Declaration of Helsinki.

Study population

Enrolled in the study were 86 patients with ulcerative colitis (men: n = 48, women: n = 38). The median age was 35 years, and the median clinical duration was 5.5 years. Six cases underwent surgery due to a toxic megacolon or cancer occurrence. Rectal inflammatory mucosal specimens were obtained from all the patients during colonoscopic biopsies and preserved at −80°C until use. Paired non-inflammatory proximal colonic mucosae were also collected from 10 cases. All UC cases were clinically in remission at the time of endoscopy. The histopathological examinations showed mild or moderate inflammation but no evidence of dysplasia or neoplasia at all the sites where the biopsies were taken. Based on appearance during endoscopy, 20 patients showed inflammatory mucosa only in the rectum, and 38 patients showed an extension of the inflammatory mucosa into the left side of the colon (sigmoid and descending colons). The remaining 38 patients showed an extension of the inflammatory mucosa into proximal sites (transverse, and ascending colons, and cecum). We also used the Mayo endoscopic subscore to evaluate the endoscopic appearance where the colonoscopic biopsy was taken [21]. Each score was based on the endoscopic findings, as follows: 0, normal or inactive disease; 1, mild disease (erythema, decreased vascular pattern, and mild friability); 2, moderate disease (marked erythema, absent vascular pattern, friability, and erosions); and 3, severe disease (spontaneous bleeding and ulcerations). This cohort was recruited from our study investigating the association between promoter DNA methylation and clinical phenotypes, [22] host genetic factors [23] and telomere length [24].

CpG methylation analysis by bisulfite pyrosequencing

DNA was extracted from the specimens by protein precipitation methods. Bisulfite-treated genomic DNA was used to evaluate the methylation status of 5 CpG island promoters by bisulfite pyrosequencing (*NEUROG1*, *CDX1*, *miR-1247*, *CDH1*, and *CDH13*). These genes have been reported to be candidate molecules in EMT. *CDH1*, encoding the transmembrane protein E-cadherin, has been known as an EMT biomarker [9,10]. A recent genome-wide association scan also identified *CDH1* as the susceptibility locus for UC [17]. *CDH13* also encodes another cadherin protein, H-cadherin, which has been shown to be methylated in colorectal cancer [18]. We also included three CpG island promoters (*NEUROG1*, *CDX1* and *miR-1247*). These genes were recently identified with candidate methylated CpG island promoters using an EMT model with the ectopic expression of the transcription factor Twist1 in immortalized human mammary epithelial cells [20]. We also evaluated the methylation status of the *LINE1* repetitive element, an indicator of global hypomethylation [25]. The bisulfite treatment of DNA was performed with an EpiTect bisulfite kit (Qiagen) according to the manufacturer's protocol. Pyrosequencing was carried out using a PSQ96 system with a Pyro-Gold reagent kit (QIAGEN), and the results were analyzed using PyroMark Q96 ID software version 1.0 (QIAGEN). The primers used for pyrosequencing are listed in Table 1.

Statistical analysis

For the paired inflammatory and non-inflammatory colonic mucosa derived from ten patients, an unsupervised hierarchical clustering analysis was used to identify distinct subgroups based on the methylation status of 5 CpG island promoters. The methylation levels between two and three groups were compared using the t-test and Kruskal-Wallis test, respectively. The correlation between the methylation levels of CpG island promoters and the *LINE1* repetitive element, age and duration was assessed using a Spearman correlation analysis. The methylation levels of the CpG island promoters and the Mayo endoscopic subscores were assessed using one-way ANOVA. A p value <0.05 was considered statistically significant.

Results

Methylation status of EMT related genes among paired samples

Fig. 1 shows the results of an unsupervised hierarchical clustering analysis using paired inflammatory and non-inflammatory colonic mucosa derived from ten patients. This analysis revealed that a majority of the inflammatory rectal mucosa was clustered as hyper methylated samples compared with the non-inflammatory proximal mucosa. One inflammatory sample (69R) was clustered as a relatively hypo methylated sample, and one non-inflammatory proximal mucosa (68N) was also clustered as a relatively hyper methylated sample. However, compared with other samples from the same patients, the inflammatory rectal samples showed hyper methylation in both cases. Therefore, hyper methylation was observed in inflammatory rectal samples compared with the non-inflammatory proximal mucosa in all ten cases. Among all genes tested, we also observed that methylation of *CDX1* was considerably higher compared to other genes (*NEUROG1*, *miR-1247*, *CDH1*, and *CDH13*) across all the samples, possibly due to the difference of methylation susceptibility in colonic tissue or UC. Association between methylation status of EMT related genes and global hypomethylation.

To determine the association between the methylation status of EMT related genes and global hypomethylation, methylation of the *LINE1* repetitive element was evaluated. Among all 5 genes, methylation of the *CDH13* promoter was significantly correlated with hypomethylation of the *LINE1* repetitive element

Table 1. Primer sequences used in pyrosequencing.

Assay name	Forward primer (1st and 2nd step PCR) sequence	Reverse primer (1st step PCR) sequence	Reverse primer (2nd step PCR) sequence	Sequencing primer sequence
LINE1	TTTTGAGTTAGGTGTGGGATATA	AAAATCAAAAAATTCCCTTTC	U-AAAATCAAAAAATTCCCTTTC	GGGTGGGAGTGAT
NEUROG	TTTGGAGAAGTTTTGGTTAGTTTAGTT	ACCCCCCAATATTTACATAATTTAT ACTC	U-ACCCCCCAATATTTACATAATTTA TACTC	GAGAAGTTTTGGTTAGTTTA
CDX1	GTAGAGGAGGTTTTAGGGTTTAGTAT	CCAAACCCAAACTAACTAACCTA	U-CCAAACCCAAACTAACTAACCTA	GTTATGTGTTGGATAAGGAT
miR1247	AGATAGTGTTTAGGGTAGTTTAGTTTT TTAGA	AAATCTCCTTTCCCCTTAAACTACAAT	U-AAATCTCCTTTCCCCTTAAACTA CAAT	TTTTTTAGAAGGGAGATAGA
CDH1	TTTGATTTTAGGTTTTAGTGAGT	ACCACAACCAATCAACAA	U-ACCACAACCAATCAACAA	TAGTAATTTTAGGTTAGAGG
CDH13	GYGAGGTGTTTATTTYGTATTTGT	AACCAACTTCCCAAATAAATCAAC	U-AACCAACTTCCCAAATAAATCAAC	TGTTATGTAAAAYGAGGG

U= biotin labeled universal primer tag: 5′-biotin-GGGACACCGCTGATCGTTTA.

($p<0.0001$), while no association was found with all the other CpG island promoters (all p values>0.1) (Fig. 2).

Association between methylation status of EMT related genes and clinical phenotypes of UC

To evaluate the association between the methylation status of EMT related genes and clinical UC phenotypes, age, duration of disease, location of inflammation, clinical course, number of hospitalizations, steroid dependency, refractory phenotype and history of surgery were included in the analysis. Of 5 CpG sites, methylation of the *CDH1* and *CDH13* promoters was significantly associated with age ($p = 0.04$, 0.03, respectively). Methylation of *CDH1* was weakly associated with the duration of disease ($p = 0.07$). Methylation of *CDH13* was more closely associated with the duration of disease ($p = 0.0002$). The mean Z score of those 2 CpG promoters was also significantly associated with the duration of disease, and this association was stronger than those with age ($p<0.00001$ *vs.* 0.005) (Fig. 3).

No significant association was found between the methylation status of 5 genes and the location of inflammation, clinical course and number of hospitalizations. On the other hand, several positive associations were found between the hypermethylation of several genes and more severe UC clinical phenotypes (Table 2 and Fig. 4). For example, the hyper methylation of *CDX1* and *miR-1247* were significantly associated with a refractory UC phenotype ($p = 0.04$ and 0.006, respectively.). A similar trend was found between *CDH1* hyper methylation and the same phenotype ($p = 0.08$). *miR-1247* and *CDH1* hyper methylation were also weakly correlated with steroid dependency (*CDH1*: $p = 0.09$) and history of surgery (*miR-1247*: $p = 0.06$). In addition, there was a significant association between *miR-1247* and *CDH1* hyper methylation and a more severe Mayo endoscopic subscore (*miR-1247*: $p = 0.0008$, *CDH1*: $p = 0.03$, mean of both: $p = 0.003$) (Fig. 4).

To further investigate the association between the methylation status of EMT related genes and clinical UC phenotypes, a severe clinical phenotype was defined as having any of following phenotypes: hospitalized more than twice, the highest Mayo endoscopic subscore, steroid dependence, refractory disease, or history of surgery. These results demonstrated that *miR-1247* hypermethylation was significantly associated with severe clinical phenotype ($p = 0.008$), and a similar trend was observed for *CDH1* hyper methylation ($p<0.1$). The mean Z score of *miR-1247* and *CDH1* hyper methylation was also associated with the same phenotype ($p<0.02$) (Fig. 5).

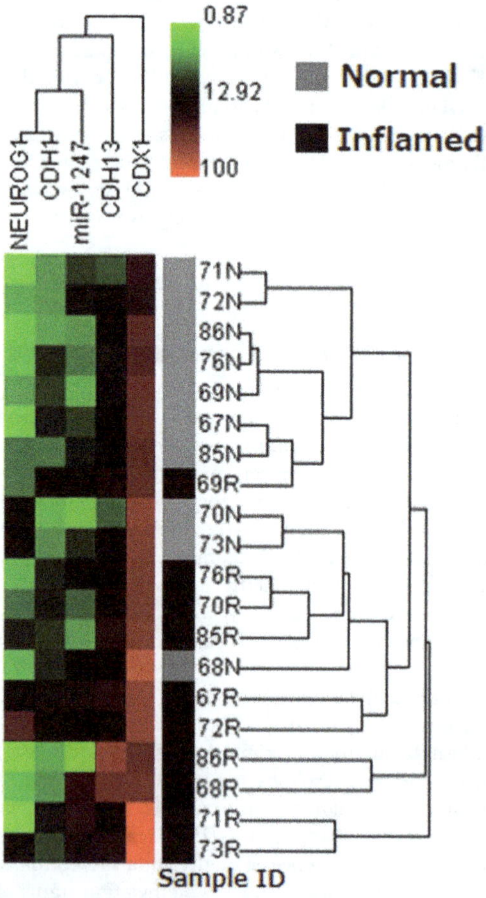

Figure 1. Unsupervised hierarchical clustering analysis using paired inflammatory and non-inflammatory colonic mucosa derived from ten patients. Black boxes, inflammatory rectal mucosa (R); grey boxes, normal proximal mucosa (N); Samples of the same ID number were obtained from the same patients.

Discussion

Our data show that rectal inflammatory mucosa in UC is characterized by hyper methylation at promoter CpG islands in EMT-related genes. Previous studies have revealed that accelerated DNA methylation is observed in both inflamed and dysplastic colonic epithelium of UC patients, especially in the age-related genes. Our result added the evidence that this methylation is also

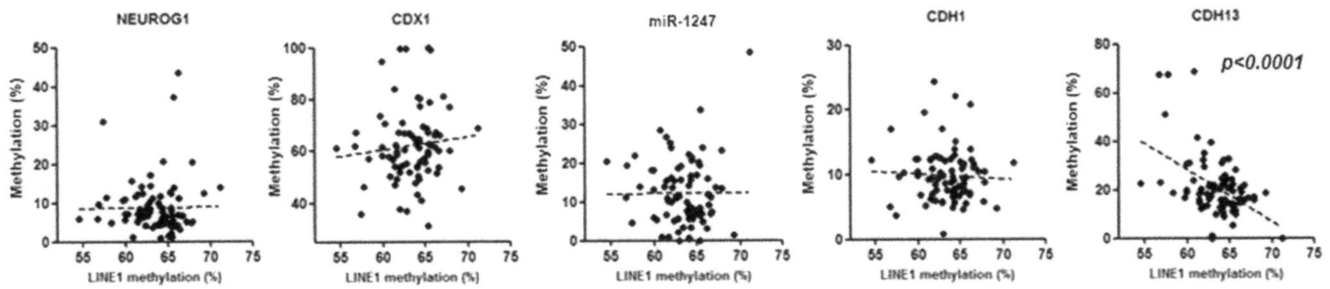

Figure 2. Association between methylation status of EMT-related genes and global hypomethylation assessed by methylation of the *LINE1* repetitive element. Statistical analysis was performed using the Spearman correlation analysis.

occurring in EMT-related genes. Recent studies suggest that EMT contributes to the pathogenesis of IBD [13,14]. One good example is reduced expression of *CDH1* encoding the epithelial cell marker E-cadherin, which may be partly explained by promoter CpG island methylation [15]. *CDH13*, encoding another cadherin protein H-cadherin, has also been reported to be methylated in colorectal cancer [18], an established complication of longstanding ulcerative colitis [19]. In this study, we also examined new candidate genes (*NEUROG1*, *CDX1* and *miR-1247*) that have recently been identified with candidate methylated CpG island promoters using an EMT human cell line model [20]. Several studies also indicate that methylation of *NEUROG1*, *CDX1* and *miR-1247* are involved in carcinogenesis in the colorectal (*NEUROG1*, *CDX1*) [26,27] and stomach (*miR-1247*) [28]. In paired colonic samples from UC patients, the inflamed rectal mucosa were well separated from the normal-appearing mucosa using the methylation status of 5 candidate genes by an unsupervised hierarchical clustering analysis. It can be speculated that the accumulation of promoter CpG island methylation of EMT-related genes affects gene expression, leading to a disturbance of intercellular adhesion in the intestinal epithelium in UC.

In inflamed and neoplastic epithelium, promoter CpG hyper methylation is closely correlated with global hypomethylation [24]. However, such an association was observed only in the *CDH13* promoter, but not for the remaining four genes, suggesting that the methylation of a majority of EMT-related genes is not linked to global hypomethylation.

We have also shown that the hypermethylation of EMT-related genes is associated with clinical UC phenotypes. The *CDH1* and *CDH13* promoters were significantly associated with patient age.

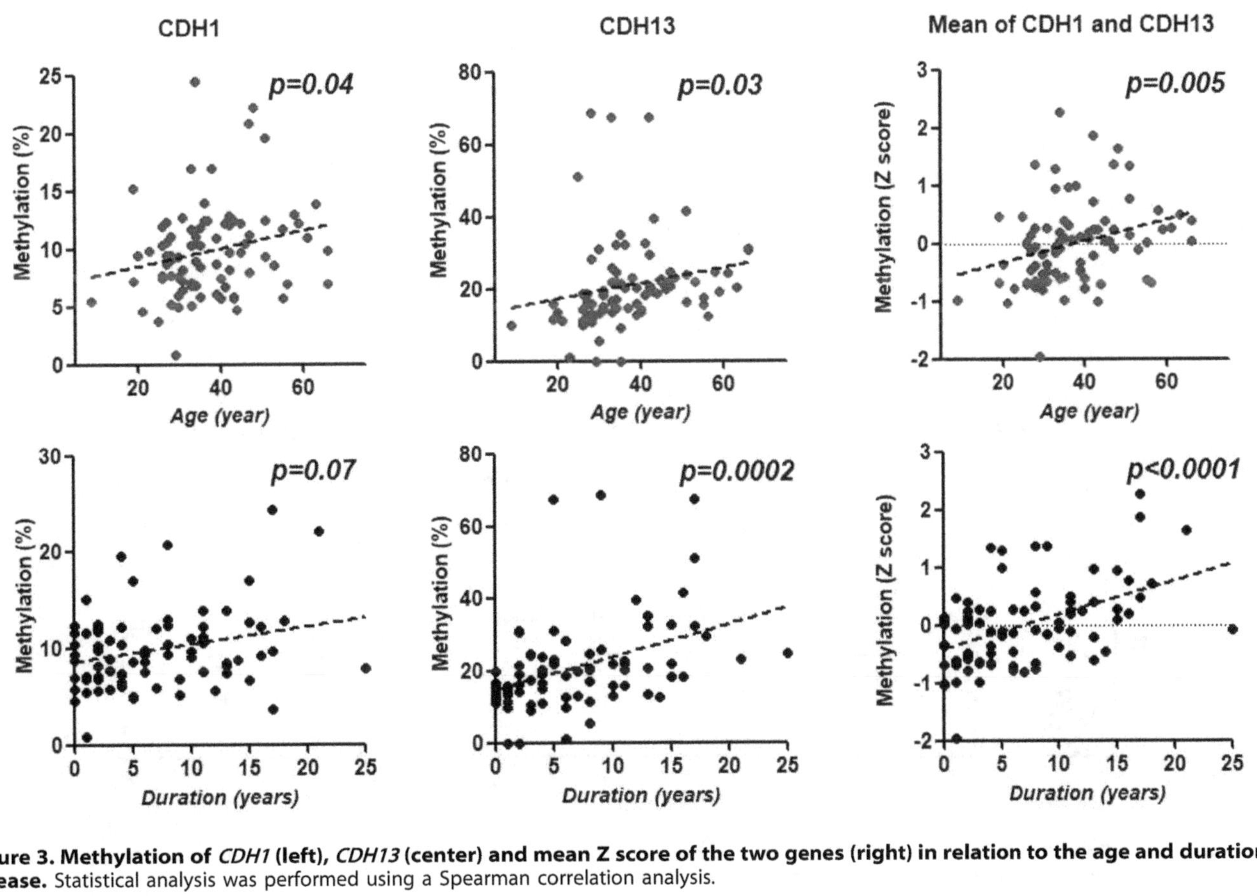

Figure 3. Methylation of *CDH1* (left), *CDH13* (center) and mean Z score of the two genes (right) in relation to the age and duration of disease. Statistical analysis was performed using a Spearman correlation analysis.

Table 2. Associations between methylation of EMT related genes and subtypes of UC.

Variables (n)	*NEUROG1* (%)	*CDX1* (%)	*miR-1247* (%)	*CDH1* (%)	*CDH13* (%)
Extension of the inflammatory lesions					
Proctitis (20)	9.6±2.0	60.9±2.9	11.0±1.9	9.7±0.8	17.9±1.4
Left sided-colitis (25)	7.5±0.7	61.1±2.7	14.5±2.0	9.5±0.8	24.7±3.8
Pancolitis (41)	9.0±1.1	63.5±2.5	11.3±1.2	10.0±0.7	20.0±1.4
Clinical courses¶					
Only one attack (9)	9.2±1.7	64.1±4.2	10.7±2.9	8.6±0.9	16.2±1.1
Relapse and remitting (38)	7.8±0.9	62.5±2.1	12.8±1.5	10.1±0.6	20.9±2
Chronic continuous (38)	9.5±1.4	61.6±2.7	11.9±1.3	9.8±0.8	22.2±2.3
Number of times hospitalized#					
0~1 (60)	8.6±0.9	61.4±1.8	11.3±0.9	9.6±0.5	21.6±1.7
2~ (23)	9.6±1.3	63.1±3.1	13.7±2.3	10.4±1.0	19.7±2.3
Steroid dependency $					
No (67)	8.3±0.8	61.3±1.7	11.9±1.1	9.4±0.4	20.2±1.4
Yes (18)	10.5±1.6	66.4±3.7	13.2±1.9	11.3±1.3	24.3±4.0
Refractory &					
No (55)	8.1±1.0	59.9±1.7	10.3±0.9	9.3±0.5	20.9±1.8
Yes (30)	10±1.1	66.8±3.0	15.6±1.9	10.9±0.8	21.1±1.9
Needing surgery*					
No (80)	8.4±0.8	61.9±1.6	11.6±0.9	9.7±0.5	21.5±1.4
Yes (6)	13.0±2.3	66.1±5.4	18.5±6.8	11.5±1.7	13.0±4.1

Note: Data are expressed as the mean ± SE. n, number of samples.
Two and three groups were compared using the t-test and Kruskal-Wallis test, respectively.
¶? #, $, & and *: Data are missing for one, three, one, and one cases, respectively.
$: *CDH1*, p=0.09, &: *CDX1*, p=0.04, *miR-1247*, p=0.006, *CDH1*, p=0.08.*: *miR-1247*, p=0.06.

Similarly, the methylation of those genes is correlated with the duration of disease, which is a well-accepted risk factor for cancer occurrence. Several positive associations were also found between the hypermethylation of EMT-related genes and more severe clinical UC phenotypes (hypermethylation of *CDX1* and *miR-1247* and refractory phenotype, hypermethylation of *miR-1247* and *CDH1* and severe Mayo endoscopic subscore). The mean Z score of *miR-1247* and *CDH1* hyper methylation was significantly associated with a severe clinical phenotype (more frequent hospitalization, the highest Mayo endoscopic subscore, steroid dependence, refractory disease, or history of surgery).

Our data suggest that there may be more variability in methylation status in the EMT-related genes during inflammation that can discriminate several phenotypic differences. UC is extremely heterogeneous in its clinical course, prognosis, and response to treatment; therefore, it is hypothesized that UC is a syndrome in which different pathogenic mechanisms lead to various clinical phenotypes, and it may be necessary to place greater emphasis on disease heterogeneity. Because severe

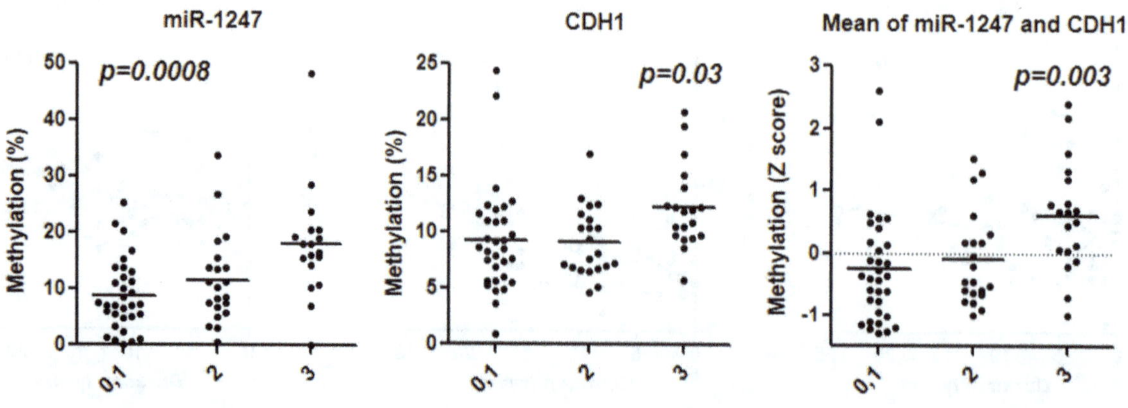

Figure 4. Methylation of *miR-1247* (left), *CDH1* (center) and mean Z score of the two genes (right) in relation to the Mayo endoscopic subscore. The statistical analysis was performed using one way ANOVA.

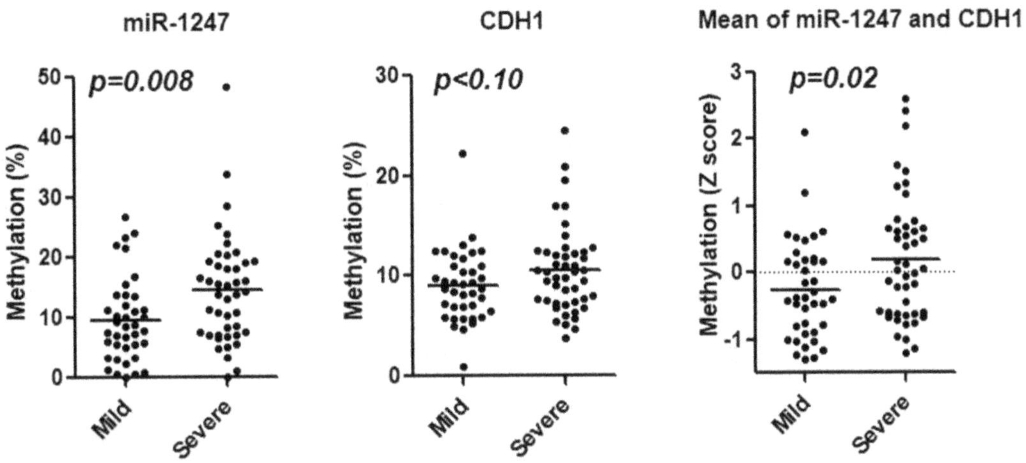

Figure 5. Methylation of *miR-1247* (left), *CDH1* (center) and mean Z score of the two genes (right) in relation to severe clinical phenotype of UC. The statistical analysis was performed using Student's t-Test.

phenotypes require more intensive clinical treatment, the results suggest that different UC subgroups have different molecular backgrounds. Our observation of an association between the hyper methylation of EMT-related genes and severe clinical UC phenotypes in the easily accessible rectum also indicates these genes' potential usefulness as molecular markers to direct more appropriate therapy that reflects an individual's pathophysiology. The findings also suggest that chronic inflammation in UC eventually leads to cancer progression [1]. Because severe inflammation characterized as having more frequent hospitalization, the highest Mayo endoscopic subscore, steroid dependence, refractory disease, or history of surgery would finally confer greater risk for developing cancer in UC, it is possible that hypermethylation predicts populations at high risk for developing colorectal cancer, which was not directly evaluated in this study. Since methylation of all genes examined have been reported to have roles in carcinogenesis in digestive tract, including colorectal and stomach. A well-designed prospective study will be needed to further clarify the clinical importance of DNA methylation in EMT-related genes as a biomarker for risk assessment of colorectal cancer in UC patients.

One limitation which should be noted is that the detailed mechanisms of how these EMT-related genes contribute to the pathogenesis of UC and/or UC-related carcinogenesis is unclear. More intensive experiment will be needed to examine the methylation of EMT-related genes in UC from the mechanistic view point including the interaction with gene expression and histone modifications etc.

Moreover, it is shown that differences in cell or tissue population will influence the nature of DNA. Since the majority of change with disease progression could occur in the epithelial DNA, it would be ideal to separate or enrich epithelial DNA from tissue. From the histological assessment from adjacent to mucosa from biopsy for DNA extraction, we confirmed that all the biopsies contained at least more than 70% of epithelial cells, however, it was not exactly same specimens used for DNA extraction. It should be therefore noted that result might be influenced depending on the difference of cell or tissue population and the methods to isolate colonic epithelium need to be considered for the future study.

Author Contributions

Not applicable. Conceived and designed the experiments: TT TS TA NO MO TI. Performed the experiments: TT. Analyzed the data: TT TA. Contributed reagents/materials/analysis tools: TT TS M. Nagasaka YN M. Nakamura NO IH TA. Wrote the paper: TT TA IH.

References

1. Head KA, Jurenka JS (2003) Inflammatory bowel disease Part I: ulcerative colitis-pathophysiology and conventional and alternative treatment options. Altern Med Rev 8: 247–283.
2. Lakatos L, Lakatos PL (2003) Etiopathogenesis of inflammatory bowel diseases. Orv Hetil 144: 1853–1860.
3. Issa JP (1999) Aging, DNA methylation and cancer. Crit Rev Oncol Hematol 32: 31–43.
4. Issa JP, Ottaviano YL, Celano P, Hamilton SR, Davidson NE, et al. (1994) Methylation of the oestrogen receptor CpG island links ageing and neoplasia in human colon. Nat Genet. 7: 536–540.
5. Maekita T, Nakazawa K, Mihara M, Nakajima T, Yanaoka K, et al. (2006) High levels of aberrant DNA methylation in Helicobacter pylori-infected gastric mucosae and its possible association with gastric cancer risk. Clin Cancer Res. 12(3 Pt 1): 989–995.
6. Issa JP, Ahuja N, Toyota M, Bronner MP, Brentnall TA (2001) Accelerated age-related CpG island methylation in ulcerative colitis. Cancer Res. 61: 3573–3577.
7. Konishi K, Shen L, Wang S, Meltzer SJ, Harpaz N, et al. (2007) Rare CpG island methylator phenotype in ulcerative colitis-associated neoplasias. Gastroenterology. 132: 1254–1260.
8. Tominaga K, Fujii S, Mukawa K, Fujita M, Ichikawa K, et al. (2005) Prediction of colorectal neoplasia by quantitative methylation analysis of estrogen receptor gene in nonneoplastic epithelium from patients with ulcerative colitis. Clin Cancer Res. 11: 8880–8885.
9. Cano A, Pérez-Moreno MA, Rodrigo I, Locascio A, Blanco MJ, et al. (2000) The transcription factor snail controls epithelial-mesenchymal transitions by repressing E-cadherin expression. Nat Cell Biol 2: 76–83.
10. Auersperg N, Pan J, Grove BD, Peterson T, Fisher J, et al. (1999) E-cadherin induces mesenchymal-to-epithelial transition in human ovarian surface epithelium. Proc Natl Acad Sci USA 96: 6249–6254.
11. Kalluri R, Neilson EG (2003) Epithelial-mesenchymal transition and its implications for fibrosis. J Clin Invest 112: 1776–1784.
12. Thiery JP (2003) Epithelial-mesenchymal transitions in development and pathologies. Curr Opin Cell Biol. 15: 740–746.
13. Scharl M, Weber A, Fürst A, Farkas S, Jehle E, et al. (2011) Potential role for SNAIL family transcription factors in the etiology of Crohn's disease-associated fistulae. Inflamm Bowel Dis 17: 1907–1916.
14. Flier SN, Tanjore H, Kokkotou EG, Sugimoto H, Zeisberg M, et al. (2010) Identification of epithelial to mesenchymal transition as a novel source of fibroblasts in intestinal fibrosis. J Biol Chem285: 20202–20212.
15. Karayiannakis AJ, Syrigos KN, Efstathiou J, Valizadeh A, Noda M, et al. (1998) Expression of catenins and E-cadherin during epithelial restitution in inflammatory bowel disease. J Pathol. 185: 413–418.

16. Saito S, Kato J, Hiraoka S, Horii J, Suzuki H, et al. (2011) DNA methylation of colon mucosa in ulcerative colitis patients: correlation with inflammatory status. Inflamm Bowel Dis. 17: 1955–1965.
17. UK IBD Genetics Consortium (2009) Genome-wide association study of ulcerative colitis identifies three new susceptibility loci, including the HNF4A region. Nat Genet. 41: 1330–1334.
18. Wang Z, Yuan X, Jiao N, Zhu H, Zhang Y, et al. (2012) CDH13 and FLBN3 gene methylation are associated with poor prognosis in colorectal cancer. Pathol Oncol Res. 18: 263–270.
19. Eaden JA, Abrams KR, Mayberry JF (2001) The risk of colorectal cancer in ulcerative colitis: a meta-analysis. Gut. 48: 526–535.
20. Malouf GG, Taube JH, Lu Y, Roysarkar T, Panjarian S, et al. (2013) Architecture of epigenetic reprogramming following Twist1-mediated epithelial-mesenchymal transition. Genome Biol. 14:R144. [Epub ahead of print].
21. Schroeder KW, Tremaine WJ, Ilstrup DM (1987) Coated oral 5-aminosalicylic acid therapy for mildly to moderately active ulcerative colitis: a randomized study. The New England Journal of Medicine. 317: 1625–1629.
22. Tahara T, Shibata T, Nakamura M, Yamashita H, Yoshioka D, et al. (2009) Promoter methylation of protease-activated receptor (PAR2) is associated with severe clinical phenotypes of ulcerative colitis (UC). Clin Exp Med. 9: 125–130.
23. Tahara T, Shibata T, Nakamura M, Okubo M, Yamashita H, et al. (2011) Association between polymorphisms in the XRCC1 and GST genes, and CpG island methylation status in colonic mucosa in ulcerative colitis. Virchows Arch. 458: 205–211.
24. Tahara T, Shibata T, Okubo M, Kawamura T, Sumi K, et al. (2014) Telomere length in non-neoplastic colonic mucosa in ulcerative colitis (UC) and its relationship to the severe clinical phenotypes. Clin Exp Med. [Epub ahead of print].
25. Estécio MR, Gharibyan V, Shen L, Ibrahim AE, Doshi K, et al. (2007) LINE-1 hypomethylation in cancer is highly variable and inversely correlated with microsatellite instability. PLoS One 2:e399
26. Shiovitz S, Bertagnolli MM, Renfro LA, Nam E, Foster NR, et al. (2014) CpG Island Methylator Phenotype Is Associated With Response to Adjuvant Irinotecan-Based Therapy for Stage III Colon Cancer. Gastroenterology. [Epub ahead of print].
27. Suh ER, Ha CS, Rankin EB, Toyota M, Traber PG (2002) DNA methylation down-regulates CDX1 gene expression in colorectal cancer cell lines. J Biol Chem. 277: 35795–35800.
28. Kim JG, Kim TO, Bae JH, Shim JW, Kang MJ, Yang K, et al. (2014) Epigenetically regulated MIR941 and MIR1247 target gastric cancer cell growth and migration. Epigenetics. [Epub ahead of print].

Myosin Light Chain Kinase Expression Induced via Tumor Necrosis Factor Receptor 2 Signaling in the Epithelial Cells Regulates the Development of Colitis-Associated Carcinogenesis

Masahiro Suzuki[1], Takashi Nagaishi[1*], Motomi Yamazaki[2], Michio Onizawa[1], Taro Watabe[1], Yuriko Sakamaki[3], Shizuko Ichinose[3], Mamoru Totsuka[4], Shigeru Oshima[1], Ryuichi Okamoto[1], Motoyuki Shimonaka[5], Hideo Yagita[6], Tetsuya Nakamura[1], Mamoru Watanabe[1*]

1 Department of Gastroenterology, Graduate School of Medical Science, Tokyo Medical and Dental University, Tokyo, Japan, **2** Department of Obstetrics and Gynecology, Nihon University School of Medicine, Tokyo, Japan, **3** Research Center for Medical and Dental Sciences, Tokyo Medical and Dental University, Tokyo, Japan, **4** Department of Applied Biological Chemistry, The University of Tokyo, Tokyo, Japan, **5** Department of Chemistry, Tokyo University of Science, Tokyo, Japan, **6** Department of Immunology, Juntendo University School of Medicine, Tokyo, Japan

Abstract

It has been suggested that prolonged inflammatory bowel diseases (IBD) may lead to colitis-associated carcinogenesis (CAC). We previously observed that the NF-κB activation in colonic epithelial cells is associated with increased tumor necrosis factor receptor 2 (TNFR2) expression in CAC development. However, the mechanism by which epithelial NF-κB activation leading to CAC is still unclear. Myosin light chain kinase (MLCK) has been reported to be responsible for the epithelial permeability associated with TNF signaling. Therefore we focused on the role of MLCK expression via TNFR2 signaling on CAC development. Pro-tumorigenic cytokines such as IL-1β, IL-6 and MIP-2 production as well as INF-γ and TNF production at the lamina propria were increased in the setting of colitis, and further in tumor tissues in associations with up-regulated TNFR2 and MLCK expressions in the epithelial cells of a CAC model. The up-regulated MLCK expression was observed in TNF-stimulated colonic epithelial cells in a dose-dependent fashion in association with up-regulation of TNFR2. Silencing TNFR2, but not TNFR1, resulted in restoration of epithelial tight junction (TJ) associated with decreased MLCK expression. Antibody-mediated blockade of TNF signaling also resulted in restoration of TJ in association with suppressed MLCK expression, and interestingly, similar results were observed with suppressing TNFR2 and MLCK expressions by inhibiting MLCK in the epithelial cells. Silencing of MLCK also resulted in suppressed TNFR2, but not TNFR1, expression, suggesting that the restored TJ leads to reduced TNFR2 signaling. Such suppression of MLCK as well as blockade of TNFR2 signaling resulted in restored TJ, decreased pro-tumorigenic cytokines and reduced CAC development. These results suggest that MLCK may be a potential target for the prevention of IBD-associated tumor development.

Editor: Emiko Mizoguchi, Massachusetts General Hospital, United States of America

Funding: This study was supported in part by Grants-in-Aid for Scientific Research (T. Nagaishi, T. Nakamura and MW), Scientific Research on Priority Areas (MW), Exploratory Research and Creative Scientific Research (MW) from the Japanese Ministry of Education, Culture, Sports, Science and Technology; the Japanese Ministry of Health, Labor and Welfare (MW); the Japan Medical Association (MW); Japan Foundation for Applied Enzymology (MO); Japan Health Sciences Foundation (MO); Memorial Fund of Nihon Univ. Medical Alumni Association (T. Nagaishi); Abbott Japan Allergy Research Award (T. Nagaishi); Foundation for Advancement of International Science (T. Nagaishi); Takeda Science Foundation (T. Nagaishi). The funders had no role in study design, data collection and analysis, decision to publish, or preparation of the manuscript.

Competing Interests: The authors have declared that no competing interests exist.

* E-mail: tnagaishi.gast@tmd.ac.jp (TN); mamoru.gast@tmd.ac.jp (MW)

These authors contributed equally to this work.

Introduction

Although the pathogenesis of inflammatory bowel disease (IBD), such as Crohn's disease and ulcerative colitis in humans, still remains unclear, chronic epithelial permeability seems to be one of the mechanisms by which extensive inflammatory factors may be introduced into the irritated intestinal tissues. Therefore, it is believed that induction of mucosal healing is critical in the management of IBD [1]. Furthermore, chronic inflammation is believed to associate with carcinogenesis, and prolonged duration of IBD likely also lead to colitis-associated cancer (CAC) [2,3,4].

Previous study had shown that activation of NF-κB in the inflamed tissue is strongly associated with carcinogenesis [5]. In this regard, we have investigated the mechanism of NF-κB activation in the colonic epithelial cells using a murine model of IBD. We have previously reported that increased expression of tumor necrosis factor (TNF) in a murine IBD model is critical for the development of CAC [6]. TNF is a pivotal cytokine associated with the continuous immune dysregulation in the inflamed tissue of IBD [7,8]. In our previous study, the specific up-regulation of the type 2 receptor for TNF (TNFR2) was also observed in the inflamed intestinal epithelial cells. This observation seems logical since the cytoplasmic domain of TNFR2 can also activate NF-κB pathway, but it lacks association with the death domains (DD) like that of TNFR1. However, the specific role of such NF-κB activation in the inflamed epithelia via TNFR2 signaling in the context of CAC has not been elucidated.

Myosin light chain kinase (MLCK) has also been reported to be expressed in the human intestinal tissue with IBD [9]. MLCK is classically known to be required for the contraction of actomyosin via the phosphorylation of myosin light chain (MLC) [10]. It is also essential to the permeability of epithelial barrier according to in vitro and in vivo studies, and it is associated with the production of pro-inflammatory cytokine, such as TNF, in the inflamed intestinal tissues [9,11]. In addition, several recent reports have implicated the role of MLCK in animal models of IBD [12,13,14]. However, the association between MLCK and CAC development has not been reported. We hypothesized that one of the roles of epithelial NF-κB activation would be the induction of MLCK in the context of IBD. We therefore examined the role of MLCK in the development of IBD-associated carcinogenesis.

Materials and Methods

Cell Culture

Murine colonic epithelial cell line, MOC1 [15], which was generated from 'non-tumor' colonic epithelia of BALB/c and transformed with SV40 large T antigen, was established by Dr. M. Totsuka (University of Tokyo, Japan) and maintained in RPMI 1640 (Sigma, St. Louis, MO) supplemented with 5% fetal bovine serum, 500 units/ml penicillin, 100 μg/ml streptomycin (Sigma) and 10 μg/ml insulin (Sigma) at 37°C in 5% CO_2. Cells were seeded at a density of 5×10^4 cells/ml in 6-well plates 24–36 h prior to the experiments with or without recombinant (r) mouse interferon (IFN)-γ and/or r mouse TNF (Peprotek, London, UK). In some experiments, cells were also incubated in the presence of either blocking anti-mouse TNF monoclonal antibody (mAb) (MP6-XT22, rat IgG1b) (DNAX Research Institute, Palo Alto, CA) [6] or MLCK inhibitor, ML-7 (Sigma).

Animals

Wild-type female C57BL/6 mice (6–8 wk old) were purchased from Japan Clea (Tokyo, Japan) and maintained under specific pathogen-free conditions in the Animal Care Facility of Tokyo Medical and Dental University (TMDU), Japan. Mice were used between 8–10 weeks of age. All animal experimentations were approved by the Animal Review Board of TMDU and were performed in accordance with institutional guidelines.

Induction of Chronic Colitis and CAC Models

Mice were randomized by body weight into three groups (n = 5) and given intraperitoneal (i.p.) 10 mg/kg of azoxymethane (AOM, Sigma) at day −7, followed by the administration of three cycles of 2.0% dextran sodium sulfate (DSS, molecular weight 10,000; Yokohama Kokusai Bio, Kanagawa, Japan) for 5 days and regular water for 16 days, and then injected i.p. with either the inhibitor against MLCK, ML-7 (2.0 mg/kg) or the vehicle control (2.0% ethanol) every 12 h from day 63 for 7 days. In some experiments, mice were injected i.p. with either 2.0 mg/kg of ML-7 every 12 h or 50 mg/kg of MP6-XT22, an anti-mouse TNF mAb, weekly starting at the end of first DSS treatment (day 5) (n = 10) and then euthanized at day 70. Mice were euthanized 11 weeks after the first injection of AOM, and colons were removed and immediately flushed with PBS. The isolated colonic epithelial samples from mice were prepared as previously described [16] for assessment of protein and/or mRNA expression in the epithelia.

Histological Scoring of Colitis and CAC

Tissues from proximal and distal colons were removed for histologic assessment. For this, the tissue samples were fixed in 10% neutral-buffered formalin. Paraffin-embedded sections (5 μm) were stained with hematoxylin and eosin (H-E). The sections were analyzed without prior knowledge of the types of treatments. The histological scoring of colitis was determined according to the previously described system with minor modifications [6,17]. Briefly, for extent of leukocyte infiltration in tissue layers, 0 points were assigned to normal appearance, or the presence of occasional inflammatory cells in the lamina propria; 1 point to increased numbers of inflammatory cells in the lamina propria; 2 points to confluence of inflammatory cells, extending into the submucosa; and 3 points to transmural extension of the infiltrate. For severity of leukocyte infiltration, 0 points were assigned to none to normal lymphoid aggregates; 1 point to mild infiltration; 2 points to moderate infiltration; 3 points to severe infiltration. For extent of leukocyte infiltration in colon, 0 points were assigned to none to occasional infiltration; 1 point to patchy (focal) infiltration; 2 points to intermediate infiltration; 3 points to diffuse (extensive) infiltration.

For tissue damage, 0 points were assigned to no mucosal damage; 1 point to discrete lymphoepithelial lesions; 2 points to surface mucosal erosion or focal ulceration; and 3 points to extensive mucosal damage and extension into deeper structures of the bowel wall. The cumulative degree of these parameters was calculated as a total histological score ranging from 0 (no changes) to 6 (extensive cell infiltration and tissue damage). For crypt abscess, the assigned points were; 0, to no crypt abscess; 1, to the presence of crypt abscess. For CAC assessment, sections (5 μm) were cut stepwise (200 μm) through the complete block and stained with H-E. Tumor numbers were counted by trained individuals blinded to the treatment group.

Western Blotting

Western blotting was performed as previously described [18,19]. Briefly, 10 to 100 μg of nucleic extracts or whole protein lysates from either the stripped epithelial samples or MOC1 cells were separated by 8–15% SDS-PAGE and each protein expressions were analyzed with following primary and secondary Abs: anti-mouse TNFR1 polyclonal Ab (pAb), anti-mouse TNFR2 pAb (R&D Systems, Minneapolis, MN), anti-phosphorylated (p)-p65 mAb at serine 536, anti-p65 pAb, anti-p-IκBα mAb at serine 32/36, anti-IκBα pAb, anti-p-MLC pAb, anti-MLC pAb (Cell Signaling Technology Inc, Beverly, MA), anti-MLCK mAb, anti-β-actin mAb (Sigma), anti-mouse IgG-HRP, anti-rabbit IgG-HRP (GE Healthcare Bio-Sciences, Piscataway, NJ) and anti-goat IgG-HRP (Santa Cruz). Signals were generated with ECL Western Blotting Detection System (GE Healthcare Bio-Sciences).

Semi-quantitative PCR (q-PCR)

Total cellular RNA was extracted from either whole colonic mucosa, isolated epithelial samples of non-tumor or tumor area removed from AOM/DSS-treated mice, or cultured MOC1 cells with RNA-Bee (Tel-Test, Inc, Friendswood, TX). Five micrograms of total RNA were subjected to reverse transcription using Superscript Reverse Transcriptase kit (Invitrogen, Carlsbad, CA). The cDNA samples were then applied for PCR with the following primer pairs: interleukin (IL)-1β, 5′-TTG ACG GAC CCA AAA GAT-3′ and 5′-GAA GCT GGA TGC TCT CAT CTG-3′; IL-6, 5′-GCT ACC AAA CTG GAT ATA ATC GGA-3′ and 5′-CCA GGT AGC TAT GGT ACT CCA GAA-3′; macrophage inflammatory protein (MIP)-2, 5′-AAA ATC ATC CAA AAG

ATA CTG AAC AA-3′ and 5′-CTT TGG TTC TTC CGT TGA GG-3′; IFN-γ, 5′-CGA CTC CTT TTC CGC TTC CTG AG-3′ and 5′-TGA ACG CTA CAC ACT GCA TCT TGG-3′; TNF, 5′-GCC ATG AGG TCC ACC ACC CTG-3′ and 5′-CTA CTG GCG CTG CCA AGG CTG T-3′; glyceraldehyde-3-phosphate dehydrogenase (G3PDH), 5′-CTA CTG GCG CTG CCA AGG CAG T-3′ and 5′-GCC ATG AGG TCC ACC ACC CTG-3′, respectively. Real time PCR was performed with QuantiTect SYBER green PCR kit (Qiagen, Venio, Netherlands) using an ABI7500 real-time PCR system and 7500 system SDS software (Applied Biosystems, Foster City, CA). mRNA was shown as the relative amount normalized to that of G3PDH.

Small Interfering (si) RNA Transfection

MOC1 cells were transfected by lipofection (Lipofectamine RNAi MAX, Invitrogen, Carlsbad, CA) with the siRNA oligomers against either mouse MLCK (Mm Mylk 9988, Sigma), TNFR1 (MSS212008), TNFR2 (MSS238548) or non-targeting control (12935-112, Invitrogen) and incubated at a density of 5×10^4 cells/ml in OPTI-MEM (Invitrogen) for 48 h.

Transmission Electron Microscopy (TEM)

TEM was performed as previously described [20]. Briefly, colonic tissues from AOM/DSS-treated mice or MOC1 cells that were seeded on the Cell Disk® (Sumitomo, Tokyo, Japan) were fixed with 2.5% glutaraldehyde in 0.1 M phosphate buffer (PB) for 2 h. The samples were washed with 0.1 M PB, post-fixed in 1.0% OsO_4 buffered with 0.1 M PB for 2 h, dehydrated in a graded series of ethanol and embedded in Epon-812. Semi-thin sections were cut at 1 μm and stained with toluidine blue. Ultrathin sections, 90 nm, were collected on copper grids, double-stained with uranyl acetate and lead citrate, and then observed using transmission electron microscopy (H-7100, Hitachi, Hitachinaka, Japan).

Statistical Analysis

The results are expressed as the mean ± standard error of the mean (SEM). Statistical significance was determined using non-parametric Mann-Whitney *U*-test, and differences were considered to be statistically significant with $p<0.05$.

Results

Secretion of Cytokines that Support Tumor Growth is Associated with Epithelial MLCK Expression in the CAC Model

We previously observed that cytokines such as IL-1β, IL-6 and MIP-2 were up-regulated in an animal model of colitis [6]. This suggested that these factors may be essential for tumor development since each had been reported to support tumor growth in such model [21,22,23,24]. However, it was unclear if these cytokines could be substantially up-regulated in the setting of CAC. In addition, it was also unclear if such elevated cytokines were mainly produced from the epithelia, since intestinal epithelial cells had been reported to be capable of expressing these molecules [25,26,27,28]. Therefore we first assessed the expression levels of these cytokines in the mucosal tissues and the isolated epithelial cells in an animal model of CAC. Wild type C57BL/6 mice were administered AOM, then treated three times with DSS to induce chronic colitis and CAC. As seen in Fig. 1A, q-PCR revealed significant up-regulation of IL-1β, IL-6 and MIP-2 in the inflamed colonic tissues when compared to the control mice. Associated with this, significant up-regulations of pro-inflammatory cytokines, such as IFN-γ and TNF, were also observed as seen in Fig. 1B. In addition, the expressions of all of these cytokines were further up-regulated in the area of tumors compared to non-tumor area. Moreover, q-PCR also indicated that these cytokines were not much expressed by the epithelial cells (Fig. 1A and B). These results imply that such increase of these cytokines are presumably produced by infiltrating cells in the tissues such as granulocytes and macrophages and may be required for the progression of CAC.

Given these results, we hypothesized that the increased pro-tumorigenic cytokines produced by the infiltrating cells in the inflamed tissues may be associated with the disrupted epithelial tight junctions (TJ), which results in bacterial translocation into the lamina propria. In addition, we have also observed that TNFR2 expression was specifically up-regulated in the inflamed epithelia [6]. In this regard, it has been reported by Wang et al. that the up-regulated MLCK in human intestinal cells is required for TNF-induced collapse of epithelial TJ by TNFR2 signaling [11,29]. Moreover, it has been reported by two groups that MLCK promoter activity is mediated by NF-κB activation [30,31,32]. Therefore, we addressed the epithelial MLCK expression in the CAC model. As seen in Fig. 1C, Western blotting revealed up-regulated MLCK expression in the epithelia from non-tumor area, and further up-regulation in that of tumor, in association with the up-regulated TNFR2 and p65. However, up-regulation of TNFR1 was not remarkable compared to that of TNFR2. These results indicate that the development of CAC may be associated with the disrupted TJ and elevated pro-tumorigenic cytokines, which are essentially induced by TNFR2 signaling and MLCK expression in the epithelia.

MLCK Expression in the Epithelial Cells is Up-regulated by the Presence of Pro-inflammatory Cytokines in vitro

Given the up-regulated TNFR2 and MLCK expressions in the epithelial cells associated with pro-tumorigenic and pro-inflammatory cytokines expressions in the mucosal tissues from chronic colitis and CAC model, it was surmised that each of these complicated phenomena may be associated with the mechanisms by which tumorigenesis is induced in the context of IBD. Especially, previous reports suggested that stimulation of human intestinal epithelial cell lines with IFN-γ results in the regulation of TNF receptors [29,33,34]. Therefore, a murine colonic epithelial cell line (MOC1) derived from colonic epithelial cell [15] was used to study the specific roles of TNFR2 and MLCK expressions in the epithelial cells in the context of inflammation. MOC1 cells were cultured in the presence of pro-inflammatory cytokines, rIFN-γ and rTNF. As seen in Fig. 2A, the up-regulations of TNFR1 and 2 were induced by rIFN-γ alone, and this is consistent with previous observations with human T84 and Caco2 cells [29,33,34]. However, the increased TNFR2 level was more remarkable compared to that of TNFR1, and such TNFR2 expression in MOC1 cells was maximal at the concentration of 1.0 ng/ml rIFN-γ (Fig. 2A).

Next, MOC1 cells were stimulated with different concentrations of rTNF together with rIFN-γ at 1.0 ng/ml. Western blotting showed that phosphorylations of p65 and IκBα were induced in these cells by the presence of rTNF in a dose-dependent manner (Fig. 2B). Moreover, the expressions of MLCK as well as TNFR2, but not much of TNFR1, were further up-regulated by the addition of rTNF in a dose-dependent fashion in collaboration with constant concentration of rIFN-γ, and these expressions were maximal at 2.5 ng/ml of rTNF (Fig. 2C). These results suggest that the pro-inflammatory cytokines, especially TNF, may be

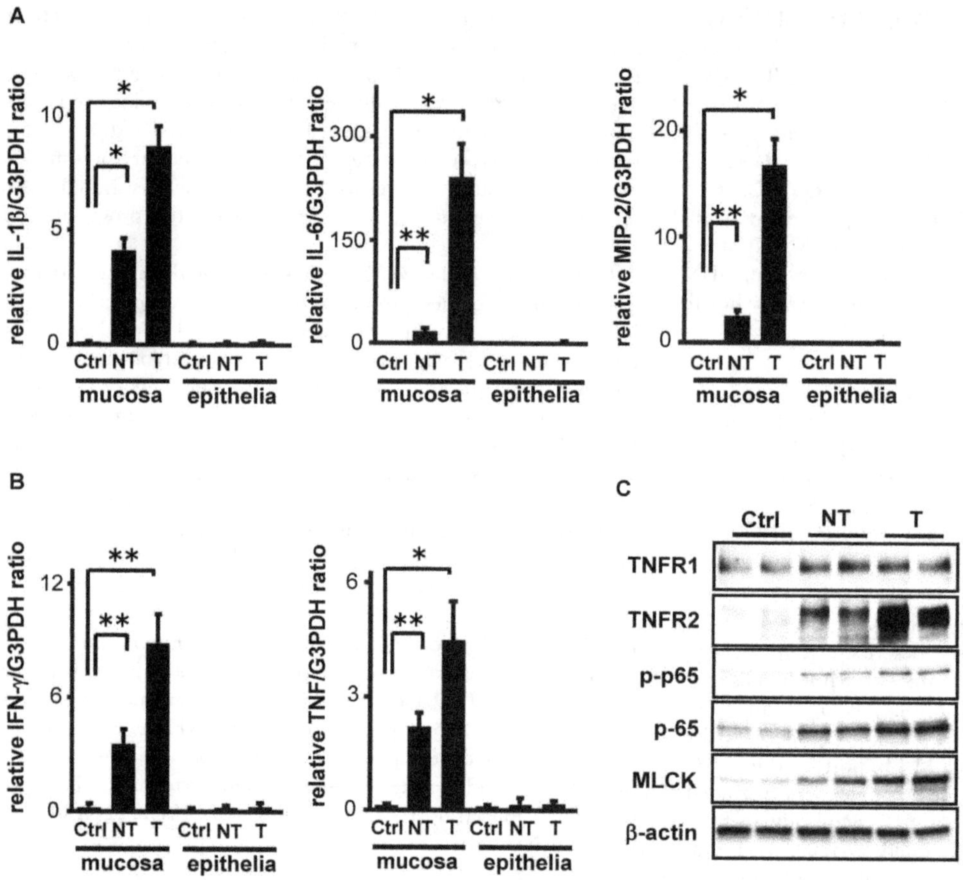

Figure 1. Pro-tumorigenic cytokines are increased in inflamed colonic mucosa, and further in tumors in AOM/DSS model. (A and B) Relative mRNA expressions for IL-1β, IL-6, MIP-2 (A), IFN-γ and TNF (B) in colonic mucosal tissues (mucosa) or isolated epithelial cells (epithelia) from either non-treated control (Ctrl), non-tumor (NT) or tumor tissues (T) in AOM/DSS treated mice are shown. Mucosal tissue samples including the epithelia and lamina propria were mechanically stripped from the whole colon to eliminate the muscularis layer, and RNA was then isolated. Mucosal tissue samples were also dissolved with 0.5 μM EDTA for 15 min, washed with PBS twice, subjected to density gradient centrifugation to isolate epithelial cells, and applied for RNA extraction. Each mRNA level was quantified by q-PCR and normalized to the level of G3PDH (n = 3). *; $p<0.01$, **; $p<0.05$. (C) Protein lysates of isolated epithelial cells from non-treated control (Ctrl), non-tumor (NT) or tumor tissues (T) were subjected to Western blotting with either anti-TNFR1, anti-TNFR2, anti-p-p65, anti-p65, anti-MLCK, or anti-β-actin Abs, respectively.

required for the induction of MLCK up-regulation via TNFR2 signaling in the colonic epithelial cells.

MLCK Expression and Disrupted Intercellular Junctions are Induced by Up-regulated TNFR2, but not TNFR1

Given the observation of up-regulated MLCK expression in association with the up-regulated TNFR2 expression in MOC1 cells, we next pursued the specific linkage between TNFR2 and MLCK in vitro. To do so, gene expressions of either TNFR1 or TNFR2 in MOC1 cells were silenced by transfection with specific siRNAs. We first confirmed the efficacies of siRNA oligomers against either TNFR1 or TNFR2 in these cells. As expected, knocked-down expressions of either TNFR1 or TNFR2 were observed with each specific siRNA (Fig. 3A). It should be noted that the endogenous expression of MLCK in MOC1 cells was not affected by the silencing of either TNFR1 or TNFR2 (Fig. 3A). We next assessed the effect of each silencing on the induction of MLCK up-regulation by pro-inflammatory cytokines in these cells. As seen in Fig. 3B, MLCK expression was up-regulated by stimulation with rIFN-γ and rTNF, and this is consistent with the results seen in Fig. 2C. In addition, the up-regulated MLCK expression in the presence of rIFN-γ and rTNF was not affected by the knocking-down of TNFR1 expression. However, such up-regulation of MLCK was remarkably suppressed by TNFR2 silencing (Fig. 3B). These results indicate that up-regulation of MLCK is specifically induced by TNFR2 signaling in the epithelial cells.

It was still unclear whether such up-regulated MLCK expression substantially affects the intestinal epithelial cells. Therefore, we next studied the morphology of MOC1 cells in the presence of rIFN-γ and rTNF. As seen in Fig. 3C, intercellular junctional complexes of these cells with intact TJ were observed using transmission electron microscopies (TEM) regardless of single stimulation with rIFN-γ. When stimulated with both rIFN-γ and rTNF, MOC1 cells showed collapsed intercellular junctional complexes with disappeared TJ, and the silencing of TNFR1 expression did not affect such features. However, the silencing of TNFR2 expression improved such disrupted intercellular junctions (Fig. 3C). Similar results were also observed using immunofluorescence microscopic studies (IFM) with anti-ZO1 pAb under confocal microscopies (data not shown). Taken together, these results suggest that the disrupted TJ among intestinal epithelial cells may be induced by TNFR2 signaling via MLCK up-regulation.

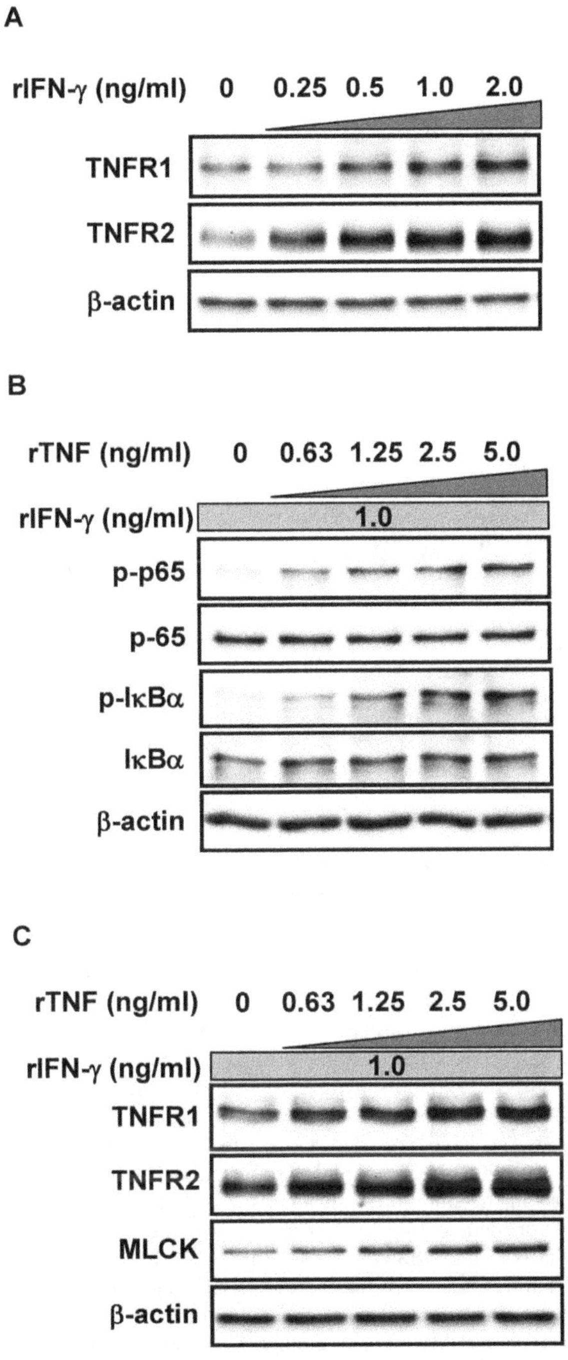

Figure 2. MLCK is up-regulated in the IFN-γ and TNF-stimulated MOC1 cells in association with NF-κB activation. (A) Protein lysates from MOC1 cells stimulated with the indicated concentration of rIFN-γ were subjected to Western blotting with either anti-TNFR1, anti-TNFR2 or anti-β-actin Abs. Representative data at 36 h after rIFN-γ stimulation are shown. (B) MOC1 cells were incubated with 1.0 ng/ml of rIFN-γ for 24 h, followed by the stimulation with the indicated concentration of rTNF, and subjected to Western blotting with either anti-p-p65, anti-p65, anti-p-IκBα, anti-IκBα or anti-β-actin Abs. Representative data at 5 min after rTNF stimulation are shown. (C) MOC1 cells were treated with 1.0 ng/ml of rIFN-γ for 24 h followed by the stimulation with the indicated concentration of rTNF and were subjected to Western blotting with anti-TNFR1, anti-TNFR2, anti-MLCK or anti-β-actin Abs. Representative data at 12 h after rTNF stimulation are shown.

The Blockade of TNF and the Suppression of MLCK Abrogate Disruption of Epithelial TJ in vitro

Given the TNFR2 signaling-dependent up-regulation of MLCK, we next assessed the effect of blocking TNF signaling in the epithelial cells on the TJ, which may be disrupted by up-regulation of MLCK. MOC1 cells were cultured in the presence of rIFN-γ to induce TNFR2 expression followed by addition of rTNF. As seen in Fig. 4A, the up-regulated MLCK expression was observed in these cells in association with remarkable TNFR2 up-regulation. In addition, such up-regulations of TNFR2 and MLCK were abrogated by the presence of MP6-XT22, a mAb against to TNF, in a dose-dependent fashion (Fig. 4A). It should be noted that slightly up-regulated TNFR1 expression by rTNF stimulation was also suppressed in the presence of MP6-XT22. Given the abrogation of MLCK up-regulation by MP6-XT22, we next studied the intercellular junctions among MOC1 cells under this condition. IFM (data not shown) and TEM (Fig. 4B) studies showed restoration of TJ in the presence of MP6-XT22. These results suggest that TNF signaling in the colonic epithelia may induce disruption of TJ via up-regulated TNFR2 and MLCK expressions. Moreover, these results also suggest that neutralization of TNF may abrogate such TJ disruption.

To confirm TJ disruption by MLCK up-regulation, rIFN-γ/rTNF-stimulated MOC1 cells were also incubated in the presence of ML-7, an MLCK inhibitor. As expected, the disturbed TJ, which was induced by the presence of rIFN-γ and rTNF, was restored by the inhibition of MLCK function (Fig. 4C). This result was originally considered to be the cause of suppressed MLCK function by ML-7. However, Western blotting showed that the up-regulated TNFR2 and MLCK expressions were interestingly suppressed by the addition of ML-7 in a dose-dependent fashion (Fig. 4D). It should be noted that the up-regulated TNFR1 expression induced by rIFN-γ and rTNF was not affected by the addition of ML-7. Given this result, MOC1 cells were also transfected with MLCK-specific siRNA. As seen in Fig. 4E, up-regulation of TNFR2 induced by rIFN-γ and rTNF was suppressed by silencing MLCK expression. Taken together, these results indicate that the disrupted TJ among intestinal epithelial cells induced by TNFR2 signaling may be restored by the suppression of MLCK function.

Suppression of MLCK Prevents the Development of CAC in Association with Restored TJ and Diminished Pro-tumorigenic Cytokine Productions in vivo

Given the disrupted TJ via TNFR2 signaling and MLCK up-regulation in vitro, we finally assessed the effect of MLCK suppression in the setting of CAC. Mice induced with CAC by AOM treatment and three cycles of DSS were injected with either vehicle control, MP6-XT22 or ML-7, and later euthanized to assess colonic inflammation and CAC development. As seen in Fig. 5A and B, the blockade of TNF in vivo, by weekly injection with MP6-XT22 throughout the entire experimental protocol, resulted in the reduction of CAC development. This result is consistent with our previous study [6]. Moreover, suppression of MLCK, by the injection with ML-7 during the entire protocol resulted in even more reduction of CAC development ('ML-7 entire' in Fig. 5A and B). In addition, administration of ML-7 at the recovering phase after the last DSS administration surprisingly revealed almost same degree of suppression on CAC development ('ML-7 final' in Fig. 5A and B). These results were relatively associated with the histological assessment of colitis in these groups, although the significances of colitis suppression with either administration of MP6-XT22 or ML-7 were not remarkable

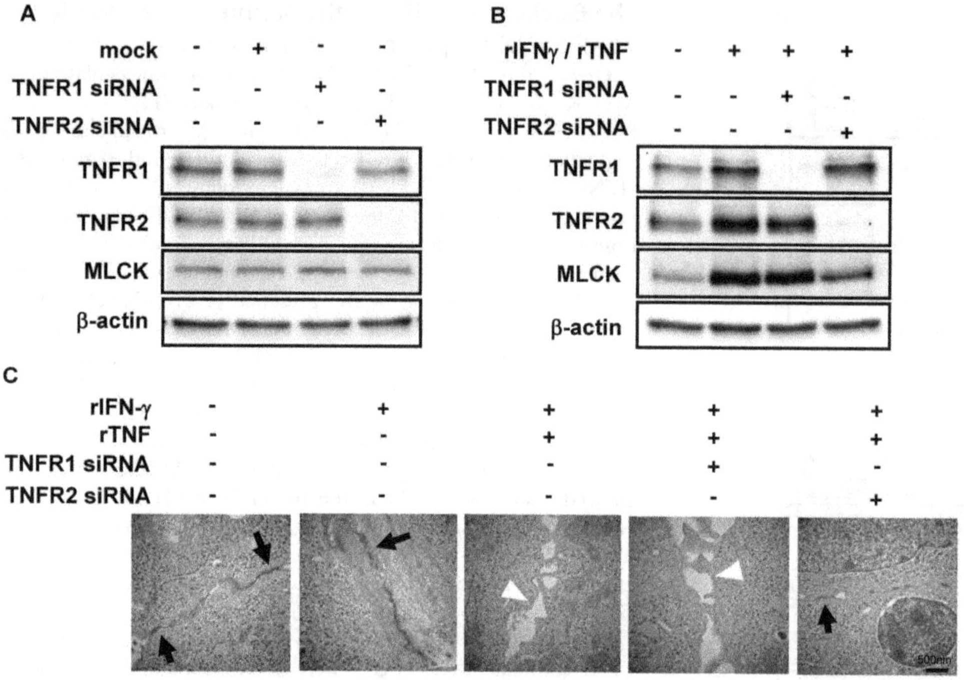

Figure 3. TNFR2-silencing in MOC1 cells diminishes TNF-induced MLCK up-regulation and disrupted epithelial tight junctions. (A) Protein lysates from MOC1 cells, which were transfected with either mock-, TNFR1- or TNFR2-targeting siRNA 36 h prior without rIFN-γ or rTNF stimulation, were subjected to Western blotting with either anti-TNFR1, anti-TNFR2, anti-MLCK or anti-β-actin Abs. (B) MOC1 cells were transfected with either mock-, TNFR1- or TNFR2-targeting siRNA, and then pre-incubated with or without 1.0 ng/ml rIFN-γ for 24 h prior to add 2.5 ng/ml rTNF for 12 h. Protein lysates from these cells were subjected to Western blotting with either anti-TNFR1, anti-TNFR2, anti-MLCK or anti-β-actin Abs. (C) MOC1 cells were transfected with either mock-, TNFR1- or TNFR2-targeting siRNA for 36 h with or without rIFN-γ and/or rTNF stimulation as indicated. Representative electron microscopic images from three experiments (n = 10) are shown. Arrows indicate fine intercellular junctional complexes including tight junctions, and arrow heads indicate disrupted intercellular junctional complexes. Scale bar indicates 500 nm.

compared to that of CAC suppression (Fig. 5C). Interestingly, q-PCR revealed that the expression levels of IL-1β, IL-6 and MIP-2 (Fig. 5D) as well as IFN-γ and TNF (data not shown) in the colonic tissue, especially in the tumor area, were suppressed by the treatment with ML-7 as well as with MP6-XT22 (Fig. 5D). In addition, the MLCK expression and MLC phosphorylation in the isolated epithelial cells from the non-tumor and tumor tissues were remarkably suppressed by the treatment with MP6-XT22 or ML-7 (Fig. 5E). It should be noted that the epithelia isolated from tumor area in each groups showed relatively higher expressions of TNFR2, p-p65, p-IκBα, MLCK and p-MLC when compared to that in non-tumor epithelia. These results are consistent with the observations of the intercellular junctional complexes among cells under TEM, since chronic inflammation in the control group induced disruption of epithelial TJ, and treatments via both TNF blockade and MLCK suppression resulted in the restoration of the disrupted TJ in the non-tumor and tumor areas and in association with reduced CAC (Fig. 5F). These results indicate that the suppression of MLCK function may contribute to reduce CAC development via restoration of the disrupted TJ.

Discussion

The etiology of IBD is considered to be associated with both epithelial permeability and dysregulated immune responses to luminal contents which include antigens derived from commensal bacteria in the gut. Regarding immune dysregulation, in patients with Crohn's disease for example, excessive amount of Th1 and Th17 cytokines, such as IFN-γ and IL-17 respectively, are secreted predominantly by the infiltrating $CD4^+$ effecter T cells in the intestinal lamina propria [19,35,36]. TNF, a pro-inflammatory cytokine produced not only by such dysregulated effecter T cells but also by macrophages and granulocytes infiltrating the inflamed intestinal tissues, is involved in the dysregulated adoptive immune responses in CD and possibly UC as well. Current therapeutic approaches in neutralizing TNF using either chimeric or humanized Abs have provided some effective therapies in the management of CD [1,37,38] and to some extent UC as well [39]. Our efforts in the study of pathogenesis of IBD have shown that TNF is expressed mainly by $F4/80^+$ macrophages rather than $CD4^+$ T cells in the DSS colitis model [6].

It is known that myeloid cell-derived macrophages and granulocytes are also capable of expressing other cytokines such as IL-1β, IL-6 and MIP-2, a homolog of IL-8 in humans. These cytokines can also induce pro-tumorigenic activities such as angiogenesis and tumor proliferation [21,22,23,24], but at the same time, these cytokine may also be expressed by intestinal epithelial cells [25,26,27,28]. In fact, we have observed in previous and current studies that the expression levels of these cytokines in colonic tissues are up-regulated in DSS colitis and further up-regulated in tumors. CAC development was suppressed by the treatment with either blocking anti-TNF mAb or MLCK inhibitor in association with reduced cytokine productions mentioned above. However, such cytokine expressions from the isolated colonic epithelial cells were not significant when compared to that of the entire colonic mucosa. Therefore, pro-tumorigenic cytokines most likely derived from the lamina propria where most macrophages reside. Others had also shown that NF-κB activation in the myeloid cells is critical for the induction of CAC [5], and

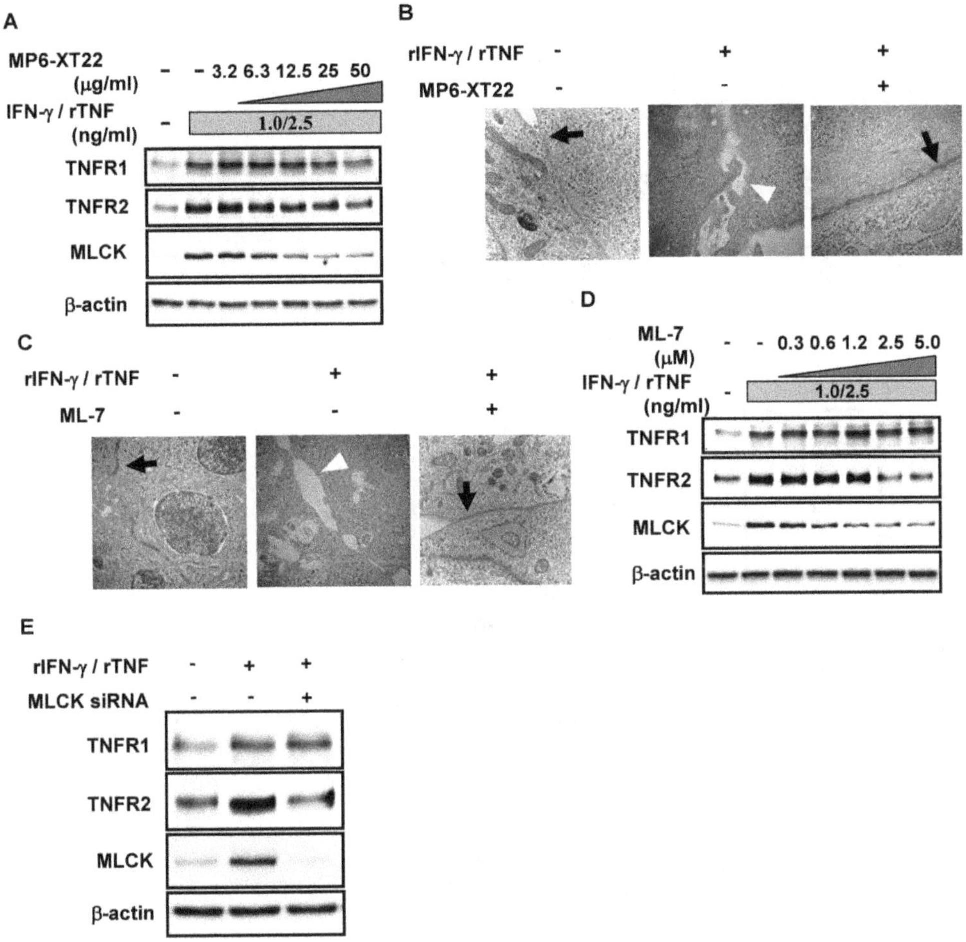

Figure 4. Suppressed MLCK functions may restore the TNF-induced disruption of intercellular junctions among MOC1 cells. (A) MOC1 cells were incubated with 1 ng/ml rIFN-γ and 2.5 ng/mL rTNF in the presence of indicated concentration of MP6-XT22. Protein lysates from these cells were subjected to Western blotting with either anti-TNFR1, anti-TNFR2, anti-MLCK, or anti-β-actin Abs. (B) MOC1 cells were incubated with rIFN-γ and rTNF in the presence or absence of 25 μg/ml MP6-XT22. Representative electron microscopic images from three experiments (n = 3) are shown. Arrows indicate fine tight junctions, and arrow heads indicate collapsed intercellular junctional complexes. (C) MOC1 cells were stimulated with rIFN-γ and rTNF, as described above, in the presence or absence of 2.5 μM ML-7. Representative electron microscopic images from three experiments (n = 3) are shown. Arrows indicate fine tight junctions and arrow heads indicate collapsed intercellular junctional complexes. (D) MOC1 cells were stimulated with rIFN-γ and rTNF, as described above, in the presence of the indicated concentration of ML-7. Protein lysates from these cells were subjected to Western blotting with either anti-TNFR1, anti-TNFR2, anti-MLCK or anti-β-actin Abs. (E) MOC1 cells were transfected with MLCK-targeting siRNA and stimulated with rIFN-γ for 24 h prior to adding rTNF for 12 h. Protein lysates from these cells were then subjected to Western blotting with either anti-TNFR1, anti-TNFR2, anti-MLCK or anti-β-actin Abs, respectively.

that NF-κB activation in myeloid cells can be induced by TNF [40].

DSS colitis is a commonly utilized murine model of IBD where a single administration of DSS can lead to acute colitis. In addition, three cycles of DSS administration can lead to chronic inflammation in the colon. Furthermore, AOM administration preceding three cycles of DSS treatment can lead to epithelial carcinogenesis and is a model of CAC [41]. By using this CAC model, Greten and colleagues showed that epithelial NF-κB activation is critical for the development of CAC [5]. However, the roles and mechanisms of epithelial NF-κB activation leading to CAC development had not previously been rigorously studied. In our previous and current studies, we demonstrated epithelial NF-κB activation in association with up-regulated TNF production by macrophages infiltrating the colonic lamina propria in the same CAC model. In addition, we showed that epithelial NF-κB activation was abrogated by neutralizing TNF with a specific mAb leading to the suppression of CAC [6]. These results suggest that the NF-κB pathway in the epithelial cells is mainly activated by the up-regulated TNF production. Previous studies by others had suggested that insufficient immunological homeostasis due to TNF production in IBD was caused by sequential activation of macrophages and neutrophils dominantly expressing TNFR1 (TNFRSF1a/p55) in the inflamed tissue [40]. However, we and other researchers had observed that intestinal epithelial cells express both TNFR1 and TNFR2 (TNFRSF1b/p75) [6,42]. There is spontaneous TNFR2 up-regulation in the epithelial cells in the setting of in vitro and in vivo inflammatory conditions [6,43]. Increased expression of TNFR2 in the epithelia was associated with CAC development [6]. These results suggest that TNF-induced epithelial NF-κB activation is associated with CAC development.

Given the results of up-regulated TNFR2 expression and NF-κB activation in the inflamed epithelial cells, we hypothesized that this may somehow be associated with reducing the recruitment of the death domains, such as FADD and TRADD, which are

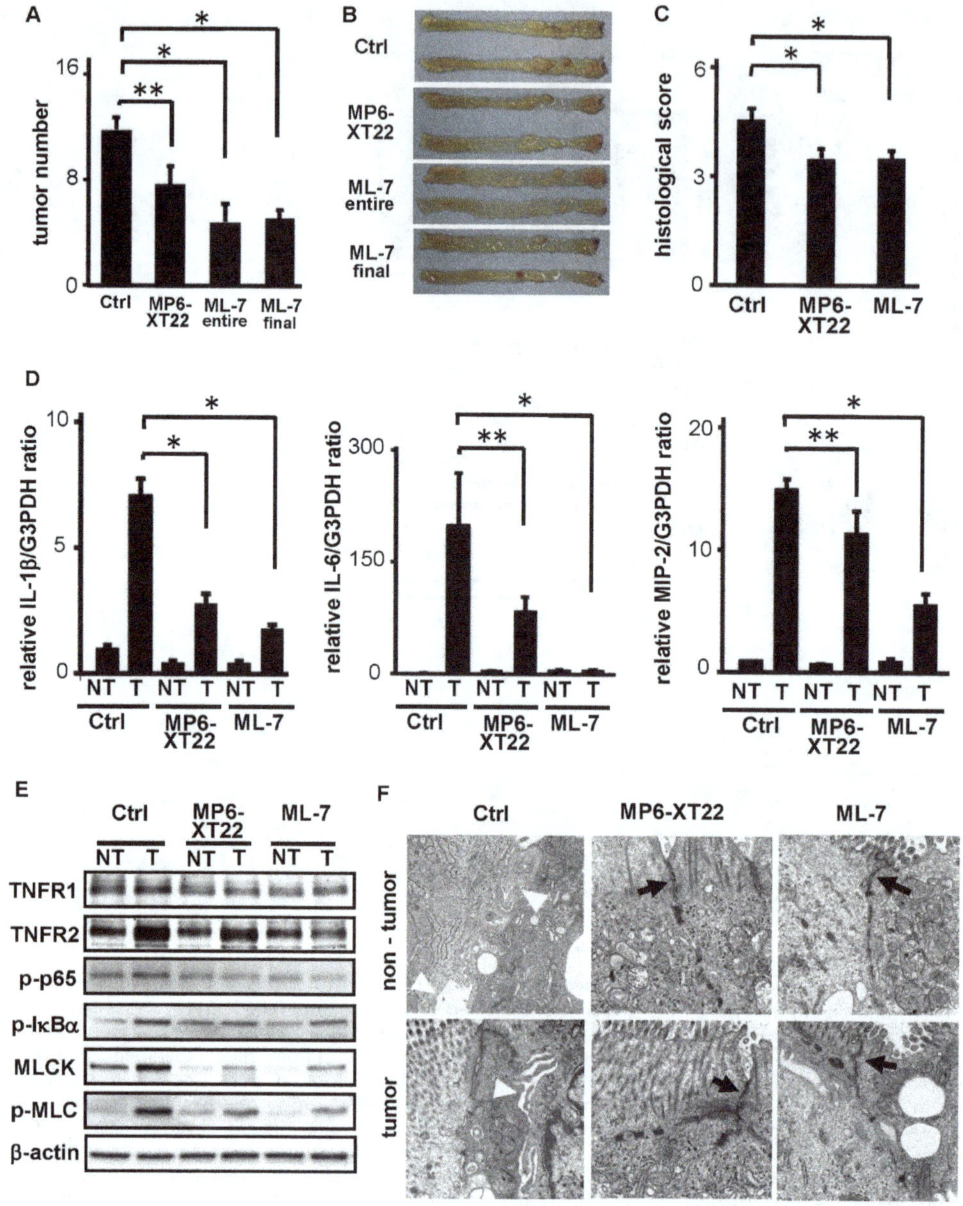

Figure 5. Treatment with ML-7, as well as with MP6-XT22, may reduce CAC development in AOM/DSS model. (A) Numbers of microscopically indicated tumors per colon in AOM/DSS-administered mice with either vehicle control (Ctrl), anti-TNF Ab (MP6-XT22), ML-7 treatment during the entire protocol (ML-7 entire), or ML-7 treatment at the final phase of protocol (ML-7 final) (n = 10) are shown. Tumors were determined under the microscope. Data are expressed as means ± SEM. *; p<0.01, **; p<0.05. (B) Macroscopic overview of representative colonic samples from each group is shown. (C) Histological assessment of colitis in mice treated with either control, MP6-XT22 or ML-7 (at the final phase) (n = 10). Data are expressed as means ± SEM. *; p<0.05. (D) Relative mRNA expressions for IL-1β, IL-6 MIP-2 and TNFR2 in inflamed mucosa from non-tumor or tumor tissues in mice treated with either control, MP6-XT22 or ML-7 (final phase) were analyzed. Each mRNA level was quantified by RT-PCR and normalized to the level of G3PDH (n = 3). *; p<0.01, **; p<0.05. (E) Protein lysates of the isolated epithelial cells from non-tumor or tumor tissues in mice administered with either control, MP6-XT22 or ML-7 (final phase) treatment were subjected to Western blotting with either anti-TNFR1, anti-TNFR2, anti-p-p65, anti-pIκBα, anti-MLCK, anti-p-MLC, or anti-β-actin Abs, respectively. (F) Electron microscopic images of representative non-tumor and tumor samples from either control, MP6-XT22 or ML-7 (final phase) treated group are shown (n = 10). Arrows indicate fine tight junction, and arrow heads indicate disrupted intercellular junctional complexes.

involved in the caspase-dependent pathway of TNFR1 signaling, so that the epithelial cells may escape apoptosis. However, the role of the epithelial NF-κB activation via TNFR2 signaling associated with CAC induction was not known previously. Therefore, we investigated whether increased expression of TNFR2 in this model leads to CAC. Using the same CAC model, TNFR2 deficient mice were used. However, CAC development was not possible due to high mortality with DSS treatment which had also been observed previously [6]. Therefore, we have utilized MOC1, which is a murine epithelial cell line derived from non-cancerous colonic epithelia transformed with SV40 large T antigen [15]. This cell line likely possess more physiological functions compared to other cell lines derived from murine colon cancer such as CT26 cells [44]. Furthermore, MOC1 cells can form confluent monolayers with epithelial TJ. Such characters of MOC1 cells allowed us to assess the collapsed TJ associated with MLCK up-regulation, because it was difficult to observe such morphologies with CT26 cells, which does not show either MLCK up-regulation or fine monolayers required for TJ observation.

It had been shown that MLCK in human intestinal cells leads to TNF-induced collapse of epithelial TJ via TNFR2 signaling [29] and that MLCK promoter activity is mediated by NF-κB [30,31,32]. Therefore, in our study, MOC1 cells were transfected with the TNRF2 siRNA to determine MLCK activities in the presence of rTNF. This resulted in the abrogation of TNF-induced TJ disruption associated with suppressed MLCK up-regulation (Fig. 3B and C), and these results are consistent with previous reports [11,29]. Moreover, we also observed that the TJ remained intact with anti-TNF treatment as well as inhibiting MLCK activity (Fig. 4B and C). In our current study, we also observed that TNFR1 expression in MOC1 cells was slightly up-regulated by addition of rTNF, and such up-regulated TNFR1 was suppressed by the presence of MP6-XT22. These results imply that presence of TNF may induce both up-regulations of TNFR1 and TNFR2 in inflamed epithelial cells as reported by Mizoguchi et al [42,43], suggesting that NF-κB activation in the epithelial cells we observed may be caused by both signaling. However, the degree of TNFR2 up-regulation was remarkably more than that of TNFR1 (Fig. 2A, 2C, 4A and 4D). Moreover, TNFR1 silencing failed to restore irritated intercellular junctions in association with not down-regulated MLCK expression (Fig. 3B and C). These results indicate that TNFR2 signaling is the key factor for MLCK-mediated epithelial permeability, as consistent with the observations by Wang et al [29]. These findings may also imply an important mechanism by which NF-κB pathway via TNFR2 signaling is regulated in the colonic epithelial cells in the setting of carcinogenesis. Thus, one potential mechanism by which TNFR2 expression in intestinal epithelial cells is associated with CAC development may be that the epithelial barrier dysfunction induced by MLCK activation via TNFR2 signaling leads to translocation of luminal bacteria into the lamina propria. Such epithelial permeability results in the stimulation of macrophages and granulocytes in mucosal tissue followed by cytokine production such as IL-1β, IL-6 and MIP-2 that are required for epithelial proliferation and tumor development. On the other hand, it should be noted that the impact of such pro-tumorigenic cytokines production, which is caused by disrupted TJ, on the severity of DSS colitis is controversial. Some recent studies have suggested that suppression of epithelial permeability by administration of MLCK inhibitors remarkably ameliorate DSS colitis [12,13]. Our current results also suggest that colitis was suppressed by ML-7 treatment, however, the impact of such treatment on the suppression of colitis was not remarkably effective compared to that on the suppression of CAC development. One reason for the different observations may be that the severity of colitis in our studies was relatively mild compared to the others, and thus, we did not observe distinct abrogation of colitis by MLCK inhibition. In addition, another recent report showed that MLCK deficient mice revealed worse DSS colitis compared to wild type [14]. These discrepant observations by others and ours suggest that another reason may be contributed by environmental factors such as the different microflora at the animal facilities that may induce different cytokine profiles.

In our current study, we observed that IFN-γ and TNF-induced up-regulation of TNFR2, and possibly MLCK, in the epithelial cells were specifically suppressed by ML-7 treatment (Fig. 4D). Up-regulation of TNFR2, but not TNFR1, was also suppressed by silencing MLCK expression (Fig. 4E). These results suggest that TJ disruption, induced by MLCK expression and MLC phosphorylation in the epithelial cells, may result in further up-regulation of TNFR2 expression in vitro. This in turn causes a vicious circle on the epithelial permeability, and such condition may promote tumor growth in the context of inflammation. Such impact of the relationship between TNFR2 and MLCK on CAC development is also suggested by the fact that the administration of ML-7, even at the final phase of CAC induction, resulted in the remarkable reduction of tumor in mice (Fig. 5A–F). In fact, ML-7 injection after final cycle of DSS treatment seemed to result in almost the same effect as the injection during the entire protocol in terms of reduction of tumor number, shown in Fig. 5A. It is suggested that colonic epithelial cells have undergone enough inflammation to initiate carcinogenesis until mice were injected with ML-7 at the final stage. One potential interpretation for this observation would be that undetectable microscopic tumors or aberrant crypt foci, which had not developed yet in the colonic epithelia, may still exist in mice treated with ML-7 only at the final phase. However, it is still suggested that the inhibition of MLCK function is absolutely effective at least for the suppression of tumor progression. In addition, we have examined whether such MLCK expression also induce up-regulation of endogenous IFN-γ and/or TNF expressions in MOC1 cells. However, neither expressions were affected regardless of MLCK expression (data not shown). Therefore, another mechanism may be involved in TNFR2 up-regulation in the irritated epithelial cells. Furthermore, our current study suggests that MLCK expression, which may be induced by TNFR2 signaling in the intestinal epithelial cells, can be a therapeutic target for the maintenance of continuous inflammation and prevention of CAC development in the setting of IBD.

Here, we demonstrate TNFR2-mediated regulation of CAC development, which is due to tumorigenic cytokines induced by MLCK-induced disruption of the TJ. This is an important mechanism that helps us understand the regulation of mucosal immune response as well as IBD- associated epithelial tumorigenesis.

Acknowledgments

We are grateful to N. Tsuge, Y. Kato, K. Mochida and Dr. Y. Saito for the technical support, Dr. H. Yagita for providing MP6-XT22 and Drs. M. Totsuka and T. Iwamoto for providing the MOC1 cells.

Author Contributions

Conceived and designed the experiments: T. Nagaishi MW. Performed the experiments: M. Suzuki T. Nagaishi MY MO YS SI. Analyzed the data: M. Suzuki T. Nagaishi MY MO. Contributed reagents/materials/analysis tools: TW MT SO RO M. Shimonaka HY T. Nakamura. Wrote the paper: M. Suzuki T. Nagaishi.

References

1. Hanauer SB, Feagan BG, Lichtenstein GR, Mayer LF, Schreiber S, et al. (2002) Maintenance infliximab for Crohn's disease: the ACCENT I randomised trial. Lancet 359: 1541–1549.
2. Ekbom A, Helmick C, Zack M, Adami HO (1990) Ulcerative colitis and colorectal cancer. A population-based study. N Engl J Med 323: 1228–1233.
3. Ekbom A, Helmick C, Zack M, Adami HO (1990) Increased risk of large-bowel cancer in Crohn's disease with colonic involvement. Lancet 336: 357–359.
4. Ekbom A, Helmick CG, Zack M, Holmberg L, Adami HO (1992) Survival and causes of death in patients with inflammatory bowel disease: a population-based study. Gastroenterology 103: 954–960.

5. Greten FR, Eckmann L, Greten TF, Park JM, Li ZW, et al. (2004) IKKbeta links inflammation and tumorigenesis in a mouse model of colitis-associated cancer. Cell 118: 285–296.
6. Onizawa M, Nagaishi T, Kanai T, Nagano K, Oshima S, et al. (2009) Signaling pathway via TNF-alpha/NF-kappaB in intestinal epithelial cells may be directly involved in colitis-associated carcinogenesis. Am J Physiol Gastrointest Liver Physiol 296: G850–859.
7. Derkx B, Taminiau J, Radema S, Stronkhorst A, Wortel C, et al. (1993) Tumour-necrosis-factor antibody treatment in Crohn's disease. Lancet 342: 173–174.
8. Pullman WE, Elsbury S, Kobayashi M, Hapel AJ, Doe WF (1992) Enhanced mucosal cytokine production in inflammatory bowel disease. Gastroenterology 102: 529–537.
9. Blair SA, Kane SV, Clayburgh DR, Turner JR (2006) Epithelial myosin light chain kinase expression and activity are upregulated in inflammatory bowel disease. Lab Invest 86: 191–201.
10. Ikebe M, Inagaki M, Kanamaru K, Hidaka H (1985) Phosphorylation of smooth muscle myosin light chain kinase by Ca2+-activated, phospholipid-dependent protein kinase. J Biol Chem 260: 4547–4550.
11. Wang F, Graham WV, Wang Y, Witkowski ED, Schwarz BT, et al. (2005) Interferon-gamma and tumor necrosis factor-alpha synergize to induce intestinal epithelial barrier dysfunction by up-regulating myosin light chain kinase expression. Am J Pathol 166: 409–419.
12. Chen C, Wang P, Su Q, Wang S, Wang F (2012) Myosin light chain kinase mediates intestinal barrier disruption following burn injury. PLoS One 7: e34946.
13. Liu X, Xu J, Mei Q, Han L, Huang J (2013) Myosin light chain kinase inhibitor inhibits dextran sulfate sodium-induced colitis in mice. Dig Dis Sci 58: 107–114.
14. Su L, Nalle SC, Shen L, Turner ES, Singh G, et al. (2013) TNFR2 activates MLCK-dependent tight junction dysregulation to cause apoptosis-mediated barrier loss and experimental colitis. Gastroenterology 145: 407–415.
15. Iwamoto T, Yamada K, Shimizu M, Totsuka M (2011) Establishment of intestinal epithelial cell lines from adult mouse small and large intestinal crypts. Biosci Biotechnol Biochem 75: 925–929.
16. Karhausen J, Furuta GT, Tomaszewski JE, Johnson RS, Colgan SP, et al. (2004) Epithelial hypoxia-inducible factor-1 is protective in murine experimental colitis. J Clin Invest 114: 1098–1106.
17. Lowe EL, Crother TR, Rabizadeh S, Hu B, Wang H, et al. (2010) Toll-like receptor 2 signaling protects mice from tumor development in a mouse model of colitis-induced cancer. PLoS One 5: e13027.
18. Brozovic S, Nagaishi T, Yoshida M, Betz S, Salas A, et al. (2004) CD1d function is regulated by microsomal triglyceride transfer protein. Nat Med 10: 535–539.
19. Nagaishi T, Pao L, Lin SH, Iijima H, Kaser A, et al. (2006) SHP1 phosphatase-dependent T cell inhibition by CEACAM1 adhesion molecule isoforms. Immunity 25: 769–781.
20. Ichinose S, Muneta T, Koga H, Segawa Y, Tagami M, et al. (2010) Morphological differences during in vitro chondrogenesis of bone marrow-, synovium-MSCs, and chondrocytes. Lab Invest 90: 210–221.
21. Driscoll KE, Hassenbein DG, Howard BW, Isfort RJ, Cody D, et al. (1995) Cloning, expression, and functional characterization of rat MIP-2: a neutrophil chemoattractant and epithelial cell mitogen. J Leukoc Biol 58: 359–364.
22. Koch AE, Polverini PJ, Kunkel SL, Harlow LA, DiPietro LA, et al. (1992) Interleukin-8 as a macrophage-derived mediator of angiogenesis. Science 258: 1798–1801.
23. Lahm H, Petral-Malec D, Yilmaz-Ceyhan A, Fischer JR, Lorenzoni M, et al. (1992) Growth stimulation of a human colorectal carcinoma cell line by interleukin-1 and -6 and antagonistic effects of transforming growth factor beta 1. Eur J Cancer 28A: 1894–1899.
24. Coussens LM, Werb Z (2002) Inflammation and cancer. Nature 420: 860–867.
25. Eckmann L, Jung HC, Schurer-Maly C, Panja A, Morzycka-Wroblewska E, et al. (1993) Differential cytokine expression by human intestinal epithelial cell lines: regulated expression of interleukin 8. Gastroenterology 105: 1689–1697.
26. Li Y, de Haar C, Chen M, Deuring J, Gerrits MM, et al. (2010) Disease-related expression of the IL6/STAT3/SOCS3 signalling pathway in ulcerative colitis and ulcerative colitis-related carcinogenesis. Gut 59: 227–235.
27. Ohno Y, Lee J, Fusunyan RD, MacDermott RP, Sanderson IR (1997) Macrophage inflammatory protein-2: chromosomal regulation in rat small intestinal epithelial cells. Proc Natl Acad Sci U S A 94: 10279–10284.
28. Prakash R, Bharathi Raja S, Devaraj H, Devaraj SN (2011) Up-regulation of MUC2 and IL-1beta expression in human colonic epithelial cells by Shigella and its interaction with mucins. PLoS One 6: e27046.
29. Wang F, Schwarz BT, Graham WV, Wang Y, Su L, et al. (2006) IFN-gamma-induced TNFR2 expression is required for TNF-dependent intestinal epithelial barrier dysfunction. Gastroenterology 131: 1153–1163.
30. Graham WV, Wang F, Clayburgh DR, Cheng JX, Yoon B, et al. (2006) Tumor necrosis factor-induced long myosin light chain kinase transcription is regulated by differentiation-dependent signaling events. Characterization of the human long myosin light chain kinase promoter. J Biol Chem 281: 26205–26215.
31. Ye D, Ma TY (2008) Cellular and molecular mechanisms that mediate basal and tumour necrosis factor-alpha-induced regulation of myosin light chain kinase gene activity. J Cell Mol Med 12: 1331–1346.
32. Ye D, Ma I, Ma TY (2006) Molecular mechanism of tumor necrosis factor-alpha modulation of intestinal epithelial tight junction barrier. Am J Physiol Gastrointest Liver Physiol 290: G496–504.
33. Fish SM, Proujansky R, Reenstra WW (1999) Synergistic effects of interferon gamma and tumour necrosis factor alpha on T84 cell function. Gut 45: 191–198.
34. Taylor CT, Dzus AL, Colgan SP (1998) Autocrine regulation of epithelial permeability by hypoxia: role for polarized release of tumor necrosis factor alpha. Gastroenterology 114: 657–668.
35. Brand S (2009) Crohn's disease: Th1, Th17 or both? The change of a paradigm: new immunological and genetic insights implicate Th17 cells in the pathogenesis of Crohn's disease. Gut 58: 1152–1167.
36. Yamaji O, Nagaishi T, Totsuka T, Onizawa M, Suzuki M, et al. (2012) The development of colitogenic CD4(+) T cells is regulated by IL-7 in collaboration with NK cell function in a murine model of colitis. J Immunol 188: 2524–2536.
37. Sands BE, Anderson FH, Bernstein CN, Chey WY, Feagan BG, et al. (2004) Infliximab maintenance therapy for fistulizing Crohn's disease. N Engl J Med 350: 876–885.
38. Targan SR, Hanauer SB, van Deventer SJ, Mayer L, Present DH, et al. (1997) A short-term study of chimeric monoclonal antibody cA2 to tumor necrosis factor alpha for Crohn's disease. Crohn's Disease cA2 Study Group. N Engl J Med 337: 1029–1035.
39. Rutgeerts P, Sandborn WJ, Feagan BG, Reinisch W, Olson A, et al. (2005) Infliximab for induction and maintenance therapy for ulcerative colitis. N Engl J Med 353: 2462–2476.
40. Popivanova BK, Kitamura K, Wu Y, Kondo T, Kagaya T, et al. (2008) Blocking TNF-alpha in mice reduces colorectal carcinogenesis associated with chronic colitis. J Clin Invest 118: 560–570.
41. Tanaka T, Kohno H, Suzuki R, Yamada Y, Sugie S, et al. (2003) A novel inflammation-related mouse colon carcinogenesis model induced by azoxymethane and dextran sodium sulfate. Cancer Sci 94: 965–973.
42. Mizoguchi E, Hachiya Y, Kawada M, Nagatani K, Ogawa A, et al. (2008) TNF receptor type I-dependent activation of innate responses to reduce intestinal damage-associated mortality. Gastroenterology 134: 470–480.
43. Mizoguchi E, Mizoguchi A, Takedatsu H, Cario E, de Jong YP, et al. (2002) Role of tumor necrosis factor receptor 2 (TNFR2) in colonic epithelial hyperplasia and chronic intestinal inflammation in mice. Gastroenterology 122: 134–144.
44. Wang M, Bronte V, Chen PW, Gritz L, Panicali D, et al. (1995) Active immunotherapy of cancer with a nonreplicating recombinant fowlpox virus encoding a model tumor-associated antigen. J Immunol 154: 4685–4692.

Permissions

All chapters in this book were first published in PLOS ONE, by The Public Library of Science; hereby published with permission under the Creative Commons Attribution License or equivalent. Every chapter published in this book has been scrutinized by our experts. Their significance has been extensively debated. The topics covered herein carry significant findings which will fuel the growth of the discipline. They may even be implemented as practical applications or may be referred to as a beginning point for another development.

The contributors of this book come from diverse backgrounds, making this book a truly international effort. This book will bring forth new frontiers with its revolutionizing research information and detailed analysis of the nascent developments around the world.

We would like to thank all the contributing authors for lending their expertise to make the book truly unique. They have played a crucial role in the development of this book. Without their invaluable contributions this book wouldn't have been possible. They have made vital efforts to compile up to date information on the varied aspects of this subject to make this book a valuable addition to the collection of many professionals and students.

This book was conceptualized with the vision of imparting up-to-date information and advanced data in this field. To ensure the same, a matchless editorial board was set up. Every individual on the board went through rigorous rounds of assessment to prove their worth. After which they invested a large part of their time researching and compiling the most relevant data for our readers.

The editorial board has been involved in producing this book since its inception. They have spent rigorous hours researching and exploring the diverse topics which have resulted in the successful publishing of this book. They have passed on their knowledge of decades through this book. To expedite this challenging task, the publisher supported the team at every step. A small team of assistant editors was also appointed to further simplify the editing procedure and attain best results for the readers.

Apart from the editorial board, the designing team has also invested a significant amount of their time in understanding the subject and creating the most relevant covers. They scrutinized every image to scout for the most suitable representation of the subject and create an appropriate cover for the book.

The publishing team has been an ardent support to the editorial, designing and production team. Their endless efforts to recruit the best for this project, has resulted in the accomplishment of this book. They are a veteran in the field of academics and their pool of knowledge is as vast as their experience in printing. Their expertise and guidance has proved useful at every step. Their uncompromising quality standards have made this book an exceptional effort. Their encouragement from time to time has been an inspiration for everyone.

The publisher and the editorial board hope that this book will prove to be a valuable piece of knowledge for researchers, students, practitioners and scholars across the globe.

List of Contributors

Yipeng Wang
Department of Gastroenterology/Hepatology, Zhongnan Hospital of Wuhan University, Wuhan, Hubei, P. R. China

Yuntao Bing and Qiao Yu
The Hubei Clinical Center & Key Laboratory of Intestinal & Colorectal Diseases, Wuhan, Hubei, P. R. China

Siying Zhu, Xiaobing Wang, Shufang Xu, Lu Song, Xintao Wang, Bing Xia, Youqing Zhu and Rui Zhou
Department of Gastroenterology/Hepatology, Zhongnan Hospital of Wuhan University, Wuhan, Hubei, P. R. China
The Hubei Clinical Center & Key Laboratory of Intestinal & Colorectal Diseases, Wuhan, Hubei, P. R. China

Masanori Kasahara, Utano Tomaru and Tomohisa Baba
Department of Pathology, Hokkaido University Graduate School of Medicine, Sapporo, Japan

Shigeru Furukawa, Naoya Sakamoto and Masahiro Asaka
Department of Gastroenterology, Hokkaido University Graduate School of Medicine, Sapporo, Japan

Takehiko Katsurada and Waka Kobayashi
Department of Pathology, Hokkaido University Graduate School of Medicine, Sapporo, Japan
Department of Gastroenterology, Hokkaido University Graduate School of Medicine, Sapporo, Japan

Akihiro Ishizu
Faculty of Health Sciences, Hokkaido University, Sapporo, Japan

Kazuyoshi Takeda
Department of Immunology, Juntendo University School of Medicine, Tokyo, Japan

Hiroshi Takeda
Department of Gastroenterology, Hokkaido University Graduate School of Medicine, Sapporo, Japan
Faculty of Pharmaceutical Sciences, Hokkaido University, Sapporo, Japan

John M. Thomson, Susan H. Berry, Mairi E. Hope, Indrani Mukhopadhya, Mairi H. McLean, Emad El-Omar and Georgina L. Hold
Gastrointestinal Research Group, Division of Applied Medicine, University of Aberdeen, Foresterhill, Aberdeen, United Kingdom

Richard Hansen
Gastrointestinal Research Group, Division of Applied Medicine, University of Aberdeen, Foresterhill, Aberdeen, United Kingdom
Child Health, University of Aberdeen, Royal Aberdeen Children's Hospital, Foresterhill, Aberdeen, United Kingdom

Graeme I. Murray
Department of Pathology, University of Aberdeen, Foresterhill, Aberdeen, United Kingdom

Zeli Shen and James G. Fox
Division of Comparative Medicine, Massachusetts Institute of Technology, Cambridge, Massachusetts, United States of America

Yanina Romero-Zerbo and Patricia Rivera
Laboratorio de Medicina Regenerativa, Hospital Carlos Haya, Mediterranean Institute for the Advance of Biotechnology and Health Research Fundación, Málaga, Spain

Lucia Márquez and Montserrat Andreu
Department of Gastroenterology, Parc de Salut Mar, Universidad Autónoma, Barcelona, Spain

Juan Suárez, Francisco J. Bermúdez-Silva and Fernando Rodríguez de Fonseca
Laboratorio de Medicina Regenerativa, Hospital Carlos Haya, Mediterranean Institute for the Advance of Biotechnology and Health Research Fundación, Málaga, Spain
El Centro de Investigación Biomédica en Red de Fisiopatología de Obesidad y Nutrición, Instituto de Salud Carlos III, Ministerio de Ciencia e Innovación, Madrid, Spain

Mar Iglesias
Department of Pathology, Parc de Salut Mar, Universidad Auto´noma, Barcelona, Spain

Linda Vong and Philip M. Sherman
Hospital for Sick Children, Research Institute, Toronto, Ontario, Canada

Neil Dufton and John L. Wallace
Farncombe Family Digestive Health Research Institute, McMaster University, Hamilton, Ontario, Canada

Jose G. P. Ferraz, Remo Panaccione and Paul L. Beck
Division of Gastroenterology, University of Calgary, Calgary, Alberta, Canada

Mauro Perretti
Centre for Biochemical Pharmacology, William Harvey Research Institute, London, United Kingdom

Ida Casorelli, Gabriele De Luca, Federica Chiera, Ivano Iavarone, Alessandro Giuliani and Margherita Bignami
Department of Environment and Primary Prevention, Istituto Superiore di Sanità, Rome, Italy

Tania Pannellini and Piero Musiani
Aging Research Center, Gabriele D'Annunzio University of Chieti, Chieti, Italy

Paolo Degan
Istituto Tumori di Genova, Genova, Italy

Alessia Butera and Monica Boirivant
Department of Infectious Parasitic and Immuno-mediated Diseases, Istituto Superiore di Sanità, Rome, Italy

Pengli Yu, Fangcheng Shen, Xiaofei Zhang, Risheng Cao, Xiaodan Zhao, Ruihua Shi and Hongjie Zhang
Department of Gastroenterology, the First Affiliated Hospital of Nanjing Medical University, Nanjing, China

Pengfei Liu
Department of Gastroenterology, the People's Hospital of Jiangyin, Jiangyin, China

Huiming Tu
Department of Gastroenterology, the Fourth People's Hospital of Wuxi, Wuxi, China

Xiaozhong Yang
Department of Gastroenterology, the First Hospital of Huaian, Huaian, China

Min Jeoung Lee, Jin-Ku Lee, Ji Won Choi Chang-Seok Lee, Chung-Hyun Cho, Myung-Hee Chung and Sang-Kyu Ye
Department of Pharmacology, Seoul National University College of Medicine, Seoul, Republic of Korea
Ischemic/Hypoxic Disease Institute, Seoul National University College of Medicine, Seoul, Republic of Korea

Ji Hyun Sim and Hang-Rae Kim
Department of Anatomy, Seoul National University College of Medicine, Seoul, Republic of Korea,

Kwang-Ho Lee
Department of Biotechnology, College of Biomedical & Health Science, Konkuk University, Chungju, Republic of Korea,

Ik-Hyun Cho
Department of Anatomy, College of Oriental Medicine, Kyung Hee University, Seoul, Republic of Korea,
Institute of Oriental Medicine, Kyung Hee University, Seoul, Republic of Korea

Xiao Feng, Hao Wang, Shicai Ye, Jiaxi Guan, Wenkai Tan, Si Cheng, Guoli Wei, Weiyun Wu and Yu Zhou
Department of Gastroenterology, The Affiliated Hospital of Guangdong Medical College, Zhanjiang, Guangdong, People's Republic of China

Feng Wu
Department of Medicine, University of Chicago, Chicago, Illinois, United States of America

Indrani Mukhopadhya, John M. Thomson, Richard Hansen, Susan H. Berry, Emad M. El-Omar and Georgina L. Hold
Gastrointestinal Research Group, Division of Applied Medicine, University of Aberdeen, Foresterhill, Aberdeen, United Kingdom

Farooq Z. Rahman, Andrew M. Smith, Bu'Hussain Hayee, Daniel J. B. Marks and Anthony W. Segal
Departments of Medicine, University College London, London, United Kingdom

Stuart L. Bloom
Department of Gastroenterology, University College London Hospital, London, United Kingdom

Stephen J. Walker
Wake Forest Institute for Regenerative Medicine, Wake Forest University Health Sciences, Winston Salem, North Carolina, United States of America,

John Fortunato
Department of Pediatrics Section on Gastroenterology, Wake Forest University Health Sciences, Winston Salem, North Carolina, United States of America

Lenny G. Gonzalez
Pediatric Gastroenterology Department, Dr. Miguel Perez Carren˜o Hospital, Caracas, Venezuela

Arthur Krigsman
Pediatric Gastroenterology Resources of New York & Texas, Far Rockaway, New York, United States of America

Radha Duttagupta, Rong Jiang, Jeremy Gollub, Jessica Kao and Keith W. Jones
Applied Reasearch Group, Affymetrix Inc, Santa Clara, California, United States of America

Jessica Bowers and Robert C. Getts
Research and Development, Genisphere LLC, Hatfield, Pennsylvania, United States of America

Sharon Di Rienzo and Tom Stamato
Lankenau Institute for Medical Research, Wynnewood, Pennsylvania, United States of America

Keith Kearney and David Rudolph
Division of Gastroenterology, Lankenau Medical Center, Wynnewood, Pennsylvania, United States of America

Noor B. Dawany and Michael K. Showe
The Wistar Institute, Philadelphia, Pennsylvania, United States of America

Boyko Kabakchiev and Mark S. Silverberg
Mount Sinai Hospital, Toronto, Ontario, Canada
University of Toronto, Toronto, Ontario, Canada

Pingzhao Hu and Anne M. Griffiths
The Hospital for Sick Children, Toronto, Ontario, Canada

Anthony R. Otley
Izaak Walton Killam Hospital, Halifax, Nova Scotia, Canada

David Mack
Children's Hospital of Eastern Ontario, Ottawa, Ontario, Canada

Jeffrey Hyams
Connecticut Children's Medical Center, Hartford, Connecticut, United States of America

James Markowitz
Schneider's Children's Hospital, New Hyde Park, New York, United States of America

Neal Leleiko
Brown University, Providence, Rhode Island, United States of America

Wallace Crandall
Columbus Children's Hospital, Columbus, Ohio, United States of America

Dan Turner
Shaare Zedek Medical Center, Jerusalem, Israel

Wei Xu
University of Toronto, Toronto, Ontario, Canada

Laura P. Hale and Paula K. Greer
Department of Pathology, Duke University Medical Center, Durham, North Carolina, United States of America

Garima Juyal, Pushplata Prasad, Sabyasachi Senapati and Thelma BK
Department of Genetics, University of Delhi, South Campus, New Delhi, India

Vandana Midha and Ajit Sood
Dayanand Medical College and Hospital, Ludhiana, Punjab, India

Devendra Amre
Department of Pediatrics, University of Montreal, Montreal, Canada
Research Center, Sainte-Justine Hospital, Montreal, Canada

Ramesh C. Juyal
National Institute of Immunology, New Delhi, India

Shigeo Koido, Toshifumi Ohkusa, Keisuke Saito, Kazuki Takakura, Shintaro Tsukinaga, Shunichi Odahara, Toyokazu Yukawa, Jimi Mitobe, Mikio Kajihara, Kan Uchiyama, Hiroshi Arakawa and Hisao Tajiri
Division of Gastroenterology and Hepatology, Department of Internal Medicine, The Jikei University School of Medicine, Tokyo, Japan

Takayuki Kajiura and Junko Shinozaki
Frontier Research Laboratories, Institute for Innovation, Ajinomoto Co., Inc., Kawasaki, Japan
Pharmaceutical Laboratories, Ajinomoto Co., Inc., Kawasaki, Japan

Manabu Suzuki
Pharmaceutical Laboratories, Ajinomoto Co., Inc., Kawasaki, Japan

Avinash Bardia, Santosh K. Tiwari, Sandeep K. Vishwakarma, Md. Aejaz Habeeb and Aleem A. Khan
Centre for Liver Research and Diagnostics, Deccan College of Medical Sciences, Kanchanbagh, Hyderabad, Andhra Pradesh, India

Pratibha Nallari
Department of Genetics, Osmania University, Hyderabad, Andhra Pradesh, India

Shaik A. Sultana and Shaik A. Pasha
College of Applied Medical Sciences, King Saud University, Riyadh, Kingdom of Saudi Arabia

Yugandhar P. Reddy
Neurobiology lab, Department of Zoology, University College of Sciences, Osmania University, Hyderabad, Andhra Pradesh, India

Jiarong Miao, Junkun Niu, Yuliang Xiao, Lifeng Zhou, Liping Duan, Shuan Li, Gang Yang, Lifang Chen, Mingxia Tong and Yinglei Miao
Department of Gastroenterology, The First Affiliated Hospital of Kunming Medical University, Kunming, P. R. China

Kunhua Wang
Department of General Surgery, The First Affiliated Hospital of Kunming Medical University, Kunming, P. R. China

Yan Du
Department of Clinical Laboratory, The First Affiliated Hospital of Kunming Medical University, Kunming, P. R. China

Li-Na Zhao, Jie-Yao Li, Tao Yu, Guang-Cheng Chen, Yu-Hong Yuan and Qi-Kui Chen
Department of Gastroenterology, Sun Yat-Sen Memorial Hospital, Sun Yat-Sen University, Guangzhou, Guangdong, People's Republic of China

Tomomitsu Tahara, Tomoyuki Shibata, Masaaki Okubo, Takamitsu Ishizuka, Mitsuo Nagasaka, Yoshihito Nakagawa, Naoki Ohmiya and Ichiro Hirata
Department of Gastroenterology, Fujita Health University School of Medicine, Toyoake, Japan

Masakatsu Nakamura and Tomiyasu Arisawa
Department of Gastroenterology, Kanazawa Medical University, Ishikawa, Japan

Masahiro Suzuki, Takashi Nagaishi, Michio Onizawa, Taro Watabe, Shigeru Oshima, Ryuichi Okamoto, Tetsuya Nakamura and Mamoru Watanabe
Department of Gastroenterology, Graduate School of Medical Science, Tokyo Medical and Dental University, Tokyo, Japan

Motomi Yamazaki
Department of Obstetrics and Gynecology, Nihon University School of Medicine, Tokyo, Japan

Yuriko Sakamaki and Shizuko Ichinose
Research Center for Medical and Dental Sciences, Tokyo Medical and Dental University, Tokyo, Japan

Mamoru Totsuka
Department of Applied Biological Chemistry, The University of Tokyo, Tokyo, Japan

Motoyuki Shimonaka
Department of Chemistry, Tokyo University of Science, Tokyo, Japan

Hideo Yagita
Department of Immunology, Juntendo University School of Medicine, Tokyo, Japan

Index

www.ingramcontent.com/pod-product-compliance
Lightning Source LLC
LaVergne TN
LVHW060605210926
848485LV00005B/1375